# ESSENTIALS OF RESTENOSIS

# CONTEMPORARY CARDIOLOGY

CHRISTOPHER P. CANNON, MD
*SERIES EDITOR*
ANNEMARIE M. ARMANI, MD
*EXECUTIVE EDITOR*

# ESSENTIALS OF RESTENOSIS

## For the Interventional Cardiologist

*Edited by*

## HENRICUS J. DUCKERS, MD, PhD

*Thoraxcenter, Erasmus Medical Center Rotterdam,*
*Rotterdam, The Netherlands*

## ELIZABETH G. NABEL, MD

*The Nabel Lab, Genome Technology Branch, NHGRI*
*Division of Intramural Research,*
*National Heart, Lung, and Blood Institute,*
*National Institutes of Health, Bethesda, MD*
*and*

## PATRICK W. SERRUYS, MD, PhD

*Thoraxcenter, Erasmus Medical Center Rotterdam,*
*Rotterdam, The Netherlands*

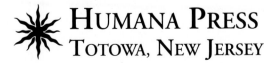

HUMANA PRESS
TOTOWA, NEW JERSEY

Production Editor: Amy Thau.

Cover design by Donna Niethe.

Cover Illustration: Top left: Fig. 4, Chapter 11, "Contribution of Circulating Progenitor Cells to Vascular Repair and Lesion Formation," by Masataka Sata and Kenneth Walsh; Top center: Fig. 7, Chapter 18, "Coronary Imaging With Multislice Spiral Computed Tomography," by Koen Nieman; Top right: Fig. 22, Chapter 22, "Clinical Data of Eluting Stents," by Marco A. Costa, Alexandre Abizaid, Amanda G. M. R. Sousa, and J. Eduardo Sousa; Lower left: Fig. 6A,B, Chapter 18; Lower center: Fig. 1, Chapter 11; Lower right: Fig. 1, Chapter 22.

# PREFACE

Restenosis remains the major obstacle in the way of the successful clinical outcome of percutaneous coronary interventions and has inspired interventional cardiologists and vascular biologists to study this complex process for the last two decades. In this book we explore the process of restenosis from bench to bedside. First, it will encompass the description of the intricate molecular and genetic basis of restenosis and will translate these findings to histomorphology, animal models, and the possible therapeutic repercussions in the diagnosis and management of the cardiovascular patient. Second, it will discuss the recent advances in invasive imaging of vascular lesions. Also, the non-invasive imaging of vascular lesions has emerged in recent years as a promising alternative to conventional angiography. This will be discussed by the very people who have pioneered this particular field of vascular imaging. Third, it will describe the exciting progress that we and others have recently achieved in the treatment of this clinical problem.

*Essentials of Restenosis: For the Interventional Cardiologist* will therefore provide a complete overview of the molecular basis and clinical approach to image, prevent, and treat this complex disease. The authors contributing to this work have pioneered the field of vascular imaging and intervention and represent the leaders in the field of interventional cardiology and vascular proliferative disease.

*Essentials of Restenosis: For the Interventional Cardiologist* is aimed at both clinicians performing vascular interventions, as well as molecular and vascular biologists. It will enable clinical cardiologists to deepen their insight in the molecular, genetic, and cellular basis of neointima formation or their application in the treatment of restenosis. It will also provide a clear perspective to the clinical application of molecular principles in vascular disease for fundamental vascular biologists.

We would like to thank the contributors for their time and efforts, for which we are greatly indebted. Without their enthusiasm and their excellent contributions, this high quality volume of the Contemporary Cardiology™ series could not have been produced.

*Henricus J. Duckers, MD, PhD*
*Elizabeth G. Nabel, MD*
*Patrick W. Serruys, MD, PhD*

# CONTENTS

# CONTRIBUTORS

ALEXANDRE ABIZAID, MD, PhD • *Institute Dante Pazzanese of Cardiology, São Paulo, Brazil*

TIMO BAKS, MD • *Thoraxcenter Rotterdam, Erasmus Medical Center, Rotterdam, The Netherlands*

MANFRED BOEHM, MD • *The Cardiovascular Branch, National Heart, Lung and Blood Institute National Institutes of Health, Bethesda, MD*

ALAIDE CHIEFFO, MD • *San Raffaele Hospital, Milan, Italy*

CAROLINE CHENG, PhD • *Thoraxcenter Rotterdam, Erasmus Medical Center, Rotterdam, The Netherlands*

ALEXANDER W. CLOWES, MD • *Section on Vascular Surgery, University of Washington School of Medicine, Seattle, WA*

ANTONIO COLOMBO, MD • *Columbus Hospital and San Raffaele Hospital, Milan, Italy*

FRANCESCO COSENTINO, MD, PhD • *Cardiovascular Research, Institute of Physiology, University of Zürich; and Cardiovascular Center, University Hospital, Zürich, Switzerland*

MARCO A. COSTA, MD, PhD • *University of Florida - Shands, Jacksonville, FL*

GEORGE DANGAS, MD, PhD • *Lenox Hill Heart and Vascular Institute of New York, Lenox Hill Hospital, Cardiovascular Research Foundation, New York, NY*

GIEDRIUS DAVIDAVICIUS, MD • *Cardiovascular Centre Aalst, OLV Hospital, Aalst, Belgium*

HENRICUS J. DUCKERS, MD, PhD • *Thoraxcenter Rotterdam, Erasmus Medical Center, Rotterdam, The Netherlands*

PIM J. DE FEYTER, MD, PhD • *Thoraxcenter, Cardiology Department, Erasmus Medical Center, Rotterdam, The Netherlands*

ALOKE V. FINN, MD • *Cardiac Unit, Department of Internal Medicine, Massachusetts General Hospital, Boston, MA*

SANTHI K. GANESH, MD • *Vascular Biology Section, Cardiovascular Branch, National Heart, Lung, and Blood Institute, NIH, Bethesda, MD*

RANDOLPH L. GEARY, MD, FACS • *Division of Surgical Sciences, Wake Forest University School of Medicine, Winston-Salem, NC*

ROBERT JAN M. VAN GEUNS, MD, PhD • *Thoraxcenter Rotterdam, Erasmus Medical Center, Rotterdam, The Netherlands*

FRANK J. H. GIJSEN, PhD • *Thoraxcenter, Cardiology Department, Erasmus Medical Center, Rotterdam, The Netherlands*

HERMAN K. GOLD, MD • *Cardiac Unit, Department of Internal Medicine, Massachusetts General Hospital, Boston, MA*

KEIJI IGAKI, PhD • *Igaki Medical Planning Co. Ltd., Kyoto, Japan*

PAT IVERSEN, PhD • *AVI Biopharma, Portland, OR*

THOMAS W. JOHNSON, BSc, MBBS, MRCP • *Bristol Heart Institute, University of Bristol, Bristol, UK*

KARL R. KARSCH, MD • *Bristol Heart Institute, University of Bristol, Bristol, UK*

NICHOLAS KIPSHIDZE, MD, PhD • *Lenox Hill Heart and Vascular Institute of New York, Lenox Hill Hospital, Cardiovascular Research Foundation, New York, NY*

VOLKER KLAUSS, MD • *Department of Cardiology, Medizinische Poliklinik–Innenstadt, University of Munich, Munich, Germany*

DOMINIQUE DE KLEIJN, PhD • *Laboratory of Experimental Cardiology, Heart Lung Institute, University Medical Center Utrecht, Utrecht, The Netherlands*

FRANK D. KOLODGIE, PhD • *Department of Cardiovascular Pathology, Armed Forces Institute of Pathology, Washington, DC*

ROB KRAMS, MD, PhD • *Thoraxcenter, Cardiology Department, Erasmus Medical Center, Rotterdam, The Netherlands*

ALEXEY KUROEDOV, MD • *Cardiovascular Research, Institute of Physiology, University of Zürich and Cardiovascular Center, University Hospital, Zürich, Switzerland*

JON D. LAMAN, PhD • *Department of Immunology, Erasmus Medical Center, Rotterdam, The Netherlands*

BURKHARD LUDEWIG, PhD, DVM • *Research Department, Kantonal Hospital St. Gallen, St. Gallen, Switzerland*

THOMAS F. LÜSCHER, MD • *Cardiovascular Research, Institute of Physiology, University of Zürich and Cardiovascular Center, University Hospital, Zürich, Switzerland*

GANESH MANOHARAN, MBBCh, MD, MRCPI • *Cardiovascular Centre Aalst, OLV Hospital, Aalst, Belgium*

ELIZABETH G. NABEL, MD • *The Nabel Lab, Genome Technology Branch, NHGRI Division of Intramural Research, National Heart, Lung, and Blood Institute, NIH, Bethesda, MD*

FRANZ-JOSEF NEUMANN, MD • *Herz Zentrum Bad Krozingen, Bad Krozingen, Germany*

KOEN NIEMAN, MD, PhD • *Thoraxcenter, Department of Cardiology and Department of Radiology, Erasmus Medical Center, Rotterdam, The Netherlands*

GERARD PASTERKAMP, PhD • *Laboratory of Experimental Cardiology, Heart Lung Institute, University Medical Center Utrecht, Utrecht, The Netherlands*

NICO H. J. PIJLS, MD, PhD • *Department of Cardiology, Catharina Hospital, Eindhoven, The Netherlands*

RAVISH SACHAR, MD • *Wake Heart and Vascular, Raleigh, NC*

MASATAKA SATA, MD, PhD • *Department of Cardiovascular Medicine, University of Tokyo Graduate School of Medicine, Tokyo, Japan*

GURPREET S. SANDHU, MD, PhD • *Division of Cardiovascular Diseases, Mayo Clinic College of Medicine, Rochester, MN*

JOHAN C. H. SCHUURBIERS, BSc • *Thoraxcenter, Cardiology Department, Erasmus Medical Center, Rotterdam, The Netherlands*

ROBERT S. SCHWARTZ, MD • *Minnesota Cardiovascular Research Institute, Minneapolis Heart Institute, Minneapolis, MN*

PATRICK W. SERRUYS, MD, PhD • *Thoraxcenter, Cardiology Department, Erasmus Medical Center, Rotterdam, The Netherlands*

GEORGIOS SIANOS, MD, PhD • *Department of Cardiology, Thoraxcenter, Erasmus Medical Center, Rotterdam, The Netherlands*

ROBERT D. SIMARI, MD • *Division of Cardiovascular Diseases, Mayo Clinic College of Medicine, Rochester, MN*

CORNELIS J. SLAGER, PhD • *Thoraxcenter, Cardiology Department, Erasmus Medical Center, Rotterdam, The Netherlands*

AMANDA G. M. R. SOUSA, MD, PhD • *Institute Dante Pazzanese of Cardiology, São Paulo, Brazil*

J. EDUARDO SOUSA, MD, PhD • *Institute Dante Pazzanese of Cardiology, São Paulo, Brazil*

BRADLEY H. STRAUSS, MD, PhD • *Department of Cardiology, St. Michael's Hospital, Toronto, Ontario, Canada*

HIDEO TAMAI, MD • *Department of Cardiology, Shiga Medical Center for Adults, Shiga, Japan*

FELIX C. TANNER, MD • *Cardiovascular Research, Institute of Physiology, University of Zürich and Cardiovascular Center, University Hospital, Zürich, Switzerland*

DENNIE TEMPEL, BSc • *Thoraxcenter, Cardiology Department, Erasmus Medical Center, Rotterdam, The Netherlands*

ATTILA THURY, MD, PhD • *Thoraxcenter, Cardiology Department, Erasmus Medical Center, Rotterdam, The Netherlands*

ERIC J. TOPOL, MD • *Department of Molecular and Experimental Medicine, Scripps Translational Science Institute, Scripps Health, Division of Cardiovascular Diseases, Scripps Clinic, The Scripps Research Institute, La Jolla, CA*

ARTURO G. TOUCHARD, MD • *Minnesota Cardiovascular Research Institute, Minneapolis Heart Institute, Minneapolis, MN*

MYKOLA TSAPENKO, MD, PhD • *Department of Medicine, Bronx VA Medical Center, New York, NY*

TAKAFUMI TSUJI, MD • *Department of Cardiology, Shiga Medical Center for Adults, Shiga, Japan*

RENU VIRMANI, MD • *Department of Cardiovascular Pathology, Armed Forces Institute of Pathology, Washington, DC*

RON WAKSMAN, MD • *Division of Cardiology, Washington Hospital Center, Washington, DC*

KENNETH WALSH, PhD • *Molecular Cardiology, Whitaker Cardiovascular Institute, Boston University School of Medicine, Boston, MA*

JOLANDA J. WENTZEL, PhD • *Thoraxcenter, Cardiology Department, Erasmus Medical Center, Rotterdam, The Netherlands*

WILLIAM WIJNS, MD, PhD • *Cardiovascular Centre Aalst, OLV Hospital, Aalst, Belgium*

ANDREW WRAGG, MD • *The Cardiovascular Branch, National Heart, Lung and Blood Institute National Institutes of Health, Bethesda, MD*

DIETLIND ZOHLNHÖFER, MD • *Deutsches Herzzentrum München, München, Germany*

# LIST OF COLOR PLATES

The color plates listed below appear following p. 226

# I  PATHOPHYSIOLOGY AND DIAGNOSIS

# 1

# Unraveling the Complex Process of Restenosis From Bench to Bedside

*Henricus J. Duckers, MD, PhD,*
*Caroline Cheng, PhD, Dennie Tempel, BSc,*
*and Patrick W. Serruys, MD, PhD*

## INTRODUCTION

The introduction of coronary balloon angioplasty in the late 1970s by Andreas Gruentzig provided an innovative, less invasive method for revascularization of patients with coronary artery disease. This has subsequently led to a rapid development of new percutaneous devices to treat atherosclerotic vasculopathies. Following its success in the initial studies, the expanded use of angioplasty in the clinic has shown that the arteries could react to angioplasty by a proliferative process similar to wound healing, a process known as restenosis. Defined as a renarrowing of the treated vessel area that equals or exceeds 50% of the lumen in the adjacent normal segment of the artery, restenosis severely limited the success of percutaneous coronary intervention. Together with the high prevalence of this vasculopathy, which ranges from 30% to 60% of lesions treated, an intensive search was prompted for interventional techniques that could minimize the risk of restenosis.

For the last two decades, intervention cardiologists and vascular biologists alike have conducted numerous studies to increase their understanding of its complex mechanism in order to cope with this new form of proliferative vascular disease. From the outcomes of these studies it has become increasingly clear that the success of any interventional method must be determined, not only by its reliability and efficiency in recovering the lumen of the diseased artery, but also by reducing its likelihood in triggering the process of restenosis.

Recently, research, diagnostics, and therapy development in restenosis have hugely advanced, with new insights of the disease emerging rapidly as vascular biologists benefit from innovative laboratory techniques that have emerged from the molecular

From: *Contemporary Cardiology: Essentials of Restenosis: For the Interventional Cardiologist*
Edited by: H. J. Duckers, E. G. Nabel, and P. W. Serruys © Humana Press Inc., Totowa, NJ

biology, cell biology, and immunology field. The application of these findings has in turn helped to design new treatments for restenosis. In addition to this, rapid advances in the development of diagnostic tools that enable early detection of restenotic lesions, and the emergence and subsequently, large-scale adaptation and refinement of (drug-eluting) stents, has pushed clinical management of this proliferative vascular disease into an innovative era, in which restenosis is adequately reduced and the healing of the arterial wall after PCI is optimized.

This book provides the practicing cardiologists and biologists an elaborate review of the current advances in the field. The process of restenosis will be explored from bench to bedside, encompassing in equal detail the newest scientific findings of the biological mechanisms as well as the progression in development of diagnostics and treatments. It also provides the reader with a basic understanding of the biological process and the latest development in diagnostics and treatments of the disease, together with an up-to-date detailed discussion of the most important recent findings. This makes it an excellent handbook for introducing the subject to new intervention cardiologists, vascular biologists, and medical students.

It will start by describing the epidemiology and the basic pathogenesis (Part I), supplying the necessary background information, and making the reader familiar with the definitions and different aspects of restenosis. It will also include chapters that encompass detailed description of the clinical manifestation and the histomorphological representation of restenosis by well-established investigators who pioneered this particular field. The mechanisms by which important factors such as shear stress and the immune system drive the pathogenesis of restenosis, are explored by experts in these particular fields. The last chapter of Part I will discuss the different animal models that are commonly used for restenosis research, providing the interested cardiologist–scientist key knowledge about the advantages, drawbacks, and limitations of each arterial injury model.

In Part II, the novel molecular biological mechanisms underlying restenosis will be discussed in depth. The reader will be introduced to the use of genomic and proteomic tools in animal and patient studies. It will provide a clear perspective to the clinical application of these molecular principles in vascular disease. The last chapters focus on the contribution of circulatory stem and progenitor cells to restenosis, vascular repair, and atherosclerosis, on cell cycle regulation, on arterial remodeling, and on the effects of endothelial nitric oxide synthase that all play significant roles in the progression of the disease.

The focus shifts in Part III to diagnostics, reviewing the recent advances in invasive and noninvasive imaging of stenotic lesions, which has emerged in the recent years as a promising alternative to conventional imaging. This will be discussed by, the very people who have pioneered this particular field of vascular imaging. The last two parts of this book explores the exciting processes, we and others recently have obtained in the treatment of this vexing clinical problem.

Part IV will discuss the clinical experience with applying pharmacotherapy, brachytherapy, eluting stents, and biodegradable stents in the prevention of restenosis. It will be then followed by chapters in Part V that describe the more daring, but nevertheless stimulating advancements in applying biotechnology in the treatment of restenosis. The chapters discuss the use of different types of vectors, transgene regulatory systems, and antisense oligonucleotides in vascular gene therapy. The use of molecular inhibitors that target restenosis by affecting the cell cycle will also be discussed. Finally, the current available methods that are suitable for local gene delivery are explored in the final chapter.

With these chapters elaboratly discussing the current understanding on the pathophysiology, molecular and genetic base, and methods of diagnosis of restenosis, and presenting the current state-of-the-art management, including pharmacotherapy and interventional percutaneous approaches using brachytherapy, gene therapy, and drug-eluting stent technology, we believe that this book provides the reader with a complete overview of the basic and applied knowledge of restenosis, leading to better insight and decision-making in clinical practice.

Finally, we would like to thank the contributors for their time and efforts. Without them, this high quality work could not have been produced.

# 2

# Epidemiology and Pathogenesis of Restenosis

*Randolph L. Geary,* MD
*and Alexander W. Clowes,* MD

### CONTENTS

## SCOPE AND EPIDEMIOLOGY OF RESTENOSIS

### Scope

Recurrent lumen narrowing has been a significant limitation of open and percutaneous methods of arterial reconstruction from their inception. The term restenosis, used in the 1950s in reference to recurrent heart valvular stenosis, was later adopted to define recurrent lumen narrowing after open arterial reconstruction such as carotid endarterectomy *(1,2)*. With the development of peripheral angioplasty by Dotter in the 1960s *(3)* and then percutaneous approaches to angioplasty of renal, coronary, and iliac arteries by Gruentzig and colleagues *(4–7)* the problem of restenosis grew exponentially. Now millions of procedures to reconstruct occlusive vascular lesions are performed worldwide each year *(8–10)*. In contrast to many hurdles overcome by the pioneers of open and percutaneous revascularization, restenosis remains a major limitation of virtually every form of arterial reconstruction (Table 1) *(2,10–23)*. The morbidity from restenosis, largely in the form of repeat interventions, has generated a health care burden presently measured in billions of dollars *(8)*.

As percutaneous coronary angioplasty became widely adopted in the 1980s, restenosis was reported in 30–60% of patients *(10,24,25)*, most presenting with recurrent symptoms 1–4 mo postprocedure *(26,27)*. Increased physician experience with angioplasty; technological refinements in equipment and imaging; and improved patient and lesion selection each reduced the frequency of restenosis slightly but a major breakthrough was not realized until stents were introduced a decade later *(28,29)*. That stents reduced coronary restenosis was established in two prospective randomized trials reported in 1994 where, compared with angioplasty, stenting reduced restenosis from

From: *Contemporary Cardiology: Essentials of Restenosis: For the Interventional Cardiologist*
Edited by: H. J. Duckers, E. G. Nabel, and P. W. Serruys © Humana Press Inc., Totowa, NJ

Table 1
Representative Restenosis Rates by Location and Intervention

| Location | Procedure | Restenosis (%) | References |
|----------|-----------|----------------|------------|
| Coronary | PTA | 21–53 (mean 40) | 10,12 |
| Coronary | Stent | 16–44 (mean 25) | 10,12 |
| Coronary | Atherectomy | 27–39 | 13,14 |
| Coronary | DES | 0–16 | 9,12 |
| Renal | PTA | 27–100 (mean 26) | 16 |
| Renal | Stent | 0–39 (mean 17) | 16 |
| Iliac | PTA | 22–34 | 11 |
| Iliac | Stent | 10–26 | 11 |
| Femoral popliteal | PTA | 39–62 | 11 |
| Femoral popliteal | Stent | 34–47 | 11,17,18 |
| Femoral popliteal | DES | 44 | 18 |
| Carotid | Endarterectomy | 1.7–9.3 | 19,20 |
| Carotid | Stent | 2.7–21 | 21–23 |

PTA, percutaneous transluminal angioplasty.

32% to 22% *(30)* and from 42% to 32% *(31)*, respectively. Stents also reduced restenosis after percutaneous coronary intervention (PCI) for chronic total occlusions, coronary vein graft stenoses, and acute myocardial infarction *(32)*. Still, the problem was not solved as explosive growth in the application of percutaneous interventions steadily increased the global burden of restenosis *(8–10)*.

Other strategies to optimize results of percutaneous interventions have flourished in the past decade only to fall short in clinical trials. Popular examples include debulking procedures with directional and rotational atherectomy catheters, lasers, and other devices *(13,14,33)*. However, there have been two significant breakthroughs since the advent of stents with high potential for reducing restenosis: brachytherapy and drug-eluting stents (DES). Brachytherapy reduced restenosis following angioplasty of *de novo* coronary lesions and treatment of in-stent restenosis, but results have been inconsistent, with late failures after angioplasty and poor outcomes in primary stenting from stent-edge restenosis and nonhealing leading to late thrombosis. Although improvements in brachytherapy devices may overcome these limitations, the expense, complexity, and stigma associated with radiation have tempered enthusiasm (*see* Chapters 23 and 24). The most significant breakthrough to date is occurring now in the form of DES (*see* Chapters 26 and 27). DES coated with sirolimus achieved near 0% restenosis in pilot studies of coronary stenting of highly selected lesions and low rates of restenosis when applied to a broader range of patients and lesions (Table 1) *(12,15)*. Although preliminary studies of sirolimus DES in peripheral arteries were also encouraging, protection from restenosis may be transient as catch-up intimal hyperplasia appears to be a problem at intermediate follow-up (superficial femoral artery restenosis at 2 yr: DES, 40% vs bare stent, 47%) *(18)*. It is with cautious optimism then that late follow-up of DES is awaited in coronary and peripheral vascular beds (*see* Chapters 21 and 22).

## *Epidemiology*

Many investigators have attempted to identify patients at high risk for restenosis after coronary angioplasty to guide recommendations for alternative treatment modalities and to enhance the understanding of underlying mechanisms. Numerous risk factors were suggested in early studies including patient, procedural, and lesion-specific characteristics but few have held up to prospective assessment or proven useful for tailoring treatment in individual patients.

Lesion and procedural risk factors for restenosis after angioplasty include small caliber arteries and longer lesion lengths; multivessel and bifurcation disease; chronic total occlusions; lesions associated with unstable angina; incomplete revascularization; absence of a focal dissection after dilation; and excessive acute elastic recoil *(34–39)*. Incomplete revascularization (i.e., significant residual stenosis or pressure gradient) is now largely of historical interest but the observation that a more complete dilation achieved a more durable result, particularly when associated with dissection *(25,38,40)*, prompted more aggressive dilation protocols. Excessive dilation created a paradoxical effect; however, increasing restenosis as higher injury to the artery wall led to a more robust hyperplastic response *(38,41)*. These observations and the problem of acute vessel closure during angioplasty contributed substantially to the impetus for stent development. Although stents reduced absolute restenosis rates by about 10%, these same risk factors, particularly small vessel caliber and longer lesion length, have also contributed to increased restenosis following coronary stenting as well *(42,43)*.

Patient demographics associated with restenosis have also been explored extensively. Race, gender *(44–46)*, smoking status, blood pressure, plasma C-reactive protein *(47)*, homocysteine *(47)*, and Lp(a) *(47)* levels were each implicated as risk factors for restenosis in early studies but have had little impact in larger statistically robust series. Nonetheless, a handful of genetic *(see* Part II) and acquired risk factors for restenosis have been identified of which diabetes is perhaps the most important *(48–53)*.

Although early reports were inconsistent in linking diabetes and restenosis it is now clearly established that diabetic patients suffer worse outcomes after PCI. The etiology is multifactorial but due in large part to increased frequency of restenosis and the associated morbidity of repeat interventions *(48,49)*. In the Bypass Angioplasty Revascularization Investigators (BARI) trial, a randomized comparison of coronary angioplasty and bypass surgery, diabetic patients on therapy were found to have significantly worse outcomes when treated with angioplasty than they did with bypass surgery. This was in contrast to roughly equivalent results for the larger study population and again was due in part to increased frequency of restenosis *(50,51)*. It was predicted that stents would improve results of coronary angioplasty in diabetic patients but this has not been the case in contemporary series *(49,52)*. However, exciting results have been obtained recently in diabetic patients undergoing coronary stenting combined with pharmacotherapies. Both the II(b)III(a) inhibitor Reopro (Lilly, Centocor) given systemically and the antiproliferative agent sirolimus delivered locally through DES have improved results of stenting in diabetic patients *(12,53)*.

Elevated plasma homocysteine, a risk factor for atherosclerosis has also been implicated in restenosis *(47,54,55)*. Treatment with a homocysteine-lowering drug regimen (folate, $B_{12}$, and pyridoxine) reduced plasma homocysteine levels and the frequency of restenosis in patients undergoing PCI *(54)*. But it is not entirely clear that the effect was linked to homocysteine lowering as observational studies have inconsistently correlated circulating homocysteine levels with restenosis following coronary interventions *(47,56,57)*. Moreover, patients with inherited polymorphisms in methylenetetrahydrofolate reducstase (MTHFR) and other genes that alter homocysteine metabolism have not been found to have increased risk for restenosis following PCI *(57)*.

As with many disorders, having had one episode of restenosis predisposes to recurrence. This association is the strongest for recurrence at the same site following repeat interventions rather than at separate sites treated on the same or later date *(39)*. Curiously, patients undergoing PCI of multiple *de novo* lesions most often develop restenosis at only one of the treated sites *(39)*. These observations suggest that inherited and acquired risk factors may have less impact on restenosis than lesion-specific or intervention-specific risk factors. It remains to be seen whether the subset of patients with multiple sites of restenosis have unique identifiable genetic or acquired risk factors to explain a more generalized phenotype.

## PATHOGENESIS OF RESTENOSIS

### *Initiation of the Injury Response*

Restenosis is the culmination of a complex series of cellular and molecular events precipitated by injury to the artery wall during reconstruction. The magnitude of this response is variable; however, and generally proportional to the magnitude of the initial injury. To assimilate and reconcile experimental and clinical data on mechanisms of lumen narrowing after PCI requires an understanding of the acute structural damage that occurs with experimental and clinical procedures used to increase lumen caliber.

The perception that inflating an angioplasty balloon increases lumen caliber by stretching the artery wall is an oversimplification. Although a normal artery wall is relatively elastic, stretching it much beyond its capacity for physiological vasodilation disrupts the syncytium of medial smooth muscle cells (SMC) and denudes endothelial cells from the lumen surface *(58)*. When modeled in normal animals a modest stretch injury that does not rupture the internal elastic lamina (IEL) results in a response that is highly reproducible with neointimal thickening over ensuing weeks consisting of cells expressing α-actin and large amounts of extracellular matrix (Fig. 1) *(58)*. If injury is minimized by simply denuding the endothelium without stretching the artery wall, the hyperplastic response is reduced but not eliminated *(59)*. Conversely, severe dilation with rupture of the IEL and tearing of the media leads to an exaggerated but less reproducible hyperplastic response.

Although much of the early biology of intimal hyperplasia was established in models of injury to normal arteries, drugs that limited hyperplasia in these models *(60,61)* consistently failed to inhibit restenosis in early clinical trials *(62–64)*. This paradox prompted a critical reappraisal of experimental models of restenosis a decade ago and it was then recognized that species differences existed in the regulation of hyperplasia *(65)* and that few models accurately depicted the contribution of advanced atherosclerotic plaques to the injury response *(66–68)*. Perhaps most importantly, during this period the concept of artery wall remodeling came to light as a key contributor to postangioplasty restenosis in coronary and peripheral arteries *(67,69–72)*.

In practice, angioplasty is applied to stenoses encompassed by advanced atherosclerotic plaque. Unlike normal artery wall these lesions are inelastic and break rather than stretch when dilated (Fig. 2) *(66–68,73–75)*. The pattern of injury in the setting of pre-existing plaque has been characterized in time-course analyses of atherosclerotic nonhuman primates undergoing angioplasty *(66–68)*. Acute structural damage to the artery wall is more extensive than in normal arteries with plaque fracture, subintimal dissection, and variable stretching, tearing or rupture of the media and adventitia (Figs. 1 and 2). Thus, the injury is transmural, influenced by plaque complexity and geometry, and closely mirrors acute damage from angioplasty to advanced human plaques *(73–75)*.

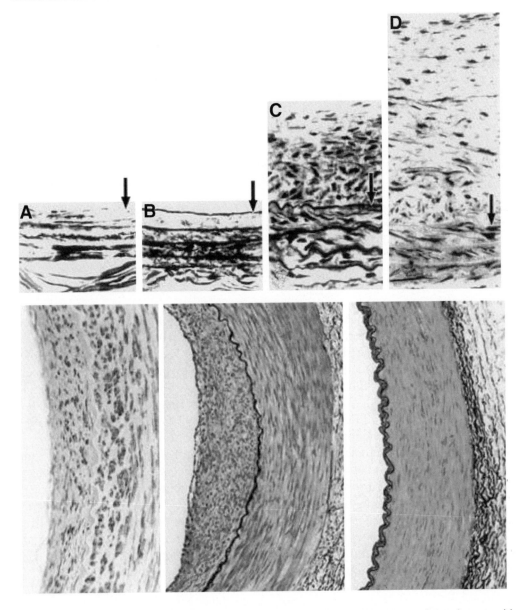

**Fig. 1.** Response to injury, normal artery wall. (Top panel) Histological cross-sections of rat carotid artery before injury (**A**), immediately after endothelial denudation with a balloon catheter (**B**), 2 wk after injury (**C**), and 12 wk after injury (**D**). Note marked intimal thickening at 2 and 12 wk. Arrows indicate IEL. Lumen is at top. (Bottom panel) Histological cross-sections of a normal baboon saphenous artery before injury (left) and 1 mo after denudation with a balloon catheter (middle). α-Actin stain demonstrates the composition of media and neointima as predominantly smooth muscle. Reprinted with permission from ref. *58*. (Please *see* insert for color version.)

As in normal arteries, neointima accumulates rapidly from 2 to 4 wk postangioplasty in atherosclerotic arteries, filling in plaque fractures and dissections created during balloon inflation (Fig. 2) *(66–68)*. Angiographic lumen diameter is the highest in this model when the balloon is maximally inflated then decreases within minutes of balloon deflation by approx 30% from acute elastic recoil. At 4 d however, average lumen area

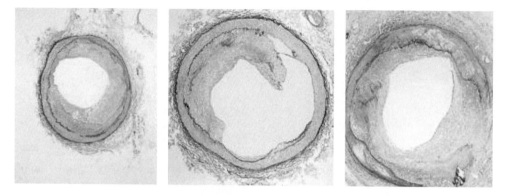

**Fig. 2.** Response to injury, atherosclerotic artery wall. Histological cross-sections of atherosclerotic primate iliac arteries before angioplasty (left), immediately after balloon inflation (middle) and 1 mo later (right). Note the acute fracture and plaque dissection on balloon deflation (middle) and the transmural injury response at 1 mo with neointima filling plaque and medial tear along with dense adventitial fibrosis (right). This response closely depicts the findings at autopsy in human beings that have undergone angioplasty *(73,75)*. (Please *see* insert for color version.)

remains about 130% larger than at baseline *(66,67)* but at 4 wk one-third of injured arteries have lost all or more of the acute gain achieved with balloon inflation *(67)*. Although virtually all injured arteries develop neointima, the extent of lumen narrowing in the atherosclerotic model does not correlate well with the extent of intimal hyperplasia but rather lumen caliber mirrors changes in artery wall size (EEL area) at 1 and 4 mo postangioplasty (Fig. 3) *(67)*. These data and serial imaging from clinical studies (*see* "Contribution of Wall Remodeling") confirm the importance of inward remodeling in restenosis following angioplasty of advanced atherosclerotic plaques.

Taken together, these data emphasize the relationship between the extent of acute injury and magnitude of the hyperplastic response and underscore two major structural determinants of lumen narrowing following PCI: accumulation of new artery wall mass (neointima) and changes in the geometry of pre-existing wall mass (inward or constrictive remodeling). Restenosis following angioplasty is in large part from excessive inward artery wall remodeling although for millions of reconstructions with stents, inward remodeling is blocked and lumen encroachment is entirely from new wall mass (Figs. 4 and 5). The remaining discussion will therefore focus on the pathogenesis of intimal hyperplasia and constrictive artery wall remodeling.

## *Contribution of New Wall Mass*

For decades the focus of restenosis research was on the biology of intimal hyperplasia, the proliferative response leading to accumulation of new cells and matrix within the artery wall. This is a generic response to virtually all forms of arterial injury (e.g., angioplasty, atherectomy, laser debridement, freezing, electrical injury, and endarterectomy) of both normal and atherosclerotic arteries. Intimal hyperplasia is not unique to the artery wall, as veins and prosthetic grafts used for bypass procedures also fail from critical stenoses caused from hyperplasia. New tissue formed by intimal hyperplasia is termed "neointima" because it generally accumulates luminally, sandwiched between endothelium and IEL (Fig. 1). However, the transmural injury caused during reconstruction of atherosclerotic arteries leads to accumulation of new tissue within the media and adventitia as well (Fig. 2).

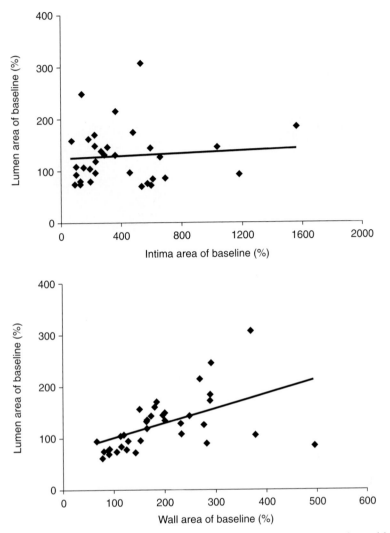

**Fig. 3.** Relationship between lumen area, intimal area, and remodeling. Scatter plots with regression lines for normalized luminal area compared with normalized intimal area (top) and with normalized artery wall size (EEL area, bottom) of iliac arteries from 37 atherosclerotic cynomolgus monkeys 1 mo after angioplasty. Lumen caliber and artery size are closely related ($r = 0.72$, $p < 0.001$), whereas a poor correlation exists between lumen caliber and intimal mass ($r = 0.10$, $p =$ not significant). Reprinted with permission from ref. *67.*

The sequence of events in forming a neointima is perhaps the most extensively characterized in the rat carotid injury model *(58–60).* Balloon inflation and withdrawal remove the endothelium and, without rupturing the IEL, stretch the media with acute loss of about 25% of SMCs (Fig. 1) *(58,59,76).* Platelets, clotting proteins, and inflammatory cells immediately adhere to the exposed subendothelium forming a thin carpet of thrombus that resolves within 48–72 h *(58,76).* Platelet degranulation releases growth and chemotactic factors onto the subendothelium and media *(77).* SMCs are also exposed to mitogenic clotting proteins and leukocyte-derived factors present in the acute thrombus. In addition, medial SMCs themselves release growth factors as a consequence of cellular injury and disruption *(78).* This confluence of diverse mitogenic

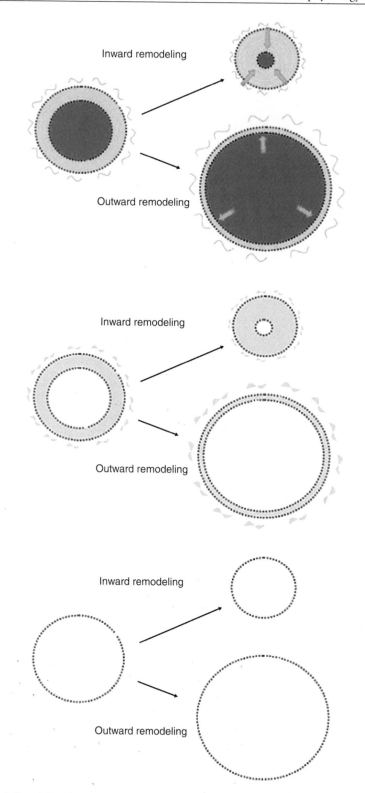

**Fig. 4.** Remodeling defined. Diagram of changes in artery wall geometry independent of changes in artery wall mass leading to inward and outward remodeling.

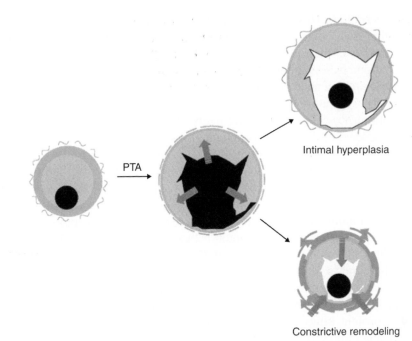

**Fig. 5.** Mechanisms of lumen narrowing following angioplasty. Diagram illustrates the early concept of restenosis after angioplasty due entirely to intimal hyperplasia (top) and the more contemporary model, which includes both neointima formation and constrictive remodeling (bottom).

stimuli initiates a marked proliferative response within 24 h of injury when fully 30% of medial SMCs have entered S-phase *(58,76)*.

A number of genes are expressed and required for SMC entry into the cell cycle and migration into the intima. For example, in the rat, c-*myc* and c-*myb* blockade with antisense oligonucleotides inhibits DNA replication and intimal hyperplasia *(79)*. Recent success of sirolimus-coated stents likely relates to interactions with critical cell-cycle proteins. Sirolimus inhibits SMC growth and migration in vitro by increasing p27$^{kip1}$, which in turn downregulates cyclin-dependent kinase activity (cdk2 and cdk4) and retinoblastoma protein phosphorylation to block the G1/S transition *(80)*. Replication continues and by 4 d both quiescent and proliferating SMCs begin migrating from the media through interstices in the IEL to form a neointima *(58,76,81,82)*. The neointima expands from continued SMC replication and production of extracellular matrix (Fig. 1) *(83)*. By 4 wk cells have largely become quiescent, intimal cell numbers remain stable and further expansion of the neointima is from additional matrix production *(58,76)*. A steady state is reached at about 3 mo when extracellular material accounts for fully 80% of lesion volume (Fig. 1) *(58,76)*.

Early studies of the injury response focused extensively on the role of platelets and thrombus based on three observations:

1. Platelets and thrombus contain potent SMC mitogens;
2. Platelet adherence and degranulation precede SMC proliferation; and
3. Thrombocytopenia attenuates intimal thickening *(77,84)*.

Rats made thrombocytopenic exhibited decreased platelet adherence to the denuded artery wall (5% of control) and neointimal formation was reduced but surprisingly medial proliferation was not *(84)*. This suggested that platelet factors primarily drove SMC migration into the neointima rather than stimulating the initial wave of replication. This hypothesis is supported by studies of platelet-derived growth factor (PDGF). In rats treated with PDGF at the time of carotid balloon injury there was little increase in medial replication but SMC migration and neointimal area increased substantially *(85)*. Conversely, blocking PDGF at the time of injury with antibody significantly reduced neointimal area without inhibiting medial replication *(86)*. Thus, PDGF and likely other platelet factors have chemotactic properties independent of the mitogens initiating medial replication.

Other coagulation factors regulating SMC growth and migration include thrombin generated acutely on the surface of the denuded artery wall. Blocking thrombin generation with hirudin or its analogs or with inhibitors of tissue factor reduces DNA synthesis after angioplasty and inhibits intimal hyperplasia *(87–89)*. A similar result is obtained in the rat model with inhibitors of the thrombin protease-activated receptors and consistent with these data, protease-activated receptor-1 knockout mice develop less neointima in response to injury than wild-type controls *(89,90)*. The anticoagulant heparin was among the first agents found to block intimal hyperplasia in animal models *(60,90)*. Heparin's mechanism of action is multimodal and incompletely defined. It inhibits thrombus formation and directly blocks rat SMC growth and migration by inhibiting activation of mitogen-activated protein kinases and cell-cycle regulatory genes (e.g., c-*myb*) *(82,90)*. Heparin also acts indirectly by inhibiting expression of proteases required for matrix degradation (e.g., plasminogen activators and matrix metalloproteinases [MMPs]) *(91)* and by dislodging matrix-bound growth factors such as basic fibroblast growth factor (bFGF, FGF2) from the extracellular matrix surrounding SMCs in the injured media *(92)*.

Given these data one would have expected clinical trials of anticoagulant and antiplatelet agents to quickly improve the problem of restenosis. In fact, the first human studies employed aspirin and coumadin in patients undergoing angioplasty but the results were disappointing *(93)*. Later trials with heparin, so effective in animal models, also failed to prevent restenosis after PCI *(62)* but there remained speculation that doses, kept low and brief to avoid bleeding complications, may have been inadequate. Moreover, none of these trials actually measured neointima, leaving open the possibility that a significant inhibitory effect was masked by adverse artery wall remodeling. Another question raised by this paradox was whether species differences existed in regulation of SMC growth. To address this question experiments were designed in primates mimicking a heparin protocol proven effective in rats. High-dose heparin was infused intravenously for 4 wk after balloon injury and, in contrast to the rat, neointimal formation in primates was not altered by heparin *(65)*. SMCs isolated from primate arteries and veins were also far less responsive than rat SMCs to heparin inhibition in vitro *(65)*, supporting the possibility that some clinical failures reflect species effects.

Enthusiasm for antiplatelet agents to inhibit restenosis was rekindled by the EPIC (Evaluation of the 7E3 for the Prevention of Ischemic Complications) trial, in which the platelet II(b)III(a) inhibitor abciximab (Reopro) significantly reduced 6 mo major adverse cardiac events following PCI *(94)*. The benefit was remarkably durable *(95)* but the underlying mechanism remained unknown until experiments in atherosclerotic primates showed Reopro had no effect on artery wall mass or remodeling following angioplasty or stenting *(96)*. These results were confirmed in later clinical trials with angiographic end points showing no improvement in lumen caliber in treated patients *(97)*. Together these studies suggest the clinical benefits of anticoagulants and platelet inhibitors are primarily resulting from prevention of acute thrombus formation at sites of injury and likely to preservation of microvascular flow downstream of PCI.

As noted earlier, a key observation in understanding the molecular regulation of inti-mal hyperplasia is the link between injury severity and magnitude of the hyperplastic response *(59)*. In the rat model a significant fraction of medial SMCs die acutely from a moderate stretch injury, releasing mitogens such as bFGF that bind to extracellular matrix, forming a reservoir for paracrine activation of surviving cells *(78,92)*. Medial replication is thus proportional to the extent of injury and can be inhibited by displac-ing bFGF from the injured artery wall with heparin or by directly neutralizing bFGF with blocking antibodies *(78,92)*. Conversely, infusing exogenous bFGF at the time of injury enhances medial SMC proliferation and neointimal thickening but surprisingly, a delayed infusion does not stimulate further replication of cells that have already arrived in the neointima *(98)*. So activation of SMCs requires context and is tightly regulated temporally and spatially after injury.

Arterial injury generally promotes spasm if the media is not disrupted and capable of vasomotor responses. Curiously, most vasoconstrictors prominent in the atherosclerotic artery wall or induced by injury are also potent SMC mitogens. Perhaps the best exam-ple of this relationship is angiotensin II *(61,99–102)*. When infused in pharmacological amounts at time of injury, angiotensin II stimulates SMC replication in the media and neointima *(99)*. Converting enzyme inhibitors, which block angiotensin II formation and inhibit kinases that degrade bradykinin, limit intimal thickening in the rat carotid injury model by inhibiting SMC migration from the media into the neointima *(61)*. Blocking angiotensin AT1 receptors with specific antagonists has a similar inhibitory effect *(102)*. Other vasoconstrictors prominent in diseased and injured arteries include endothelin-1, norepinephrine, thrombin, thromboxane A2, and serotonin, and each of these has been shown to possess mitogenic and/or chemotactic effects toward SMCs *(103)*. The corol-lary that vasodilators are generally growth inhibitors, may also be true. Nitric oxide (NO) is an important example. Treatment with NO donors or overexpression of NO syn-thases (NOS) can inhibit intimal hyperplasia as discussed later *(104–106)*.

Extracellular matrix accumulating at sites of injury contributes up to 80% of neointi-mal mass. The amount of new matrix elaborated is influenced significantly by growth factors such as transforming growth factor (TGF)-β and angiotensin II *(107,108)*. TGF-β is a pleiotropic stimulant for SMCs in culture but it is not entirely clear whether SMC replication or migration are enhanced or inhibited in vivo. Intimal thickening can be blocked with neutralizing antibodies to TGF-β and a soluble TGF receptor used as a blocking reagent reduced lumen narrowing carotid ligation in mice *(107)*. The latter effect appears to be primarily from improved remodeling however, as neointimal area was unaltered *(107)*. Overexpression of TGF-β in the artery wall of swine with a viral vector increased neointimal growth primarily by driving excessive matrix syn-thesis *(108)*.

In addition to adding mass to the neointima directly, the altered composition of pericellu-lar matrix at sites of injury facilitates SMC replication and migration. The existing pericel-lular matrix is fragmented by angioplasty when the wall is disrupted and then further by leukocyte and SMC proteases induced as cells begin to divide. Matrix-degrading proteases upregulated during the first 2 wk following injury include the plasminogen activators uPA and tissue plasminogen activator (tPA) *(109,110)*. Inhibition with tranexamic acid or local overexpression of the gene encoding plasminogen-activator inhibitor-1 suppresses SMC migration without affecting replication *(109–112)*. Intimal hyperplasia is reduced in uroki-nase plasminogen activator and tPA-receptor null mice; increased in plasminogen-activator inhibitor-1 null mice; but unaltered in the tPA knockout *(110)*. MMP activity also increases rapidly after injury as SMCs upregulate expression of gelatinase B (MMP-9) and stromelysin-1 (MMP-3) whereas gelatinase A (MMP-2) is expressed constitutively before the injury *(112–115)*.

Blocking MMP activity pharmacologically or with vectors expressing endogenous inhibitors (e.g., tissue inhibitor of metalloproteinases-1) suppresses intimal thickening by blocking SMC migration. The effects of pharmacological MMP inhibitors have often been transient; however, with "catch up" growth of neointima after treatment is stopped. Certain species also show less of an effect *(116)* and preliminary results of clinical studies employing stents coated with the broad-spectrum MMP inhibitor batimastat have been disappointing with no decrease in neointimal accumulation. New matrix elaborated in early neointima has a composition distinct from the quiescent uninjured media, a proteoglycan-rich mix of versican and hyaluronan (HA) with vitronectin, fibronectin, and matricellular proteins such as osteopontin *(68,83,117,118)*. These and other molecules create a substrate, conducive to cell movement and tissue remodeling mediated by cell–matrix adhesive interactions. Ligation of specific matrix receptors, for example, integrins, CD44, and receptor for hyaluronic-mediated motility, initiate autocrine and paracrine signaling that contribute to first wave replication and migration *(119–121)*.

Although there is a great deal of knowledge about factors that promote SMC replication, migration, and matrix production, much less is known about negative regulators of SMC growth. In fact, medial SMC replication in mature arteries is less than 0.01%/d and these cells normally turn over only once every two to three decades! So although mechanical injury can induce SMCs to enter the cell cycle within 24 h they are normally refractory to transient mitogenic stimuli. Indeed, an intravenous bolus or local infusion of a potent mitogen such as bFGF has no stimulatory effect on the uninjured artery wall *(122,123)*. Thus, the normal artery wall possesses very efficient mechanisms of negative growth regulation. Two features that contribute to growth inhibition within intact arteries include the normal pericellular matrix and a functional endothelium.

As discussed earlier, the matrix composition changes dramatically after angioplasty and continues to evolve as healing progresses. As neointima matures new signals are generated that may play an important role in returning the artery wall to quiescence. For example, versican and HA are prominent in the initial stages of neointimal development but versican is present only transiently whereas HA persists for months *(68)*. Conversely, elastin is absent from the neointima at 1 mo, but distinct lamellae are present at 4 mo after angioplasty in atherosclerotic primates *(68)* and elastin production has been associated with cessation of SMC replication in vitro and after injury *(124)*. Polymerized interstitial collagen also suppresses SMC growth by inducing endogenous cyclin inhibitors *(125)*. Despite expression of type-I procollagen message during all stages of neointimal development mature collagen fiber deposition is a very late event as measured by picrosirius red staining *(68)*. These changes are consistent with induction and maintenance of SMC quiescence through altered matrix composition over time.

In the rat-carotid injury model SMC replication and neointimal accumulation cease in regions that rapidly re-endothelialize *(58)*. An intact endothelium, in addition to providing a physical barrier between SMCs and blood also produces key inhibitory factors including NO, prostaglandins, heparan sulfate, and others *(104,105,126,127)*. NO generated by endothelial NOS (eNOS, NOSIII) contributes to growth inhibition by directly inhibiting SMC replication and by blocking-platelet activation and leukocyte recruitment at sites of injury *(126)*. Endothelial cyclooxygenases are also important in regulating synthesis of inhibitory prostaglandins such as prostaglandin I2 from arachidonic acid *(127)*. Experimental models in which NO is overexpressed have shown reduced intimal hyperplasia whereas lesions are exacerbated in eNOS knockout mice *(104)*.

Although accumulation of SMCs within the neointima requires replication it is also dependent on the balance with cell death (apoptosis). Apoptosis is an important event in vasculogenesis and vascular remodeling and prominent during intimal thickening after injury *(128–131)*. Even though SMCs continue to replicate at the surface of stable neointimal lesions lacking endothelium, no net increase in SMC number occurs and apoptotic cells are readily detected in this region. Mechanisms regulating apoptosis in the context of vascular injury are still being defined but involve activation of death receptors (e.g., Fas, TNFR) or intracellular stresses that alter the balance of pro- and antiapoptotic signals leading to caspase activation *(130–131)*. The events initiating apoptosis in whole vessels are not well defined but include an increase in certain growth inhibitors (e.g., NO) or a decrease in growth/survival factors (e.g., PDGF, angiotensin II) *(131)*.

### *Contribution of Wall Remodeling*

The early focus of restenosis research was logically on intimal hyperplasia and controlling SMC replication but despite more than a decade of bench research and clinical trials little progress was made at inhibiting restenosis until the breakthrough with stents. Stents were designed to counteract acute elastic recoil on balloon deflation and to maintain higher postprocedural lumen caliber than could be achieved safely with angioplasty alone. A remarkable paradox discovered in early stent studies was that lumen caliber was improved and restenosis reduced despite the fact that stents caused more intimal hyperplasia than angioplasty alone *(29,42,132)*. These observations helped to introduce artery wall remodeling as a key mechanism in the pathogenesis of restenosis.

Discussions of remodeling can be confusing without clear definitions and terminology. For the author's purposes, remodeling will refer to a change in artery wall caliber achieved through a change in the geometry of wall elements (intima, media, and adventitia) independent of a change in wall mass (Fig. 4). An increase in artery wall caliber will be referred to as "outward remodeling" whereas a decrease will be referred to as "inward" or "constrictive remodeling." In experimental studies of remodeling, changes in wall caliber are generally measured histologically by the area bounded by the external elastic lamina (EEL area), recognizing that adventitia is the true outer wall boundary but its margins are not well defined. Clinically, remodeling is assessed with serial imaging such as intravascular ultrasound (IVUS), which can measure changes in artery wall caliber at the medial-adventitial interface as well as changes in composite wall area *(69,70,133)*. In the context of lumen narrowing after angioplasty, it is easier to conceptualize remodeling in isolation from intimal hyperplasia but these processes are clearly linked (Fig. 5).

Angioplasty-induced remodeling begins with balloon inflation, which acutely redistributes artery wall mass outward and longitudinally by variably compressing, extruding, stretching, and tearing plaque, media, and adventitia to achieve a larger lumen. Restenosis would largely be prevented if the artery wall simply maintained the new geometry achieved with balloon inflation. Data supporting this argument come from experimental time-course studies as outlined earlier *(66,67)* and clinical studies employing serial angiography or IVUS early after angioplasty and stenting *(69,70)*. Acute elastic recoil on balloon deflation decreases lumen diameter 10–15% on average unless a stent is deployed *(27,34)*. IVUS data estimate changes in wall geometry then contribute 60–80% of late lumen loss after angioplasty whereas new wall mass contributes 20–40% *(69)*.

In fact, few arteries demonstrate further outward remodeling after angioplasty and most exhibit loss of wall caliber from variable inward remodeling *(67)*.

The molecular regulation of inward remodeling remains poorly defined but clues have come from histological assessment of animal and human lesions examined temporally following angioplasty *(66–68,73,75)*. A popular view of remodeling has emerged from these studies equating constrictive reorganization of cells and extracellular matrix material in the injured artery wall to wound healing, wound contraction, and fibrosis. In cutaneous wounds left to heal by secondary intension, the sequence of cellular events is analogous in many ways to healing of the artery wall after angioplasty *(68,134–137)*. A platelet fibrin plug forms to stop hemorrhage, which then serves as provisional matrix for the influx of leukocytes and subsequent out growth of fibroblasts from damaged wound edges. Fibroblasts dedifferentiate into myofibroblasts, which like SMCs express α-actin and are capable of contracting in response to vasoconstrictors *(135)*. As inflammatory cells remove clot and wound debris myofibroblasts replicate and produce new wound matrix rich in proteoglycans to form granulation tissue. Wound contraction then begins as fibroblasts reorganize and apply traction to the new matrix to bring wound edges together. Subsequent matrix turnover with a change in composition to a more collagen-rich material heralds fibrosis and progression to mature scar. Scar maturation evolves over many months until a final result is achieved beyond 1 yr.

Parallels occur in atherosclerotic arteries wounded by angioplasty where thrombus forms within fractures, clefts and dissections providing provisional scaffolding for the influx of leukocytes *(66,68)*. As in wounds, neutrophils are present during the first 48 h after which monocytes and lymphocytes predominate *(66,68)*. A transient but intense wave of proliferation occurs in all wall layers, peaking at 4 d and then subsides as actin-positive cells move luminally into areas of injury at 7 d *(66)*. These new cells rapidly replace leukocytes and the thrombus scaffolding with new matrix material rich in proteoglycans, filling in plaque and medial fractures with neointima. The neointima thickens substantially between 14 and 28 d whereas at the same time the adventitia exhibits an increase in cellularity and fibrosis (Fig. 2). Constrictive remodeling of the artery wall, perhaps from tension created in reorganization of new matrix, is often dramatic during this time frame *(67,68)*.

Given matrix accounts for more than 60% of artery wall mass constrictive remodeling of the artery wall must involve reorganization of extracellular matrix by SMCs and perhaps adventitial fibroblasts. Matrix reorganization is dependent on cell–matrix adhesive interactions, matrix degradation by proteases, and new matrix synthesis. As in healing wounds the composition of the new matrix material is distinct from that in the pre-existing artery wall *(68,83,117,118,138,139)*. The normal medial matrix is rich in collagen types I and III and elastin with a lesser contribution from proteoglycans *(117)*. As outlined in the previous section neointimal matrix is quite different, rich in proteoglycans and glycosaminoglycans including versican and HA, respectively, matrices prominent in early wounds. Procollagen message expression is also induced at sites of injury but curiously message does not correlate well with the appearance of collagen fibers, which is extensive in adventitia but not neointima one month after injury *(68)*.

HA is a large hydrophilic polymer of repeating disaccharides commonly associated with tissue remodeling in embryogenesis, wound healing, and neoplasia *(140,141)*. Although its role in wound healing is incompletely defined HA is also associated with scarless healing in the embryo and improved collagen reorganization and re-epithelialization when applied exogenously to cutaneous wounds in mature animals. Versican binds along the HA backbone changing its physical-chemical properties, increasing viscoelasticity and together they provide hydrated space favorable for cell movement, invasion, and replication *(137,141)*. The ratio of HA and structural matrix proteins (collagen and elastin) alters matrix reorganization in culture and likely within the healing artery wall *(142)*. HA is expressed in all artery wall layers after angioplasty most prominently the adventitia and neointima *(68,139)*. Colocalization of collagen and HA in the fibrotic adventitia suggests an important interaction supported by in vitro studies of collagen reorganization. Adventitial fibroblasts and medial SMCs cultured from primate aorta use β1 integrins to contract three dimensional collagen gels *(142–144)*. Adding HA significantly enhances collagen reorganization, accelerating gel contraction, and pericellular condensation of collagen fibers *(142)*. This effect is dependent on CD44, an important HA receptor induced in the injured artery wall *(119,142)*. Thus, HA could enhance constrictive reorganization of collagen in the adventitia and inward remodeling.

Although MMPs are important for SMC migration in vitro and expression is upregulated by injury their role in constrictive remodeling is less clear. MMPs have been strongly implicated in the most severe form of outward remodeling—aneurysm formation *(145–148)*. Activity of MMP-2 and MMP-9 is highly increased in the aneurysmal artery wall *(145–148)* and inhibitors prevent aneurysm expansion and rupture in animal models *(148–151)*. Clinical trials of long-term treatment with oral MMPs inhibitors to prevent aneurysm expansion are ongoing. Extending the aneurysm analogy to the injured artery wall suggests that increased MMP activity should lead to favorable outward artery remodeling rather than inward or constrictive remodeling. Experiments in animals are conflicting, however. Mini swine treated with batimastat after iliac angioplasty showed improved remodeling after 6 wk *(152)*. Although arteries were not significantly larger in treated animals the extent of artery shrinkage measured by IVUS was reduced. In contrast, a larger study in atherosclerotic nonhuman primates documented that a 4-wk infusion with a broad-spectrum MMP inhibitor had no effect on artery wall remodeling or intimal hyperplasia after iliac angioplasty *(116)*. This was despite significant plasma MMP inhibitory activity and a marked inhibition of angiogenesis in the same animals *(116)*.

TGF-β and connective tissue growth factor (CTGF) have both been implicated in matrix contraction during wound healing *(153–155)* and CTGF is prominently upregulated in neointima formed in nonhuman primates after aortic reconstruction *(154)*. CTGF stimulates SMC growth and migration and mediates enhanced collagen reorganization by fibroblasts in vitro in response to TGF-β *(153)*. Blocking TGF-β with a soluble receptor has been shown to reduced lumen narrowing after carotid ligation in mice by limiting inward remodeling *(107)*.

More recently, reactive oxygen species (ROS) have been implicated in inward artery wall remodeling. Angioplasty induces an immediate increase in ROS throughout the artery wall that is transient. A second delayed increase in ROS occurs as neointima is enlarging. NADPH oxidases contribute superoxide ($O_2-$), which in turn can react with NO to form peroxynitrite and reduce NO bioavailability *(156)*. Superoxide dismutase (SOD) helps maintain the redox balance by catalyzing the reaction of $O_2-$ to $H_2O_2$, which in turn preserves NO. In a recent study of rabbits undergoing iliac angioplasty, SOD activity was sharply decreased after injury as constrictive remodeling contributed to lumen renarrowing *(156)*. By enhancing SOD with exogenous administration of endothelial cell superoxide dismutase lumen caliber was improved as constrictive remodeling was reduced by 59%. Treatment also significantly increased nitrate levels in the injured artery suggesting improved remodeling was because of increased NO, likely derived from inducible nitric oxide synthase *(156)*. In addition to limiting intimal hyperplasia, NO has been shown in previous studies to improve outward remodeling or limit inward remodeling after angioplasty *(106)*.

## DISCUSSION

Although the number of catheter-based interventions continues to grow in response to an aging population; refinements in technology; societal demands for minimally invasive, cutting edge health care; and marketing pressures from a multibillion dollar industry, recent breakthroughs provide a sense of optimism that the cycle of reintervention for restenosis may be broken in the near future. At present, optimal results from PCI can be achieved through careful patient and lesion selection and complete revascularization using appropriate combinations of angioplasty, stents, and pharmaceuticals. Ideally, treatments to prevent restenosis should target the two major underlying pathological mechanisms: intimal hyperplasia and constrictive remodeling. That emerging technologies such as DES hold such promise should not be surprising when considering they address both mechanisms to enhance the durability of PCI.

## REFERENCES

1. Stoney RJ, String ST. Recurrent carotid stenosis. Surgery 1976;80:705–710.
2. Cossman D, Callow AD, Stein A, Matsumoto G. Early restenosis after carotid endarterectomy. Arch Surg 1978;113:275–278.
3. Dotter CT, Judkins MP. Transluminal treatment of arteriosclerotic obstruction: description of a new technic and a preliminary report of its application. Circulation 1964;3:654–670.
4. Gruntzig A, Kuhlmann U, Vetter W, Lutolf U, Meier B, Siegenthaler W. Treatment of renovascular hypertension with percutaneous transluminal dilatation of a renal-artery stenosis. Lancet 1978;1:801–802.
5. Gruntzig A. Transluminal dilatation of coronary-artery stenosis. Lancet 1978;1:263.
6. Gruntzig A, Kumpe DA. Technique of percutaneous transluminal angioplasty with the Gruntzig balloon catheter. AJR Am J Roentgenol 1979;132:547–552.
7. Gruntzig AR, Senning A, Siegenthaler WE. Nonoperative dilatation of coronary-artery stenosis: percutaneous transluminal coronary angioplasty. N Engl J Med 1979;301:61–68.
8. Topol E, Ellis S, Cosgrove D, et al. Analysis of coronary angioplasty practice in the United States with an insurance-claims data base. Circulation 1993;87:1489–1497.
9. Thom T, Haase N, Rosamond W, et al. Heart disease and stroke statistics—2006 update: A report from the American Heart Association statistics committee and stroke statistics subcommittee. Circulation 2006;113:85–151.
10. Moliterno DJ, Topol EJ. Restenosis: Epidemiology and Treatment. In: Topol EJ, ed. Textbook of Cardiovascular Medicine, 2nd ed. Lippincott-Raven, Philadelphia, 2002, pp. 1715–1750.
11. Dormandy JA, Rutherford RB. Management of peripheral arterial disease (PAD). TASC Working Group. TransAtlantic Inter-Society Concensus (TASC). J Vasc Surg 2000;31:S1–S296.
12. Moses JW, Leon MB, Popma JJ, et al. Sirolimus-eluting stents versus standard stents in patients with stenosis in a native coronary artery. N Engl J Med 2003;349:1315–1323.
13. Stankovic G, Colombo A, Bersin R, et al. Comparison of directional coronary atherectomy and stenting versus stenting alone for the treatment of de novo and restenotic coronary artery narrowing. Am J Cardiol 2004;93:953–958.
14. Bittl JA, Chew DP, Topol EJ, Kong DF, Califf RM. Meta-analysis of randomized trials of percutaneous transluminal coronary angioplasty versus atherectomy, cutting balloon atherotomy, or laser angioplasty. J Am Coll Cardiol 2004;43:936–942.
15. Colombo A, Drzewiecki J, Banning A, et al. Randomized study to assess the effectiveness of slow- and moderate-release polymer-based paclitaxel-eluting stents for coronary artery lesions. Circulation 2003;108:788–794.
16. Leertouwer TC, Gussenhoven EJ, Bosch JL, et al. Stent placement for renal arterial stenosis: where do we stand? A meta-analysis. Radiology 2000;216:78–85.

17. Becquemin JP, Favre JP, Marzelle J, Nemoz C, Corsin C, Liezorovicz A. Systematic versus selective stent placement after superficial femoral artery balloon angioplasty: a multicenter prospective randomized study. J Vasc Surg 2003;37:487–494.

18. Drug-elluting stent update. Endovasc Today 2004;3:28–29.

19. Katras T, Baltazar U, Rush DS, Sutterfield WC, Harvill LM, Stanton PE, Jr. Durability of eversion carotid endarterectomy: comparison with primary closure and carotid patch angioplasty. J Vasc Surg 2001;34:453–458.

20. Archie JP, Jr. A fifteen-year experience with carotid endarterectomy after a formal operative protocol requiring highly frequent patch angioplasty. J Vasc Surg 2000;31:724–735.

21. Shawl FA. Carotid artery stenting: acute and long-term results. Curr Opin Cardiol 2002;17:671–676.

22. Khan MA, Liu MW, Chio FL, Roubin GS, Iyer SS, Vitek JJ. Predictors of restenosis after successful carotid artery stenting. Am J Cardiol 2003;92:895–897.

23. Lal BK, Hobson RW, 2nd, Goldstein J, et al. In-stent recurrent stenosis after carotid artery stenting: life table analysis and clinical relevance. J Vasc Surg 2003;38:1162–1168.

24. Thornton MA, Gruentzig AR, Hollman J, King SB, 3rd, Douglas JS. Coumadin and aspirin in prevention of recurrence after transluminal coronary angioplasty: a randomized study. Circulation 1984;69:721–727.

25. Holmes DR, Jr, Vlietstra RE, Smith HC, et al. Restenosis after percutaneous transluminal coronary angioplasty (PTCA): a report from the PTCA Registry of the National Heart, Lung, and Blood Institute. Am J Cardiol 1984;53:77C–81C.

26. Serruys PW, Luijten HE, Beatt KJ, et al. Incidence of restenosis after successful coronary angioplasty: a time-related phenomenon. A quantitative angiographic study in 342 consecutive patients at 1, 2, 3, and 4 months. Circulation 1988;77:361–371.

27. Nobuyoshi M, Kimura T, Nosaka H, et al. Restenosis after successful percutaneous transluminal coronary angioplasty: serial angiographic follow-up of 229 patients. J Am Coll Cardiol 1988;12: 616–623.

28. Sigwart U, Puel J, Mirkovitch V, Joffre F, Kappenberger L. Intravascular stents to prevent occlusion and restenosis after transluminal angioplasty. N Engl J Med 1987;316:701–706.

29. Puel J, Juilliere Y, Bertrand ME, Rickards AF, Sigwart U, Serruys PW. Early and late assessment of stenosis geometry after coronary arterial stenting. Am J Cardiol 1988;61:546–553.

30. Serruys PW, de Jaegere P, Kiemeneij F, et al. A comparison of balloon-expandable-stent implantation with balloon angioplasty in patients with coronary artery disease. N Engl J Med 1994;331:489–495.

31. Fischman DL, Leon MB, Baim DS, et al. A randomized comparison of coronary-stent placement and balloon angioplasty in the treatment of coronary artery disease. N Engl J Med 1994;331:496–501.

32. Levine GN, Kern MJ, Berger PB, et al. Management of patients undergoing percutaneous coronary revascularization. Ann Intern Med 2003;139:123–136.

33. Hinohara T, Selmon MR, Robertson GC, Braden L, Simpson JS. Directional atherectomy. New approaches for treatment of obstructive coronary and peripheral vascular disease. Circulation 1990;81(3 Suppl):IV79–IV91.

34. Sanders M. Angiographic changes thirty minutes following percutaneous transluminal coronary angioplasty. Angiology 1985;36:419–424.

35. Califf RM, Fortin DF, Frid DJ, et al. Restenosis after coronary angioplasty: an overview. J Am Coll Cardiol 1991;17:2B–13B.

36. Weintraub WS, Kosinski AS, Brown CL, 3rd, King SB, 3rd. Can restenosis after coronary angioplasty be predicted from clinical variables? J Am Coll Cardiol 1993;21:6–14.

37. Leimgruber PP, Roubin GS, Hollman J, et al. Restenosis after successful coronary angioplasty in patients with single-vessel disease. Circulation 1986;73:710–717.

38. Rensing BJ, Hermans WR, Vos J, et al. Angiographic risk factors of luminal narrowing after coronary balloon angioplasty using balloon measurements to reflect stretch and elastic recoil at the dilation site. Am J Cardiol 1992;69:584–591.

39. DiSciascio G, Cowley MJ, Vetrovec GW. Angiographic patterns of restenosis after angioplasty of multiple coronary arteries. Am J Cardiol 1986;58:922–925.

40. Leimgruber PP, Roubin GS, Anderson HV, et al. Influence of intimal dissection on restenosis after successful coronary angioplasty. Circulation 1985;72:530–535.

41. Beatt KJ, Serruys PW, Luijten HE, et al. Restenosis after coronary angioplasty: the paradox of increased lumen diameter and restenosis. J Am Coll Cardiol 1992;19:258–266.

42. Cutlip DE, Chauhan MS, Baim DS, et al. Clinical restenosis after coronary stenting: perspectives from multicenter clinical trials. J Am Coll Cardiol 2002;40:2082–2089.

43. Ruygrok PN, Webster MW, Ardill JJ, et al. Vessel caliber and restenosis: a prospective clinical and angiographic study of NIR stent deployment in small and large coronary arteries in the same patient. Catheter Cardiovasc Interv 2003;59:165–171.

44. Bell MR, Grill DE, Garratt KN, Berger PB, Gersh BJ, Holmes DR, Jr. Long-term outcome of women compared with men after successful coronary angioplasty. Circulation 1995;91:2876–2881.

45. Trabattoni D, Bartorelli AL, Montorsi P, et al. Comparison of outcomes in women and men treated with coronary stent implantation. Catheter Cardiovasc Interv 2003;58:20–28.

46. Mehilli J, Kastrati A, Bollwein H, et al. Gender and restenosis after coronary artery stenting. Eur Heart J 2003;24:1523–1530.

47. Zairis MN, Ambrose JA, Manousakis SJ, et al. The impact of plasma levels of C-reactive protein, lipoprotein (a) and homocysteine on the long-term prognosis after successful coronary stenting: The Global Evaluation of New Events and Restenosis After Stent Implantation Study. J Am Coll Cardiol 2002;40:1375–1382.

48. Stein B, Weintraub WS, Gebhart SP, et al. Influence of diabetes mellitus on early and late outcome after percutaneous transluminal coronary angioplasty. Circulation 1995;91(4):979–989.

49. Mathew V, Gersh BJ, Williams BA, et al. Outcomes in patients with diabetes mellitus undergoing percutaneous coronary intervention in the current era: a report from the Prevention of REStenosis with Tranilast and its Outcomes (PRESTO) trial. Circulation 2004;109:476–480.

50. BARI Investigators. Comparison of coronary bypass surgery with angioplasty in patients with multi-vessel disease. N Engl J Med 1996;335:217–225.

51. Ferguson JJ. NHLI BARI clinical alert on diabetics treated with angioplasty. Circulation 1995;92:3371.

52. Huynh T, Eisenberg MJ, Deligonul U, et al. Coronary stenting in diabetic patients: Results from the ROSETTA registry. Am Heart J 2001;142:960–964.

53. Marso SP, Lincoff AM, Ellis SG, et al. Optimizing the percutaneous interventional outcomes for patients with diabetes mellitus: results of the EPISTENT (Evaluation of platelet IIb/IIIa inhibitor for stenting trial) diabetic substudy. Circulation 1999;100:2477–2484.

54. Schnyder G, Roffi M, Pin R, et al. Decreased rate of coronary restenosis after lowering of plasma homocysteine levels. N Engl J Med 2001;345:1593–1600.

55. Schnyder G, Roffi M, Flammer Y, Pin R, Hess OM. Effect of homocysteine-lowering therapy with folic acid, vitamin B12, and vitamin B6 on clinical outcome after percutaneous coronary interven-tion: the Swiss Heart study: a randomized controlled trial. JAMA 2002;288:973–979.

56. Kojoglanian SA, Jorgensen MB, Wolde-Tsadik G, Burchette RJ, Aharonian VJ. Restenosis in Intervened Coronaries with Hyperhomocysteinemia (RICH). Am Heart J 2003;146:1077–1081.

57. Koch W, Ndrepepa G, Mehilli J, et al. Homocysteine status and polymorphisms of methylenetetrahy-drofolate reductase are not associated with restenosis after stenting in coronary arteries. Arterioscler Thromb Vasc Biol 2003;23:2229–2234.

58. Clowes AW, Reidy MA, Clowes MM. Kinetics of cellular proliferation after arterial injury. I. Smooth muscle growth in the absence of endothelium. Lab Invest 1983;49:327–333.

59. Fingerle J, Au YP, Clowes AW, Reidy MA. Intimal lesion formation in rat carotid arteries after endothelial denudation in absence of medial injury. Arteriosclerosis 1990;10:1082–1087.

60. Clowes AW, Karnovsky MJ. Suppression by heparin of smooth muscle cell proliferation in injured arteries. Nature 1977;265:625–626.

61. Powell JS, Clozel JP, Muller EKM, et al. Inhibitors of angiotensin-converting enzyme prevent myoin-timal proliferation after vascular injury. Science 1989;245:186–188.

62. Faxon DP, Spiro TE, Minor S, for the ERA Investigators. Low molecular weight heparin in prevention of restenosis after angioplasty: Results of enoxaparin restenosis (ERA) trial. Circulation 1994;90:908–914.

63. MERCATOR Study Group. Does the new angiotensin converting enzyme inhibitor cilazapril prevent restenosis after percutaneous transluminal coronary angioplasty? Results of the MERCATOR study: A multicenter, randomized, double-blind placebo-controlled trial. Circulation 1992;86:100–110.

64. Faxon DP. Effect of high dose angiotensin-converting enzyme inhibition on restenosis: Final results of the MERCATOR study, a multicenter, double-blind, placebo-controlled trial of cilazapril. J Am Coll Cardiol 1995;25:362–369.

65. Geary RL, Koyama N, Wang TW, Vergel S, Clowes AW. Failure of heparin to inhibit intimal hyper-plasia in injured baboon arteries: The role of heparin-sensitive and heparin-insensitive pathways in the stimulation of smooth muscle cell migration and proliferation. Circulation 1995;91:2972–2981.

66. Geary RL, Williams JK, Golden D, Brown DG, Benjamin ME, Adams MR. Time course of cellular proliferation, intimal hyperplasia, and remodeling following angioplasty in monkeys with estab-lished atherosclerosis: A nonhuman primate model of restenosis. Arterioscler Thromb Vasc Biol 1996;16:34–43.

67. Mondy JS, Williams JK, Adams MR, Dean RH, Geary RL. Structural determinants of lumen narrowing after angioplasty in atherosclerotic nonhuman primates. J Vasc Surg 1997;26:875–883.

68. Geary RL, Nikkari ST, Wagner WD, Williams JK, Adams MR, Dean RH. Wound healing: a paradigm for lumen narrowing following arterial reconstruction. J Vasc Surg 1998;27:96–108.

69. Mintz GS, Popma JJ, Pichard AD, et al. Arterial remodeling after coronary angioplasty. A serial intravascular ultrasound study. Circulation 1996;94:35–43.

70. Lansky AJ, Mintz GS, Popma JJ, et al. Remodeling after directional coronary atherectomy (with and without adjunct percutaneous transluminal coronary angioplasty): a serial angiographic and intravascular ultrasound analysis from the Optimal Atherectomy Restenosis Study. J Am Coll Cardiol 1998;32:329–337.

71. Post MJ, Borst C, Kuntz RE. The relative importance of arterial remodeling compared with intimal hyperplasia in lumen renarrowing after balloon angioplasty: A study in the normal rabbit and the hypercholesterolemic Yucatan micropig. Circulation 1994;89:2816–2821.

72. Kakuta T, Currier JW, Haudenschild CC, Ryan TJ, Faxon DP. Differences in compensatory vessel enlargement, not intimal formation, account for restenosis after angioplasty in the hypercholesterolemic rabbit model. Circulation 1994;89:2809–2815.

73. Ueda M, Becker AE, Tsukada T, Numano F, Fujimoto T. Fibrocellular tissue response after percutaneous transluminal coronary angioplasty: An immunocytochemical analysis of the cellular composition. Circulation 1991;83:1327–1332.

74. Zarins CK, Lu CT, Gewertz BL, Lyon RT, Rush DS, Glagov S. Arterial disruption and remodeling following balloon dilatation. Surgery 1982;92:1086–1095.

75. Kohchi K, Takebayashi S, Block PC, Hiroki T, Nobuyoshi M. Arterial changes after percutaneous transluminal coronary angioplasty: results at autopsy. J Am Coll Cardiol 1987;10:592–599.

76. Clowes AW, Reidy MA, Clowes MM. Mechanisms of stenosis after arterial injury. Lab Invest 1983;49:208–215.

77. Ross R, Glomset J, Kariya B, Harker L. A platelet-dependent serum factor that stimulates the proliferation of arterial smooth muscle cells in vitro. Proc Natl Acad Sci USA 1974;71:1207–1210.

78. Lindner V, Reidy MA. Proliferation of smooth muscle cells after vascular injury is inhibited by an antibody against basic fibroblast growth factor. Proc Natl Acad Sci USA 1991;88:3739–3743.

79. Baek S, March KL. Gene therapy for restenosis—Getting nearer the heart of the matter. Circ Res 1998;82(3):295–305.

80. Marx SO, Marks AR. Bench to bedside: the development of rapamycin and its application to stent restenosis. Circulation 2001;104:852–855.

81. Clowes AW, Schwartz SM. Significance of quiescent smooth muscle migration in the injured rat carotid artery. Circ Res 1985;56:139–145.

82. Majesky MW, Schwartz SM, Clowes MM, Clowes AW. Heparin regulates smooth muscle S phase entry in the injured rat carotid artery. Circ Res 1987;61:296–300.

83. Nikkari ST, Järveläinen HT, Wight TN, Ferguson M, Clowes AW. Smooth muscle cell expression of extracellular matrix genes after arterial injury. Am J Pathol 1994;144:1348–1356.

84. Fingerle J, Johnson R, Clowes AW, Majesky MW, Reidy MA. Role of platelets in smooth muscle cell proliferation and migration after vascular injury in rat carotid artery. Proc Natl Acad Sci USA 1989;86:8412–8416.

85. Jawien A, Bowen-Pope DF, Lindner V, Schwartz SM, Clowes AW. Platelet-derived growth factor promotes smooth muscle migration and intimal thickening in a rat model of balloon angioplasty. J Clin Invest 1992;89:507–511.

86. Ferns GAA, Raines EW, Sprugel KH, Motani AS, Reidy MA, Ross R. Inhibition of neointimal smooth muscle accumulation after angioplasty by an antibody to PDGF. Science 1991;253:1129–1132.

87. Sarembock IJ, Gertz SD, Thome LM, et al. Effectiveness of hirulog in reducing restenosis after balloon angioplasty of atherosclerotic femoral arteries in rabbits. J Vasc Res 1996;33:308–314.

88. Walters TK, Gorog DA, Wood RFM. Thrombin generation following arterial injury is a critical initiating event in the pathogenesis of the proliferative stages of the atherosclerotic process. J Vasc Res 1994;31:173–177.

89. Cheung WM, D'Andrea MR, Andrade-Gordon P, Damiano BP. Altered vascular injury responses in mice deficient in protease-activated receptor-1. Arterioscler Thromb Vasc Biol 1999;19:3014–3024.

90. Hedin U, Daum G, Clowes AW. Heparin inhibits thrombin-induced mitogen-activated protein kinase signaling in arterial smooth muscle cells. J Vasc Surg 1998;27:512–520.

91. Kenagy RD, Nikkari ST, Welgus HG, Clowes AW. Heparin inhibits the induction of three matrix metalloproteinases (stromelysin, 92-kD gelatinase, and collagenase) in primate arterial smooth muscle cells. J Clin Invest 1994;93:1987–1993.

92. Lindner V, Olson NE, Clowes AW, Reidy MA. Inhibition of smooth muscle cell proliferation in injured rat arteries. Interaction of heparin with basic fibroblast growth factor. J Clin Invest 1992;90:2044–2049.

93. Schwartz L, Bourassa MG, Lesperance J, et al. Aspirin and dipyridamole in the prevention of restenosis after percutaneous transluminal coronary angioplasty. N Engl J Med 1988;318:1714–1749.

94. The EPIC Investigation. Use of a monoclonal antibody directed against the platelet glycoprotein IIb/IIIa receptor in high-risk coronary angioplasty. N Engl J Med 1994;330:956–961.

95. The EPILOG Investigators. Platelet glycoprotein IIb/IIIa receptor blockade and low-dose heparin during percutaneous coronary revascularization. N Engl J Med 1997;336:1689–1696.

96. Deitch JS, Williams JK, Adams MR, et al. Effects of beta3-integrin blockade (c7E3) on the response to angioplasty and intra-arterial stenting in atherosclerotic nonhuman primates. Arterioscler Thromb Vasc Biol 1998;18:1730–1737.

97. The ERASER Investigators. Acute platelet inhibition with abciximab does not reduce in-stent restenosis (ERASER study). Circulation 1999;100:799–806.

98. Lindner V, Majack RA, Reidy MA. Basic fibroblast growth factor stimulates endothelial regrowth and proliferation in denuded arteries. J Clin Invest 1990;85:2004–2008.

99. Daemen MJAP, Lombardi DM, Bosman FT, Schwartz SM. Angiotensin II induces smooth muscle cell proliferation in the normal and injured rat arterial wall. Circ Res 1991;68:450–456.

100. Dzau VJ, Gibbons GH, Pratt RE. Molecular mechanisms of vascular renin-angiotensin system in myointimal hyperplasia. Hypertension 1991;18(Suppl 4):II100–II105.

101. Van Kleef EM, Smits JFM, De Mey JGR, et al. a1-Adrenoreceptor blockade reduces the angiotensin II- induced vascular smooth muscle cell DNA synthesis in the rat thoracic aorta and carotid artery. Circ Res 1992;70:1122–1127.

102. Griendling KK, Lassegue B, Alexander RW. Angiotensin receptors and their therapeutic implications. Annu Rev Pharmacol Toxicol 1996;36:281–306.

103. Owens GK. Role of contractile agonists in growth regulation of vascular smooth muscle cells. Adv Exp Med Biol 1991;308:71–79.

104. Yogo K, Shimokawa H, Funakoshi H, et al. Different vasculoprotective roles of NO synthase isoforms in vascular lesion formation in mice. Arterioscler Thromb Vasc Biol 2000;20:E96–E100.

105. Janssens S, Flaherty D, Nong Z, et al. Human endothelial nitric oxide synthase gene transfer inhibits vascular smooth muscle cell proliferation and neointima formation after balloon injury in rats. Circulation 1998;97:1274–1281.

106. Baek SH, Hrabie JA, Keefer LK, et al. Augmentation of intrapericardial nitric oxide level by a prolonged-release nitric oxide donor reduces luminal narrowing after porcine coronary angioplasty. Circulation 2002;105:2779–2784.

107. Ryan ST, Koteliansky VE, Gotwals PJ, Lindner V. Transforming growth factor-beta-dependent events in vascular remodeling following arterial injury. J Vasc Res 2003;40:37–46.

108. Nabel EG, Shum L, Pompili VJ, et al. Direct transfer of transforming growth factor beta 1 gene into arteries stimulates fibrocellular hyperplasia. Proc Natl Acad Sci USA 1993;90:10,759–10,763.

109. Clowes AW, Clowes MM, Au YPT, Reidy MA, Belin D. Smooth muscle cells express urokinase during mitogenesis and tissue-type plasminogen activator during migration in injured rat carotid artery. Circ Res 1990;67:61–67.

110. Carmeliet P. Insights from gene-inactivation studies of the coagulation and plasminogen. Fibrinolysis 1997;11:181–191.

111. Hasenstab D, Lea H, Clowes AW. Local plasminogen activator inhibitor type 1 overexpression in rat carotid artery enhances thrombosis and endothelial regeneration while inhibiting intimal thickening. Arterioscler Thromb Vasc Biol 2000;20(3):853–859.

112. Hasenstab D, Forough R, Clowes AW. Plasminogen activator inhibitor type 1 and tissue inhibitor of metalloproteinases-2 increase after arterial injury in rats. Circ Res 1997;80(4):490–496.

113. Webb KE, Henney AM, Anglin S, Humphries SE, McEwan JR. Expression of matrix metalloproteinases and their inhibitor TIMP-1 in the rat carotid artery after balloon injury. Arterioscler Thromb Vasc Biol 1997;17(9):1837–1844.

114. Bendeck MP, Irvin C, Reidy MA. Inhibition of matrix metalloproteinase activity inhibits smooth muscle cell migration but not neointimal thickening after arterial injury. Circ Res 1996;78:38–43.

115. Forough R, Koyama N, Hasenstab D, et al. Overexpression of tissue inhibitor of matrix metalloproteinase-1 inhibits vascular smooth muscle cell functions in vitro and in vivo. Circ Res 1996;79(4):812–820.

116. Cherr GS, Motew SJ, Travis JA, et al. Metalloproteinase inhibition and the response to angioplasty and stenting in atherosclerotic primates. Arterioscler Thromb Vasc Biol 2002;22:161–166.

117. Raines EW. The extracellular matrix can regulate vascular cell migration, proliferation, and survival: relationships to vascular disease. Int J Exp Pathol 2000;81:173–182.

118. Wight TN, Merrilees MJ. Proteoglycans in Atherosclerosis and Restenosis: Key Roles for Versican. Circ Res 2004;94:1158–1167.

119. Jain M, He Q, Lee WS, et al. Role of CD44 in the reaction of vascular smooth muscle cells to arterial wall injury. J Clin Invest 1996;97:596–603.

120. Savani RC, Wang C, Yang B, et al. Migration of bovine aortic smooth muscle cells after wounding injury. The role of hyaluronan and RHAMM. J Clin Invest 1995;95:1158–1168.

121. Skinner MP, Raines EW, Ross R. Dynamic expression of $\alpha1\beta1$ and $\alpha2\beta1$ integrin receptors by human vascular smooth muscle cells: $\alpha2\beta1$ integrin is required for chemotaxis across type I collagen-coated membranes. Am J Pathol 1994;145:1070–1081.

122. Reidy MA. Neointimal proliferation: The role of basic FGF on vascular smooth muscle cell proliferation. Thromb Haemost 1993;70:172–176.

123. Cuevas P, Gonzalez AM, Carceller F, Baird A. Vascular response to basic fibroblast growth factor when infused onto the normal adventitia or into the injured media of the rat carotid artery. Circ Res 1991;69:360–369.

124. Belknap JK, Grieshaber NA, Schwartz PE, Orton EC, Reidy MA, Majack RA. Tropoelastin gene expression in individual vascular smooth muscle cells. Relationship to DNA synthesis during vascular development and after arterial injury. Circ Res 1996;78:388–394.

125. Koyama H, Raines EW, Bornfeldt KE, Roberts JM, Ross R. Fibrillar collagen inhibits arterial smooth muscle proliferation through regulation of Cdk2 inhibitors. Cell 1996;87(6):1069–1078.

126. Schäfer A, Wiesmann F, Neubauer S, Eigenthaler M, Bauersachs J, Channon KM. Rapid Regulation of Platelet Activation In Vivo by Nitric Oxide. Circulation 2004;109:1819–1822.

127. Topper JN, Cai JX, Falb D, Gimbrone MA, Jr. Identification of vascular endothelial genes differentially responsive to fluid mechanical stimuli: Cyclooxygenase-2, manganese superoxide dismutase, and endothelial cell nitric oxide synthase are selectively up-regulated by steady laminar shear stress. Proc Natl Acad Sci USA 1996;93(19):10,417–10,422.

128. Perlman H, Maillard L, Krasinski K, Walsh K. Evidence for the rapid onset of apoptosis in medial smooth muscle cells following balloon injury. Circulation 1997;95:981–987.

129. Walsh K, Smith RC, Kim HS. Vascular cell apoptosis in remodeling, restenosis, and plaque rupture. Circ Res 2000;87:184–188.

130. Mallat Z, Tedgui A. Apoptosis in the vasculature: mechanisms and functional importance. Br J Pharmacol 2000;130:947–962.

131. Pollman MJ, Yamada T, Horiuchi M, Gibbons GH. Vasoactive substances regulate vascular smooth muscle cell apoptosis—Countervailing influences of nitric oxide and angiotensin II. Circ Res 1996;79(4):748–756.

132. Kimura T, Nosaka H, Yokoi H, Iwabuchi M, Nobuyoshi M. Serial angiographic follow-up after Palmaz-Schatz stent implantation: comparison with conventional balloon angioplasty. J Am Coll Cardiol 1993;21:1557–1563.

133. Pasterkamp G, Mali WP, Borst C. Application of intravascular ultrasound in remodelling studies. Semin Interv Cardiol 1997;2:11–18.

134. Martin P. Wound healing-aiming at perfect skin regeneration. Science 1997;276:75–81.

135. Gabbiani G, Hirshcel BJ, Ryan GB, Statkov PR, Majno G. Granulation tissue as a contractile organ. J Exp Med 1972;135:719–733.

136. Scott PG, Dodd CM, Tredget EE, Ghahary A, Rahemtulla F. Immunohistochemical localization of the proteoglycans decorin, biglycan and versican and transforming growth factor-$\beta$ in human postburn hypertrophic and mature scars. Histopathology 1995;26:423–431.

137. Oksalo O, Salo T, Tammi R, et al. Expression of proteoglycans and hyaluronan during wound healing. J Histochem Cytochem 1995;43:125–135.

138. Hedin U, Roy J, Tran PK, Lundmark K, Rahman A. Control of smooth muscle cell proliferation—the role of the basement membrane. Thromb Haemost 1999;82(Suppl 1):23–26.

139. Riessen R, Wight TN, Pastore C, Henley C, Isner JM. Distribution of hyaluronan during extracellular matrix remodeling in human restenotic arteries and balloon-injured rat carotid arteries. Circulation 1996;93:1141–1147.

140. Fraser JRE, Laurent TC, Laurent UBG. Hyaluronan: its nature, distribution, functions and turnover. J Intern Med 1997;242:27–33.

141. Knudson CB, Knudson W. Hyaluronan-binding proteins in development, tissue homeostasis, and disease. FASEB J 1993;7:1233–1241.

142. Travis JA, Hughes MG, Wong JM, Wagner WD, Geary RL. Hyaluronan enhances contraction of collagen by smooth muscle cells and adventitial fibroblasts: role of CD44 and implications for constrictive remodeling. Circ Res 2001;88:77–83.

143. Gotwals PJ, Chi-Rosso G, Lindner V, et al. The $\alpha 1\beta 1$ integrin is expressed during neointima formation in rat arteries and mediates collagen matrix reorganization. J Clin Invest 1996;97:2469–2477.

144. Schiro JA, Chan BMC, Roswit WT, et al. Integrin $\alpha 2\beta 1$ (VLA-2) mediates reorganization and contraction of collagen matrices by human cells. Cell 1991;67:403–410.

145. Knox JB, Sukhova GK, Whittemore AD, Libby P. Evidence for altered balance between matrix metalloproteinases and their inhibitors in human aortic diseases. Circulation 1997;95:205–212.

146. Irizarry E, Newman KM, Gandhi RH, et al. Demonstration of interstitial collagenase in abdominal aortic aneurysm disease. J Surg Res 1993;54:571–574.

147. Newman KM, Ogata Y, Malon AM, et al. Identification of matrix metalloproteinases-3 (stromelysin-1) and -9 (gelatinase B) in abdominal aortic aneurysm. Arterioscler Thromb 1994;14:1315–1320.

148. Thompson RW, Parks WC. Role of matrix metalloproteinases in abdominal aortic aneurysms. Ann NY Acad Sci 1996;800:157–174.

149. Allaire E, Forough R, Clowes M, Starcher B, Clowes AW. Local over-expression of TIMP-1 prevents aortic aneurysm degeneration and rupture in a rat model. J Clin Invest 1998;102:1413–1420.

150. Bigatel DA, Elmore JR, Carey DJ, Cizmeci-Smith G, Franklin DP, Youkey JR. The matrix metalloproteinase inhibitor BB-94 limits expansion of experimental abdominal aortic aneurysms. J Vasc Surg 1999;29:130–139.

151. Mason DP, Kenagy RD, Hasenstab D, et al. Matrix metalloproteinase-9 overex-pression enhances vascular smooth muscle cell migration and alters remodeling in the injured rat carotid artery. Circ Res 1999;85:1179–1185.

152. de Smet BJ, de Kleijn D, Hanemaaijer R, et al. Metalloproteinase inhibition reduces constrictive arterial remodeling after balloon angioplasty: a study in the atherosclerotic Yucatan micropig. Circulation 2000;101:2962–2967.

153. Daniels JT, Schultz GS, Blalock TD, et al. Mediation of transforming growth factor-beta(1)-stimulated matrix contraction by fibroblasts: a role for connective tissue growth factor in contractile scarring. Am J Pathol 2003;163:2043–2052.

154. Geary RL, Wong JM, Rossini A, Schwartz SM, Adams LD. Expression profiling identifies 147 genes contributing to an unique primate neointimal smooth muscle cell phenotype. Arterioscler Thromb Vasc Biol 2002;22:2010–2016.

155. Kingston PA, Sinha S, Appleby CE, et al. Adenovirus-mediated gene transfer of transforming growth factor-beta3, but not transforming growth factor-beta1, inhibits constrictive remodeling and reduces luminal loss after coronary angioplasty. Circulation 2003;108:2819–2825.

156. Leite PF, Danilovic A, Moriel P, et al. Sustained decrease in superoxide dismutase activity underlies constrictive remodeling after balloon injury in rabbits. Arterioscler Thromb Vasc Biol 2003;23: 2197–2202.

# 3    Clinical Presentation of Restenosis

*Ganesh Manoharan, MBBCh, MD, MRCPI,*
*Giedrius Davidavicius, MD,*
*and William Wijns, MD, PhD*

## CONTENTS

## INTRODUCTION

Coronary artery disease remains a major cause of mortality and morbidity. Unstable angina and non-Q-wave myocardial infarction (MI) account for approx 2–2.5 million hospitalizations worldwide *(1)*. Furthermore, unstable angina is associated with a high risk of MI or death if treated inadequately *(2)*. Advances in clinical therapeutics and the introduction of percutaneous coronary therapy by Grüntzig and coworkers in the late 1970s have revolutionized the way ischemic heart disease is managed in clinical practice *(3)*. Percutaneous coronary intervention (PCI) is now the primary mode of treatment for managing occlusive coronary disease in symptomatic patients. However, the practice of using stand-alone balloon angioplasty has largely been superseded by the addition of stent deployment to improve procedural success and outcome *(4–7)*. The advent of the stent era and improvements in stent technology has enabled treatment of more complex and difficult coronary lesions, with multivessel stenting and techniques such as direct stenting *(8)*, increasing in frequency.

Despite these technological advances, restenosis remains a major issue with PCI. Although the mechanistic progression of restenosis that occurs following stand-alone balloon angioplasty *(9)* differs from that observed following stent implantation *(10,11)*, the clinical impact on patients remains. The clinical presentation of restenosis varies widely ranging from silent ischemia, progressive angina, unstable angina, and MI to sudden death. Although numerous predictors of restenosis have been suggested (Tables 1 and 2), relating symptoms to severity of restenosis may be difficult, because the disease process is largely progressive and patients may develop atherosclerotic lesions in nonculprit sites *(12,13)*.

From: *Contemporary Cardiology: Essentials of Restenosis: For the Interventional Cardiologist*
Edited by: H. J. Duckers, E. G. Nabel, and P. W. Serruys © Humana Press Inc., Totowa, NJ

Table 1
Clinical, Hematological, and Biochemical Predictors of Restenosis

| Predictors | References |
|---|---|
| Diabetes Mellitus | 14,72–78 |
| Elevated blood insulin level | 79 |
| Lower BMI in diabetics | 77 |
| Male gender | 31,49,79–81 |
| Previous history of restenosis | 82,83 |
| Absence of CABG | 14 |
| Overweight | 14 |
| Unstable angina at presentation | 31,49,79,80,83 |
| Smoking | 31,59,79 |
| Chronic renal failure | 84,85 |
| Allergy to Nickel and Molybdenum | 86 |
| PI[A] polymorphism of glycoprotein IIIa | 87 |
| Polymorphism of angiotensin I-converting enzyme | 88,89 |
| Increased circulating monocytes | 90 |
| Increased plasma monocyte chemoattractant protein-1 | 91,92 |
| Elevated whole blood tissue factor procoagulant activity | 93 |
| Elevated serum homocysteine | 94 |

Table 2
Angiographic Predictors of Restenosis

| Angiographic predictors | References |
|---|---|
| Left main stem lesion | 83 |
| Venous graft stenosis | 49,79,81,83 |
| Chronically occluded vessel | 79,81,83 |
| Significant dissection | 79,83 |
| Postprocedure stenotic gradient ≥15–20 mmHg | 49,79 |
| Preprocedure stenotic gradient ≥40 mmHg | 49 |
| Lesion in branch vessel | 79 |
| Larger final diameter stenosis | 31,79,80 |
| Thrombus | 79 |
| Long stents | 81 |
| Severity of stenosis | 31,49 |
| Multiple stents | 81,95 |
| Long lesion | 31,79,95 |
| Multiple lesions | 83 |
| Proximal anterior descending artery stenosis | 31,79,83 |
| Restenotic lesion | 80,83 |
| Suboptimal result | 83 |
| Small postprocedure mean luminal diameter | 80,81 |
| Small vessel | 80,81 |

## TIMING OF RESTENOSIS

When compared with stand-alone balloon angioplasty, the introduction of bare metal stents has reduced the risk of restenosis in patients, ranging from 19 to 40% at 6 mo (5–7,14–17). Furthermore, recent data have shown significant reductions in the incidence of in-stent restenosis with the use of drug-eluting stents (DES) *(18–28)*. As the mechanisms of restenosis differ between stand-alone balloon angioplasty vs stenting, the timing of restenosis appears to develop later for the stented segment, when assessed by angiography.

In the era of stand-alone balloon angioplasty, it has been suggested that the timing of restenosis at PCI sites tends to occur within 3–9 mo of the procedure *(29–31)*. Nobuyoshi and coworkers *(29)* studied 229 patients following successful percutaneous transluminal coronary angioplasty (PTCA) by prospective angiography at 1, 3, 6, and 12 mo. Using quantitative measurements of coronary stenosis recorded with cinevideo-densitometric analysis, the authors demonstrated that the restenosis was most prevalent between 1 and 3 mo, and rarely beyond this period. Actuarial restenosis rates observed for the 1, 3, 6, and 12 mo were 12.7, 43, 49.4, and 52.5%, respectively. A similar peak in progressive incidence of restenosis was observed between 3 and 4 mo, depending on the criterion used to define restenosis, by Serruys and coworkers *(30)*.

Neointimal proliferation within stented segments, however, has been shown to peak at approx 6 mo *(32,33)*. Kimura and coworkers demonstrated, following implantation of Palmaz-Schatz stents and angiographic follow-up up to 3 yr, a decrease in minimal luminal diameter (MLD) from $2.54 \pm 0.44$ mm immediately poststent to $1.87 \pm 0.56$ mm at 6 mo, but with no further reduction at 1 yr. On the contrary, a significant increase in MLD, from $1.94 \pm 0.48$ mm at 6 mo to $2.09 \pm 0.48$ mm at 3 yr, was observed in patients with paired angiograms ($p < 0.001$).

More recently, Kimura and coworkers *(34)* suggested, following clinical and angiographic follow-up of patients between 7 and 11 yr that the luminal response post-PCI tended to follow a triphasic route, in that there is a early restenosis phase (until 6 mo), an intermediate regression phase (from 6 mo to 3 yr), and a late renarrowing phase beyond 4 yr.

A variant form of restenosis, described as aggressive or "malignant," has been suggested to present earlier, with patients more likely to be symptomatic when compared with nonaggressive lesions *(35)*. Predictors of an aggressive restenosis process, by multivariate logistic regression, include female gender, a large baseline MLD, a shorter baseline lesion length, and a greater stent to lesion ratio *(35)*.

Conversely, the use of brachytherapy to treat in-stent restenosis tends to delay the reoccurrence of restenosis by 1–3 yr *(36)*. A similar very late presentation is likely to be observed with DES. The 4-yr follow-up of the *first in man* trial using sirolimus eluting stents (slow and fast release formulation) suggested that although the benefits of DES were maintained, there is a gradual progression of percent in-stent stenosis, with an initial regression of the stenosis observed at 2-yr for the slow release but an eventual gradual increase at 4-yr (immediately postprocedure: slow = 5% and fast = 4.2%; 1-yr: slow = 6.6% and fast = 4.9%; 2-yr: slow = 1.4% and fast = 14.6%; 4-yr: slow=11.1% and fast = 14.2%) (presented at the American College of Cardiology Scientific Meeting, 2004 by Dr Sousa JE, MD, PhD).

Despite these angiographic parameters and variations in timing of restenosis, correlation to clinical symptoms of chest pain remains elusive, as will become apparent next.

## SILENT ISCHEMIA

Numerous large clinical trials have demonstrated that the drive for repeat target vessel revascularization tends to be guided more by angiographic features than by clinical symptoms. Angiographic features associated with silent restenosis are listed in Table 3. From large-scale clinical studies, asymptomatic restenosis tends to occur in approx 48–58% of patients undergoing PCI (Fig. 1). Although some studies have reported

Table 3
Angiographic Features Associated With Asymptomatic Restenosis

| Angiographic features | References |
| --- | --- |
| Significant or occluded culprit vessel | 40 |
| Presence of collateral flow | 40,41 |
| Left anterior descending lesions | 96 |
| Single vessel disease | 37,41 |
| More complete revascularization | 37,96 |
| Larger reference vessel diameter | 38 |
| Lower lesion severity | 38 |

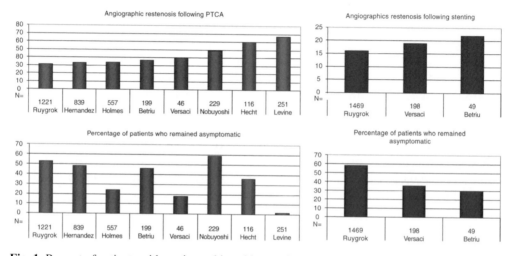

**Fig. 1.** Percent of patients with angiographic evidence of restenosis following PTCA only and stenting (upper panel), with percent of these patients who remained asymptomatic (lower panel). Definition of restenosis and method of assessing for restenosis, however, were not similar among the studies. (References: Ruygrok [38], Hernandez [37], Holmes [81], Betriu [5], Versaci [110], Nobuyoshi [29], Hecht [99], Levine [111].)

lower rates of asymptomatic restenosis (Fig. 1), these tended to have study design limitations, smaller cohort of patients, variable angiographic follow-up, differing criteria for restenosis, and incomplete angiographic follow-up.

Hernandez and coworkers (37) demonstrated in 277 consecutive patients, where restenosis (>50% lumen narrowing) was documented 6–9 mo after PTCA, that 48% of patients were asymptomatic. The authors further concluded that a normal blood pressure, previous history of MI, single vessel disease, and a short duration of symptoms were independent correlates to asymptomatic restenosis.

A comprehensive assessment of 10 PCI studies, where use of coronary stents were a feature in nine of the studies, was performed by Ruygrok and coworkers (38) to investigate clinical and angiographic factors associated with asymptomatic restenosis. Of the 1469 patients who received stents, 16% had in-stent restenosis, of whom 58% were asymptomatic. Multivariate analysis of this group suggested unstable angina at time of screening and absence of nitrate use were associated with silent restenosis. However, multivariate analysis of the whole cohort of patients suggested male sex, reference diameter at follow-up, and lesser lesion severity at 6 mo to be predictors. Despite these high rates of silent restenosis, what, if any, is the impact on prognosis?

The impact of silent ischemia in patients who have not had PCI has been shown to be detrimental. The asymptomatic cardiac ischemia pilot study showed both death (4%) and the combination of death or MI (9%) at 1 yr to be significantly higher in patients who were treated by symptoms guided medical treatment rather than revascularization *(39)*. Whether a similar trend accompanies patients post-PCI, especially in the stent era has not been fully evaluated. Despite some earlier studies suggesting a more favorable outcome for patients *(37,40)*, more recent studies suggest otherwise.

An observational study, by Pfisterer and coworkers *(41)*, documented consecutive series of 490 patients 6 mo following successful PTCA by thallium-201 scintigraphy. Ischemia was noted in 112 of 405 patients, with 60% being asymptomatic. The degree of restenosis was similar between the symptomatic ($80 \pm 16\%$) and asymptomatic ($81 \pm 21\%$) patients. The long-term prognosis between the two groups was also noted to be identical.

During a mean follow-up of $40 \pm 13$ mo after thallium single-photon emission computed tomography in patients who underwent prior PCI, Cottin and coworkers *(42)* observed a significantly higher major cardiac event rates in the 31% of patients who had evidence of silent ischemia compared with patients without evidence of reversible ischemia (28% vs 3%, respectively; $p < 0.001$). The proportion of patients who received stents was equal between the two groups (46% vs 45%, respectively). This prognostic evaluation was further strengthened by the findings of Zellweger and coworkers *(43)*. In this study, follow-up (mean $4.1 \pm 0.3$ yr) of 356 patients following PCI and stenting showed 62% of patients had evidence of silent ischemia on perfusion imaging at 6 mo. Furthermore, the prognosis of patients with silent ischemia, although tended to be better than those with symptoms, was worse than those without evidence of ischemia (Fig. 2), with the composite end point (death, nonfatal MI, and late revascularization) of 38% for ischemic and 17% for nonischemic patients ($p = 0.001$, Fig. 2).

Based on these findings and as some authors have suggested routine angiographic follow-up following PCI *(44)*, should angiographic follow-up at 6 mo or later be recommended to all patients who undergo PCI? In the Benestent II study, where patients were randomized to stenting or conventional balloon angioplasty, a subrandomization allocated patients to 6-mo clinical follow-up (349 patients) or clinical and angiographic follow-up (357 patients) *(45)*. This substudy demonstrated that patients who had routine angiography were more likely to undergo repeat PCI or coronary artery bypass graft surgery (44 vs 21 patients, $p = 0.003$, Fig. 3). Patients in the angiography subgroup were also more likely to be symptomatic, although the authors concluded that this increase might have been influenced by investigator bias and that the increase in intervention may be more of an "occulostenotic reflex" phenomena (Fig. 4).

Furthermore, it has been shown both angiographically and by angioscopic studies that there is a tendency for moderate stenosis severity to spontaneously regress after PCI. Kimura and coworkers *(32)* observed late improvement in luminal diameter in a 3-yr angiographic follow-up of patients following implantation of the Palmaz-Schatz stent. This improvement tended to occur between 6 mo and 3 yr (Fig. 5). This observation was supported by findings of Hermiller and coworkers, following implantation of the Gianturco Roubin stents *(46)*. A similar finding was observed by Ormiston and coworkers *(47)* following stand-alone balloon angioplasty in a 5-yr angiographic follow-up of patients postprocedure, where late regression was found to be related to stenosis

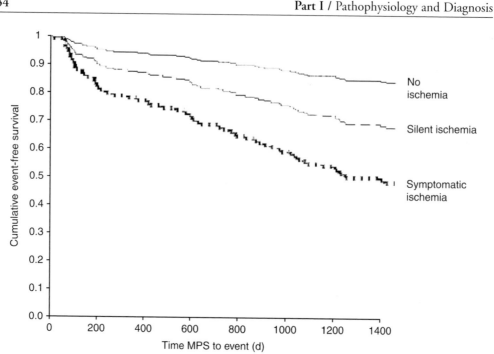

**Fig. 2.** Kaplan-Meier event-free survival curves by symptomatic status. Patients without ischemia ($n = 242$) had significantly lower event rates than patients with silent ($n = 44$) or symptomatic ischemia ($n = 21$; $p = 0.006$, and $p < 0.0001$, respectively); patients with silent ischemia tended to have lower event rates than patients with symptomatic ischemia ($p = 0.12$). MPS = myocardial perfusion single photon emission computed tomography. Reproduced with permission from Zellweger et al. *(43)*.

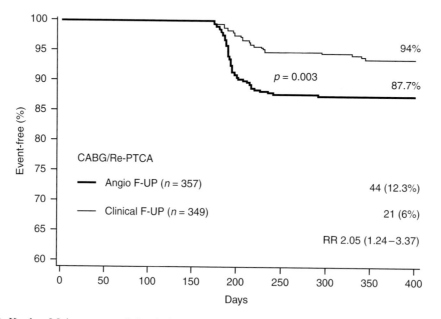

**Fig. 3.** Kaplan-Meier curves of the timing of (first) repeat revascularization procedures 6–12 mo after intervention for the clinical and angiography groups. Reproduced with permission from Ruygrok et al. *(45)*.

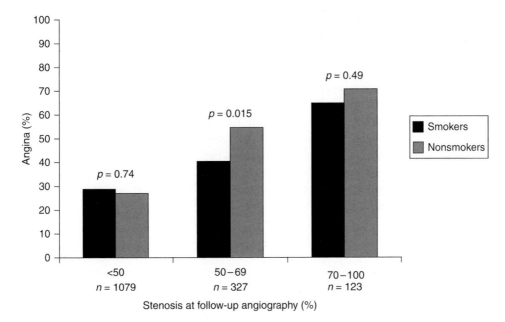

**Fig. 4.** Relationship between follow-up diameter stenosis and angina (CCS class 1 through 4), according to smoking status in angiographic cohort. Among patients with 50–69% diameter stenosis by quantitative angiography, smokers were less likely to report angina than nonsmokers. Reproduced with permission from Cohen et al. *(59)*.

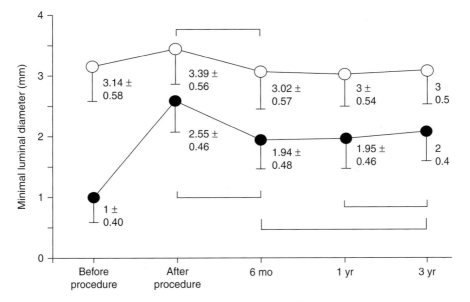

**Fig. 5.** Serial changes in the mean (±SD) MLD of 72 lesions for which sequential studies over a 3-yr period were completed (●), as compared with a reference diameter (○). Significant improvement in MLD during the period from 1 to 3 yr after implantation of the stent was observed. $p < 0.001$ for comparison between the points linked by brackets. Reproduced with permission from kimura et al. *(32)*.

severity at early angiography (at ~6 mo). Asakura and coworkers *(48)* further observed by angioscopy that the neointima became thick and nontransparent until 6 mo and then became thin and transparent by 3 yr, concluding that neointimal remodeling exists following stenting and contributes to the alteration of coronary luminal diameter after stenting. However, some investigators have suggested that the progression of restenosis tends to increase from 4 yr onwards *(34)*.

Thus, the practice of routine angiography on all patients may not actually identify those presenting with late restenosis but may subject some to undergo repeat percutaneous coronary intervention, when this may not be clinically necessary. The evidence for the presence of asymptomatic restenosis is clear and the evidence for adverse impact of asymptomatic ischemia on prognosis is mounting. Perhaps the old saying, "what you don't see will not hurt" does not apply in the setting of silent ischemic restenosis.

## CHEST PAIN

In clinical practice, reoccurrence of symptoms is one of the most common reasons to reinvestigate a patient, either invasively or by noninvasive means, for evidence of restenosis. However, it has been suggested by several investigators that chest pain, as opposed to patients presenting with unstable angina, is a poor marker of restenosis (Table 4).

Data from the PTCA registry of the National Heart, Lung and Blood Institute, however, suggests that patients with symptomatic restenosis tend to present with chest pain within 4–5 mo of the procedure *(49)*. Although approx 45% of patients who present with chest pain from the same registry did not have any angiographic evidence of restenosis following PCI. Development of chest pain after 9 mo tends to be more often because of disease progression at new sites *(12,50)*, with rates of disease progression at new sites approaching 7% per annum *(12,13)*.

Studies following stand-alone balloon angioplasty have repeatedly shown that restenosis tends to present predominantly as progressive exertional angina *(51–55)*. Despite these findings, some investigators have suggested that unstable angina is a common presentation of restenosis *(56)*.

Walters and coworkers *(56)* compared the clinical presentation of in-stent restenosis in 262 (191 patients with stent deployment during PCI) consecutive patients at repeat angiography. Recurrent clinical ischemia developed at a mean of $5.5 \pm 4.6$ mo for the stented patients and $6.5 \pm 7.2$ mo for the PTCA only group. Angina Braunwald class II or III were present in 48% of stented and 32% of PTCA patients ($p = 0.032$). Explanations provided by the authors for the difference from what is believed to be the norm for presentation of restenosis, in that it does not present as unstable angina *(57)*, are that patients with asymptomatic restenosis or those with symptomatic restenosis treated medically without repeat catheterization were not included in the study. The findings of Walters and coworkers, however, concur with that observed by Bossi and coworkers, where 42.8% of patients presented with stable angina and 53.7% with unstable angina *(58)*.

The impact of smoking on angiographic and clinical restenosis following PCI was addressed by Cohen and coworkers *(59)* using pooled data from 8671 patients in nine multicenter clinical trials. Angiographic restenosis was evaluated in 2989 patients, whereas clinical restenosis was assessed in 5682 patients. Of those assigned to clinical follow-up only, target lesion revascularization was lower among smokers compared with nonsmokers (6.6% smokers and 10.1% nonsmokers, $p < 0.001$), whereas, no difference in rates of restenosis was observed between the smoker and nonsmoker in the

**Table 4**
**Accuracy of Chest Pain as Predictor of Restenosis**

| First author | References | Total patients | Sensitivity (%) | Specificity (%) | Positive predictive value (%) | Negative predictive value (%) | Accuracy (%) |
|---|---|---|---|---|---|---|---|
| Holmes | 81 | 524 | 79 | 68 | 56 | 86 | 72 |
| Nobuyoshi[a] | 29 | 229 | 41 | 95 | 91 | 59 | 66 |
| Hecht | 98 | 116 | 64 | 34 | 59 | 39 | 52 |
| Hernández[b] | 37 | 839 | 52 | – | – | – | – |
| Legrand | 99 | 325 | 56 | 86 | 51 | 89 | 80 |
| Ruygrok | 38 | 2690 | 45 | – | – | – | – |

Table adapted from Giedd and Bergeman (97).
Unless stated, data reflect 6-mo symptom and angiographic findings.
[a]1-yr data.
[b]6–9 mo data.

Table 5

Overview of Drug Eluting Stent Studies

| Author | References | Pub year | Acronym | Total patients | Stent | Stent coating | Follow-up (months) | Angiographic in-stent restenosis (%) | MI (n) | Death (n) | Stent thrombosis (n) | TLR (n) |
|---|---|---|---|---|---|---|---|---|---|---|---|---|
| Morice M-C | 20 | 2002 | RAVEL | 238 | Bx Velocity | Sirolimus | A = 6 C = 1, 6, and 12 | Control = 26.6 DES = 0 | Control = 5[a] DES = 4 | Control = 2[a] DES = 2 | Control = 0 DES = 0 | Control = 27[b] DES = 0 |
| Colombo | 28 | 2003 | TAXUS II | 536 | NIR | Paclitaxel | A = 6 C = 1, 6, and 12 | Control SR = 17.9 TAXUS SR = 2.3 Control MR = 20.2 TAXUS MR = 4.7 | Control SR = 7 TAXUS SR = 3 Control MR = 7 TAXUS MR = 5 | Control SR = 2 TAXUS SR = 0 Control MR = 0 TAXUS MR = 0 | Control SR = 0[c] TAXUS SR = 2 Control MR = 0 TAXUS MR = 1 | Control SR = 17 TAXUS SR = 6 Control MR = 21 TAXUS MR = 5 |
| Moses | 21 | 2003 | SIRIUS | 1058 | Bx Velocity | Sirolimus | A = 8 C = 1, 3, 6, and 9 | Control = 35.4 DES = 3.2 | Control = 17[d] DES = 15 | Control = 3 DES = 5 | Control = 4[d] DES = 2 | Control = 87 DES = 22 |
| Park SJ | 70 | 2003 | ASPECT | 177 | Cook | Paclitaxel | A = 6 C = 1 and 6 | Control = 27 Low dose = 12 High dose = 4 | Control = 1[e] Low dose = 1 High dose = 2 | Control = 0[f] Low dose = 1 High dose = 0 | Control = 0[f] Low dose = 1 High dose = 3 | Control = 2 Low dose = 2 High dose = 2 |
| Schofer | 22 | 2003 | E-SIRIUS | 352 | Bx Velocity | Sirolimus | A = 8 C = 9 | Control = 41.7 DES = 3.9 | Control = 4[g] DES = 8 | Control = 1 DES = 2 | Control = 0[g] DES = 2 | Control = 37 DES = 7 |
| Stone | 23 | 2004 | TAXUS IV | 1314 | EXPRESS | Paclitaxel | A = 9 C = 9 | Control = 24.4 DES = 5.5 | Control = 24[h] DES = 23 | Control = 7 DES = 9 | Control = 5[h] DES = 4 | Control = 74[h] DES = 20 |
| Gershlick | 26 | 2004 | ELUTES | 190 | V-Flex Plus | Paclitaxel | A = 6 C = 1, 3, 6, and 12 | Control = 33.9[i] DES = 14.2 | Control = 0[i] DES = 2 | Control = 0[i] DES = 1 | Control = 33.9[i] DES = 14.2 | Control = 33.9[i] DES = 14.2 |

| Author | | Year | Trial | N | Stent | Drug | | | | | | | |
|---|---|---|---|---|---|---|---|---|---|---|---|---|---|
| Schampaert | 25 | 2004 | C-SIRIUS | 100 | Bx Velocity | Sirolimus | A = 8, C = 9 | Control = 45.5, DES = 0 | – | Control = 2[j], DES = 1 | Control = 0, DES = 0 | Control = 1[j], DES = 1 | Control = 2[j], DES = 9 |
| Holmes | 27 | 2004 | SIRIUS | 1058 | Bx Velocity | Sirolimus | C = 9 and 12 | Control = 18, DES = 16 | Control = 18, DES = 7 | Control = 4, DES = 7 | Control = 4[k], DES = 2 | Control = 105[k], DES = 26 | |

MI, Myocardial infarction; TLR, Target lesion revascularization; A, angiographic; C, clinical; DES, drug-eluting stent.

[a]MI occurred during stent implantation in three patients in each group. Deaths in the control group were because of MI and gastrointestinal hemorrhage and in DES, which were noncardiac in origin.

[b]Revascularization performed because of angina or abnormal stress test (16 patients) and angiographic restenosis (11 patients).

[c]One periprocedure in-stent thrombosis occurred in TAXUS SR and the rest were assumed to be the cause of MI (6–12 mo) as stent were patent on angiography post-thrombolytic therapy.

[d]Majority of MIs were non-Q-wave in nature (control = 15 and DES = 11). All stent thrombosis were subacute (one in each group) or late (three in control and one in DES). Cumulative frequency of stent thrombosis was 0.4% in sirolimus stent and 0.8% in standard stent.

[e]All events (non-Q-MI only) occurred within 1 mo in one patient in the paclitaxel/aspirin/thienopyridine group and three in those receiving cilostazol.

[f]Events occurred in the paclitaxel group treated with aspirin and cilostazol within 1 mo.

[g]Majority of MIs were non-Q-wave. Thromboses were subacute with no late observed.

[h]Majority of MIs were non-Q-wave. Stent thrombosis presented as subacute or late. TLR was clinically driven.

[i]Polymer free stent used. Percent restenosis is for the 2.7 μg/mm$^2$ paclitaxel dosage. All MIs were non-Q-wave (one for 0.7 μg/mm$^2$ and one for the 2.7 μg/mm$^2$ dosage). Death and stent thrombosis occurred in the 2.7 μg/mm$^2$. All TLR were symptom driven.

[j]All MIs were non-Q-wave. In-stent thrombosis were subacute (DES) and late (control). All TLR were symptom driven.

[k]Rate of stent thrombosis unchanged from initial SIRIUS data. The TLR were all clinically driven (Recurrent angina for 81% of control and 96.2% of sirolimus group). A positive functional test contributed toward decision for TLR (19% of controls and 15.4% of sirolimus group).

angiographic cohort. This dissociation in smokers between angiographic and clinical restenosis was explained in part by the reduced sensitivity to restenosis and greater reluctance of smokers to seek medical help despite recurrent angina (Fig. 3). Therefore, in this subset of patients, who tend to have a worse long-term prognosis post-PCI *(60)*, require close follow-up, especially if PCI of unprotected left main or in the setting of severe left ventricular dysfunction was performed where restenosis may be fatal *(61)*.

In the drug-eluting stent era, with paclitaxel and sirolimus, the overall angiographic restenosis rates are significantly lower than with bare metal stents (Table 5). The pattern of in-stent restenosis, furthermore, appears to be more focal, which tends to be associated with discontinuity in stent coverage *(62)*. Although the rates of in-stent restenosis is low, of those who did present with symptoms, the majority appeared to present with non-Q-wave MI (Table 5).

Although chest pain *per se* is a poor indicator of restenosis, nevertheless, patients who were initially asymptomatic postprocedure, but presented with new symptoms, those presenting with worsening angina within 6–9 mo of the procedure and those in the high-risk category for restenosis should be monitored for evidence of restenosis, as this is related to poor overall outcome.

## MI AND DEATH

The catastrophic outcomes of MI and sudden death post-PCI have fortunately been reduced significantly in the modern era of coronary revascularization and therapeutics. The incidence of stent thrombosis, giving rise to MI and/or sudden death has been reported to be approx 1% *(63)*. Despite this, subacute closure of the target vessel or lesion remains the major cause of mortality post-PCI *(64,65)*. Numerous predictors for stent thrombosis have been suggested; broadly they can be categorized as technical/stent issues, procedural issues, and patient/target lesion factors (Table 6).

In a retrospective study of 4509 patients who underwent successful PCI by Orford and coworkers *(66)*, showed a 0.51% (23 patients) rate of stent thrombosis (95% CI:0.32–0.76%). All were treated with aspirin and ticlopidine or clopidogrel for 2–4 wk. The authors found that the number of stents placed was the only independent predictor of thrombosis. Of the 23 patients with stent thrombosis, the frequency of death and nonfatal MI was 48 and 39%, respectively.

More recently, Farb and coworkers evaluated the predictors for late stent thrombosis ($\geq 30$ d), following postmortem analysis of stented coronary segments *(67)*. Of the 13 cases analyzed, the cause of death was sudden cardiac death ($n = 10$), acute MI ($n = 2$), and heart failure ($n = 1$). The pathological mechanisms include stenting across branch ostia, adjacent vulnerable plaque disruption, radiation therapy, extensive in-stent restenosis, and extensive plaque prolapse. Importantly, underlying in-stent restenosis was evident in only four of the 13 cases. Clinical studies have also demonstrated, albeit a small percent, MI as the presenting symptom for late thrombosis *(68,69)*.

Despite the significant improvements observed with DES in reducing the rates of in-stent restenosis, the rates of stent thrombosis appears to be similar to bare metal stents (Table 5). However, the events tend to present later as "subacute" or "late" in-stent thrombosis. The risk of thrombosis also appears to be associated with the type of concomitant medications used. Increased rates of subacute thrombosis observed in the ASPECT trial were exclusively in patients who received paclitaxel stent in combination with aspirin and cilostazol. None were observed in those treated with aspirin and a thienopyridine *(70)*.

Table 6
Predictors of Stent Thrombosis

| Predictors | References |
|---|---|
| Diabetes Mellitus | 100–102 |
| Poor ventricular function | 100,102 |
| Older age | 100,102 |
| Echolucent and poorly calcified plaques | 103 |
| Stent length | 100,102,104 |
| Stent diameter | 100,102 |
| Stent under deployment | 103,105 |
| Multiple stents | 66 |
| Stent overlap | 104 |
| Bailout stenting | 106 |
| Smaller balloon size | 106 |
| Stenting across side branch | 67 |
| Suboptimal result | 100,107 |
| Smaller lumen dimension | 108 |
| Dissection | 103–105 |
| Low maximal inflation pressure | 109 |
| Presence of thrombus | 103,105 |
| Intrastent tissue prolapse | 103 |
| Stent thrombogenecity | 4,54 |
| Inadequate pharmacotherapy | 4,54 |
| Local radiotherapy | 67 |

Furthermore, the risk of thrombosis may also be dependent on the dosage and the delivery system of the eluting agent. Doses up to 4000 µg of paclitaxel derivative delivered through acrylate polymer sleeves for up to 6 mo (Quanam QuaDDS stent system, Quanam Medical Corp.) was associated with an increased incidence of acute, subacute, and late stent thrombosis (SCORE trial) *(71)*. The overall risk of in-stent thrombosis following implantation of commercially available DES is low and comparable with bare-metal stents. In addition, 4-yr follow-up of the RAVEL study confirmed that no new evidence of in-stent thrombosis was observed in patients who received sirolimus-coated stents (presented at the American College of Cardiology Scientific Meeting, 2004 by Dr W Wijns, MD, PhD).

The significant advances already made in the field of therapeutics, stent technology, and procedural techniques has resulted in marked reductions in procedural-related morbidity and mortality. However, the risk of restenosis with thrombotic occlusion and neointimal proliferation still remains, with devastating outcome for the patient. Attention and research to potential causes should continue, with optimization of procedural outcomes and therapeutics in order to reduce and ultimately eliminate this iatrogenic complication.

## CONCLUSIONS

- Asymptomatic restenosis rate remains high and is associated with a worse prognosis.
- Chest pain is a common but poor marker of restenosis.
- Patients with new onset symptoms post-PCI or worsening angina within 6–9 mo of PCI require coronary angiography.

- Large percent of patients who present with thrombotic occlusion follow on to have a MI and/or death in the modern era of PCI.
- Early detection tools, ideally noninvasively, are required to identify those who develop restenosis, although preventing or halting the process is preferred.
- Advances in PCI technology, particularly with the use of bioactive stents such as DES, will undoubtedly continue to alter the time-course of restenosis and its presentation.

# REFERENCES

1. Braunwald E, Antman EM, Beasley JW, et al. ACC/AHA guidelines for the management of patients with unstable angina and non-ST-segment elevation myocardial infarction: a report of the American College of Cardiology/American Heart Association Task Force on Practice Guidelines (Committee on the Management of Patients with Unstable Angina). J Am Coll Cardiol 2000;36:970–972.
2. Collinson J, Flather MD, Fox KAA, et al. Clinical outcomes, risk stratification and practice patterns of Unstable angina and myocardial infarction without ST elevation: Prospective Registry of acute ischaemic syndromes in the UK (PRAIS-UK). Eur Heart J 2000;21:1450–1457.
3. Grüntzig AR, Senning Ä, siegenthaler WE. Nonoperative dilatation of coronary-artery stenosis: percutaneous transluminal coronary angioplasty. N Engl J Med 1979;301:61–68.
4. Sigwart U, Puel J, Mirkovitch V, et al. Intravascular stents to prevent occlusion and restenosis after transluminal angioplasty. N Eng J Med 1987;316:701–706.
5. Betriu A, Masotti M, Serra A, et al. Randomised comparison of coronary stent implantation and balloon angioplasty in the treatment of de novo coronary artery lesions (START): a four-year follow-up. J Am Coll Cardiol 1999;34:1498–1506.
6. Serruys PW, de Jaegere P, Kiemeneij F, et al. A comparison of balloon expandable stent implantation with balloon angioplasty in patients with coronary artery disease: the BENESTENT study group. N Eng J Med 1994;331:489–495.
7. Fischman DL, Leon MB, Baim DS, et al. A randomised comparison of stent placement and balloon angioplasty in the treatment of coronary artery disease: Stent Restenosis Study Investigators. N Eng J Med 1994;331:496–501.
8. Barbato E, Marco J, Wijns W. Direct stenting. Eur Heart J 2003;24:394–403.
9. Mintz GS, Popma JJ, Pichard AD, et al. Arterial remodelling after coronary angioplasty: a serial intravascular ultrasound study. Circulation 1996;94:35–43.
10. Hoffman R, Mintz GS, Dussaillant GR, et al. Patterns and mechanisms of in-stent restenosis: a serial intravascular ultrasound study. Circulation 1996;94:1247–1254.
11. Virmani R, Farb A. Pathology of in-stent restenosis. Curr Opin Lipidol 1999;10:499–506.
12. Guiteras P, Tomas L, Varas C, et al. Five years of angiographic and clinical follow-up after successful percutaneous transluminal coronary angioplasty. Eur Heart J 1989;10(Suppl G):42–48.
13. Kober G, Vallbracht C, Kadel C, et al. Results of repeat angiography up to eight years following percutaneous transluminal angioplasty. Eur Heart J 1989;10(Suppl G):49–53.
14. Mercado N, Boersma E, Wijns W, et al. Clinical and quantitative coronary angiographic predictors of coronary restenosis: a comparative analysis from the balloon-to-stent-era. J Am Coll Cardiol 2001;38:645–652.
15. Martnez-Elbal L, Ruiz-Nodar JM, Zueco J, et al. Direct coronary stenting versus stenting stenting with balloon predilatation: mmediate and follow-up results of a multicentre, prospective randomised study. The DISCO trial. Eur Heart J 2002;23:633–640.
16. Mudra H, di Mario C, de Jaegere, et al. Randomised comparison of coronary stent implantation under ultrasound or angiographic guidance to reduce stent restenosis (OPTICUS Study). Circulation 2001;104:1343–1349.
17. Mehilli J, Kastrati A, Dirschinger J, et al. A randomised trial comparing the hand-mounted JoStent with the premounted Multi-Link Duet stent in patients with coronary artery disease. Catheter Cardiovasc Interv 2001;54:414–419.
18. Babapulle MN, Eisenberg MJ. Coated stents for the prevention of restenosis: PartI. Circulation 2002;106:2734–2743.
19. Babapulle MN, Eisenberg MJ. Coated stents for the prevention of restenosis: Part II. Circulation 2002;106:2859–2866.
20. Morice MC, Serruys PW, Sousa JE, et al. A randomised comparison of a sirolimus-eluting stent with a standard stent for coronary revascularisation. N Eng J Med 2002;346:1773–1780.

21. Moses JW, Leon MB, Popma JJ, et al. Sirolimus-eluting stents versus standard stents in patients with stenosis in a native coronary artery. N Eng J Med 2003;349:1315–1323.
22. Schofer J, Schlüter M, Gershlick AH, et al. Sirolimus-eluting stents for treatment of patients with long atherosclerotic lesions in small coronary arteries: double-blind, randomised controlled trial. (E-SERIUS). Lancet 2003;362:1093–1099.
23. Stone GW, Ellis SG, Cox DA, et al. A polymer-based, paclitaxel-eluting stent in patients with coronary artery disease. N Eng J Med 2004;350:221–231.
24. Serruys PW, Degertekin M, Tanabe Kengo, et al. Vascular responses at proximal and distal edges of paclitaxel-eluting stents: serial intravascular ultrasound analysis from the TAXUS II trial. Circulation 2004;109:627–633.
25. Schampaert E, Cohen EA, Schlüter M, et al. The Canadian study of the sirolimus-eluting stent in the treatment of patients with long de novo lesions in small native coronary arteries (C-SIRIUS). J Am Coll Cardiol 2004;43(6):1110–1115.
26. Gershlick A, de Scheerder I, Chevalier B, et al. Inhibition of restenosis with a paclitaxel-eluting, polymer-free coronary stent: (ELUTES Trial). Circulation 2004;109:487–493.
27. Holmes DR, Jr, Leon MB, Moses JW, et al. Analysis of 1-year clinical outcomes in the SIRIUS trial. A randomised trial of a serolimus-eluting stent versus a standard stent n patients at high risk for coronary restenosis. Circulation 2004;109:634–640.
28. Colombo A, Drzewiecki J, Banning A, et al. for the TAXUS II Study group. Randomised study to assess the effectiveness of slow- and moderate release polymer-based paclitaxel-eluting stents for coronary artery lesions. Circulation 2003;108:788–794.
29. Nobuyoshi M, Kimura T, Nosaka H, et al. Restenosis after successful percutaneous coronary angioplasty: serial angiographic follow-up of 229 patients. J Am Coll Cardiol 1988;12:616–623.
30. Serruys PW, Luijten HE, Beatt KJ, et al. Incidence of restenosis after successful coronary angioplasty: a time-related phenomena. A quantitative angiographic study in 342 consecutive patients at 1, 2, 3 and 4 months. Circulation 1988;77:361–371.
31. Califf RM, Fortin DF, Frid DJ, et al. Restenosis after coronary angioplasty: an overview. J Am Coll Cardiol 1991;17:2B–13B.
32. Kimura T, Yokoi H, Nakagawa Y, et al. Three-year follow-up after implantation of metallic coronary-artery stents. N Engl J Med 1996;334:561–566.
33. Hoffmann R, Mintz GS. Coronary in-stent restenosis—predictors, treatment and prevention. Eur Heart J 2000;21:1739–1749.
34. Kimura T, Abe K, Shizuta S, et al. Long-term clinical and angiographic follow-up after coronary stent placement in native coronary arteries. Circulation 2002;105:2986–2991.
35. Goldberg SL, Loussararian A, De Gregorio J, et al. Predictors of diffuse and aggressive intra-stent restenosis. J Am Coll Cardiol 2001;37:1019–1025.
36. Brenner DJ, Miller RC, Hall EJ. The radiobiology of intravascular irradiation. Int J Radiat Oncol Biol Phys 1996;36:805–810.
37. Hernández RA, Macaya C, Iñiguez A, et al. Midterm outcome of patients with asymptomatic restenosis after coronary balloon angioplasty. J Am Coll Cardiol 1992;19:1402–1409.
38. Ruygrok PN, Webster MWI, de Valk V, et al. Clinical and angiographic factors associated with asymptomatic restenosis after percutaneous coronary intervention. Circulation 2001;104:2289–2294.
39. Rogers WJ, Bourassa MG, Andrews TC, et al. Asymptomatic Cardiac Ischaemia Pilot (ACIP) study: outcome at 1 year for patients with asymptomatic cardiac ischaemia randomised to medical therapy or revascularisation. J Am Coll Cardiol 1995;26:594–605.
40. Popma JJ, van de Berg EK, Dehmer GJ. Long term outcome of patients with asymptomatic restenosis after percutaneous transluminal coronary angioplasty. Am J Cardiol 1988;62:1298–1299.
41. Pfisterer M, Rickenbacher P, Kiowski W, et al. Silent ischaemia after percutaneous coronary angioplasty: incidence and prognostic significance. J Am Coll Cardiol 1993;22:1446–1454.
42. Cottin Y, Rezaizedah K, Touzery C, et al. Long-term prognostic value of $^{201}$Tl single-photon emission computed tomographic myocardial perfusion imaging after coronary stenting. Am Heart J 2001;141:999–1006.
43. Zellweger MJ, Weinbacher M, Zutter AW, et al. Long-term outcome of patients with silent versus symptomatic ischaemia six months after percutaneous coronary intervention and stenting. J Am Coll Cardiol 2003;42:33–40.
44. Rupprecht HJ, Espinola-Klein C, Erbel R, et al. Impact of routine angiographic follow-up after angioplasty. Am Heart J 1998;136:613–619.

45. Ruygrok PN, Melkert R, Morel M-AM, et al. Does angiography six months after coronary intervention influence management and outcome? J Am Coll Cardiol 1999;34:1507–1511.
46. Hermiller JB, Fry ET, Peters TF, et al. Late coronary artery stenosis regression within the Gianturco Roubin intracoronary stent. Am J Cardiol 1996;77:247–251.
47. Ormiston JA, Stewart FM, Roche AHG, et al. Late regression of the dilated site after coronary angioplasty. Circulation 1997;96:468–474.
48. Asakura M, Ueda Y, Nanto S, et al. Remodeling of in-stent neointima, which became thinner and transparent over 3 years. Serial angiographic and angioscopic follow-up. Circulation 1998;97: 2003–2006.
49. Holmes DR, Jr, Vliestra RE, Smith HC, et al. Restenosis after percutaneous transluminal coronary angioplasty (PTCA): a report from the PTCA Registry of the National Heart, Lung and Blood Institute. Am J Cardiol 1984;53:77C–81C.
50. Suresh CG, Grant SCD, Henderson RA, et al. Late symptom recurrence after successful coronary angioplasty: angiographic outcome. Int J Cardiol 1993;42:257–262.
51. Mata LA, Bosch X, David PR, et al. Clinical and angiographic assessment 6 months after double vessel percutaneous coronary angioplasty. J Am Coll Cardiol 1985;6:1239–1244.
52. Gruentzig AR, King SB III, Schlumpf M, et al. Long-term follow-up after percutaneous transluminal coronary angioplasty. The early Zurich experience. N Eng J Med 1987;316:1127–1132.
53. Kent KM, Bentivoglio LG, Block PC, et al. Long-term efficacy of percutaneous transluminal coronary angioplasty (PTCA): report from the National Heart, Lung and Blood Institute PTCA Registry. Am J Cardiol 1984;53:27C–31C.
54. Serruys PW, Strauss BH, Beatt KJ, et al. Angiographic follow-up after placement of a self expanding coronary artery stent. N Eng J Med 1991;324:13–17.
55. Schatz RA, Baim DS, Leon M, et al. Clinical experience with the Palmaz-Schatz coronary stent. Initial results of a multicentre study. Circulation 1991;83:148–161.
56. Walters DL, Harding SA, Walsh CR, et al. Acute coronary syndrome is a common clinical presentation of in-stent restenosis. Am J Cardiol 2002;89:491–494.
57. Miller JM, Ohman EM, Moliterno DJ, Califf RM. Restenosis the clinical issues. In: Topol EJ, ed. Textbook of Interventional Cardiology, 3rd ed. WB Saunders, Philadelphia, PA, 1999, pp. 379–415.
58. Bossi I, Klersy C, Black AJ, et al. In-stent restenosis: lont-term outcome and predictors of subsequent target lesion revascularisation after repeat ballon angioplasty. J Am Coll Cardiol 2000;35: 1569–1576.
59. Cohen DJ, Doucet M, Cutlip DE, et al. Impact of smoking on clinical and angiographic restenosis after percutaneous coronary intervention. Another smoker's paradox? Circulation 2001;104:773–778.
60. Hasdai D, Garratt KN, Grill DE, et al. Effect of smoking status on the long-term outcome after successful percutaneous coronary revascularization. N Eng J Med 1997;336:755–761.
61. Ellis SG, Tamai H, Nobuyoshi M, et al. Contemporary percutaneous treatment of unprotected left main coronary stenosis: initial results from a multicentre registry analysis, 1994–1996. Circulation 1997;96:3867–3872.
62. Lemos PA, Saia F, Ligthart JMR, et al. Coronary Restenosis after sirolimus-eluting stent implantation. Morphological description and mechanistic analysis from a consecutive series of cases. Circulation 2003;108:257–260.
63. Honda Y, Fitzgerald PJ. Stent thrombosis: an issue revisited in a changing world. Circulation 2003;108:2–5.
64. Haude M, Erbel R, Issa H, et al. Subacute thrombotic complications after intracoronary implantation of Palmaz-Schatz stents. Am Heart J 1993;126:15–22.
65. Malenka DJ, O'Rourke D, Miller MA, et al. Cause of in-hospital death in 13,232 consecutive patients undergoing percutaneous transluminal coronary angioplasty. Am Heart J 1999;137:632–638.
66. Orford JL, Lennon R, Melby S, et al. Frequency and correlates of coronary stent thrombosis in the modern era. Analysis of a single centre registry. J Am Coll Cardiol 2002;40:1567–1572.
67. Farb A, Burke AP, Kolodgie FD, et al. Pathological mechanisms of fatal late coronary stent thrombosis in humans. Circulation 2003;108:1701–1706.
68. Dadenberg HD, Lotan C, Hasin Y, et al. Acute myocardial infarction—a late complication of intracoronary stent placement. Clin Cardiol 2000;23:376–378.
69. Heller LI, Shemwell KC, Hug K. Late stent thrombosis in the absence of prior intracoronary brachytherapy. Catheter Cardiovasc Interv 2001;53:23–28.
70. Park SJ, Shim WH, Ho DS, et al. A paclitaxel-eluting stent for the prevention of coronary restenosis. N Eng J Med 2003;348:1537–1545.

71. Kataoka T, Grube E, Honda Y, et al. 7-Hexanoyltaxol-eluting stent for prevention of neointimal growth: an intravascular ultrasound analysis from the Study to Compare Restenosis rate between QueST and QuaDS-QP2 (SCORE). Circulation 2002;106:1788–1793.

72. Stein B, Weintroub WS, Gebhart SP, et al. Influence of diabetes mellitus on early and late outcomes after percutaneous transluminal coronary angioplasty. Circulation 1995;91:979–989.

73. Kornowski R, Mintz GS, Kent KM, et al. Increased restenosis in diabetes mellitus after coronary interventions is due to exaggerated intimal hyperplasia: a serial intravascular ultrasound study. Circulation 1997;95:1366–1369.

74. Abizaid A, Kornowski R, Mintz GS, et al. The influence of diabetes mellitus on acute and late outcomes following coronary stent implantation. J Am Coll Cardiol 1998;32:584–589.

75. Elezi S, Kastrati A, Pache J, et al. Diabetes mellitus and the clinical and angiographic outcome after coronary stent placement. J Am Coll Cardiol 1998;32:1866–1873.

76. Van Belle E, Perie M, Braune D, et al. Effects coronary stenting on vessel patency and long-term clinical outcome after percutaneous coronary revascularisation in diabetic patients. J Am Coll Cardiol 2002;40:410–417.

77. West NEJ, Ruygrok PN, Disco CMC, et al. Clinical and angiographic predictors of restenosis after stent deployment in diabetic patients. Circulation 2004;109:867–873.

78. Mathew V, Gersh BJ, Williams BA, et al. Outcomes in patients with diabetes mellitus undergoing percutaneous coronary intervention in the current era: a report from the prevention of restenosis with tranilast and its outcomes (PRESTO) trial. Circulation 2004;109:476–480.

79. Smith SC, Dove JT, Jacobs AK, et al. ACC/AHA guidelines for percutaneous coronary intervention: a report of the American College of Cardiology/American Heart Association Task force on Practice Guidelines (Committee to Revise the 1993 Guidelines for Percutaneous Transluminal Coronary Angioplasty). J Am Coll Cardiol 2001;37(8):2215–2239.

80. Mintz GS, Hoffmann R, Mehran R, et al. In-stent restenosis: the Washington Hospital Center experience. Am J Cardiol 1998;81(7A):7E–13E.

81. Lowe HC, Oesterle SN, Khachigian LM. Coronary in-stent restenosis: current status and future strategies. J Am Coll Cardiol 2002;39:183–193.

82. Mittal S, Weiss DL, Hirshfeld JWJ, et al. Comparison of outcome after stenting for de novo versus restenotic narrowings in native coronary arteries. Am J Cardiol 1997;80:711–715.

83. Holmes DR, Schwartz RS, Webster MWI, et al. Coronary restenosis: what have we learned from angiography? J Am Coll Cardiol 1991;17:14B–22B.

84. Khan JK, Rutherford BD, McConahay DR, et al. Short- and long-term outcome of percutaneous transluminal coronary angioplasty in chronic dialysis patients. Am Heart J 1990;119:484–489.

85. Schoebel FC, Gradaus F, Ivens K, et al. Restenosis after elective coronary balloon angioplasty in patients with end-stage renal disease: a case control study using quantitative coronary angiography. Heart 1997;78:337–442.

86. Koster R, Vieluf D, Kiehn M, et al. Nickel and molybdenum contact allergies in patients with coronary in-stent restenosis. Lancet 2000;356:1895–1897.

87. Kastrati A, Schömig A, Seyfarth M, et al. PI$^A$ polymorphism of platelet glycoprotein IIIa and risk of restenosis after coronary stent placement. Circulation 1999;99:1005–1010.

88. Ribichini F, Steffenino G, Dellavalle A, et al. Plasma activity and insertion/deletion polymorphism of angiotensin I-converting enzyme. Circulation 1998;97:147–154.

89. Jørgensen E, Kelbaek H, Helqvist S, et al. Predictors of coronary in-stent restenosis: importance of angiotensin-converting enzyme gene polymorphism and treatment with angiotensin-converting enzyme inhibitors. J Am Coll Cardiol 2001;38:1434–1439.

90. Fukuda D, Shimada K, Tanaka A, et al. Circulating monocytes and in-stent neointima after coronary stent implantation. J Am Coll Cardiol 2004;43:18–23.

91. Cipollone F, Marini M, Fazia M, et al. Elevated circulating levels of monocyte chemoattractant protein-1 in patients with restenosis after coronary angioplasty. Arterioscler Thromb Vasc Biol 2001;21:327–334.

92. Hokimoto S, Ogawa H, Saito T, et al. Increased plasma antigen levels of monocyte chemoattractant protein-1 in patients with restenosis after percutaneous transluminal coronary angioplasty. Jpn Circ J 2000;64:831–834.

93. Tutar E, Ozcan M, Kilickap M, et al. Elevated whole-blood tissue factor procoagulant activity as a marker of restenosis after percutaneous transluminal coronary angioplasty and stent implantation. Circulation 2003;108:1581–1584.

94. Kojoglanian SA, Jorgensen MB, Wolde-Tsadik G, et al. Restenosis in intervened coronaries with hyperhomocysteinemia (RICH). Am Heart J 2003;146:1077–1081.

95. Bauters C, Hubert E, Prat A, et al. Predictors of restenosis after coronary stent implantation. J Am Coll Cardiol 1998;31:1291–1298.

96. Marie PY, Danchin N, Karcher G, et al. Usefulness of exercise SPECT-thallium o detect asymptomatic restenosis in patients who had angina before coronary angioplasty. Am Heart J 1993;126: 571–577.

97. Giedd KN, Bergmann SR. Myocardial perfusion imaging following percutaneous coronary intervention. The importance of restenosis, disease progression and directed reintervention. J Am Coll Cardiol 2004;43:328–336.

98. Hecht HS, Shaw RE, Chin HL, et al. Silent ischaemia after coronary angioplasty: evaluation of restenosis and extent of ischaemia in asymptomatic patients by tomographic thallium-201 exercise imaging and comparison with symptomatic patients. J Am Coll Cardiol 1991;17:670–677.

99. Legrand V, Raskinet B, Laarman G, et al. Diagnostic value of exercise electrocardiography and angina after coronary artery stenting. Am Heart J 1997;133:240–248.

100. Moussa I, Mario CD, Reimers B, et al. Subacute stent thrombosis in the era of intravascular ultrasound-guided coronary stenting without anticoagulation: frequency, predictors and clinical outcome. J Am Coll Cardiol 1997;29:6–12.

101. Silva JA, Ramee SR, White CJ, et al. Primary stenting acute myocardial infarction: influence of diabetes mellitus in angiographic results and clinical outcome. Am Heart J 1999;138:446–455.

102. Cutlip DE, Baim DS, Kalon KL, et al. Stent thrombosis in the modern era: a pooled analysis of multicentre coronary stent clinical trials. Circulation 2001;103:1967–1971.

103. Cheneau E, Leborgne L, Mintz GS, et al. Predictors of subacute stent thrombosis: Results of a systematic intravascular ultrasound study. Circulation 2003;108:43–47.

104. Schuhlen H, Kastrati A, Dirschinger J, et al. Intracoronary stenting and risk of major adverse cardiac events during the first month. Circulation 1998;98:104–111.

105. Uren NG, Schwarzacher SP, Metz JA, et al. Predictors and outcomes of stent thrombosis: an intravascular ultrasound registry. Eur Heart J 2002;23:124–132.

106. Karrillon GJ, Morice MC, Benveniste E, et al. Intracoronary stent implantation without ultrasound guidance and with replacement of conventional anticoagulation by antiplatelet therapy: 30-day clinical outcome of the French Multicentre Registry. Circulation 1996;94:1519–1527.

107. Nakamura S, Colombo A, Gaglione A, et al. Intracoronary ultrasound observations during stent implantation. Circulation 1994;89:2026–2034.

108. Werner GS, Gastmann O, Ferrari M, et al. Risk factors for acute and subacute stent thrombosis after high-pressure stent implantation: a study by intracoronary ultrasound. Am Heart J 1998;135:300–309.

109. De Servi S, Repetto S, Klugmann S, et al. Stent thrombosis: incidence and related factors in the RISE Registry (Registro Impianto Stent Endocoronarico). Catheter Cardiovasc Interv 1999;46:13–18.

110. Versaci F, Gaspardone A, Tomai F, et al. A comparison of coronary artery stenting with angioplasty for isolated stenosis of the proximal left anterior descending coronary artery. N Eng J Med 1997;336:817–822.

111. Levine S, Ewels CJ, Rosing DR, et al. Coronary angioplasty: clinical and angiographic follow-up. Am J Cardiol 1985;55:673–676.

# 4 Pathological Anatomy of Restenosis

*Renu Virmani, MD, Frank D. Kolodgie, PhD, Aloke V. Finn, MD, and Herman K. Gold, MD*

## CONTENTS

## INTRODUCTION

Until recently, in-stent restenosis remained the "Achilles Heal" for interventional cardiologists. The introduction of drug-eluting stents (DES) [CYPHER, Cordis J&J, NJ (sirolimus) and TAXUS, Boston Scientific Corp. Boston (paclitaxel)] however, has made a tremendous impact on rates of in-stent restenosis with dramatic reductions from 30 to 40% in bare metal stent to 0 to 9% with DES *(1–4)*. The compelling results from large clinical trial with DES stents involve mostly simple lesion morphologies with follow-up of only 6–12 mo; it is still unclear whether a sustained benefit will be reached in more complex lesions and high-risk patients such as diabetics *(5)*. In this review, the stages of healing in response to bare metal stents implants in animals and humans will be discussed as a bases for understanding the localized effects of polymers and/or drugs on these natural biological processes.

From: *Contemporary Cardiology: Essentials of Restenosis: For the Interventional Cardiologist*
Edited by: H. J. Duckers, E. G. Nabel, and P. W. Serruys © Humana Press Inc., Totowa, NJ

# BARE METAL STENTS AND VASCULAR HEALING
# IN ANIMAL MODELS

Negative remodeling rather than increased tissue burden causes restenosis associated with balloon angioplasty *(6)*. Although, stenting prevents negative remodeling, the incidence of restenosis remains unacceptably high from excessive in-stent neointimal hyperplasia *(7)*. When bare metal stents are implanted in porcine coronary or rabbit iliac arteries there is an immediate accumulation of platelets surrounding the stent struts, which reaches a maximum at 24–48 h *(8–10)*. This response is accompanied by infiltration of acute inflammatory cells within the thrombus and injured medial and adventitial layers. Macrophage infiltration follows and is maximal at 5–7 d combined with fibrin accumulation around stent struts. At this time smooth muscle cell (SMC) proliferation peaks in the neointima whereas in the media this response occurs at 3 d. At 14 d, most of the stents are covered by a neointima rich in SMCs, proteoglycans, and type III collagen. Persistent fibrin around stent struts may be present; however, inflammation is generally absent and sparse if present. The rate of SMC proliferation is approximately half of that at 7 d and at 28 d the neointima is fully healed with negligible cell proliferation and little or no fibrin or inflammatory cells. Re-endothelialization of the luminal surface begins as early as 24 h and is 80% complete by 7 d in normal animal arteries. At 28 d, stents are fully covered by endothelium. Although in animals the neointima is completely healed by 28 d, wound retraction does not occur until 3 mo when type III collagen is replaced by type I collagen causing tissue shrinkage *(11)*. SMCs at this point are concentrated around the lumen where they are densely packed.

# HEALING IN HUMAN STENTED CORONARY ARTERIES

Vascular responses to stenting in humans occur at much slower rates although the healing phase is similar to animals. The earliest change is deposition of thrombus (platelet aggregates) in the first 24–48 h. Platelet adherence is generally observed in 72% of stent sections within 3 d and the lack of platelets may represent aggressive antiplatelet therapy. A similar percentage of sections show the persistence of platelets up to 11 d, but thereafter it decreases to 24%, and stents beyond 30 d lack evidence of platelets. Fibrinogen is essential for platelet aggregation, and when platelets are activated, the platelet glycoprotein IIb/IIIa integrin binds fibrinogen, which serves as a bridge between activated platelets. Acute inflammatory cells (polymorphonuclear leukocytes) are present within the thrombus around the stent struts in 79% of arterial sections and in 85% of stents in place for less than or equal to 3 d. These cells persist for up to 11 d and then decline in frequency till their absence beyond 30 d. Inflammatory cells are maximal at sites of medial injury and where stent struts have penetrated the necrotic core; very few inflammatory cells are found at sites of fibrous plaque (Fig. 1).

In contrast, chronic inflammation (macrophages, T-, and rare B- lymphocytes) in human stented arteries occurs at all phases of healing: 82% of sections at less than or equal to 3 d; 67% at 4–11 d; 97% at 12–30 d; and in 85% beyond 30 d *(12)*. The persistence of chronic inflammation beyond 90 d is associated with increased neointimal thickness and restenotic lesions have higher numbers of chronic inflammatory cells than nonrestenotic lesions *(13)*. Multinucleated giant cells are also observed but are only found beyond 11 d and only in 10% of sections (Fig. 2). The number of giant cells around stent struts increases to 30% in implants >30 d *(14)*.

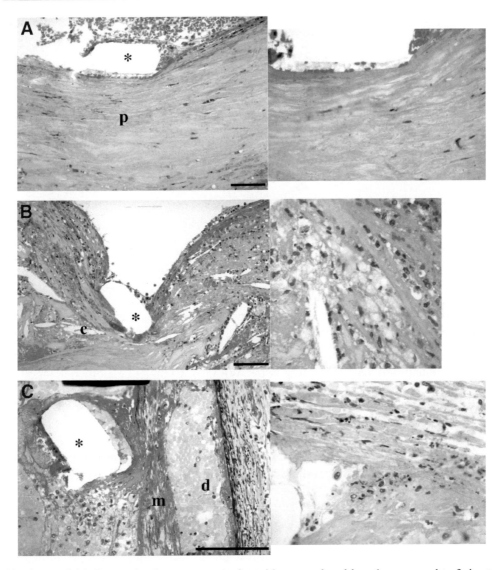

**Fig. 1.** Arterial inflammation in coronary arteries with stents placed less than or equal to 3 d ante-mortem: Movat pentachrome stain (left panel) with higher power H&E (right panel) from same section. In **(A)**, few inflammatory cells are present adjacent to Palmaz-Schatz strut (*) in contact with fibrous plaque (p). In **(B)**, increased numbers of inflammatory cells are associated with a Palmaz Schatz strut (*) that penetrates into a necrotic core (c). In **(C)**, a Palmaz Schatz strut (*) is in contact with damaged media (m) with dissection (d) and associated inflammatory cells. Reproduced with permission from *(14)*. (Please *see* insert for color version.)

Many investigators have documented the absence of an intact endothelium soon after stenting native coronary arteries or venous bypass grafts *(15)*. However, as early as 3 wk after stenting, Anderson et al. *(16)* showed the presence of an endothelial lining both by scanning electron microscopy and immunohistochemistry using antibodies directed against von Willebrand Factor. At 3 mo after stenting of vein bypass grafts, polygonal shaped endothelial cells are found with loose intercellular junctions and surface leuko-cytes. In contrast, stents in native coronary arteries demonstrate the persistence of fibrin

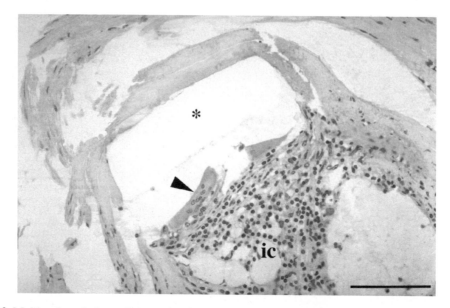

**Fig. 2.** Multinucleated giant cell (arrowhead) and numerous chronic inflammatory cells (ic) associated with Palmaz-Schatz stent strut (*) placed 70 d antemortem in the left anterior descending coronary artery. Reproduced with permission *(14)*.

beyond 60 d and only partial staining with vWF *(15)*. Complete endothelialization of stented native coronary arteries is likely to take at least 90 d (Fig. 3), depending on the type of underlying plaque *(17)*.

The appearance of neointimal SMCs in human stents is evident beyond 11 d with approx 50% of cases showing SMCs between 12 and 30 d; however, after 30 d, SMCs are always present (Fig. 4). The spindle shaped cells that initially invade the thrombus within 30 d are negative for markers of α-actin such as HHF-35 and 1A4 *(17,18)*, whereas beyond 30 d, α-actin positive SMCs are clearly identifiable in the neointima *(15)*.Thus, the early spindle-shaped cells represent dedifferentiated SMCs, which over time gradually redifferentiate into α-actin positive SMCs. Later, SMCs become circularly aligned near the lumen, which may be 15–30 layers thick by 3–6 mo. The adjacent middle neointimal layer is less cellular with scattered SMCs and proteoglycan matrix. The few SMCs close to the stent struts show marked intercellular interdigitations *(17)*.

## SMC PROLIFERATION

Cell proliferation studies in atherectomy specimens of human restenotic coronary tissue retrieved from a few days to just beyond 1 yr typically show low-proliferation rates with no characteristic peak as exemplified in animal models *(18–20)*. Clearly, significantly more rapid proliferative events appear to occur in animals as distinguished from human restenotic coronary arteries. Further, smooth muscle-cell migration from within the plaque or media to the expanding neointima may be the more dominant factor contributing to in-stent restenosis in humans.

## THE EXTRACELLULAR MATRIX

The fact that at least 40% of the neointima following stenting is made up of extra-cellular matrix is underappreciated *(18)*. The extracellular matrix, made up of initially proteoglycans and type III collagen, is gradually replaced by type I collagen. Recently

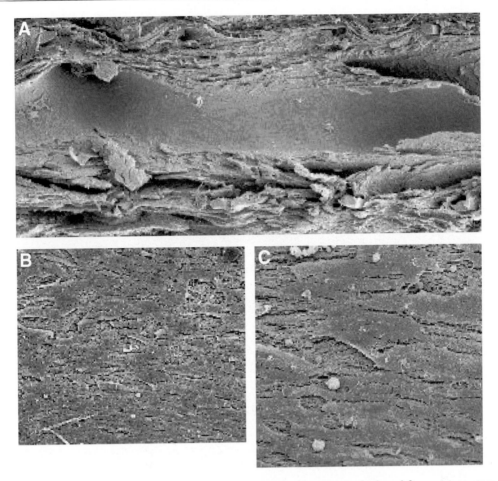

**Fig. 3.** Scanning electron microscopy of human coronary artery stent deployed 3 mo antemortem. The stent surface is covered by endothelial cells (**A**). At high power, poorly formed intercellular junctions are focally present (**B**) and rare adherent platelets and leukocytes are seen (**C**).

several extracellular matrix molecules were characterized in autopsy specimens of stented human coronary arteries based on the age of the implant (3–9 mo, >9–18 mo, and >18 mo) *(13)*. The two principle matrix molecules of the early neointima, which are present up to at least 18 mo, are versican-hyaluronan. In contrast, decorin begins to appear after 9 mo but significant accumulation occurs only after18 mo. Other early matrix components include type III collagen although beyond 18 mo, type I collagen predominates. Morphometric analysis has shown that neointimal area is not significantly different among 3–9 mo and more than 9–18 mo stents but is significantly less in stents >18 mo most likely resulting from the crosslinking of type I collagen leading to shrinkage of the neointima *(13)*. In addition, SMCs' density in lesions >18 mo may also contribute to a decrease in neointimal area.

## DIFFERENCE IN ARTERIAL HEALING BETWEEN HUMANS AND ANIMALS

One obvious explanation for delayed healing of humans stents is contingent on the underlying atherosclerotic plaque, which usually manifests in the fifth to sixth decade of life *(10)*. Preclinical studies in animal models are typically performed in young

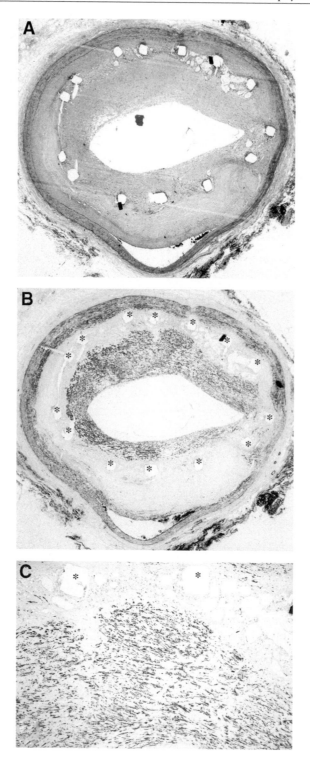

**Fig. 4.** In-stent restenosis. A 69-yr-old woman with coronary atherosclerosis underwent right coronary artery stenting 4 mo before presenting with angina. Coronary angiography demonstrated in-stent restenosis, and the patient died 1 d postcoronary artery bypass surgery. The right coronary artery (**A**) shows neointimal thickening within the stent (green color on Movat stain) to the

adults in normal vessels unburdened by inflammation and the absence of atherosclerotic disease likely contributes to the more predictable healing response. In contrast, at least 70% of the stented human coronary arteries are in direct contact with an underlying lesion *(12,14)*. Arterial healing is likely influenced by physical components of the plaque relative to the position of the stent. For example, stent struts in proximity to a necrotic core are exposed to only a limited number of SMCs and thus, heal slower than stents in direct contact with areas of adaptive intimal thickening, which contain an abundance of SMCs *(12)*. Similarly, stents overlying calcified and densely fibrotic plaques also take longer to develop a neointima as these are relatively hypocellular lesions.

The differential rate of healing between animals and humans may also be proportional to the longevity of the species. The typical life-span of a human is >70 yr; in contrast, pigs have a life-span of 16 yr, and rabbits 5–6 yr. The concept that biological differences in rates of healing are age-dependent is exemplified in animal models of cutaneous wounds. This analogy may be appropriate to in-stent restenosis because the developing neointima is considered a response to traumatic injury. For example, the extent of cutaneous re-epithelialization declines with age partly because of a decrease in the expression of growth factors *(21)*. Further, wound contraction (analogous to "remodeling" in the stent) is markedly accelerated in juvenile as compared with adult pigs. The extent of injury is another consideration; wound healing is delayed in traumatic as compared with surgically-induced injury and if the injury site is large vs small *(22,23)*. Human coronary stenting is often associated with extensive local trauma characterized by plaque splitting and medial disruption. Conversely, most stents in animals are deployed in normal arteries with 1.1:1 stent to artery ratio producing only mild arterial injury *(8)*.

## INFLAMMATION AND RESTENOSIS: THE RELATIONSHIP TO VESSEL INJURY AND PLAQUE TYPE

The inflammatory reaction that ensues after arterial injury is another critical factor that influences the extent of neointimal growth *(24)*. Although macrophages are abundant after stenting, acute inflammation representing neutrophils precedes the arrival of macrophages with simple balloon injury *(25)*. Anti-inflammatory molecular targets that prevent in-stent restenosis include Mac-1 (CD11b/CD18, $\alpha_M\beta_2$), which is responsible for firm leukocyte adhesion to platelets and fibrinogen at injured vessels *(26)*. The selective inhibition of neutrophils by high-affinity antibodies against Mac-1 (M1/70 or 8B2) when administered to rabbits after stenting results in a significant inhibition neointimal growth coinciding with inhibition of medial SMC proliferation at 3 d *(25,26)*. Similarly, administration of recombinant interleukin-10 a potent monocyte deactivator has been shown to reduce neointimal thickening after angioplasty or stent implantation in hypercholesterolemic rabbits *(27)*. In human stent implants more than 90 d, morphological studies from this laboratory demonstrate that neointimal growth correlates with

---

**Fig. 4.** *(Continued)*   extensive deposition of proteoglycan matrix resulting in in-stent restenosis. In **(B)**, a section stained with antibody to α-actin, shows that the neointima contains a large number of smooth muscle cells. **(C)** is a high power view of the in-stent neointima showing spindle shaped α-actin positive cells arranged parallel to the lumen. The "*" marks the location of stent struts. Reproduced with permission *(50)*. (Please *see* insert for color version.)

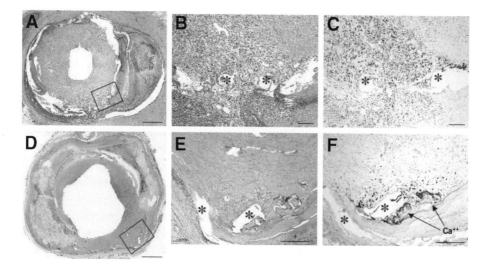

**Fig. 5.** Neointimal macrophages and neointimal growth. (**A**) shows in-stent restenosis of a left circum-flex artery stent placed 6 mo antemortem. A hypercellular neointima (**B**) surrounds stents struts (*), and KP-1 immunohistochemistry (**C**) identifies numerous brown-staining macrophages. Fewer intimal macrophages are associated with the widely patent left anterior coronary artery stent deployed 4 mo antemortem (**D–F**). Peri-strut calcium ($Ca^{++}$) deposits are indicated in **panel F**. Increased neointi-mal macrophage content is associated with in-stent restenosis (G). Neo, Neointima. Reproduced with permission *(12)*. (Please *see* insert for color version.)

the extent of chronic inflammation (lymphocytes and macrophages) around stent struts ($r^2 = 0.24$, $p < 0.0001$). Further, the percentage of the neointimal area occupied by macrophages was threefold higher in stents with restenosis vs no-restenosis (Fig. 5) *(12)*. Similar finding of the influence of macrophages on restenosis have been reported in atherectomy specimens from cases of coronary angioplasty *(28)*.

## ANGIOGENESIS AND NEOINTIMAL FORMATION AND INFLAMMATION

Neointimal angiogenesis occurs early with balloon arterial injury in animal models *(29)*. Angiogenesis is also a recognized feature of atherosclerotic lesions and is pro-portional to the underlying plaque burden *(30)* and symptomatology and plaque morphology in human coronary arteries *(31,32)*. Peri-strut neoangiogenesis correlates weakly but significantly with mean in-stent neointimal thickness, and increased inflammatory-cell density *(12)*. Struts associated with medial disruption also have higher neovascular density. Brasen et al. *(33)* have shown multiple capillaries around stent struts with abundant iron deposition as late as 2 yr following stenting. Immunostaining for platelet-derived growth factor was observed in the macrophages and giant cells close to the stent struts and in SMCs close to the luminal surface. Vascular endothelial growth factor-A expression colocalized in areas containing macrophages and endothelial cells and was much less intense in regions containing SMCs. The authors postulate that microhemorrhages play an important role in the development of neointimal formation, which may present a useful target for the prevention and treatment of in-stent resteno-sis. In addition, persistent fibrin has been shown around stent struts correlates with restenosis *(12)*. Although the mechanism(s) of fibrin-induced neointimal growth are speculative, fibrin degradation products have been shown to promote SMC proliferation *(34,35)*, migration *(36)*, and neoangiogenesis *(37)*.

## PLAQUE CHARACTERISTICS AND RESTENOSIS

### *Native Coronary Arteries*

In an effort to determine specific component of the atherosclerotic plaque that are crucial to the development of in-stent restenosis histomorphometric analysis was performed on stented human coronary arteries implanted for ≥90 d *(12)*. Surprisingly, neither the necrotic core area, extent of calcification, nor degree of inflammation was predictive of restenosis. On the other hand, stent strut penetration into the necrotic core accompanied by plaque prolapse was associated with increased neointimal thickness. Moreover, the size of the necrotic core and percentage of plaque occupied was a determinant of strut penetration. In addition, necrotic core penetration resulted in higher number of inflammatory cells around stent struts.

### *Saphenous Vein Grafts*

Atherosclerotic lesions in venous bypass grafts typically show larger necrotic cores and higher concentrations of foam cells than native coronaries. Although there is an initial high-clinical success rate in stented atherosclerotic vein grafts these results are encumbered by higher long-term restenosis rates than stents implanted in native coronary arteries *(38)*. Additional mechanisms such as progression of atherosclerosis within the stented lumen and late graft thrombosis may effect the patency of stented vein grafts beyond neointimal hyperplasia *(39)*. In atherosclerotic vein bypass grafts, leukocytes, platelets, and fibrin have been shown to be present at 3–14 d after stenting *(40)*. In a recent study of human stents lipid core penetration was more frequent in saphenous vein graft atherosclerosis than in native disease (48% vs 29%) *(41)*. Lipid core penetration by stent struts in vein grafts is associated with a high frequency of thrombotic occlusion (80% vs 0%) and an increase in the percentage of cross-sectional area narrowing (87% vs 47%) than in patients without necrotic core penetration, respectively *(41)*.

## THE INFLUENCE OF DIABETES ON RESTENOSIS

Diabetic patients treated with balloon angioplasty or stenting have higher rates of restenosis and target vessel revascularization than nondiabetics. The underlying mechanisms may be related to the rapid progression of the atherosclerotic disease in this population *(5)*. Insulin-dependent diabetes mellitus patients are at higher risk for in-hospital mortality and subsequent target vessel revascularization, and as a result have a significantly lower cardiac event-free survival rate *(42)*. In a diabetic pig model, Carter et al. *(43)* showed a higher rate of thrombosis than nondiabetic pigs but neointimal formation was similar. The experience with stents in human diabetic patients has failed to show higher restenosis or any morphological parameters, which would distinguish, diabetic from nondiabetic restenotic lesions (RV, unpublished observation, 2006). However, compared with native coronary arteries in nondiabetics, there are larger necrotic cores in diabetics, and a higher rate of SMC and macrophage apoptosis *(44)*.

## DES AND HEALING IN PRECLINICAL STUDIES

Preclinical studies of DES loaded with immunosuppressant and chemotherapeutic agents at 28 d show delayed healing characterized by persistent fibrin, sustained rates of SMC proliferation, inflammation, and incomplete endothelialization *(9,45,46)*. These results are similar to 7 d morphology of bare stainless steel stents *(8)*. Animal studies with sirolimus-eluting stents at 3 and 6 mo show a return of neointimal growth with complete healing and absence of fibrin *(10)*. Selective cytotoxic drugs may lead to even higher neointimal formation if accompanied by necrosis and inflammation, as reported with actinomycin-D *(47)*. Clearly, preclinical animal studies highly suggest that the effectiveness of the current generation of DES extends from a delay healing response and sustained suppression of neointimal growth is lost when the drug concentrations inevitably reaches a critical low.

Some polymers designed for drug delivery promote inflammation around stent struts as shown in implants at 28- and 90-d. As many as 12.5% to 35% of polymer-coated stents at 3 mo show inflammation characterized by granulomas and extensive eosinophilic infiltration *(48)*. The degree of inflammation may be further impacted at sites of stent overlap. Similar inflammatory reactions occur in stainless steel stents but to a lesser degree. The mechanism(s) of granuloma formation in stents remains poorly understood and it is important to emphasize that granulomas are a potential complication of all types of stents regardless of whether there is polymer/drug *(49)*. Increased inflammation in DES with specific involvement of eosinophils, however, suggests that polymers and/or drugs may be responsible for the hypersensitivity *(48)*.

## REFERENCES

1. Morice MC, Serruys PW, Sousa JE, et al. A randomized comparison of a sirolimus-eluting stent with a standard stent for coronary revascularization. N Engl J Med 2002;346:1773–1780.
2. Park SJ, Shim WH, Ho DS, et al. A paclitaxel-eluting stent for the prevention of coronary restenosis. N Engl J Med 2003;348:1537–1545.
3. Moses JW, Leon MB, Popma JJ, et al. Sirolimus-eluting stents versus standard stents in patients with stenosis in a native coronary artery. N Engl J Med 2003;349:1315–1323.
4. Popma JJ, Leon MB, Moses JW, et al. Quantitative assessment of angiographic restenosis after sirolimus-eluting stent implantation in native coronary arteries. Circulation 2004;110:374–379.
5. Loutfi M, Mulvihill NT, Boccalatte M, Farah B, Fajadet J, Marco J. Impact of restenosis and disease progression on clinical outcome after multivessel stenting in diabetic patients. Catheter Cardiovasc Interv 2003;58:451–454.
6. Bennett MR, O'Sullivan M. Mechanisms of angioplasty and stent restenosis: implications for design of rational therapy. Pharmacol Ther 2001;91:149–166.
7. Froeschl M, Olsen S, Ma X, O'Brien ER. Current understanding of in-stent restenosis and the potential benefit of drug eluting stents. Curr Drug Targets Cardiovasc Haematol Disord 2004;4:103–117.
8. Carter AJ, Laird JR, Farb A, Kufs W, Wortham DC, Virmani R. Morphologic characteristics of lesion formation and time course of smooth muscle cell proliferation in a porcine proliferative restenosis model. J Am Coll Cardiol 1994;24:1398–1405.
9. Farb A, John M, Acampado E, Kolodgie FD, Prescott MF, Virmani R. Oral everolimus inhibits in-stent neointimal growth. Circulation 2002;106:2379–2384.
10. Virmani R, Kolodgie FD, Farb A, Lafont A. Drug eluting stents: are human and animal studies comparable? Heart 2003;89:133–138.
11. Finn AV, Gold HK, Tang A, et al. A novel rat model of carotid artery stenting for the understanding of restenosis in metabolic diseases. J Vasc Res 2002;39:414–425.
12. Farb A, Weber DK, Kolodgie FD, Burke AP, Virmani R. Morphological predictors of restenosis after coronary stenting in humans. Circulation 2002;105:2974–2980.
13. Farb A, Kolodgie FD, Hwang J-Y, et al. Extracellular matrix changes in stented human coronary arteries. Circulation 2004;110:940–947.

14. Farb A, Sangiorgi G, Carter AJ, et al. Pathology of acute and chronic coronary stenting in humans. Circulation 1999;99:44–52.

15. Komatsu R, Ueda M, Naruko T, Kojima A, Becker AE. Neointimal tissue response at sites of coronary stenting in humans: macroscopic, histological, and immunohistochemical analyses. Circulation 1998;98:224–233.

16. Anderson PG, Bajaj RK, Baxley WA, Roubin GS. Vascular pathology of balloon-expandable flexible coil stents in humans. J Am Coll Cardiol 1992;19:372–381.

17. Grewe PH, Deneke T, Machraoui A, Barmeyer J, Muller KM. Acute and chronic tissue response to coronary stent implantation: pathologic findings in human specimen. J Am Coll Cardiol 2000;35:157–163.

18. Chung IM, Gold HK, Schwartz SM, Ikari Y, Reidy MA, Wight TN. Enhanced extracellular matrix accumulation in restenosis of coronary arteries after stent deployment. J Am Coll Cardiol 2002;40:2072–2081.

19. Pickering JG, Weir L, Jekanowski J, Kearney MA, Isner JM. Proliferative activity in peripheral and coronary atherosclerotic plaque among patients undergoing percutaneous revascularization. J Clin Invest 1993;91:1469–1480.

20. O'Brien ER, Alpers CE, Stewart DK, et al. Proliferation in primary and restenotic coronary atherectomy tissue. Implications for antiproliferative therapy. Circ Res 1993;73:223–231.

21. Yao F, Visovatti S, Johnson CS, et al. Age and growth factors in porcine full-thickness wound healing. Wound Repair Regen 2001;9:371–377.

22. Forrester JS, Fishbein M, Helfant R, Fagin J. A paradigm for restenosis based on cell biology: clues for the development of new preventive therapies. J Am Coll Cardiol 1991;17:758–769.

23. Schwartz RS, Huber KC, Murphy JG, et al. Restenosis and the proportional neointimal response to coronary artery injury: results in a porcine model. J Am Coll Cardiol 1992;19:267–274.

24. Welt FG, Rogers C. Inflammation and restenosis in the stent era. Arterioscler Thromb Vasc Biol 2002;22:1769–1776.

25. Welt FG, Edelman ER, Simon DI, Rogers C. Neutrophil, not macrophage, infiltration precedes neointimal thickening in balloon-injured arteries. Arterioscler Thromb Vasc Biol 2000;20: 2553–2558.

26. Inoue T, Uchida T, Yaguchi I, Sakai Y, Takayanagi K, Morooka S. Stent-induced expression and activation of the leukocyte integrin Mac-1 is associated with neointimal thickening and restenosis. Circulation 2003;107:1757–1763.

27. Feldman LJ, Aguirre L, Ziol M, et al. Interleukin-10 inhibits intimal hyperplasia after angioplasty or stent implantation in hypercholesterolemic rabbits. Circulation 2000;101:908–916.

28. Piek JJ, van der Wal AC, Meuwissen M, et al. Plaque inflammation in restenotic coronary lesions of patients with stable or unstable angina. J Am Coll Cardiol 2000;35:963–967.

29. Pels K, Labinaz M, Hoffert C, O'Brien ER. Adventitial angiogenesis early after coronary angioplasty: correlation with arterial remodeling. Arterioscler Thromb Vasc Biol 1999;19:229–238.

30. Winter PM, Morawski AM, Caruthers SD, et al. Molecular imaging of angiogenesis in early-stage atherosclerosis with alpha(v)beta3-integrin-targeted nanoparticles. Circulation 2003;108:2270–2274.

31. McCarthy MJ, Loftus IM, Thompson MM, et al. Angiogenesis and the atherosclerotic carotid plaque: an association between symptomatology and plaque morphology. J Vasc Surg 1999;30:261–268.

32. Mofidi R, Crotty TB, McCarthy P, Sheehan SJ, Mehigan D, Keaveny TV. Association between plaque instability, angiogenesis and symptomatic carotid occlusive disease. Br J Surg 2001;88:945–950.

33. Brasen JH, Kivela A, Roser K, et al. Angiogenesis, vascular endothelial growth factor and platelet-derived growth factor-BB expression, iron deposition, and oxidation-specific epitopes in stented human coronary arteries. Arterioscler Thromb Vasc Biol 2001;21:1720–1726.

34. Sturge J, Carey N, Davies AH, Powell JT. Fibrin monomer and fibrinopeptide B act additively to increase DNA synthesis in smooth muscle cells cultured from human saphenous vein. J Vasc Surg 2001;33:847–853.

35. Naito M, Stirk CM, Smith EB, Thompson WD. Smooth muscle cell outgrowth stimulated by fibrin degradation products. The potential role of fibrin fragment E in restenosis and atherogenesis. Thromb Res 2000;98:165–174.

36. Kodama M, Naito M, Nomura H, et al. Role of D and E domains in the migration of vascular smooth muscle cells into fibrin gels. Life Sci 2002;71:1139–1148.

37. Stirk CM, Reid A, Melvin WT, Thompson WD. Locating the active site for angiogenesis and cell proliferation due to fibrin fragment E with a phage epitope display library. Gen Pharmacol 2000;35:261–267.

38. Le May MR, Labinaz M, Marquis JF, et al. Predictors of long-term outcome after stent implantation in a saphenous vein graft. Am J Cardiol 1999;83:681–686.
39. Pratsos A, Fischman DL, Savage MP. Restenosis in Saphenous Vein Grafts. Curr Interv Cardiol Rep 2001;3:287–295.
40. van Beusekom HM, van der Giessen WJ, van Suylen R, Bos E, Bosman FT, Serruys PW. Histology after stenting of human saphenous vein bypass grafts: observations from surgically excised grafts 3 to 320 days after stent implantation. J Am Coll Cardiol 1993;21:45–54.
41. Pessanha BS, Farb A, Weber DK, Burke AP, Virmani R. Accelerated atherosclerotic change in saphenous vein bypass graft restenosis: Importance of the lipid core. J Am Coll Cardiol 2002;39:33A.
42. Tarantini G, Briguori C, Stankovic G, et al. Insulin-treated diabetes mellitus and predictors of midterm clinical outcome after percutaneous coronary interventions with stent implantation. Ital Heart J 2003;4:843–849.
43. Carter AJ, Bailey L, Devries J, Hubbard B. The effects of uncontrolled hyperglycemia on thrombosis and formation of neointima after coronary stent placement in a novel diabetic porcine model of restenosis. Coron Artery Dis 2000;11:473–479.
44. Burke AP, Kolodgie FD, Zieske A, et al. Morphologic findings of coronary atherosclerotic plaques in diabetics: a postmortem study. Arterioscler Thromb Vasc Biol 2004;24:1266–1271.
45. Farb A, Heller PF, Shroff S, et al. Pathological analysis of local delivery of paclitaxel via a polymer-coated stent. Circulation 2001;104:473–479.
46. Suzuki T, Kopia G, Hayashi S, et al. Stent-based delivery of sirolimus reduces neointimal formation in a porcine coronary model. Circulation 2001;104:1188–1193.
47. Serruys PW, Ormiston J, Degertekin M, et al. Actinomycin-eluting stent for coronary revascularization: A randomized feasibility and safety study (The ACTION Trial). J Am Coll Cardiol 2004; (in press).
48. Virmani R, Guagliumi G, Farb A, et al. Localized hypersensitivity and late coronary thrombosis secondary to a sirolimus-eluting stent: should we be cautious? Circulation 2004;109:701–705.
49. Kornowski R, Hong MK, Virmani R, Jones R, Vodovotz Y, Leon MB. Granulomatous foreign body reactions contribute to exaggerated in-stent restenosis. Coron Artery Dis 1999;10:9–14.

# 5

# The Influence of Shear Stress on Restenosis

*Attila Thury, MD, PhD,*
*Jolanda J. Wentzel, PhD,*
*Frank J. H. Gijsen, PhD,*
*Johan C. H. Schuurbiers, Bsc,*
*Rob Krams, MD, PhD,*
*Pim J. de Feyter, MD, PhD,*
*Patrick W. Serruys, MD, PhD,*
*and Cornelis J. Slager, PhD*

## CONTENTS

## SHEAR STRESS AND VASCULAR (PATHO) BIOLOGY

### Hemodynamic Forces Acting on the Vessel Wall

Wall shear stress (WSS) is the (tangential) drag force acting on the luminal wall, induced by blood flow, normalized to wall area. As WSS is defined as force/area, its dimension equals that of pressure, i.e., $N/m^2$ or Pa. An older, frequently used unit for shear stress, i.e., $dyne/cm^2$ relates to Pa according to $1\ Pa = 10\ dyne/cm^2$. WSS on the endothelium (Fig. 1) can be calculated from the local shear rate ($s^{-1}$) times blood viscosity ($\mu$) (Pa/s). Shear rate is the spatial blood velocity gradient ([m/s]/m). Especially near the vessel wall, generally large velocity gradients between adjacent fluid layers exist and the shear stress is at its highest value. In a simple straight tube the Hagen-Poiseuille formula (WSS = $4\mu Q/\pi R^3$, with $\mu$ viscosity, R tube radius and Q flow) can be applied for steady laminar viscous flow. A normal WSS range of $0.68 \pm 0.2$ Pa was derived from Doppler based velocity measurements in angiographically normal coronary

From: *Contemporary Cardiology: Essentials of Restenosis: For the Interventional Cardiologist*
Edited by: H. J. Duckers, E. G. Nabel, and P. W. Serruys © Humana Press Inc., Totowa, NJ

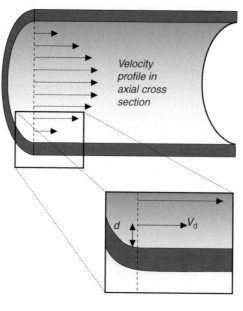

Wall shear rate ≈ $V_d/d$

Wall shear stress = Wall shear rate * Viscosity

**Fig. 1.** Top: flow velocity profile in axial cross-section. Over a very small distance (bottom) velocity increases linearly with distance and wall shear rate (velocity difference/distance) approaches $v_d/d$.

arteries of 21 patients *(1)*. Considering the fact that the flow in the investigated branches varied from 6 to 123.2 mL/min, while blood viscosity was assumed constant (3.5 mPa/s), the surprisingly narrow range of shear stress values clearly demonstrates the efficacy of the regulation of coronary lumen size by WSS.

From a mechanical point of view, it is important to realize that WSS, when increased above normal levels, has an extremely small magnitude and therefore is not likely to have direct mechanical consequences that would impair the endothelium by wear out or erosion. As an example, normal arterial WSS is less than the shear stress (~2–3 Pa) acting on the adhesive strip of a Post-it™ note pulled down by its weight when stuck to a vertical surface.

### Arterial Adaptation to Shear Stress

Arteries sensitively respond both in short- and long-term to WSS changes in order to keep the local WSS in a narrow range. Therefore, it is generally accepted that a negative feedback loop exists between WSS and the vessel lumen dimensions with WSS as the controlling variable *(2)*. The shear stress imposed on the endothelium by the movement of blood deforms the endothelial cells (ECs) to a microscopically small amount, but stimulates shear stress sensing elements in the ECs. These sensors induce the activation of second messenger systems (Fig. 2), which ultimately results in a biological response *(3)*.

It has been well established *(4)* that the vessel dilates under the influence of an acute increment in flow, thereby controlling the WSS in an artery (flow-dependent vasodilatation). A variety of vasoactive substances are produced by the endothelium under the influence of WSS *(5,6)*. The best-studied factor is endothelium-derived relaxing factor *(7)* that appeared to be nitric oxide *(8)* and which is produced in a WSS dependent way *(9)*. The

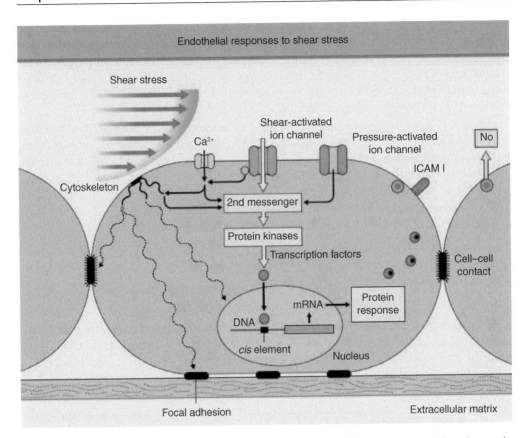

**Fig. 2.** Endothelial responses to shear stress. The endothelium rapidly responds to sudden changes in WSS, with changes in membrane potential and in intracellular calcium concentration. These induce the cell-signaling cascades within the endothelial cells including activation of the mitogen-activated protein kinase (MAP kinase) signaling cascade. There are also changes within the cytoskeleton of the cell and the cell membrane, both of which are likely to facilitate the release of nitric oxide and other vasodilators, including prostacyclin. These immediate changes are followed within a few hours by changes in the regulation of a subset of genes. Intercellular adhesion molecule-I.

endothelium also produces, as a response to alterations of WSS, prostacyclin and endothelin-1 *(5,10)*. After sustained periods of WSS alterations the ECs accommodate to the new environment through several genes *(11)*, including those of intercellular cell adhesion molecule-1, vascular cell adhesion molecule-1, and platelet derived growth factor (PDGF)-β. It has been shown that the regulation of some of these genes is dependent on shear responsive elements *(12)*. More sustained stimulation with WSS remodels the organization of F-actin microfilaments and aligns the ECs to the streamlines of the flow *(12)*. Furthermore, integrins in the cell membrane tend to cluster after chronic WSS increments, which ultimately enable the EC to adapt its shape and phenotype to local flow conditions *(9)*. The mechanisms described previously involve many other aspects, which exceed the scope of this chapter. However, it is clear that acute and chronic adaptation of the arterial wall, are WSS (flow) dependent processes.

### Role of Shear Stress in Localization of Atherosclerosis

The systemic nature of atherosclerotic risk factors cannot explain the observation that atherosclerosis occurs predominantly at certain locations in the arterial tree including bifurcations and near the junction sites of side branches (13). As these predilection sites are associated with deviations of the normal velocity field, it has been postulated that flow-induced shear stress, acting on the ECs, plays an important role in plaque localization and plaque growth (14,15). Indeed, low or oscillating WSS results in cellular (e.g., monocyte) adhesion onto the vascular wall, lipid accumulation and oxidation, release of vasoactive substances, induction of growth factors, and smooth muscle cell proliferatory characteristics (16,17). It has not unequivocally been shown whether spatial gradients in WSS or low oscillatory WSS is the main modulator of atherogenesis, although most evidences point to the latter (13,18,19). For example, the carotid arteries are often unilaterally involved in atherosclerosis, with the affected region displaying lower mean WSS (15). In diabetics the common carotid arteries have a lower mean WSS than that found in normoglycemic individuals, with unilateral lesions again associated with localized areas of low WSS (20).

## SHEAR STRESS IN PATIENTS

### Computational Fluid Dynamics: In Vivo Application in Human Coronary Arteries

In vivo accurate measurement of the wall shear rate is difficult and at this moment it cannot be applied to map WSS distributions in human coronary arteries. Therefore, to determine the local wall WSS in these arteries, computational fluid dynamics is applied (21). As a first step, a computational grid fitting in a three dimensions (3D) reconstructed lumen of human coronary arteries is generated (Fig. 3). Next, measured flow rate and patient specific blood viscosity data are transformed to the appropriate boundary conditions. The computational grid and the input conditions are subsequently fed into a numerical code to solve the Navier-Stokes equations and the continuity equation. This procedure renders the local velocity and WSS distribution at any point in the computational grid of the reconstructed human coronary artery. This method has been applied for various relevant hemodynamical problems (21–26).

### Atherosclerosis, Vascular Remodeling, and Shear Stress

Vascular remodeling has been observed in physiological conditions in response to changes in WSS, where it is aimed at restoring the original values of WSS (27). WSS acting on ECs is a major regulator of remodeling in developing blood vessels (28) and in blood vessels affected by atherosclerotic lesions (14). This is of importance, as it has been shown that the endothelium plays an essential role in vascular remodeling (29).

During early atherosclerosis, the control of lumen dimensions by WSS is still operable (30). Hence, Glagov et al. (31) suggested that WSS control might explain his observations on lumen preservation by compensatory enlargement of arteries during early plaque accumulation. Only if the plaque area exceeded 40% of the intima-bounded area was lumen narrowing observed (31). A consequence of lumen preservation by compensatory enlargement is that plaque buildup remains clinically and angiographically unnoticed until this compensation gradually fails or acute coronary syndromes occur. Prolonged plaque accumulation at persisting low WSS predilection locations explains a negative relation between wall thickness (WT) and WSS (21).

Until recently, there has been no data on the relation between WT and WSS when lumen narrowing and loss of compensatory remodeling commence. The authors investigated (32)

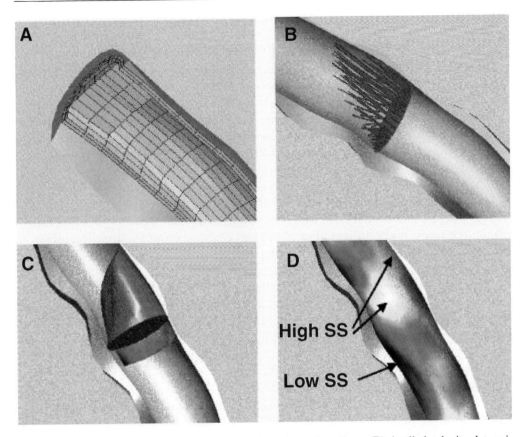

**Fig. 3. (A)** After lumen meshing, computational flow dynamics allows **(B)** detailed velocity determination at any cross-section. From this **(C)** the local velocity profile and wall WSS (colored band) are derived. Ultimately, **(D)** WSS is calculated at any location of the lumen wall as shown in color-code. Note, that in general at the outer curve of this human coronary example WT is smallest and WSS highest, whereas the reverse can be noticed at the inner vessel curve. (Please *see* insert for color version.)

angiographically normal arteries (stenosis <50%) of 14 patients with ANGiography and ivUS (ANGUS) to provide 3D lumen and wall geometry *(33)*. WSS of 25 segments was calculated by computational fluid dynamics. For segments of preserved lumens axially averaged WT and WSS were negatively related and positive vascular remodeling was observed. Narrowed segments showed no relation between WT and WSS or vascular remodeling. It was concluded *(32)* that in a patient with coronary arteries, the often-reported negative WT-WSS relationship appears restricted to lumen preservation and positive vascular remodeling. Its disappearance with lumen narrowing suggests a growing importance of non-WSS-related plaque progression.

Recently, Stone et al. *(34)* studied six native arteries of patients by 3D reconstruction and intravascular flow profiling at baseline and after 6-mo follow-up. Regions of abnormally low baseline WSS exhibited a significant increase in plaque thickness and enlargement of the outer vessel wall, such that lumen radius remained unchanged (outward remodeling). Regions of physiological WSS showed little change. Regions with increased WSS exhibited outward remodeling with normalization of WSS *(34)*.

## SHEAR STRESS AND RESTENOSIS AFTER BALLOON ANGIOPLASTY

### *Vascular Changes After Balloon Angioplasty*

Early balloon injury denudation models provided important insights into the mechanisms of restenosis after angioplasty. Kohler and Jawien *(35)* examined the effects of blood flow on intimal hyperplasia after balloon catheter injury of the rat common carotid artery. By ligation of the ipsilateral carotid artery they obtained 35% decrease in blood flow and corresponding mean blood velocity. They found that early (2–4 wk after the injury) neointimal hyperplasia (NIH) increased when flow was reduced, and related it to alteration of smooth muscle cell migration *(35)*. Thus, it is readily suggestive that evolution of the healing reaction is sensitive to flow and thereby to WSS *(36)*.

Immediately after balloon angioplasty the endothelium is damaged and also after regeneration the endothelial layer may be dysfunctional *(29)*. Balloon dilatation causes plaque fractures, breaks, dissection clefts and cracks extending from the lumen to resulting in injury to the intima *(37)*. Owing to these spatial changes of the intimal surface, major changes in local WSS take place. In addition, localized medial dissection, stretching of the plaque-free wall and combination of plaque stretching and compression, result in geometrical transitions that are also responsible for alterations in wall shear and tensile stresses. As blood flow is determined by dimensional adaptations to WSS and wall tensile stress (WS, force acting perpendicularly to a surface, normalized to area), a reasonable hypothetical paradigm has been set forth by Glagov *(36)*. This describes the sequence of adaptive functional responses underlying outcomes after interventional injury of arteries; after modification of WSS and WS, these regulate the healing tissue responses (cell proliferation and matrix biosynthesis) until baseline (stable) levels of these stresses are re-established. If these levels are established, it will result in arrest of intimal thickening thus maintaining lumen patency. If it fails, persistent intimal proliferation or negative remodeling (considered to be the predominant cause of restenosis after angioplasty *[38,39]*) will cause restenosis. This hypothesis is descriptive, however, the causative factor for distinguishing between these two processes is not clarified. Below, arguments and findings further describing this hypothesis are given.

### *Low Shear Stress Related to Restenosis*

Segmental coronary blood flow may remain impaired after angioplasty *(40)* because of microvascular dysfunction, infarction of some of the tissue downstream, or the presence of persistent competing collateral circulation. Increased incidence of restenosis in patients has been repeatedly associated with reduced flow *(41,42)* and abnormally low flow reserve *(43)*. The mechanisms by which these hemodynamic forces may modulate the vascular smooth muscle cells (VSMC) proliferative and migratory responses in vivo include induction of mitogenic cytokines, such as PDGF. PDGF contributes to these responses, as both PDGF and its receptor ($\beta$-type) are upregulated by injury *(44)*. Other mediators, such as matrix metalloproteinases are also involved *(45)*.

As WSS and WS have been implicated as regulators of vascular remodeling during physiological conditions, the authors evaluated their role in vascular remodeling after balloon angioplasty in a well-accepted pig model *(46)*. It was argued that if WSS and/or WS are important regulators in vascular remodeling after balloon angioplasty then they should comply with the following criteria. First, WSS or WS will change after balloon angioplasty, second, the change of WSS or WS induced by balloon angioplasty should be predictive of vascular remodeling, and third, vascular remodeling should arrest when WSS and WS have been returned to "normal values."

The results showed (46) that a significant decrease in WSS and increase in WS after balloon angioplasty was reached and these changes measured at baseline were predictive for vascular remodeling at 6 wk follow-up. Moreover, data showed that the WSS and WS were returned to the reference values. As all data in respect to the values of reference segments were normalized, results were fully independent of the assumed inflow conditions for the WSS calculation. Hence, from these results it can be concluded that in the Yucatan atherosclerotic pig model, vascular remodeling after gentle balloon angioplasty is controlled by a WSS and a WS negative feedback mechanism, aiming at keeping WSS and WS constant (Fig. 4).

Because the integrity of the endothelial layer is damaged directly after balloon angioplasty pathways other than the endothelium might get activated. Sterpetti et al. (47) reported that VSMCs also sense WSS and that increasing WSS directly inhibits whereas decreasing WSS facilitates VSMC proliferation. Recent studies indicate that when cultured VSMCs are in the synthetic phenotype, they respond to WSS in an analogous manner to the endothelium, altering their production of growth factors (48). In the balloon catheter–injured and de-endothelialized rat carotid artery, the VSMCs that migrate through the internal elastic lamina to form the neointima rapidly change to the synthetic phenotype, and they maintain phenotypic modulation until at least 2 wk after injury (49). Thus, it is possible that juxtaluminal synthetic VSMCs could respond to abnormal shear forces in a manner similar to the endothelium and hence potentially influence inward remodeling.

Ward et al. (41) examined how increases or decreases in blood flowthrough balloon catheter–injured rat carotid arteries affected vessel morphometry, cell migration, and levels of promigratory mRNAs. After 28 d, the luminal area in vessels with low blood flow was significantly smaller than in those with normal and high blood flow, predominantly because of accentuated inward remodeling. Low flow also enhanced VSMC migration 4 d after injury by 90% above normal and high flows. They concluded (41) that low blood flow might promote restenosis after angioplasty because of its adverse effect on vascular remodeling, and its association with the augmented expression of multiple genes central to cell migration and restenosis.

However, other than negative remodeling, additional potential mechanisms for restenosis after angioplasty should be mentioned. Bassiouny et al. (45) found that platelet activation after experimental arterial injury as measured by thromboxane $B_2$ levels was greater with injured arteries subjected to reduced flow compared with normal and increased flow conditions. This suggests that platelet adhesion to regions of injury is enhanced in a low-flow and low-shear environment. Activated platelets release many growth factors, including PDGF, basic fibroblast growth factor, and transforming growth factor. These factors play an important role in regulating VSMC migration and proliferation (50). Conclusively, studies point at low WSS leading to inward remodeling after balloon angioplasty ultimately resulting in restenosis. However, the reason why the physiological feedback mechanism (i.e., process to restore normal range of WSS) passes the point of the normal lumen settings and fails by further lumen loss is not yet clear.

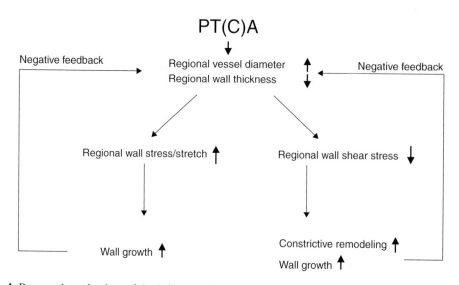

**Fig. 4.** Proposed mechanism of the influence of geometry on control mechanisms during the follow-up period after PT(C)A.

## *Flow Eddies After Balloon Angioplasty and Restenosis*

It has been suggested that apart from uniform sluggish laminar flow, irregular flow patterns including eddies that result from high average flow velocities and irregular lumen may also predict restenosis after angioplasty *(51)*. Similarly, after balloon angioplasty, mild residual stenosis with complex ultrastructure of intimal flaps and cracks may be optimal for development of local small oscillating flow patterns, which might arise within the "normal" range of brisk blood flow.

The authors published an appealing finding *(52)* when average WSS was calculated from the gross blood velocity using a Doppler wire proximal to, in and distal to the lesion after angiographically successful balloon dilatation. The Hagen-Poiseuille formula was applied and volumetric blood flow and lumen radius were derived from Doppler velocities and videodensitometric cross-sectional areas. Postprocedural proximal and in-lesion WSS values were higher in vessels that developed restenosis ($n = 72$; $1.2 \pm 0.6$ and $3.6 \pm 2.4$ N/m$^2$, respectively) than those without ($n = 130$, $1.1 \pm 0.5$ N/m$^2$ and $2.5 \pm 1.4$, respectively, $p < 0.05$). In-lesion WSS was predictive of restenosis, whereas WSS of the proximal segment was associated with an increased rate of target lesion revascularization (odds ratio = 2.33, $p < 0.005$). Moreover, proximal high WSS was the only independent predictor when entered with known predictors as diameter stenosis and coronary flow reserve (odds ratio was 2.15, $p < 0.05$). This paradoxical finding raised the following arguments as theoretical explanations *(52)*. Although high average WSS values for the entire cross-section were calculated in the patient group, no certainty about the spatial distribution of the WSS could be investigated. Indeed, it is possible that next to a high average lumen WSS, in the adjacent wall regions of flaps and cracks low WSS zones exist. These zones of low WSS can also coexist with flow separation zones inducing strong secondary and oscillatory flows *(53)*. It might be that especially these regions are prone to the evolvement of restenosis: possibly the patients that developed restenosis had more severe vessel injury after angioplasty, with more flow separation and more regions of secondary flow and localized low WSS. One might

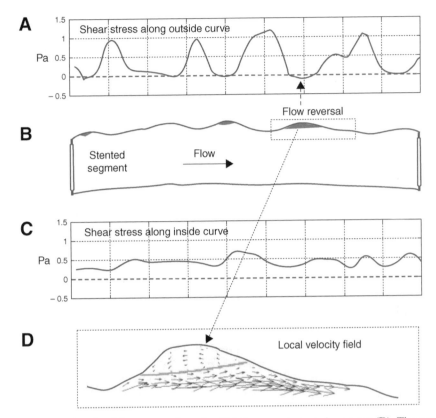

**Fig. 9.** Two-dimensional axial cross-section of a slightly curved stented segment (**B**). The results of a computation of velocity and WSS distribution in this segment at follow-up show regions with low WSS (**A**) that coincide with the shallow pits in B. Along the inner curve, the region with lower WSS, the pits are virtually absent and WSS distribution is much more homogeneous (**C**). In some of the pits along the outside curve B, flow reversal can be observed (inset and **D**). The areas containing reversed axial velocity are indicated by the shaded boxed regions in B.

This is in good accordance with the earlier-described finding of the step-up phenomenon and further encourages the acknowledgment of low WSS as a causative mechanism for enhanced neointimal growth. One might speculate that in case of stent oversizing by 15% (as group 1 in the study of Sick et al. *[96]*), which approximately lowers WSS (proportional to 1/diameter$^3$) by 39%, might have been indeed associated with the increased NIH in the long-term. Similarly, undersizing by 15% enhances WSS by approx 63%, thus providing a strong inhibitory effect for neointimal growth. Thus, it might be concluded that oversizing of stents is no longer necessary with current standards of antiplatelet treatment.

### ENHANCEMENT OF SHEAR STRESS: FLOW DIVIDER

In line with the earlier-described research on Wallstents, a new therapeutic experimental device was developed to increase WSS aiming at reduction of neointimal formation. This device *(97)* (Endoart, Lausanne, Switzerland) consists of a small cylinder (1 mm diameter) placed in the middle of a (stented) arterial segment and divides the flow, thereby increasing WSS while keeping the pressure drop below 1 mmHg. The authors performed *(97)* an animal study to evaluate the possible therapeutic application of the flow divider. In this investigation, the iliac arteries of nine rabbits were stented.

One of the stented arteries was randomly equipped with the flow divider, whereas the other artery served as a control. In the arteries with flow divider, CFD computations indicated that the WSS in the stented segment increased by 100%. The resulting neointimal formation in the stented arteries with the flow divider was compared with the stented segments without the device. Histological analysis showed *(97)* that the presence of the flow divider reduced neointimal formation by approx 40% (Fig. 10). This large effect identifies WSS as a major independent modulating factor in restenosis and merits further research on methods to, at least temporarily, create a local increase of WSS to suppress NIH.

### ENHANCEMENT OF SHEAR STRESS: PHYSICAL EXERCISE

The notion that regular aerobic exercise reduces cardiovascular morbidity and mortality in the general population as well as in patients with coronary artery disease is strongly supported by evidence derived from epidemiological studies *(98)*. More recently, exercise-induced increases in blood flow and WSS have been observed to enhance vascular function and structure *(99)*. Quantitative angiographic studies *(100,101)* have revealed that exercise programs reduce the progression of coronary artery disease and even showed superiority over percutaneous intervention in a certain patient subset in a recent study *(102)*. These observations provided the basis for the hypothesis that exercise may also induce changes in lumen diameter in patients after coronary angioplasty. Indeed, patients randomized to a 12-wk intervention program consisting of daily exercise after balloon angioplasty enjoyed a significantly lower rate of restenosis than patients in the control group *(103)*. A recent study of Indolfi et al. *(104)* showed a significant reduction of both NIH after stenting and negative remodeling 14 d after balloon injury in trained compared with sedentary rats. L-NMMA administration eliminated the benefits of physical training on vessel wall after balloon dilation, which signifies that increase in WSS related eNOS expression and activity might contribute to the potential beneficial effects of exercise. Moreover, they demonstrated *(104)* that exercise training produced accelerated re-endothelialization of the balloon injured arterial segments compared with sedentary. It can partly be attributed to a very recent finding of Laufs et al. *(105)* who demonstrated that physical activity increases the production and circulating numbers of endothelial progenitor cells (EPCs). Concerning the general beneficial effect of exercise training on cardiovascular events, a new study *(106)* revealed a possible mechanism: in the apoE-deficient mice, exercise training reduced neointimal growth and even stabilized vascular lesions after injury. This was based on the reduction of the number of Mac-3–positive, oxidized LDL-containing macrophages in the vessel wall and the increased content of collagen fibers. Plasminogen activator inhibitor-1, tissue factor, and fibrinogen were all significantly reduced in the lesions of trained mice *(106)*. These observations further encourage population-based studies to establish the optimal duration and intensity of exercise, which should, preferably be individually recommended for each patient.

### PROGRAMMABLE DES

A next-generation coronary drug delivery system (Conor MedStent™) has recently been proposed as being engineered specifically to allow programmable control over spatial and temporal release kinetics of different drugs and to enhance drug-loading capacity *(107)*. This stent has relatively large reservoirs (holes) being able to elute any drug (micro to macro molecules), oligonucleotides, microspheres, cDNA toward the wall and the lumen in a coronary artery. However, the transport of certain materials by blood and uptake into the vessel wall are complex processes *(108)* and found to be

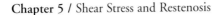

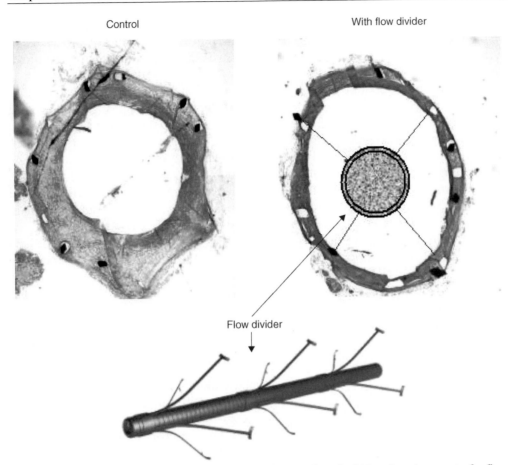

**Fig. 10.** Cross-sectional histological specimens of iliac arteries of rabbits after placement of a flow divider in the center of a stent that increases WSS at the stent surface. This resulted in a reduced intimal hyperplasia as described in the text.

dependent on the nature of the flow in the vessel and blood rheological properties including the red cell concentration *(109)*. One of the promising perspectives is to address the treatment of distal vulnerable plaque or diffuse disease by long time drug delivery to the lumen distal of the stent. However, because of the complex process of endothelialization and drug diffusion from the possibly tissue covered reservoirs the feasibility of drug delivery over a long time period is yet unknown. Extensive studies are needed to test the theory and efficacy of such a therapy with various agents.

## STENTS SEEDED WITH EPCs

In order to enhance rapid re-endothelialization, early attempts were reported *(110,111)* using ECs. However, difficulty of harvesting autologous ECs from patients has hampered clinical usage of this method *(112)*. Recently, EPCs have been used for fabrication of new cell-seeded stents *(113)*. Circulating EPCs have been demonstrated in the peripheral blood and shown to differentiate into a functional EC type, along with the ability to traffic to damaged vasculature *(114)*. Moreover, impaired adhesion and reduced numbers of circulating EPCs in patients with diffuse in-stent restenosis was detected *(115)*. Another problem to solve is how to achieve a stent surface properly seeded with a sufficient number of ECs/EPCs, capable of withstanding balloon trauma at implantation. This issue has been recently addressed with the newly designed Genous™ Bio-engineered Surface (Orbus Medical Technologies, Inc. FL). This utilizes antibodies to capture the patient's own circulating EPCs.

Blood flow most certainly plays a crucial rule when attachment of EPCs to antibodies and their differentiation into mature EC lining are considered. Intuitively, two opposing effects of the magnitude of WSS at a certain location of the stented surface take place. Low WSS by increasing near-wall residence time of any particle or cell favors EPC capture. A proof for this was elegantly presented in a recent report *(116)* by establishing a representative quantitative correlation between monocyte deposition and residence time. On the other hand, low WSS may stimulate thrombosis possibly covering the antibodies. High shear rate causing short residence time and increased detachment force might prevent EPCs to be arrested by antibodies *(117)*. Maintenance of the EC monolayer is also dependent on physiologically relevant (high) WSS conditions *(118,119)*. EPCs are more sensitive to WSS than matured ECs *(120)* and moreover, WSS was shown to stimulate EPC proliferation and their alignment in the direction of flow *(120)*. One might consider these mechanisms to be hardly optimally distributed at all locations of the stent struts. Further studies are encouraged to investigate the delicate WSS related processes of EPC capturing and proliferation.

## CONCLUSIONS

WSS is of paramount importance in vascular biology because of its multiple effects on EC. WSS explains the local and eccentric nature of atherosclerosis and vascular remodeling. With advanced technologies it became feasible to investigate these mechanisms and its effect after vascular intervention. Low and oscillating WSS have been associated with restenosis after balloon angioplasty and stent implantation. The process of neointima growth has many WSS related facets. The manipulation of WSS might have future clinical implications as has been already shown in the case of the flow divider.

## REFERENCES

1. Doriot PA, Dorsaz PA, Dorsaz L, et al. In-vivo measurements of wall shear stress in human coronary arteries. Coron Artery Dis 2000;11:495–502.
2. Kamiya A, Togawa T. Adaptive regulation of wall shear stress to flow change in the canine carotid artery. Am J Physiol 1980;239:H14–H21.
3. Fisher AB, Chien S, Barakat AI, et al. Endothelial cellular response to altered shear stress. Am J Physiol Lung Cell Mol Physiol 2001;281:L529–L533.
4. Lie M, Sejersted OM, Kiil F. Local regulation of vascular cross section during changes in femoral arterial blood flow in dogs. Circ Res 1970;27:727–737.
5. Davies PF, Tripathi SC. Mechanical stress mechanisms and the cell. An endothelial paradigm. Circ Res 1993;72:239–245.
6. McIntire LV. 1992 ALZA Distinguished Lecture: bioengineering and vascular biology. Ann Biomed Eng 1994;22:2–13.
7. Furchgott RF, Zawadzki JV. The obligatory role of endothelial cells in the relaxation of arterial smooth muscle by acetylcholine. Nature 27 1980;288(5789):373–376.
8. Furchgott RF, Jothianandan D. Endothelium-dependent and -independent vasodilation involving cyclic GMP: relaxation induced by nitric oxide, carbon monoxide and light. Blood Vessels 1991;28:52–61.
9. Malek AM, Alper SL, Izumo S. Hemodynamic shear stress and its role in atherosclerosis. JAMA 1999;282:2035–2042.

10. Redmond EM, Cahill PA, J.V. S. Flow-mediated regulation of endothelium receptors in cocultured vascular smooth muscle cells: an endothelium-dependent effect. Vasc Res 1997;34:425–435.

11. Gimbrone MA Jr, Nagel T, Topper JN. Biomechanical activation: an emerging paradigm in endothelial adhesion biology. J Clin Invest 1997;100:S61–S65.

12. Resnick N, Yahav H, Khachigian LM, et al. Endothelial gene regulation by laminar shear stress. Anal Quantitative Cardiol 1997;13:155–164.

13. VanderLaan PA, Reardon CA, Getz GS. Site specificity of atherosclerosis: site-selective responses to atherosclerotic modulators. Arterioscler Thromb Vasc Biol 2004;24:12–22.

14. Zarins CK, Giddens DP, Bharadvaj BK, et al. Carotid bifurcation atherosclerosis. Quantitative correlation of plaque localization with flow velocity profiles and wall shear stress. Circ Res 1983;53:502–514.

15. Gnasso A, Irace C, Carallo C, et al. In vivo association between low wall shear stress and plaque in subjects with asymmetrical carotid atherosclerosis. Stroke 1997;28:993–998.

16. Khachigian LM, Anderson KR, Halnon NJ, et al. Egr-1 is activated in endothelial cells exposed to fluid shear stress and interacts with a novel shear-stress-response element in the PDGF A-chain promoter. Arterioscler Thromb Vasc Biol 1997;17:2280–2286.

17. Hagiwara H, Mitsumata M, Yamane T, et al. Laminar shear stress induced GRO mRNA and protein expression in endothelial cells. Circulation 1998;98:2584–2590.

18. Friedman MH, Deters OJ, Bargeron CB, et al. Shear-dependent thickening of the human arterial intima. Atherosclerosis 1986;60:161–171.

19. Giddens DP, Zarins CK, Glagov S. The role of fluid mechanics in the localization and detection of atherosclerosis. J Biomech Eng 1993;115:588–594.

20. Irace C, Carallo C, Crescenzo A, et al. NIDDM is associated with lower wall shear stress of the common carotid artery. Diabetes 1999;48:193–197.

21. Krams R, Wentzel J, Oomen J, et al. Evaluation of endothelial shear stress and 3D geometry as factors determining the development of atherosclerosis and remodeling in human coronary arteries in vivo. Combining 3D reconstruction from angiography and IVUS (ANGUS) with computational fluid dynamics. Arterioscler Thromb Vasc Biol 1997;17:2061–2065.

22. Wentzel JJ, Whelan MD, van der Giessen WJ, et al. Coronary stent implantation changes 3-D vessel geometry and 3-D shear stress distribution. J Biomech 2000;33:1287–1295.

23. Wentzel JJ, Krams R, Schuurbiers JC, et al. Relationship between neointimal thickness and shear stress after Wallstent implantation in human coronary arteries. Circulation 2001;103:1740–1745.

24. Thury A, Wentzel JJ, Vinke RV, et al. Images in cardiovascular medicine. Focal in-stent restenosis near step-up: roles of low and oscillating shear stress? Circulation 11 2002;105:E185–E187.

25. Gijsen FJ, Oortman RM, Wentzel JJ, et al. Usefulness of shear stress pattern in predicting neointima distribution in sirolimus-eluting stents in coronary arteries. Am J Cardiol 2003;92:1325–1328.

26. Gijsen FJ, Allanic E, van de Vosse FN, et al. The influence of the non-Newtonian properties of blood on the flow in large arteries: unsteady flow in a 90 degrees curved tube. J Biomech 1999;32:705–713.

27. Zarins CK, Bomberger RA, Glagov S. Local effects of stenoses: increased flow velocity inhibits atherogenesis. Circulation 1981;64:II221–II227.

28. Cho A, Mitchell L, Koopmans D, et al. Effects of changes in blood flow rate on cell death and cell proliferation in carotid arteries of immature rabbits. Circ Res 1997;81:328–337.

29. Shimokawa H, Flavahan NA, Vanhoutte PM. Natural course of the impairment of endothelium-dependent relaxations after balloon endothelium removal in porcine coronary arteries. Possible dysfunction of a pertussis toxin-sensitive G protein. Circ Res 1989;65:740–753.

30. Zarins CK, Zatina MA, Giddens DP, et al. Shear stress regulation of artery lumen diameter in experimental atherogenesis. J Vasc Surg 1987;5:413–420.

31. Glagov S, Weisenberg E, Zarins CK, et al. Compensatory enlargement of human atherosclerotic coronary arteries. N Engl J Med 1987;316:1371–1375.

32. Wentzel JJ, Janssen E, Vos J, et al. Extension of increased atherosclerotic wall thickness into high shear stress regions is associated with loss of compensatory remodeling. Circulation 2003;108:17–23.

33. Slager CJ, Wentzel JJ, Schuurbiers JC, et al. True 3-dimensional reconstruction of coronary arteries in patients by fusion of angiography and IVUS (ANGUS) and its quantitative validation. Circulation 2000;102:511–516.

34. Stone PH, Coskun AU, Kinlay S, et al. Effect of endothelial shear stress on the progression of coronary artery disease, vascular remodeling, and in-stent restenosis in humans: in vivo 6-month follow-up study. Circulation 29 2003;108:438–444.

35. Kohler TR, Jawien A. Flow affects development of intimal hyperplasia after arterial injury in rats. Arterioscler Thromb 1992;12:963–971.
36. Glagov S. Intimal hyperplasia, vascular modeling, and the restenosis problem. Circulation 1994;89:2888–2891.
37. Waller BF. Coronary luminal shape and the arc of disease-free wall: morphologic observations and clinical relevance. J Am Coll Cardiol 1985;6:1100–1101.
38. Mintz GS, Popma JJ, Pichard AD, et al. Arterial remodeling after coronary angioplasty: a serial intravascular ultrasound study. Circulation 1996;94:35–43.
39. Pasterkamp G, de Kleijn DP, Borst C. Arterial remodeling in atherosclerosis, restenosis and after alteration of blood flow: potential mechanisms and clinical implications. Cardiovasc Res 2000;45:843–852.
40. Uren NG, Crake T, Lefroy DC, et al. Delayed recovery of coronary resistive vessel function after coronary angioplasty. J Am Coll Cardiol 1993;21:612–621.
41. Ward MR, Tsao PS, Agrotis A, et al. Low blood flow after angioplasty augments mechanisms of restenosis: inward vessel remodeling, cell migration, and activity of genes regulating migration. Arterioscler Thromb Vasc Biol 2001;21:208–213.
42. Stankovic G, Manginas A, Voudris V, et al. Prediction of restenosis after coronary angioplasty by use of a new index: TIMI frame count/minimal luminal diameter ratio. Circulation 2000;101:962–968.
43. Serruys PW, di Mario C, Piek J, et al. Prognostic value of intracoronary flow velocity and diameter stenosis in assessing the short- and long-term outcomes of coronary balloon angioplasty: the DEBATE Study (Doppler Endpoints Balloon Angioplasty Trial Europe). Circulation 18 1997;96:3369–3377.
44. Majesky MW, Reidy MA, Bowen-Pope DF, et al. PDGF ligand and receptor gene expression during repair of arterial injury. J Cell Biol 1990;111:2149–2158.
45. Bassiouny HS, Song RH, Hong XF, et al. Flow regulation of 72-kD collagenase IV (MMP-2) after experimental arterial injury. Circulation 1998;98:157–163.
46. Wentzel JJ, Kloet J, Andhyiswara I, et al. Shear-stress and wall-stress regulation of vascular remodeling after balloon angioplasty: effect of matrix metalloproteinase inhibition. Circulation 2001;104:91–96.
47. Sterpetti AV, Cucina A, D'Angelo LS, et al. Shear stress modulates the proliferation rate, protein synthesis, and mitogenic activity of arterial smooth muscle cells. Surgery 1993;113:691–699.
48. Ueba H, Kawakami M, Yaginuma T. Shear stress as an inhibitor of vascular smooth muscle cell proliferation. Role of transforming growth factor-beta 1 and tissue- type plasminogen activator. Arterioscler Thromb Vasc Biol 1997;17:1512–1516.
49. Thyberg J, Blomgren K, Hedin U, et al. Phenotypic modulation of smooth muscle cells during the formation of neointimal thickenings in the rat carotid artery after balloon injury: an electron-microscopic and stereological study. Cell Tissue Res 1995;281:421–433.
50. Jawien A, Bowen-Pope DF, Lindner V, et al. Platelet-derived growth factor promotes smooth muscle migration and intimal thickening in a rat model of balloon angioplasty. J Clin Invest 1992;89:507–511.
51. Kinlay S, Grewal J, Manuelin D, et al. Coronary flow velocity and disturbed flow predict adverse clinical outcome after coronary angioplasty. Arterioscler Thromb Vasc Biol 2002;22:1334–1340.
52. Thury A, van Langenhove G, Carlier SG, et al. High shear stress after successful balloon angioplasty is associated with restenosis and target lesion revascularization. Am Heart J 2002;144:136–143.
53. Asakura T, Karino T. Flow patterns and spatial distribution of atherosclerotic lesions in human coronary arteries. Circ Res 1990;66:1045–1066.
54. Smedby O. Do plaques grow upstream or downstream?: an angiographic study in the femoral artery. Arterioscler Thromb Vasc Biol 1997;17:912–918.
55. Seiler C. The human coronary collateral circulation. Heart 2003;89:1352–1357.
56. van Royen N, Piek JJ, Buschmann I, et al. Stimulation of arteriogenesis; a new concept for the treatment of arterial occlusive disease. Cardiovasc Res 2001;49:543–553.
57. Werner GS, Emig U, Mutschke O, et al. Regression of collateral function after recanalization of chronic total coronary occlusions: a serial assessment by intracoronary pressure and Doppler recordings. Circulation 2003;108:2877–2882.
58. Watanabe N, Yonekura S, Williams AG, Jr., et al. Regression and recovery of well-developed coronary collateral function in canine hearts after aorta-coronary bypass. J Thorac Cardiovasc Surg 1989;97:286–296.

59. Werner GS, Bahrmann P, Mutschke O, et al. Determinants of target vessel failure in chronic total coronary occlusions after stent implantation. The influence of collateral function and coronary hemodynamics. J Am Coll Cardiol 2003;42:219–225.

60. Holmes DR Jr, Hirshfeld J Jr, Faxon D, et al. ACC Expert Consensus document on coronary artery stents. Document of the American College of Cardiology. J Am Coll Cardiol 1998;32:1471–1482.

61. Virmani R, Farb A. Pathology of in-stent restenosis. Curr Opin Lipidol 1999;10:499–506.

62. Schwartz RS, Huber KC, Murphy JG, et al. Restenosis and the proportional neointimal response to coronary artery injury: results in a porcine model. J Am Coll Cardiol 1992;19:267–274.

63. Hehrlein C, Zimmermann M, Metz J, et al. Influence of surface texture and charge on the biocompatibility of endovascular stents. Coron Artery Dis 1995;6:581–586.

64. Gyongyosi M, Yang P, Khorsand A, et al. Longitudinal straightening effect of stents is an additional predictor for major adverse cardiac events. Austrian Wiktor Stent Study Group and European Paragon Stent Investigators. J Am Coll Cardiol 2000;35:1580–1589.

65. Garasic JM, Edelman ER, Squire JC, et al. Stent and artery geometry determine intimal thickening independent of arterial injury. Circulation 22 2000;101:812–818.

66. Rogers C, Edelman ER. Endovascular stent design dictates experimental restenosis and thrombosis. Circulation 15 1995;91:2995–3001.

67. Gunn J, Arnold N, Chan KH, et al. Coronary artery stretch versus deep injury in the development of in-stent neointima. Heart 2002;88:401–405.

68. Peacock J, Hankins S, Jones T, et al. Flow instabilities induced by coronary artery stents: assessment with an in vitro pulse duplicator. J Biomech 1995;28:17–26.

69. Tominaga R, Kambic HE, Emoto H, et al. Effects of design geometry of intravascular endoprostheses on stenosis rate in normal rabbits. Am Heart J 1992;123:21–28.

70. Berry JL, Santamarina A, Moore JE Jr, et al. Experimental and computational flow evaluation of coronary stents. Ann Biomed Eng 2000;28:386–398.

71. Robaina S, Jayachandran B, He Y, et al. Platelet adhesion to simulated stented surfaces. J Endovasc Ther 2003;10:978–986.

72. Kohler TR, Kirkman TR, Kraiss LW, et al. Increased blood flow inhibits neointimal hyperplasia in endothelialized vascular grafts. Circ Res 1991;69:1557–1565.

73. Salam T, Lumsden A, Suggs W, et al. Low shear stress promotes intimal hyperplasia thickening. J vasc invest 1996;2:12–22.

74. Kraiss LW, Geary RL, Mattsson EJ, et al. Acute reductions in blood flow and shear stress induce platelet-derived growth factor-A expression in baboon prosthetic grafts. Circ Res 1996;79:45–53.

75. Mattsson EJ, Kohler TR, Vergel SM, et al. Increased blood flow induces regression of intimal hyperplasia. Arterioscler Thromb Vasc Biol 1997;17:2245–2249.

76. Liu SQ. Prevention of focal intimal hyperplasia in rat vein grafts by using a tissue engineering approach. Atherosclerosis 1998;140:365–377.

77. Sprague EA, Luo J, Palmaz JC. Human aortic endothelial cell migration onto stent surfaces under static and flow conditions. J Vasc Interv Radiol 1997;8:83–92.

78. Van Belle E, Bauters C, Asahara T, et al. Endothelial regrowth after arterial injury: from vascular repair to therapeutics. Cardiovasc Res 1998;38:54–68.

79. Fontaine AB, Spigos DG, Eaton G, et al. Stent-induced intimal hyperplasia: are there fundamental differences between flexible and rigid stent designs? J Vasc Interv Radiol 1994;5:739–744.

80. Prati F, Di Mario C, Moussa I, et al. In-stent neointimal proliferation correlates with the amount of residual plaque burden outside the stent: an intravascular ultrasound study. Circulation 1999;99:1011–1014.

81. Vorwerk D, Redha F, Neuerburg J, et al. Neointima formation following arterial placement of self-expanding stents of different radial force: experimental results. Cardiovasc Intervent Radiol 1994;17:27–32.

82. Richter GM, Palmaz JC, Noeldge G, et al. Relationship between blood flow, thrombus, and neointima in stents. J Vasc Interv Radiol 1999;10:598–604.

83. de Smet BJ, Kuntz RE, van der Helm YJ, et al. Relationship between plaque mass and neointimal hyperplasia after stent placement in Yucatan micropigs. Radiology 1997;203:484–488.

84. Lemos PA, Serruys PW, Sousa JE. Drug-eluting stents: cost versus clinical benefit. Circulation 2003;107:3003–3007.

85. Serruys PW, Degertekin M, Tanabe K, et al. Intravascular ultrasound findings in the multicenter, randomized, double-blind RAVEL (Randomized study with the sirolimus-eluting Velocity balloon-expandable stent in the treatment of patients with de novo native coronary artery Lesions) trial. Circulation 2002;106:798–803.

86. Yatscoff RW, Fryer J, Thliveris JA. Comparison of the effect of rapamycin and FK506 on release of prostacyclin and endothelin in vitro. Clin Biochem. Oct 1993;26:409–414.

87. Morice MC, Serruys PW, Sousa JE, et al. A randomized comparison of a sirolimus-eluting stent with a standard stent for coronary revascularization. N Engl J Med 2002;346:1773–1780.

88. Suzuki T, Kopia G, Hayashi S, et al. Stent-based delivery of sirolimus reduces neointimal formation in a porcine coronary model. Circulation 2001;104:1188–1193.

89. Hwang CW, Wu D, Edelman ER. Physiological transport forces govern drug distribution for stent-based delivery. Circulation 2001;104:600–605.

90. Rassaf T, Preik M, Kleinbongard P, et al. Evidence for in vivo transport of bioactive nitric oxide in human plasma. J Clin Invest 2002;109:1241–1248.

91. Degertekin M, Serruys PW, Tanabe K, et al. Long-term follow-up of incomplete stent apposition in patients who received sirolimus-eluting stent for de novo coronary lesions: an intravascular ultrasound analysis. Circulation 2003;108:2747–2750.

92. Moses JW, Leon MB, Popma JJ, et al. Sirolimus-eluting stents versus standard stents in patients with stenosis in a native coronary artery. N Engl J Med 2003;349:1315–1323.

93. Serruys PW, Degertekin M, Tanabe K, et al. Vascular responses at proximal and distal edges of paclitaxel-eluting stents: serial intravascular ultrasound analysis from the TAXUS II trial. Circulation 2004;109:627–633.

94. Kuntz RE, Safian RD, Carrozza JP, et al. The importance of acute luminal diameter in determining restenosis after coronary atherectomy or stenting. Circulation 1992;86:1827–1835.

95. Serruys PW, Kay IP, Disco C, et al. Periprocedural quantitative coronary angiography after Palmaz-Schatz stent implantation predicts the restenosis rate at six months: results of a meta-analysis of the Belgian Netherlands Stent study (BENESTENT) I, BENESTENT II Pilot, BENESTENT II and MUSIC trials. Multicenter Ultrasound Stent In Coronaries. J Am Coll Cardiol 1999;34:1067–1074.

96. Sick P, Huttl T, Niebauer J, et al. Influence of residual stenosis after percutaneous coronary intervention with stent implantation on development of restenosis and stent thrombosis. Am J Cardiol 2003;91:148–153.

97. Carlier SG, van Damme LC, Blommerde CP, et al. Augmentation of wall shear stress inhibits neointimal hyperplasia after stent implantation: inhibition through reduction of inflammation? Circulation 2003;107:2741–2746.

98. Ekelund LG, Haskell WL, Johnson JL, et al. Physical fitness as a predictor of cardiovascular mortality in asymptomatic North American men. The Lipid Research Clinics Mortality Follow-up Study. N Engl J Med 1988;319:1379–1384.

99. Clarkson P, Montgomery HE, Mullen MJ, et al. Exercise training enhances endothelial function in young men. J Am Coll Cardiol 1999;33:1379–1385.

100. Haskell WL, Alderman EL, Fair JM, et al. Effects of intensive multiple risk factor reduction on coronary atherosclerosis and clinical cardiac events in men and women with coronary artery disease. The Stanford Coronary Risk Intervention Project (SCRIP). Circulation 1994;89:975–990.

101. Schuler G, Hambrecht R, Schlierf G, et al. Regular physical exercise and low-fat diet. Effects on progression of coronary artery disease. Circulation 1992;86:1–11.

102. Hambrecht R, Walther C, Mobius-Winkler S, et al. Percutaneous coronary angioplasty compared with exercise training in patients with stable coronary artery disease: a randomized trial. Circulation 2004;109:1371–1378.

103. Kubo H, Yano K, Hirai H, et al. Preventive effect of exercise training on recurrent stenosis after percutaneous transluminal coronary angioplasty (PTCA). Jpn Circ J 1992;56:413–421.

104. Indolfi C, Torella D, Coppola C, et al. Physical training increases eNOS vascular expression and activity and reduces restenosis after balloon angioplasty or arterial stenting in rats. Circ Res 2002;91:1190–1197.

105. Laufs U, Werner N, Link A, et al. Physical training increases endothelial progenitor cells, inhibits neointima formation, and enhances angiogenesis. Circulation 20 2004;109:220–226.

106. Pynn M, Schafer K, Konstantinides S, et al. Exercise training reduces neointimal growth and stabilizes vascular lesions developing after injury in apolipoprotein e-deficient mice. Circulation 2004;109:386–392.

107. Finkelstein A, McClean D, Kar S, et al. Local drug delivery via a coronary stent with programmable release pharmacokinetics. Circulation 2003;107:777–784.

108. Tarbell JM. Mass transport in arteries and the localization of atherosclerosis. Annu Rev Biomed Eng 2003;5:79–118.

109. Turitto VT, Baumgartner HR. Platelet interaction with subendothelium in flowing rabbit blood: effect of blood shear rate. Microvasc Res 1979;17:38–54.

110. van der Giessen W, Serruys P, Visser W, et al. Endothelization of intravascular stents. J Interven Cardiol 1988;1:109–120.

111. Rogers C, Parikh S, Seifert P, et al. Endogenous cell seeding. Remnant endothelium after stenting enhances vascular repair. Circulation 1996;94:2909–2914.

112. Parikh SA, Edelman ER. Endothelial cell delivery for cardiovascular therapy. Adv Drug Deliv Rev 2000;42:139–161.

113. Shirota T, Yasui H, Shimokawa H, et al. Fabrication of endothelial progenitor cell (EPC)-seeded intravascular stent devices and in vitro endothelialization on hybrid vascular tissue. Biomaterials 2003;24:2295–2302.

114. Hristov M, Erl W, Weber PC. Endothelial progenitor cells: mobilization, differentiation, and homing. Arterioscler Thromb Vasc Biol 2003;23:1185–1189.

115. George J, Herz I, Goldstein E, et al. Number and adhesive properties of circulating endothelial progenitor cells in patients with in-stent restenosis. Arterioscler Thromb Vasc Biol 2003;23:E57–E60.

116. Longest PW, Kleinstreuer C, Truskey GA, et al. Relation between near-wall residence times of monocytes and early lesion growth in the rabbit aorto-celiac junction. Ann Biomed Eng 2003; 31:53–64.

117. van Kooten TG, Schakenraad JM, van der Mei HC, et al. Fluid shear induced endothelial cell detachment from glass—influence of adhesion time and shear stress. Med Eng Phys 1994;16:506–512.

118. Reinhardt PH, Kubes P. Differential leukocyte recruitment from whole blood via endothelial adhesion molecules under shear conditions. Blood 15 1998;92:4691–4699.

119. Braddon LG, Karoyli D, Harrison DG, et al. Maintenance of a functional endothelial cell monolayer on a fibroblast/polymer substrate under physiologically relevant shear stress conditions. Tissue Eng 2002;8:695–708.

120. Yamamoto K, Takahashi T, Asahara T, et al. Proliferation, differentiation, and tube formation by endothelial progenitor cells in response to shear stress. J Appl Physiol 2003;95:2081–2088.

# 6

# The Immune System in the Pathogenesis of Vascular Proliferative Disease

*Jon D. Laman, PhD*
*and Burkhard Ludewig, PhD, DVM*

## CONTENTS

During the recent years, cardiovascular and immunological research has provided profound experimental and clinical evidence supporting the notion that inflammation and immune responses are crucial components of vascular proliferative diseases. This chapter aims to provide a state-of-the-art overview of this concept. In doing so, we discuss a number of novel developments in the highly dynamic field of immunology,

From: *Contemporary Cardiology: Essentials of Restenosis: For the Interventional Cardiologist*
Edited by: H. J. Duckers, E. G. Nabel, and P. W. Serruys © Humana Press Inc., Totowa, NJ

with particular emphasis on their relevance for cardiovascular disease. These include functional subsets of macrophages and T-lymphocytes, newly identified receptors for pathogens, the reciprocal regulation of lipid metabolism, inflammation and infection, and the hygiene hypothesis.

## INTRODUCTION: THE INTERVENTIONAL CARDIOLOGIST AND MODERN IMMUNOLOGY

Why would or should an interventional cardiologist care about the immune system? In short, because modern immunology and cardiovascular research demonstrate pivotal roles of immunity in vascular injury, tissue remodeling, lipid metabolism, atherosclerosis, and plaque instability. Hence, insight into immune reactivity improves understanding of vascular disease pathogenesis and provides exciting new inroads to diagnosis and intervention. Figure 1, which is referred to throughout this chapter, provides an overview of the main cellular and molecular players in the formation of atherosclerotic plaques.

Immunology as a discipline may easily come across as a conspiracy against the interested outsider. Although this perhaps is true for any professional field, immunology may be worse because of its rapid development, the relatively abstract nature of some of its central tenets (e.g., self vs nonself recognition, tolerance vs autoreactivity), the extreme variation in specificity of T and B lymphocyte clonotypic receptors as generated by gene rearrangement, the hundreds of cellular surface markers in the cluster of differentiation (CD) classification system, and last but not least the equally abundant cytokines and chemokines with pleiotropic and redundant functions.

Therefore, this chapter aims to provide a concise background overview of state of the art immunology relevant to vascular disease. Longstanding and novel controversies in immunology will be briefly outlined when useful to interpret recent developments with potentially far reaching implications for pathogenesis, diagnosis, and treatment. To these ends, sacrificing immunological detail for clarity, this chapter offers means of categorization for functionality of concepts, cell subsets and molecules, and it provides inroads to more detailed literature, including excellent comprehensive recent reviews on separate topics. It is trusted that the instant reward for spending an hour reading this chapter will be a (more) lucid overview of immunity's impact on vascular disease. If even an hour is not readily available, scrutiny of figures, tables, and keypoints (p. 122) provides a worthwhile summary of this chapter. Abbreviations are listed on p. 123.

## ATHEROSCLEROSIS AS AN INFLAMMATORY DISEASE

As with many scientific concepts, the notion that atherosclerosis is an inflammatory disease emerged several times during the last 100 yr (*see* ref. *1*). Only in more recent times did this concept gain a strong foothold, because of contributions from researchers like George Wick, Peter Libby, Joseph Witztum, Daniel Steinberg, Christoph Binder, Christopher Glass, Yehuda Schoenfeld, Göran Hansson, and the late Russel Ross, to name but a few whose work is cited here extensively. For a long time, atherosclerosis was seen only as a lipid metabolism and storage disease based on the association with elevated blood-cholesterol lipid. Accumulation of lipid in the arterial well was presumed to be responsible for vascular hardening, stenosis, and other disease sequelae, and hence likened to a "plumbing problem" *(2)*. For a while the "response to injury" hypothesis stating that atherosclerosis was a result of damage to endothelium *(1)*. Currently, the inflammation hypothesis is the leading concept in the field, with the understanding that

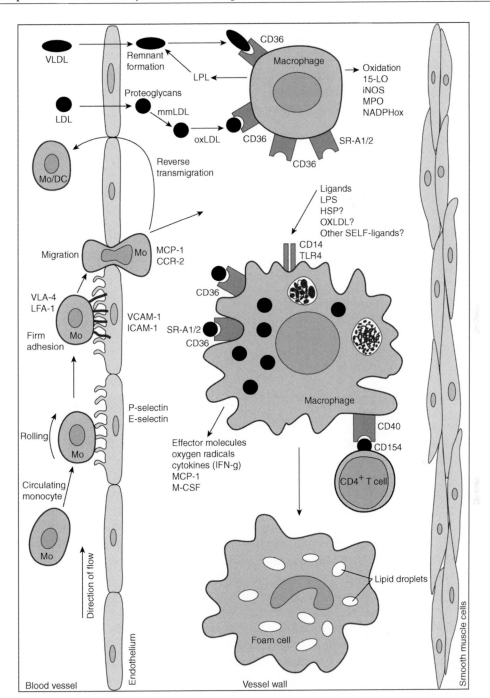

**Fig. 1.** Macrophages, T-cells, and foam cells in lesion development. The left hand side of the figure summarizes monocyte migration from the artery over the endothelium into the vessel wall. Access of very low-density lipoprotein (VLDL) and LDL from the blood is also depicted. Lipid accumulation, stimuli from microbial antigens as well as self ligands, and interaction with CD4+ T-cells jointly lead to formation of macrophage-derived foam cells, of large irregular shape and filled with lipid droplets. Plaque growth leads to stenosis, and late stage plaques have necrotic cores (to which local death of foam cells contributes), and caps, which provoke thrombolic events and which eventually may rupture (not shown).

Table 1
Comparison of Innate and Adaptive Antigen Receptors

| Receptor characteristic | Innate immunity | Adaptive immunity |
|---|---|---|
| Specificity ready encoded by intact gene | Yes | No |
| Expressed by all cells of a subset | Yes | No |
| Can respond immediately | Yes | No, takes days |
| Recognizes broad classes of pathogens through a molecular pattern | Yes | No |
| Encoded in multiple gene segments | No | Yes |
| Requires gene rearrangement | No | Yes |
| Clonally distributed: inherited by daughter cells on clonal expansion | No | Yes |
| Able to recognize a wide variety of molecular structures | No | Yes |
| Estimated number of potential receptors and hence specificities | ~100 | $10^{14}$ for B-cells $10^{18}$ for T-cells |

Table modified and extended from ref. *160*.

first, lipid metabolism clearly is a critical factor closely intertwined in multiple ways with inflammation, and second that diverse microbial infections are beginning to emerge as plausible cofactors.

## IS THE IMMUNE SYSTEM INVOLVED IN VASCULAR DISEASE?

Although the question whether the immune system is involved in occurrence and progression of vascular afflictions is fully justified and apparently unambiguous, it is argued that research and interpretation can benefit considerably from systematic phrasing and breakdown into testable questions. Historically, loose use of immunological definitions and continuously emerging novel findings requiring reassessment of dogmas necessitate careful delineation of critical items. A first item is to distinguish between activities of the immune system per distinct event in the pathogenic cascade, for instance, formation of the initial fatty streak vs rupture of an end stage plaque. Key points (listed on p. 122) on plaque aspects provide a listing of relevant aspects of plaque physiology, and the relevant cellular players from the vascular tissue as well as the immune system. A second item is whether the role of the immune system in such a distinct event is causal, or acts as a cofactor, or whether it might even be just a secondary or epiphenomenon irrelevant to the disease, for instance, evoked by tissue damage.

Importantly, much confusion comes about from the equation of immunity with adaptive immunity, i.e., T and B lymphocytes generating antigen-specific receptors through gene rearrangement (up to $10^{18}$ and $10^{12}$ specificities, respectively). This equation of immunity with only adaptive immunity is incorrect, as the innate immunity arm consists of a wide array of physical, chemical, and cellular barriers provided by stromal cells and leukocytes, which are critical for protection of the host against infection as well as for homeostasis and tissue repair. By definition, innate immunity does not require gene rearrangement. Its receptors (~100 different ones) with limited to exquisite specificity are ready encoded in the genome by intact genes, and are often expressed by leukocytes and stromal cells constitutively. Table 1 compares antigen receptors in innate and adaptive responses.

An explosion of exciting studies in the past decade has revived interest in innate immunity, the driving force being the identification of the family of Toll-like receptor (TLR) molecules recognizing typical molecular patterns on pathogens (*see* Table 2, discussed in detail later). Not surprising in hindsight, the distinction between innate and adaptive immunity is an artificial one (albeit useful) to which nature is oblivious: innate immunity is fully geared toward interaction with adaptive immunity. The innate immune system prevents and responds to insults instantaneously. In contrast, adaptive immunity takes days to weeks to develop, which is way too slow to fend off invaders by itself. On the other hand, adaptive immunity provides exquisite specificity, memory responses of lymphocytes leading to much swifter and more effective protection on second exposure. A telling example of the clinical relevance of the adaptive/innate dichotomy is rheumatoid arthritis (RA).

Decades of intense research focused on $CD4^+$ T-helper (Th1) cells recognizing autoantigens in the joints as the initiators of disease and the optimal target for therapy. However, immunotherapeutic strategies based on that concept all failed thus far. Instead, highly successful therapy in approximately two-thirds of patients (but not always without side effects) neutralizes the proinflammatory cytokine tumor necrosis factor (TNF)-$\alpha$ as produced by infiltrating macrophages and synoviocytes *(3)*. This does not exclude a role for adaptive $CD4^+$ Th1-cells or the eventual identification of a true autoantigen, but the race for the first successful immunotherapy was won on the basis of innate immune effector function.

A general argument for immune system engagement in atherosclerosis is the predictive value of soluble inflammatory markers, such as P-selectin, soluble intercellular adhesion molecule (ICAM)-1, interleukin (IL)-6, and TNF-$\alpha$. The most promising of these markers is C-reactive protein (CRP), an acute phase reactant involved in recognition of pathogens, complement activation, and Fc-receptor binding. Joint use of cholesterol and CRP readings is a very good predictor of disease and cardiovascular disease-related death (reviewed by Blake and Ridker *[4]*). By comparison, CRP is still one of the best serological markers for chronic inflammation in RA despite decades of research into more disease-specific tests.

## SELECTED IMMUNE SYSTEM BASICS

Expanding on the previous section, a selection of immune system basics is briefly discussed, some of which have been recently revised or developed, as they are helpful for interpretation of subsequent sections. The immune system has evolved specialized and elaborate cellular and soluble effector systems to protect against four classes of pathogens being

1. Extracellular bacteria, parasites, and fungi (e.g., pneumonia, tetanus);
2. Intracellular bacteria and parasites (e.g., leprosy, malaria);
3. Intracellular viruses (flu, pox, AIDS); and
4. Extracellular parasitic worms (e.g., ascariasis).

### *Innate Immunity Mechanisms*

An important part of innate immunity is the epithelial barriers limiting infection. Mechanical components include tight junctions of epithelial cells as well as flow of air, fluid, and mucus, the latter assisted by cilia. Chemical components include bacteriolytic and bacteriostatic enzymes in secretions, such as saliva and stomach, acidic pH,

Table 2
Toll-Like Receptors

| TLR location | Ligands | Source | Signaling pathways | Cooperating receptors |
|---|---|---|---|---|
| TLR1 surface | Triacyl lipopeptides (Pam$_3$CSK$_4$) | Bacteria, mycobacteria | MyD88 and TRAF6→NF-κB activation | TLR2 |
| TLR2 surface | Peptidoglycan, bacterial lipoproteins, lipoteichoid acid, porins, zymosan | Gram-positive bacteria, *Neisseria*, fungi | MyD88, Mal/TIRAP, and TRAF6→ NF-κB activation | TLR1 or TLR6 |
| TLR3 endosomal | Double-stranded RNA | Virus | MyD88, TICAM-1/TRIF, TRAF-6→ NF-κB activation | |
| TLR4 surface | LPS, Taxol (only in mouse), HSP60? HSP70? | Gram-negative bacteria, plant | MyD88, Mal/TIRAP, and TRAF6→ NF-κB activation | MD-2 and CD14 |
| TLR5 surface | Flagellin | Gram-negative bacteria | MyD88, Mal/TIRAP, and TRAF6→ NF-κB activation | |
| TLR6 surface | Diacyl lipopeptides (MALP-2) | Mycoplasma | MyD88, Mal/TIRAP, and TRAF6→ NF-κB activation | TLR2 |
| TLR7 endosomal | Single-stranded RNA (ssRNA) Small antiviral molecules (imidazolquinolones) Mouse TLR7 detects viral U-rich ssRNA | Virus synthetic | MyD88, Mal/TIRAP, and TRAF6→ NF-κB activation | |
| TLR8 surface | ssRNA Small antiviral molecules (imidazolquinolones). Human TLR8 detects viral ssRNA | Virus synthetic | MyD88, Mal/TIRAP, and TRAF6 → NF-κB activation | |
| TLR9 endosomal | Unmethylated CpG dinucleotides in prokaryotic DNA. Host DNA bound to histones or antihistone autoantibody. | Bacteria, virus, synthetic | MyD88, Mal/TIRAP, and TRAF6→ NF-κB activation | |

*(continued)*

Table 2 *(Continued)*

| TLR location | Ligands | Source | Signaling pathways | Cooperating receptors |
|---|---|---|---|---|
| TLR10 | ? | ? | ? | |
| TLR11 surface | PAMP not conclusively identified, but may be a flagellin-like protein in fimbriae in view of similarity between TLR5 and TLR11 | *E. coli* uropathogenic bacteria | | |

*Legend:* This table is based on refs. *111,161,162. See also* Fig. 2 for TLR signaling.

*Abbreviations:* DC, dendritic cells; LPS, lipopolysaccharide; Mal, MyD88-adapter-like; MALP-2, mycoplasmal macrophage-activating lipopeptide-2kD; MyD88, myeloid-differentiation protein 88; TRIF, TIR domain-containing adapter inducing IFN-β; TICAM-1, TIR-containing adapter molecule-1; TIRAP, Toll-IL-1R domain-containing adapter; TRAF6, TNF receptor-associated factor 6.

and elaboration of antibacterial peptides in the skin and the gut. The next barrier for pathogens is provided by phagocytic cells, macrophages and neutrophils, which effectively recognize and ingest microorganisms using a series of innate (i.e., intact genes ready in the genome) antigen receptor molecules (*see* Table 3). Macrophages and granulocytes kill and degrade microorganisms using several mechanisms including intracellular acidification, toxic oxygen-derived products (superoxide, hydrogen peroxide, singlet oxygen, and so on), antimicrobial peptides (defensins and cationic proteins), enzymes (lysozyme degrading the bacterial cell wall compound peptidoglycan, acid hydrolases), and competitors for pathogen nutrients (e.g., lactoferrin sequestering away iron ions).

Another major player in innate immunity is the complement system of soluble proteins, which acts by itself and also crucially assists phagocytes. Three pathways are now known to engage complement: the classical pathway starts with antigen–antibody complexes, whereas the mannose/mannan-binding lectin pathway is recruited by mannose/mannan-binding lectin binding to mannose on pathogen surfaces. The alternative pathway is recruited by spontaneously activated complement components to pathogen surfaces. All three pathways converge in production of C3 convertase, which in turn can lead to three types of effector functions:

1. Phagocyte recruitment and production of peptide mediators of inflammation;
2. Opsonization of pathogens (through C3b binding to complement receptors on phagocytes) and removal of immune complexes; and
3. Formation of the membrane attack complex consisting of C5b–9, leading to lysis of pathogens and cells.

## *Innate Antigen Receptors*

For rapid recognition of infectious agents, approx 100 types of antigen receptors are available, differentially expressed on cellular subsets (*see* Table 2). The late Charles A. Janeway has developed the concept that these molecules are pattern recognition receptors, which recognize pathogen-associated molecular patterns (PAMP). Janeway and Medzhitov validated this concept by showing that the TLR4 is the pattern recognition receptor recognizing lipopolysaccharide (LPS) on Gram-negative bacteria as a signature molecular pattern (reviewed in ref. 5). The demonstration by Beutler [6] that the C3H/HeJ mouse strain long known to be unresponsive to LPS have a spontaneous mutation in the *TLR4* gene provided the molecular explanation to a long-standing mystery for immunologists. A true explosion of studies by these groups and others, notably Akira and colleagues, led to identification and functional characterization of 11 members of the TLR family (Table 2), and the molecular signaling pathways involved (Fig. 2).

With respect to protection against extracellular vs intracellular pathogens, it is of note that some TLR are surface expressed, whereas others are expressed on the intracellular membrane of the phagosome allowing monitoring of the cell interior. An interesting aspect is whether some TLR can be activated by self-components from the host. There are claims that heat shock protein (HSP) 60 or breakdown products of the extracellular matrix productively engage TLR, possibly coinvolving other cellular receptors. However, this field is wrought with contaminated studies in the double sense of the word, as undue trace amounts of other TLR ligands (e.g., LPS) for instance, HSP preparations can inadvertently render experiments completely meaningless.

Other recently discovered intracellular innate antigen receptors are the Nod1 (nucleotide-binding oligomerization domain) and Nod2 molecules (also known as CARD4

Table 3

Antigen and Scavenging Receptors (Potentially) Involved in Atherosclerosis Immunity

| Receptor | Expressed by | Ligands | Function |
|---|---|---|---|
| SR-A1/2 | Macrophages | LPS, lipoteichoic acid, bacteria, acetylated LDL, oxLDL, apoptotic cells | Phagocytosis, scavenging. Inadvertent foam cell formation[a] |
| CD36 | Macrophages | oxLDL | Phagocytosis, scavenging. Inadvertent foam cell formation[a] |
| SR-B1 mu CLA-1 hu | | HDL, LPS | Mediates reverse cholesterol transport Mediates transfer of HDL-bound LPS into the cell |
| MARCO | Macrophages | Bacteria | Phagocytosis, scavenging |
| CD14 | Macrophages, neutrophils, immature DC | LPS, peptidoglycan, oxLDL | Binding and transfer to signaling receptors, such as TLR2 and TLR4. No signaling as a transmembrane domain is lacking |
| LBP | Secreted adaptor protein in plasma | LPS | Efficient transfer and clearance of LPS |
| MD-2 | Secreted adaptor protein in plasma | LPS | Associates with TLR4 on cell surface Enhances LPS response. Deficiency of MD-2-like proteins leads to lipid metabolism disorders, such as Tay-Sachs and Newman-Pick |
| CD68 | Macrophages | oxLDL | Phagocytosis, scavenging |
| LOX-1 | Vascular endothelium, macrophages | oxLDL, advanced glycation end products, anionic phospholipids | Phagocytosis, scavenging |
| SR-PSOX | Macrophages | Phosphatidylserine, oxLDL | Phagocytosis, scavenging |
| Galectin 3 | Macrophages | oxLDL, acetylated LDL, advanced glycation end product-LDL | |
| G2A | T-cells, lesional macrophages | lysophosphatidylcholine (hence also oxLDL?) | G protein-coupled. Ligation induces proinflammatory activity |

*(Continued)*

93

Table 3 (Continued)

| Receptor | Expressed by | Ligands | Function |
|---|---|---|---|
| ZAG zinc α2-glycoprotein | Macrophages | Polyunsaturated fatty acids | Homeostasis of lipid stores. May present lipid to T-cells because of homology to MHC/HLA/CD1 molecules |
| Nod1 | Endosomal, mostly in epithelial cells | Sensor of Gram-negative bacteria through binding of peptidoglycan motif containing DAP | General intracellular sensor of Gram-negative bacteria |
| Nod2 | Endosomal, mostly in myeloid cells | Molecular pattern in peptidoglycan of all bacteria | General intracellular sensor of bacteria |

*Legend*: The upper part of this table is mostly based on refs. *14,163,164*.

[a]In vitro, receptors SR-A and CD36 jointly account for approx 90% of oxLDL uptake by macrophages and are hence presumed to be the key molecules in foam cell formation in vivo. Other than the phagocytosis of apoptotic cells, uptake of bacteria through these receptors triggers proinflammatory responses.

*Abbreviations*: LBP, lipopolysaccharide binding protein; Nod, nucleotide-binding oligomerization domain; SR, scavenger receptor-A; LOX, lectin-like oxidized low-density lipoprotein receptor; SR-PSOX, scavenger receptor tozphosphatidylserine and oxidized lipoprotein.

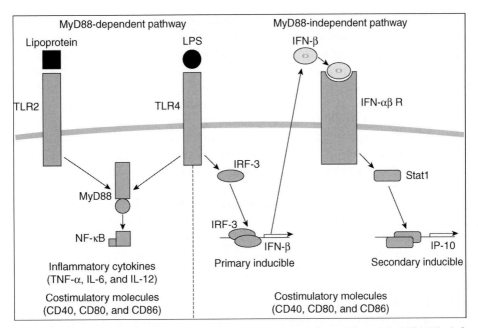

**Fig. 2.** Two broad routes of TLR signaling. This figure is adapted from Akira et al., 2004. The left part demonstrates that in general the TLR act through the general pathway with the adaptor protein MyD88 and activating the NF-κB pathway to induce inflammatory cytokines and expression of important costimulatory molecules (*see* also Table 2). The MyD88-independent pathway utilizes the transcription factor IRF-3 (IFN regulatory factor 3) to induce the cytokine IFN-β, which then secondarily can mediate cytokine and chemokine induction, and costimulatory molecules. Adapted from ref. *161*.

and CARD15). Nod1 is expressed mostly in epithelial cells whereas Nod2 is expressed prominently in myeloid cells. These molecules have exquisite pattern specificity for peptidoglycan molecular composition, allowing distinction between subtly different fragments of peptidoglycan. Nod1 is a general sensor for both Gram-positive and Gram-negative bacteria, as it recognizes muramyldipeptide, which is a minimal motif in peptidoglycans of all bacteria. In addition, Nod2 detects muramyl-tri-lysine, but not muramyl-tri-diaminopimelic acid (DAP). In contrast to Nod2, Nod1 only senses the DAP-type of peptidoglycan in form of the GM-tri-DAP fragment, which is produced by Gram-negative bacteria only during their normal metabolism *(7,8)*. Interestingly, genetic polymorphism in Nod2 is associated with Crohn's disease, and it is hypothesized that such polymorphisms affect inflammatory activity in atherosclerosis, in analogy to those in TLR4.

Receptors for which the involvement in atherosclerosis is much more established than for the TLR include CD36, one of the receptors for oxidized low-density lipoprotein (oxLDL), and the scavenger receptor SR-A types 1 and 2 (*see* Table 3), which are expressed by macrophages and the related foam cells within lesions. Could some components recognized by scavenger receptors be classified as foreign, i.e., nonself? Although LDL clearly is a self-component, oxLDL could be regarded as nonself or at least as an undesirable neoantigen. The role of oxLDL in immune reactivity during atherosclerosis is further discussed below.

## *Functional T-Lymphocyte Subsets*

T-cell precursors from the bone marrow further develop in the thymus where they are selected for proper affinity and specificity to limit autoreactivity, and mature into

CD8 and CD4 subsets expressing the α–β chain T-cell receptor specific for antigenic peptide. Functional definition of the CD8 subset is fairly straightforward, because these T-cells are cytotoxic, monitoring intracellular infection, and killing the body's own cells when these display pathogen-derived peptides. Such peptides are generated intracellulary where they associate with the major histocompatibility complex (MHC) class I antigen presenting molecule, which is surface-expressed by all nucleated cells. The human counterpart of MHC is called human leukocyte antigen (HLA). The clonally distributed T-cell receptor of CD8$^+$ T-cells recognizes this peptide in context of MHC class I and exerts cytolytic function, if appropriate costimulatory molecules and cytokines are also provided (see "Costimulatory Molecules (Signal 2) Assist and Regulate Cell Interactions").

Functional definition of the CD4 subset is more complex. Table 4 provides a simplified overview. CD4$^+$ T-helper cells are crucial in assisting many different types of immune processes, emphasized by the generalized immunodeficiency in AIDS, where this subset is depleted through HIV-1 infection. T-helper cells stimulate B-cell maturation, isotype switching and antibody responses, activate macrophages, and support CD8-mediated cytotoxicity. A driving paradigm in immunology for the last 15 yr has been the Th1–Th2 paradigm, the functional specialization of CD4 subsets based on differential cytokine production. Th1 cells producing interferon (IFN)-γ, IL-2, lymphotoxin, and IL-12 support cellular immunity, including function of macrophages and CD8$^+$ cytotoxic T-cells. In this way, Th1 cells protect against intracellular bacteria, fungi, and protozoa. In contrast, Th2 cells producing IL-4, -5, -6, -9, -10, and -13 support humoral (antibody) responses, providing protection against extracellular pathogens, such as helminths.

For a long time, the Th1–Th2 paradigm was used over strictly by some to categorize many diseases as being purely driven by Th1 (diabetes, RA, multiple sclerosis) or Th2 pathways (asthma). It is also helpful to realize Th1–Th2 responses are not identically regulated in man and mice. For instance, in mice the immunoglobulin (Ig)G2a antibody subclass is driven by Th1 activity, whereas this subclass has no direct counterpart in humans. The role of T-cells in atherosclerosis is briefly reviewed by de Boer et al. (9). The main candidate antigens for T-cells in atherosclerosis are oxLDL, platelet β2-glycoprotein1b, and pathogen antigens. Interestingly, antigen-independent activation of T-cells can be brought about by IL-15, which is produced in the plaque.

More recently, a major development has been the functional and molecular characterization of regulatory T-helper cell subsets (Th3, Tr1, T regulatory [Treg]) (see Table 4), which can modulate and restrain physiological immune responses as well as diseases (10,11). One of the promises of this concept is that chronic inflammation, such as occurring in atherosclerosis, can be approached as being a result from a lack of counterregulation, instead of (only) resulting from undue immune activation. Expectations in this research field are high and further characterization will reduce confusion about true existence of distinct types of regulatory T-cells as well as their functional relationships.

### B Lymphocytes and Antibodies

B-cells and antibodies are relatively inconspicuous in atherosclerosis research thus far, but the group of Wick (1) provides evidence for a role of antibodies against HSP in atherosclerosis. B-cells mature in the bone marrow and seed secondary lymphoid organs (lymph nodes and spleen), where complex interactions with pathogens, antigen

**Table 4**
**Functional T-Cell Subsets**

| T-cell subset | Subdivision | MHC restriction | Function | Products |
|---|---|---|---|---|
| CD8 | Cytotoxic T lymphocyte | MHC class I, monitors intracellular infection | Cytoxicity against infected host cells | IFN-γ, granzymes, perforins |
| CD4 | T-helper 1 | MHC class II, monitors extracellular milieu | Cell-mediated immunity: inflammation, delayed type hypersensitivity (DTH), cytotoxicity. Protection against intracellular bacteria, fungi, protozoa inadvertently: autoimmunity | IFN-γ, TNF-β, IL-2, -12, -10 (in man) |
| | T-helper 2 | MHC class II, monitors extracellular milieu | Humoral (antibody) immunity against parasites. Protection against Helminths. Inadvertently: allergic disease | IL-4, -5, -6, -9, -10, -13 (in mouse and man) |
| | Treg | Debated | Regulation of CD4+ activity | IL-10, transforming growth factor (TGF)β, other? |

*Legend: see* refs. *10,11* for extensive reviews on the rapidly evolving field of regulatory CD4+ T-cells.

presenting cells (APC), and T-cells lead to differentiation into plasma cells, which secrete specific antibody. These plasma cells migrate to areas of inflammation and infection, but also take up residence in the bone marrow, maintaining long-term anti-body production leading to protective antibody titer. It is useful to realize that immunoglobulins come in five isotypes (IgD, IgM, IgA, IgG, IgE), and in subclasses (human: IgA1 and 2, IgG1, 2, 3, and 4; mouse IgG1, IgG2a, IgG2b, IgG3). Antibodies are Y-shaped molecules forming a soluble flexible adapter between the pathogen and the immune system. An epitope of the pathogen (or derived molecule, like a toxin) is recognized by the two tops of the Y having identical antigen-binding specificity. This bivalency may lead to bridging of two pathogens and can thereby limit the spread of the invader. The tail of the Y, the Fc-part is the opposite end of the bridge engaging other immune effector functions. In general, antibody works by four main ways:

1. Extracellular neutralization of toxin followed by phagocyte ingestion;
2. Opsonization of pathogens for ingestion facilitated by Fc-receptors expressed by phagocytes;
3. Complement activation leading to lysis of the pathogen as well as improved ingestion; and
4. Finally, lysis of the body's own cells when coated with antibody and complement by macrophages in a process called antibody-dependent cellular cytotoxicity.

The Fc-tail of the different subclasses determines if, and what effector functions are being engaged. This is based on factors like complement-activating ability and binding to the different types of Fc-receptors (of which one actually deactivates the phagocyte) as well as to complement receptors. Still it is not completely known which cytokine and costimulatory signals drive isotype switching in man vs other species. Many simply equate an IgM response with a primary response, lack of somatic mutation in anti-body genes and absence of memory. This assumption is not fully correct, and for instance, IgM memory B-cells have been described in several studies. Similarly, the conclusion that CD4 T-cell help must have occurred if any of the IgG subclasses are found remains to be fully substantiated (12).

### Functional Macrophage Subsets: Relations to Foam Cells?

Monocytes differentiate into macrophages on transmigrating the vascular endothe-lium. Within the plaque, these macrophages are crucial to the disease process, because accumulating lipids, they transform into foam cells, a process that is closely related to lesion growth (Fig. 1). On activation, macrophages and foam cells can secrete a wide array of cytokines (e.g., IFN-γ) and other compounds (e.g., matrix metallopro-teinase [MMP]) contributing to lesion activity, tissue remodeling, stenosis, and thrombotic as well as plaque-rupture events. A detailed discussion of lipid metabo-lism with respect to atherosclerosis is beyond the scope of this chapter, and instead can be found in refs. 13–15.

In the past decade, the concept of functionally distinct macrophage subsets has been developed, known as M1/M2 or classical vs alternatively activated macrophages (for recent reviews see refs. 16–19). Table 5 lists properties and functions of these macrophage subsets: in broad terms, classically activated macrophages have antimicro-bial function and mediate tissue damage, whereas alternatively activated macrophages act against parasites and promote tissue repair, and may act to counterregulate immune activation. The concept of classic/alternative activation may have relevance for athero-sclerosis. For instance, one pathway for development of alternatively activated macrophages is uptake of apoptotic cells, oxLDL, and glucocerebrosides.

**Table 5**
**Functional Macrophage Subpopulations**

| Parameter | Classically activated macrophage | Alternatively activated macrophage |
|---|---|---|
| Function | Microbicidal | Humoral immunity |
| | Tissue damage | Allergic and antiparasite responses |
| | Cellular immunity | |
| | DTH | |
| | Matrix degradation | Tissue repair (arginase expression) |
| | | −matrix synthesis and stabilization |
| | | −induction of cell survival and proliferation |
| | | −angiogenesis |
| | Production of proinflammatory cytokines and chemokines | Production of anti-inflammatory cytokines and chemokines |
| | Phagocytosis of debris | Phagocytosis of debris |
| | Phagocytosis of apoptotic cells | Phagocytosis of apoptotic cells |
| | Presentation of antigen | Presentation of antigen |
| In vitro induction by | IFN-$\gamma$, TNF-$\alpha$ | IL-4, IL-13, glucocorticoids |
| Surface markers | MHC class II, CD80, CD86 | Mannose receptor, SR-A, SR-B, CD23, CD163, CD13 (aminopeptidase inactivating inflammatory mediators) |
| Cytokines | TNF-$\alpha$, IL-12, IL-1, IL-6 | IL-10, IL-1ra, TGF-$\beta$ |
| Chemokines | IL-8/CXCL8 | MDC/CCL22 |
| | IP-10/CXCL10 | PARC/CCL18 |
| | MIP-1$\alpha$/CCL3 | TARC/CCL17 |
| | MCP-1/CCL2 | |

*(Continued)*

99

**Table 5 (Continued)**

| Parameter | Classically activated macrophage | Alternatively activated macrophage |
|---|---|---|
| Respiratory burst killer molecules | $NO$, $O_2^-$ | None |
| Miscellaneous | MMP-1, -2, -7, -9, -12 (degrading collagen, elastin, fibronectin) | Ym1, Ym2, chitotriosidase (chitinases with antifungal action) |
| | | PDGF, IGF (promote cell proliferation) fibronectin |
| | | Transglutaminase (matrix crosslinking) |
| | | Osteopontin (cell adhesion to matrix) |

*Legend*: This table is mostly based on refs. *16–19*.

*Abbreviations*: IP-10, IFN-inducible protein 10; IGF, insulin growth factor; MCP-1, monocyte chemoattractant protein-1; MIP-1α, macrophage inflammatory protein-1α; PDGF, platelet-derived growth factor.

100

In addition, a subset of macrophages in atherosclerotic plaques produces chitotriosi-dase *(20)*, an enzyme-degrading chitin in fungi, which is now recognized as prototypi-cal for alternatively activated macrophages. As this field is fairly new, consensus on nomenclature and functional definitions of these macrophage subsets is quite far, also because much of this work is based on in vitro data. As macrophages are very sensitive responders to local conditions, it is conceivable that the in vivo extremes of M1 and M2 adopt subtle differences in chronically inflamed tissues. One example is Gaucher dis-ease in which a genetic defect in glucocerebrosidase leads to storage of high amounts of lipids, leading to a foamy appearance, and a phenotype of splenic macrophages most compatible with the M2/alternatively activated macrophage but lacking the typical expression of the mannose receptor *(21)*.

## *APC Come in Many Flavors*

A common source of confusion is the term APC: this is not one cell type, but an oper-ational definition of any cell capable of initiating an adaptive immune response of lym-phocytes. Such responses rely on expression of antigenic peptide in the context of MHC class I (for CD8 cytotoxic T-cells) or MHC class II (for CD4 helper T-cells and B-cells) with appropriate costimulatory molecules and cytokines. It is imperative to discriminate between the first exposure of antigenic peptide to a naive (i.e., antigen-inexperienced) lymphocyte leading to clonal expansion, and secondary exposure to antigen leading to effector function. All nucleated cells express MHC class I, which makes perfect sense as all cell types are potential targets of intracellular infection. Hence, all cells in principle can act as APC in the secondary response of cytotoxic T-cells, leading to elimination of the infected cell. On the other hand, activation of primary cytotoxic T cells is brought about by dendritic cells (DC) in the secondary lymphoid organs.

In contrast, MHC class II is only expressed by many nonimmune cells under inflam-matory conditions, with IFN-γ being the main stimulatory cytokine. Given such a proin-flammatory milieu, highly diverse cell types express MHC class II plus costimulatory molecules, and examples relevant to atherosclerosis include endothelial cells, (myo)fibroblasts, and smooth muscle cell (SMC). This allows antigen-specific interac-tion with infiltrating T-cells expressing a T-cell receptor recognizing peptide in context of MCH class II. In view of the central role of MHC in protection of pathogens, it is not surprising that coevolution of pathogens and host has led to multiple mechanisms by which pathogens corrupt MHC expression and function *(22)*.

In contrast to nonimmune cells able to become APC under specific conditions, three types of professional APC are usually discriminated: B-cells, macrophages, and DC. The differential characteristics of these cell types collectively allows effective dealing with the four main types of pathogens mentioned in "Selected Immune System Basics."

B-cells effectively recognize and concentrate their complementary antigen by means of the specific membrane immunoglobulin. Subsequent antigen processing and presen-tation of antigenic peptide in context of MHC class II allows the B-cell to recruit its own peptide-specific CD4 T-cell help for further activation and differentiation to anti-body-producing plasma cells. Macrophages are specialized to effectively ingest partic-ulate pathogen, especially when opsonized by antibody and complement. Macrophages are thought to more effectively present to already antigen-experienced T-cells.

Finally, DC are highly effective APC for primary T-cells. Specialized forms of DC are found in many organ systems as organized networks of sentinel cells using their dendrites to capture pathogens and self-antigens alike, and to transport these to draining lymph nodes for interaction with T-cells. For instance, the Langerhans cells of the skin monitor the outside environment, and migrate through the lymph vessel system as veiled cells toward the lymph node. In the gut, DC are able to sample the gut content to maintain homeostasis by regulating mucosal antibody production keeping the normal gut flora at bay *(23–25)*. Morphological and functional DC subsets exist and this is a dynamically developing area *(26,27)*. Although most attention thus far has focused on the role of DC in priming of naive T-cells, it is becoming increasingly clear that DC are also locally involved in chronic inflammatory responses, for instance, in the lung during allergic asthma *(28)* and multiple sclerosis *(29)*. In view of their functions, DC are avidly investigated for immunostimulatory therapy in cancer *(30)* and tolerance induction in autoimmune disease and transplantation *(31)*.

APC and especially DC are integrators of innate and adaptive immunity, in view of their differential expression of innate antigen receptors, such as C-type lectin receptor (e.g., mannose receptor) and TLR (e.g., TLR4 for LPS). It has been shown that titration of TLR agonists affects Th1 vs Th2 signature of responses in vitro *(32)* and in vivo *(33)*.

### Costimulatory Molecules (Signal 2) Assist and Regulate Cell Interactions

For productive antigen-specific interactions between APC and lymphocytes, two signals are needed (*see* Fig. 3). The first is presentation of a peptide in the context of MHC class I (presentation to CD8$^{(}$ cytotoxic T-cells) or MHC class II (presentation to CD4$^+$ T-helper cells). The second signal is provided by membrane expressed receptor-ligand pairs, the so-called costimulatory molecules, and/or soluble molecules, i.e., immunostimulatory cytokines, such as IL-2. Only if both signals are provided full activation of the lymphocyte as well as the APC occurs as a result of crosstalk of a series of these molecules. Figure 3 summarizes current insight into costimulatory molecule function. When MHC-associated peptides (signal 1) are presented to lymphocytes in the absence of appropriate costimulation, functional unresponsiveness can ensue, which may be a mechanism to maintain tolerance against self-components.

It is generally thought that the requirement for costimulatory molecules and cytokines is a means to prevent autoimmunity, as peptides and other components from the host itself can also be presented by MHC molecules to autoreactive lymphocytes present in the circulating repertoire. Such T lymphocytes carrying receptors, specific for self-components, occur despite the existence of deletional mechanisms in the primary lymphoid organs, thymus, and bone marrow, respectively. The family of cell-surface-associated costimulatory molecules is ever-expanding. In order to allow fine-tuning and eventual resolution of APC-lymphocyte interactions, some of these receptor-ligand pairs can inhibit cellular activation (Fig. 4).

### CD40–CD154 Costimulatory Interactions as a Therapeutic Target

The relevance of costimulatory interactions for atherosclerosis pathophysiology is underscored by a series of studies on the CD40–CD154 system. CD40 is expressed on activated APC, whereas its ligand CD154 is transiently expressed on recently activated CD4$^+$ T-cells (extensively reviewed in ref. *34*). The interaction between these molecules has a wide array of functions, such as immunoglobulin isotype switching from IgM to IgG subclasses, and B-cell memory formation. Furthermore, CD154 expressing T-helper cells can interact with CD40-expressing endothelial cells and fibroblasts to increase expression of adhesion molecules and elicit cytokine production. Similarly, even in its soluble trimeric

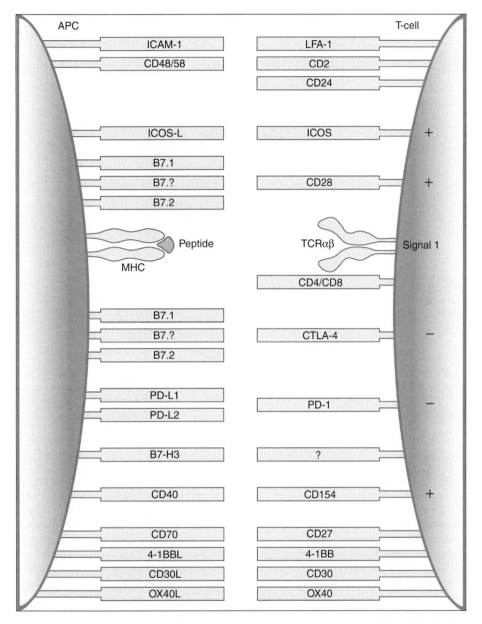

**Fig. 3.** Overview of costimulatory molecules regulating interactions between APC and T-cell. Signal 1 (center) in the interaction between T-cell and APC is provided by MHC containing the binding complementary peptide. The specific T-cell receptor recognizes the joint surface provided by MHC plus peptide *(recognition of peptide in context of MHC)*. A large series of cell surface- expressed costimulatory receptor-ligand systems provides the necessary signal 2 for activation (indicated by +) of both APC and T-cell in a reciprocal fashion. Hence, cell activation is licensed by the appropriate expression of costimulatory molecules as induced by microbial antigens or cytokines. This is generally thought to act as a failsafe mechanism reducing the risk of autoimmune disease as self-peptides can also bind to MHC. Some costimulatory molecules downregulate activation (indicated by −) to fine tune the response of both APC and T-cell.

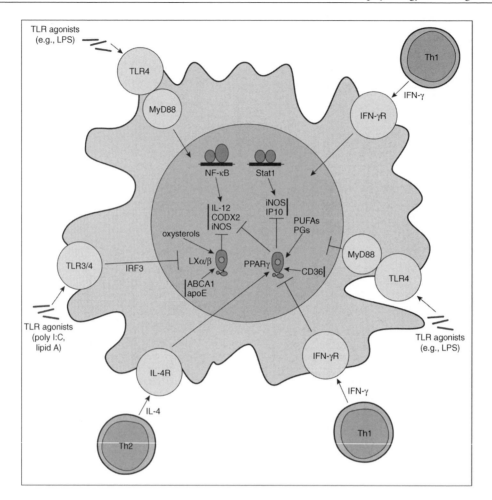

**Fig. 4.** Reciprocal regulation of TLR and PPAR/LXR signaling in macrophages. This figure is based on refs. *16,157,159*, integrating a number of recent concepts on macrophage signaling and atherogenesis. The broad interpretation is that immunity against pathogens and lipid metabolism reciprocally influence each other. PPAR-γ and LXR are nuclear transcription factors activated by ligands: oxysterols for LXR and polyunsaturated fatty acids and prostaglandins for PPAR-γ. In the figure, the macrophage is exposed to two types of outside signals, namely Th-cells (either Th1 or Th2 type), and to microbial compounds triggering TLR. Th1 cells stimulate inflammation by IFN-γ secretion, which increases protective function against infection, including expression of inflammatory molecules like inducible nitric oxide synthase and the chemokine IP-10/CXCL10 (upper right). Simultaneously, Th1 cells repress activity of PPAR-γ (lower right), relieving its counter regulation of these inflammatory molecules. In contrast, Th2 cells stimulate PPAR-γ, thereby limiting expression of inflammatory molecules. TLR agonists also stimulate inflammation by the MyD88 pathway (upper left, and *see* also Fig. 2). In addition, these TLR agonists simultaneously inhibit PPAR-γ (middle right), relieving its block on synthesis of inflammatory molecules. However, TLR ligands employing the MyD88-independent pathway plus the transcription factor IRF3 may act proatherogenic by blocking LXR, limiting expression of the cholesterol transporter ATP-binding cassette 1, and hence limiting cholesterol efflux leading to lipid accumulation.

form CD154 can activate macrophages to enhance costimulatory molecule expression, and to elaborate inflammatory cytokines, inducible nitric oxide synthase, and MMP's.

A role of this receptor-ligand pair in atherosclerosis was predicted to be based on the expression of CD40 by foam cells and fibroblasts in plaques *(35)* and simultaneously functionally demonstrated in animal models *(36)*. Genetic knockout (KO) of CD154 in apolipoprotein E (ApoE)-deficient mice lead to reduced plaque area, less lipid, increased collagen content, and stable plaque phenotype with a paucity of T-cells and macrophages *(37)*. Treatment with monoclonal antibody (Mab) against CD154 in ApoE KO induced a stable plaque phenotype *(38)*. Similarly, Mab treatment of low-density lipoprotein receptor-deficient mice limited lesion progression and favored plaque stability.

These in vivo studies were supported by extensive in vitro analysis of CD40–CD154 interactions. Interestingly, elevation of soluble CD154 indicates an increased risk of cardiovascular events *(39)*. Under inflammatory conditions, CD40 can be expressed by many different cell types including major players in vascular disease (endothelium, SMC, macrophages, myofibroblast). Functional effects of CD40 ligation by CD4$^+$ Th cells expressing CD154 include induction of proinflammatory cytokines; costimulatory molecules and adhesion molecules; stimulation of cell survival; induction COX-2 and prostaglandins; synthesis of enzymes modifying the extracellular matrix, such as MMP; and procoagulant activity *(40,41)*.

Clearly, interfering with CD40–CD154 pathways acts at multiple anatomic levels and on multiple effector pathways, involved in both inflammation and tissue dynamics. Interestingly, therapeutic Mab are under clinical development, which block either CD154 on activated CD4$^+$ T-cells or CD40 on activated APC preventing productive interactions. Such Mab can potentially be applied in atherosclerosis but also in other chronic inflammatory diseases, such as morbus Crohn and multiple sclerosis *(42–45)*. Despite thrombo-embolic complications in the trials of one of the anti-CD154 Mab, alternative Mab are under active development. It is important to stress that such Mab can interfere with antigen-specific interactions between APC and lymphocytes, but can also block the general activating effect that surface-expressed or soluble CD154 exerts on APC without a requirement for cognate interactions driven by MHC-binding peptides. Side effects from long-term therapy with such Mab may be reduced immune competence. However, in adults much of the immunity against prevalent pathogens has already been established, and relies on responses of CD8$^+$ cytotoxic memory T-cells and memory B-cells, which may not be depressed to a major extent by interfering with CD40–CD154 interactions.

## *Adhesion and Migration*

A large set of receptor-ligand pairs regulates migration of leukoctes, adhesion to cellular barriers, such as endothelium, subsequent transendothelial migration, and interaction with other cell types *(see* Fig. 1). Here only those molecules, currently thought to be crucial in recruitment of leukocytes to atherosclerotic plaques, are briefly touched on. This process is usually subdivided into initial interactions leading to leukocyte tethering and rolling mediated by selectins, subsequent firm adhesion mediated by integrins, and diapedesis occurring after activation through chemokines. P-selectin and E-selectin on the activated endothelium mediate rolling by interaction with P-selectin glycoprotein ligand-1 on the monocyte. Firm adhesion is brought about by vascular cellular adhesion molecule-1 and ICAM-1 on the endothelium, respectively interacting with very late antigen (VLA)-4 and lymphocyte function-associated antigen 1 on the monocyte.

The chemokine monocyte chemoattractant protein (MCP)-1/C-C chemokine ligand 2 (monocyte chemotactic protein 1) locally produced by endothelial cells, macrophages, and SMC, engages its receptor C-chemokine receptor (CCR2) on the monocyte, leading to activation and migration *(46)*. In the atherosclerotic plaque, the growth factor (macrophage colony stimulating factor) stimulates local proliferation and differentiation of macrophages. T-cells use similar mechanisms to gain access to the plaque. Intriguingly, a very recent study demonstrates that monocytes can also emigrate out of plaques, in a process called reverse transmigration. On exit, these cells acquire an intermediate phenotype of macrohages and DC, and can subsequently gain access to lymph nodes (*see* also Subheading "Prevailing Dogma: Activation of Primary Lymphocytes in the Lymph Node"). Lipid mediators involved in atherosclerosis prevent this exit, implying that progressive vs regressive plaque character is codependent on migration *(47,48)*.

Novel therapeutic approaches use, for instance, Mab to block VLA-4 on leukocytes, in an attempt to limit multiple sclerosis plaque progression and activity *(49)*. The obvious payoff is reduced migration to leukocytes where they are needed to fight off infection.

### *Paths Through the "Kine"-Jungle: Cytokines–Chemokines–Interleukins*

To the outsider but also to immunologists, the number of soluble signaling molecules is appallingly large, and all the more so far their functions are redundant and pleiotropic. Obviously, "kine" refers to kinesis, and accordingly cytokines are "cell-movers," chemokines are chemical movers and ILs are the soluble signals between leukocytes. A new addition to this list is adipokine for signaling molecules regulating fat metabolism, in keeping with the notion that fat tissue functions as endocrine organ in addition to its storage capability. Here, some simple means of broad "kine"-categorization according to recent reviews are provided *(50,51)*. Table 6 provides an overview of selected cytokines, chemokines, and adipokines important in atherosclerosis. Afficionados will find an excellent and fully comprehensive review of pathophysiological and therapeutical features of "kines" in Von der Thüsen et al. *(50)*.

One means of categorization is their division into six families of ILs, TNF family, IFNs, colony-stimulating factors, growth factors, and chemokines. However, these families clearly overlap in many ways. A second means of broad division is homology in the receptor sequence homology as that relates to functional outcome of cytokine binding. A third way is to distinguish between pro- vs anti-inflammatory activity, with on the one hand TNF, IL-12, IL-18, and IFN-γ, and on the other IL-4, -10, -13, and -1 receptor antagonist (IL-1ra). However, this dichotomy has proven to be oversimplified, as several cytokines have a Janus face in inflammation, dependent on many factors, such as local concentrations, participating cell types, receptor modulation, and so on. Having said that it is still safe to state that IL-10 and IL-1ra are anti-inflammatory. A fourth division of cytokines is as produced by Th1 vs Th2 cells (Table 4). A final categorization is based on major functions, such as chemoattraction (e.g., MCP-1/CCL2 for macrophages, IL-8/CXCL8 for neutrophils), homeostasis, inflammation, angiogenesis, and hematopoiesis.

All of these classifications are hampered to some extent by the functional redundancy of cytokines, and their pleiotropic action (productive interaction with diverse cell types). Within the class of chemokines, distinction is made between those having a single amino acid between the two amino terminal cysteine residues (CXC chemokines) and those lacking a separating amino acid (CC chemokines).

## PREVAILING DOGMA: ACTIVATION OF PRIMARY LYMPHOCYTES IN THE LYMPH NODE

An overwhelming body of evidence argues that activation of primary T-cells only effectively occurs in the highly organized anatomical compartments of the secondary lymphoid organs, lymph nodes, and spleen. Specialized areas contain B-cells with

Table 6

Selected Cytokines and Chemokines Relevant in Atherosclerosis Immunity

| Cytokine/chemokine/adipokine | Receptor/ligand | Function | Atherogenic |
|---|---|---|---|
| IL-1 | IL-1 R | Increases expression of cytokines, adhesion molecules, MMP. Macrophage recruitment and differentiation | Pro |
| IL-1ra | IL-1 R | Counteracts activity of IL-1 | Anti |
| IL-4 | IL-4 R | Th2 signature cytokine | Pro/anti |
| IL-10 | IL-10 R | Anti-inflammatory activity | Anti |
| TGF-β (types 1, 2, 3) | TGF-β R | Anti-inflammatory activity | Anti |
| TNF-α | TNF-α R | Promotes anorexia and weight loss. Th1 cytokine involved in immunity and autoimmunity. Promotes macrophage activity and protects from infection | Pro |
| IFN-γ | IFN-γ R | Promotes anorexia and weight loss. Th1 cytokine involved in immunity and autoimmunity. Promotes macrophage activity and protects from infection | Pro |
| IL-6 | IL-6 R | Promotes anorexia and weight loss. Acute phase reactant promoting CRP | Pro |
| IL-8/CXCL8 | CXCR1 | Promotes monocyte endothelial adhesion. Neutrophil chemo-attractant | Pro |
| IL-12 | IL-12 R | Proinflammatory cytokine of Th1 cells | Pro |
| IL-18 | IL-18 R | Induction of IFN-γ | Pro |
| MCP-1/CCL2 | CCR2 | Monocyte transendothelial migration | Pro |
| M-CSF | M-CSF R | Growth and differentiation factor for macrophages | Pro |
| MIP-1α/CCL3 | CCR1, CCR5 | Monocyte chemotaxis | Pro |
| CD154 (soluble) (=CD40L) | CD40 | Expressed by T-cells: broad activation of APC | Pro |
| Leptin | Leptin R | Inhibits food intake. Promotes Th1 cytokines | Pro/anti |
| Insulin | Insulin R | Glucose regulation. Promotes T-cell activation | Pro/anti |
| Corticotropin-releasing hormone | Corticotropin-releasing hormone R | Increases energy expenditure and catabolism. Inhibits inflammatory and delayed type hypersensitivity responses | Anti? |
| α-Melanocyte-stimulating hormone | α-melanocyte-stimulating hormone R | Inhibits food intake, increases catabolism. Inhibits inflammatory responses and promotes Treg function | Anti? |

*Legend*: This table is partly compiled from refs. *50,51,165*. The latter review provides an extensive and insightful overview of this broad subject. The last part of the table describes molecules, which are not formally "kines," such as insulin and hormones.

107

dedicated APC and other supportive subsets (follicles with follicular DCs, DC, and T-helper cells), mostly T-cells with DC (e.g., paracortical areas in the lymph node and periarteriolar lymphocyte sheath in the spleen). Functional interactions between helper T-cells and B-cells specifically occur at the borders of T- and B-cell areas *(52,53)*.

State of the art functional organization of secondary lymphoid organs is reviewed concisely in ref. *54*. The lymph nodes bring together a number of dynamic critical parameters required for lymphocyte activation: rare numbers of clonally distributed antigen receptor on recirculating T and B lymphocytes; concentration of antigen by transport of soluble compounds in the lymph, and carried by phagocytes or DC. Chances of rare lymphocyte specificities and complementary antigen meeting are highly increased by unique features of DC, as demonstrated by elegant imaging techniques of intact lymph nodes by Cahalan, Campbell, and colleagues *(55,56)*.

Although DC are not very migratory when in the lymph node, they are extremely motile increasing their "swept volume" by continuously throwing around their dendrites. Their resulting surface area of 2400 $\mu m^2$ is about 20-fold that of T-cells. DC can scan up to 5000 T-cells per hour so that 250 T-cells are in contact with each DC. Hence, 200 DC need 1 h to scan all $10^6$ T-cells in a mouse lymph node. A practical but in the author's opinion crucial corollary of the lymph node paradigm is that both animal and patient studies should assess lesional activity in direct conjunction with the lymph node station draining the vessel of interest, as a major part of immune regulation occurs there.

However, despite all evidence supporting the dogma of conditional priming of lymphocytes in the lymphoid organs, it remains conceivable that under some conditions naive T-cells and B-cells can be activated by APC located outside the secondary lymphoid organs, for instance, in the neoformations of lymphoid tissues as found in some chronic inflammatory conditions (e.g., B-cell germinal centers in joints of RA patients) *(57)*.

## PLAQUE TYPE AND VASCULAR-ASSOCIATED LYMPHOID TISSUE

An extensive discussion of plaque diversity and vulnerability is beyond the scope of this chapter, and can be found in refs. *58–61*. Clearly, plaque location, composition, and vulnerability are all parameters that need to be weighed carefully when adressing issues of inflammation and immune reactivity (*see* also Key Points). Recent work by the groups of Wick and Bobryshev has significantly advanced understanding of leukocyte distribution in vessels during health and disease (reviewed in refs. *62,63*). Within the healthy artery intima (but not of veins) a network of DC expressing CD1a is present, very similar to the Langerhans cells of the skin, thought to be sentinels detecting damage and infection early on. DC are in close contact with the endothelial cells, and it is suggested that they may sample the bloodstream by extending dendrites between endothelial cells, analogous to the situation in the gut *(23,24)*. At plaque predilection sites, these DC accumulate together with activated T-cells, macrophages, with few mast cells, and hardly any B-cells. This accumulation is accompanied by a higher density of selected extracellular matrix components as well as endothelial expression of vascular cellular adhesion molecule-1 and P-selectin. Wick et al. *(62)* dubbed these mononuclear cell infiltrations vascular-associated lymphoid tissue, in analogy to bronchus-, gut-, and nasal-associated lymphoid tissues. Interestingly, a limited number of foam cells are derived from DC. Within the plaque there are two regions where DC frequently colocalize with T-cells, which they might activate: the area of neovascularization associated with inflammatory infiltrates, and the area around inflamed vasa vasorum.

## EVIDENCE FROM ANIMAL MODELS FOR IMMUNE SYSTEM INVOLVEMENT

The limits of human experimentation including ethical constraints and extended time frame of lesion formation strongly call for appropriate small animal models to dissect immune system contributions to vascular disease. This field has seen major progress through the general advent of genetic engineering for tissue- and cell-specific transgenic mice and genetic KO *(64)* as well as more classic analysis of interbred mouse strains *(65)*. Importantly, the availability of ApoE as well as LDLR genetic KO has provided a tremendous boost. These models now provide opportunities to assess dietary influence, interactions of immune system and lipid metabolism, and development of experimental immunotherapy.

However, no convincing models of plaque rupture are available as yet, and the study of infectious agents in mice is limited by pathogen–host species compatibility. Of course differences between mouse and man extend to immunity *(66)*. Table 7 *(67)* lists a summary of the evidence from a large series of animal studies on adaptive immune system involvement. Recombinase-activating gene (RAG)-deficient mice were used as these animals lack T and B lymphocytes, hence lacking adaptive immunity. All in all, current collective interpretation of these studies is that: there is no evidence thus far that immune mechanisms are the primary cause of atherosclerosis; the influences of diverse immune system activities are complex, ranging from protective to proatherogenic; under high and long-term atherogenic pressure, T and B-cells are not required for lesion initiation of progression; when less atherogenic pressure is maintained, lymphocytes do affect lesion development; gender influences outcome; cytokines promoting, and limiting inflammation similarly promote and limit atherosclerosis.

In addition, Table 7 also lists examples of innate immunity molecules and mechanisms presumed to be involved in atherosclerosis, including CRP and complement, but also the enzyme cathepsin S, which degrades elastin and hence may be involved in leukocyte transmigration through the subendothelial basement membrane and damage to the elastic lamina of the aorta.

## ROLE OF NONPATHOGENIC MICROBES AND INFECTIONS

### *Nonpathogenic Microbes*

When considering infections and microbes, it is of crucial importance to distinguish infectious pathogens from nonpathogenic bacteria present in the normal flora of the human skin, and all mucosal membranes including the respiratory tract, and notably the gastrointestinal tract with its staggering numbers of commensals, outnumbering the body's own cell number 100-fold (*see* review *[68]*). The normal flora provides a continuous lifelong presence of strongly proinflammatory compounds including LPS (coengaging TLR4), lipopeptides and lipoteichoic acid (TLR2), GpC dinucleotide repeats (TLR9), and peptidoglycan (TLR2) (*see* Table 2). An intricate and only partly understood system of innate and adaptive mechanisms allows the host to "keep little friends at bay" *(25)*, confined to the exterior at the epithelial barriers to prevent undue bacterial translocation and inflammation, whereas taking full advantage of metabolic contributions to host physiology.

Research in this area is hampered by the extreme complexity of the gut flora (estimated between 500 and 1000 species in man), the density (up to $10^{12}$ microbes/mL in

Table 7

Evidence for Involvement of the Adaptive and Innate Immune System in Atherosclerosis

| Defect or treatment | Immunological effect | Atherosclerosis | Model | Diet | References |
|---|---|---|---|---|---|
| $Rag1^{-/-} Rag2^{-/-}$ | T- and B-cell defect | ↓ | $Apoe^{-/-}$ | Chow diet | 166,167 |
| $Rag1^{-/-} Rag2^{-/-}$ | T- and B-cell defect | No effect | $Apoe^{-/-}$ | High-fat diet | 166,168 |
| $Rag1^{-/-}$ | T- and B-cell defect | ↓ (early) | $Ldlr^{-/-}$ | High-fat diet | 169 |
| Anti-CD154 | No CD40 signaling | ↓ | $Ldlr^{-/-}$ | High-fat diet | 36,37,170 |
| $CD154^{-/-}$ | No CD40 signaling | ↓ | $Apoe^{-/-}$ | Chow diet | 38 |
| $IFN-\gamma R^{-/-}$ | No IFN-γ effects | ↓ | $Apoe^{-/-}$ | High-fat diet | 171 |
| IFN-γ treatment | More IFN-γ effects | ↑ | $Apoe^{-/-}$ | Chow diet | 172 |
| IL-10 transgenic | More IL-10 by T-cells | ↓ | $Ldlr^{-/-}$ | High-fat diet | 173 |
| IL-12 treatment | More IL-12 effects | ↑ | $Apoe^{-/-}$ | High-fat diet | 174 |
| IL-18 treatment | More IFN-γ effects | ↑ | $Apoe^{-/-} \times IFN-\gamma^{-/-}$ | Chow diet | 175 |
| Anti-TGF-β1, -2, -3 | No TGF-β signaling | ↑ | $Apoe^{-/-}$ | Chow diet | 176,177 |
| Polyspecific IgG | Immunosuppression | ↓ | $Apoe^{-/-}$ | High-fat diet | 178 |
| Hsp65 | Vaccination | ↑ | $Ldlr^{-/-}$ | Chow diet | 179 |
| oxLDL | Vaccination | ↓ | $Ldlr^{-/-}$ | High-fat diet | 180 |
| oxLDL | Vaccination | ↓ | $Apoe^{-/-}$ | High-fat diet | 181,182 |
| Complement C3$^{-/-}$ | No complement activation | Altered plaque composition | $Ldlr^{-/-} \times C3^{-/-}$ | High-fat diet | 183 |
| CRP injection | Increased local CRP concentration | ↑ | Coronary infarct normal | | 133 |
| Neutrophil elastase (NE) | remodeling, cytokine activation | ? | Expression in human samples | | 184 |

| | | | | |
|---|---|---|---|---|
| Cathepsin S (elastase) | Migration ↓ elastin degradation ↓ | → | Ldlr$^{-/-}$ × Cathepsin S$^{-/-}$ High fat diet | 185 |
| TLR4$^{-/-}$ | No TLR4 signaling by LPS or HSP neointima formation | → | Femoral artery cuff, LPS in TLR4$^{-/-}$ | 116 |
| TLR4$^{-/-}$ | No TLR4 signaling by LPS or HSP outward arterial remodel | → | Femoral artery cuff, LPS in TLR4$^{-/-}$ | 117 |

*Legend*: The upper part of this table is adapted from ref. *67*. The lower part of this table is not exhaustive but shows selected examples of innate immunity molecules demonstrated to be relevant. Mice lacking RAG cannot recombine functional T and B-cell receptors and hence lack lymphocytes of the adaptive immune system.

*Abbreviations*: RAG; recombinase-activating gene. SCID, severe combined immunodeficiency; Anti-CD154, antibody against CD154 (CD40Ligand [CD40L]); IFN-γ R, IFN-γ receptor; Anti-TGF-β1,2,3, antibody against TGF-β1,2,3.

the distal gut) the difficulties in culturing anaerobic species, and the technical challenges in maintaining germfree mouse colonies. In addition, a frequent misconception
is that germfree mice are also free of microbial antigens: this is wrong when animals
are fed irradiated normal mouse chow as this is full of microbial antigens, albeit non-
replicating. Only when carefully controlled synthetic low-molecular-weight compounds
are fed, an environment devoid of microbial compounds is truly approximated *(68)*.

There is some evidence from animal studies that the gut flora indeed affects atherosclerotic disease. For instance, Mallat et al. *(69)* addressed the role of the anti-inflammatory
cytokine IL-10, which deactivates macrophages and T-cells. Mice genetically deficient for
IL-10 fed an atherogenic diet had a threefold increase in lipid accumulation, increased
T-cell infiltration and IFN-γ production, concomitant with decreased collagen content,
when they were kept under specific pathogen-free conditions. Susceptibility to atherosclerosis showed a 30-fold increase when animals were housed under conventional conditions,
demonstrating that altered microflora can affect lesion formation at distal sites.

It has been demonstrated that bacterial peptidoglycan, a major proinflammatory cell
wall compound, which acts through CD14 and TLR2 engagement on phagocytes, is
present intracellularly in human atherosclerotic plaques. The number of cells containing peptidoglycan was significantly higher in vulnerable plaques *(70)*. In addition, the
level of serum IgM against peptidoglycan was inversely correlated with the extent of
atherosclerotic disease in a cross-sectional study, suggesting that IgM may be involved
in immune exclusion, i.e., keeping bacterial antigens at the mucosa *(71)*. Interestingly,
as DC can sample gut contents and subsequently redistribute microbes, but also breakdown products, they may carry peptidoglycan to inflammatory plaques without a need
for local replication of bacteria. In addition, as peptidoglycan from all pathogenic and
commensal bacterial species similarly stimulates inflammation, both pathogens and gut
commensals may contribute to inflammatory activity, in keeping with the pathogen
burden hypothesis (*see* Subheadings "Infectious Pathogens" and "Infectious Burden").

### The Hygiene Hypothesis: Its Appeal and Dirty Secrets

The hygiene hypothesis has attracted major scientific and popular attention and
deserves some attention here because of its promise, also for cardiovascular disease, and
its potential pitfalls. Critical concise *(68,72)* and more extensive reviews have been published elsewhere *(73)*. In 1989, Strachan *(74)* posed the idea that infections protect against
the development of asthma and allergies, as the risk of developing asthma and allergies is
negatively correlated with the number of children in a family. This would be caused by
the higher incidence of infections going around larger families. The general concept now
holds that a hygienic environment would direct the immune system into a T-helper cell
type 2 (Th2) pathway, typified by cytokines, such as IL-4, -5, and -13, resulting in
enhanced development of asthma, allergies, and eczema. A Westernized lifestyle, use of
antibiotics, vaccination, and other factors would promote this. On the other hand, a poorly
hygienic environment with early childhood infections (hepatitis, tuberculosis), high
microbial exposure, older siblings, daycare exposure, farming exposure, and contacts
with pets would favor protective responses against asthma, allergies, and eczema.

However, recent mouse studies using flu in relation to asthma clearly argue against
at least parts of the hygiene hypothesis: acute influenza infection strongly increased
allergic and respiratory responses *(75)*. Another counter argument is that autoimmune
diseases are thought to be caused by the Th1-pathway are also increasing in the
Western world. Furthermore, in Third World countries, the occurrence of parasitic

worm infections stimulating Th2 type of responses is not accompanied by allergy, but instead a robust anti-inflammatory network with a prominent role of IL-10 is operational *(73)*. In an insightful comment, Umetsu concludes that clearly, abandoning good hygiene and use of antibiotics and vaccines should not be considered in an attempt to stave off allergy.

Furthermore, it is possible that a few specific infectious pathogens and/or commensal bacteria, and certain less hygienic conditions limit development of asthma. Umetsu mentions hepatitis A virus and *Toxoplasma gondii,* which are associated with reduced asthma and allergy, and the same is true for colonization of the gut with *Bifidobateria* or *Lactobacillus* strains. Although controversial, there is some evidence for causal links between bacteria-mediating chronic inflammation of the gingiva and atherosclerotic disease *(see* ref. *76* for data in ApoE-deficient mice and references therein).

## *Infectious Pathogens*

The possible involvement of pathogens in maintaining a state of chronic inflammation in atherosclerosis and contributing to stenosis and lesion formation is being actively pursued. Obstacles are the high prevalence of several of these candidate pathogens in the population and the obvious multifactorial origin of atherosclerosis and stenosis. A particularly promising approach as pioneered by Stephen E. Epstein is the analysis of infectious burden, i.e., all pathogens by which the host is (latently) infected or has recently encountered. This approach is in line with the concept of polymicrobial disease causation where multiple pathogens and potentially also bacteria of the normal mucosal flora collectively stimulate inflammation through several mechanisms *(77)*.

Later three selected infectious pathogens were discussed, which are prime suspects, and studies analyzing infectious burden. Here it is important to distinguish studies using late-stage atherothrombotic disease including plaque rupture, thrombotic events, myocardial infarction, and cardiac arrest, from those assessing earlier stages of atherogenesis (often lesion formation and activity in animal models) or endothelial dysfunction.

## *Human Cytomegalovirus*

Several members of the herpesvirus family infect cells of the cardiovascular system. Already in 1978 it was shown that acute arteritis and atherosclerotic changes in chicken can be induced by infection with a γ-herpesvirus *(78)*. The β-herpesvirus Human Cytomegalovirus (HCMV) infects 50–100% of humans during early childhood. HCMV is associated with human vasculitides and atherosclerosis based on serological studies *(79,80)*. In addition, HCMV DNA is frequently present in abdominal aortic aneurysms (AAA) *(81)* and in lesions from patients with coronary artery disease (CAD) *(82,83)*.

Interestingly, impaired vascular function of asymptomatic individuals is associated with serological evidence for HCMV. This virus infects all cell types of the vascular wall, including endothelial cells and SMC. Endothelial cells can be lysed but HCMV can also take up latent residence *(84)*. SMC are stimulated by HCMV to produce reactive oxygen species and nuclear factor-κB (NF-κB) activation leading to production of atherogenic cytokines and chemokines *(see* Table 6) *(85)*. An intriguing mechanism is the action of the *US28* gene product of HCMV: this molecule is a viral chemokine receptor, which stimulated migration of SMC in response to the inflammatory chemokines RANTES/CCL5 and MCP-1/CCL2. This may promote neointima formation.

## Helicobacter pylori

*Helicobacter pylori* is a Gram-negative bacterial species infecting human gastric epithelium, and notorious for its association with ulcers and gastric cancer. There is some evidence for the presence of *H. pylori* in atherosclerotic plaques *(86)*, supported by some *(87,88)* but not all *(89)* serological studies. Recent studies claim that *H. pylori* strains with certain virulence factors, such as the cytotoxin-associated gene A codetermine risk of atherosclerosis. Hence, further analysis of *H. pylori* including the mechanisms of how it would affect plaque activity is warranted.

## Chlamydia pneumoniae

*Chlamydia pneumoniae* is a Gram-negative bacterium growing intracellularly in macrophages and inducing respiratory disease. Interestingly, recent studies claim associations between *C. pneumoniae* and chronic inflammatory disease of organs other than the airways, including the brain *(90–92)*. In vitro, *C. pneumoniae* infects cell types relevant to plaque formation: macrophages, endothelial cells, and SMC of the aorta *(93)*. Atheromatous lesions can contain *C. pneumoniae* antigens and DNA *(83)*. In addition, bacteria have been cultured from lesions *(94)*. It seems unlikely that *C. pneumoniae* is cytopathic to vascular wall cells, but infection of endothelial cells may stimulate production of factors promoting SMC proliferation *(95)*.

C. pneumoniae serology in relation to atherosclerotic disease is controversial *(96–98)*, and it does not reliably predict the presence of this pathogen in atherosclerotic lesions *(99)*. There is promise in molecular detection of *C. pneumoniae* DNA in peripheral blood mononuclear cells *(100)*. It will be worthwhile to further explore contributions of *C. pneumoniae* to vascular disease using such methods.

## *Infectious Burden*

Epstein *(101)* has proposed that the "impact of infection on atherogenesis is related to the aggregate number of pathogens with which an individual is infected, a concept referred to as pathogen burden." The rationale for selection of the pathogens CMV, hepatitis A virus, herpes simplex virus-1, *H. pylori*, and *C. pneumoniae* in some of these studies was that they are obligate intracellular pathogens, and elicit lifelong immune responses, as measured by serology for antibody levels. In one study, CAD was assessed by coronary angiography in relation to five of these pathogens: the number of seropositive responses increased with CRP levels and prevalence of CAD *(102)*. An increase in pathogen burden as reflected by specific IgG antibody was also shown to correlate with endothelial dysfunction as an early readout of atherosclerosis *(103)*. Two prospective studies indicated that pathogen burden predicted cardiovascular event rate *(104,105)*. Further evidence for infectious burden was provided in refs. *106,107*. However, there are also studies with negative results. For instance, in (working) men with stable coronary heart disease, there was no association between inflammatory biomarkers and seropositivity for *H. pylori*, *C. pneumoniae*, CMV, and EBV, whereas CRP was increased *(108)*.

Hence, infectious burden may be a predictor of CAD (mainly because of plaque rupture and thrombosis) as well as initiation of atherosclerotic lesions. However, as pointed out in critical reviews *(101)* the hypothesis that infection contributes has not been fully proven despite the convincing evidence accrued, and the seroepidemiological cross-sectional studies used, suffer from confounding factors, such as socioeconomic status, smoking, and publication bias toward positive outcomes *(109)*. Continued well-controlled prospective studies are required in close conjunction with advanced animal models.

For instance, Wright et al. *(110)* further addressed whether infectious agents are required for atherogenesis in elegant experiments using ApoE-deficient mice on a high-fat western diet. These mice were backcrossed to animals deficient for TLR4, the LPS receptor, and atherosclerosis was not different in double-deficient animals. Using germ-free ApoE-deficient mice free of all bacterial, viral, and fungal microbial agents, atherosclerosis was again not different than animals with normal exposure to agents in an animal facility.

Apparently in this model, infectious agents are not necessary for initiation, progression, or distribution of lesions. As the authors point out high levels of cholesterol in this model are sufficient to drive lesion formation, and this model does not investigate plaque rupture, thrombotic events, or myocardial infarction. They further indicate that infection may indirectly affect metabolism and known risk factors: infection stress affects insulin resistance and hyperglycemia, increase in plasma triglycerides, increased leukocyte count, elevated acute phase proteins including CRP and fibrinogen, and finally reduced high-density lipoprotein (HDL) cholesterol. It will be of great interest to further pursue this approach using other mouse models less dependent on high-cholesterol levels, such as the LDLR-deficient mice and multiple (human) pathogens.

## MECHANISMS BY WHICH MICROBES AND INFECTION MAY AFFECT ATHEROSCLEROSIS

### *Overview of Distal vs Local Effects*

Table 8 provides a listing of mechanisms linking atherosclerosis to microbial influence. As mentioned earlier, effects of infectious agents should be separated into local effects in the lesion because of local replication or presence/persistence of microbial compounds in the absence of replication vs effects on the lesion as a result of distal infection/replication. Distal effects are likely to be brought about by soluble compounds, such as cytokines/chemokines (e.g., IL-1, IL-6, TNF-α, IFN-γ), (crossreactive) antibodies, acute phase reactants (e.g., CRP, fibrinogen), insulin resistance, hyperglycemia, elevated plasma triglycerides, reduced HDL, and increased numbers of leukocytes.

### *Relevance of TLR in Atherosclerosis*

As discussed earlier and shown in Table 2, the TLR recognize components of pathogens, and possibly also self-components: therefore these two sources of TLR ligands need to be considered for atherosclerosis. The interaction between DC and T-cells (Fig. 3) relies on maturation of the DC by TLR ligation such that costimulatory signals can be provided (signal 2), in addition to MHC-peptide (signal 1). TLR regulate the adaptive immune response by controlling the expression of costimulatory molecules, production of cytokines, and by relieving the suppression exerted on effector T-cells by regulatory T-cells (*see* review *[111]*). The intracellular signaling pathways of TLR are largely overlapping but partly distinct: this is schematically summarized in Fig. 3 where the MyD88-dependent and independent routes are emphasized.

Several studies have demonstrated TLR expression in plaques, including TLR1, -2, and -4 *(43,112,113)*. In addition, the TLR4 Asp299Gly polymorphism, which attenuates receptor signaling and limits inflammation is associated with a decreased risk of atherosclerosis *(114)*, but an increased risk of severe infections. Mechanistically, this is not

Table 8
Distal and Local Mechanisms by Which Microbes May Affect Atherosclerosis

Systemic induction of acute phase reactants, for example, IL-6, CRP.
Systemic and local induction of proinflammatory cytokines and MMP, including those
    affecting plaque stability.
Insulin resistance, hyperglycemia, elevated plasma triglycerides, reduced HDL.
Increased numbers of circulating leukocytes.
Direct infection of key cellular players in plaque formation (endothelium, SMC, T-cells,
    DC, macrophages, foam cells).

  • For instance, pathogens can infect endothelial cells, increase synthesis of tissue factor,
    cell-surface thrombin expression, platelet adherence, expression of adhesion mole-
    cules, cytokines and growth factors, and decrease prostacyclin release.

Redistribution of inflammatory microbial compounds from site of infection to
    inflammatory plaque by DC and macrophages.
Increased SR expression by macrophages leading to enhanced uptake of lipid compounds and
    foam cell formation.
Enhanced procoagulant activity.
Increased vascular adhesion molecule expression induced by HSP.
Increased SMC migration and proliferation.
Molecular mimicry

  • Pathogen molecules mimicking self components, induce B and/or T lymphocytes with
    crossreactive antigen-receptors.
  • Autoantibodies against HSP: heat-stressed endothelial cells carry HSP-derived peptides
    rendering them susceptible to complement-dependent lytic effects of antibodies.

*Legend*: The table is compiled from many studies cited in this review. Please also refer to Fig. 5 for a
further comparison of direct cytopathicity and molecular mimicry.

very well understood as good evidence is lacking that macrophages with this polymorphism respond differently to LPS, and hence other TLR4 ligands may be involved *(115)*.
    In some support of this, very recently, functional evidence for TLR involvement in
atherosclerosis was obtained in mice double-deficient for ApoE and the TLR adaptor
protein MyD88, and hence deficient in signaling for TLRs and for IL-1 and IL-18. A
marked reduction in early atherosclerosis was seen, concomitant with a reduction in
chemokines involved in macrophage recruitment. Apparently, defective recruitment of
macrophages resulted from a noninfectious inflammatory stimulus. MyD88 did not
appear to be involved in foam cell generation. In contrast, mice double-deficient for
ApoE and CD14, a coreceptor for LPS had no decrease in early lesion development.
    On the other hand, it remains very clear that microbial compounds activate TLR and
may therefore contribute to local inflammation and vascular proliferation. Arterial remodeling can be increased by LPS ligating TLR4 by using a periadventitial cuff around the
femoral artery of mice. TLR4-deficient animals had reduced neointima formation *(116)*.
Also outward arterial modeling is promoted by TLR4 ligation *(117)*. For instance,
Chlamydial HSP60 activates macrophages and endothelial cells employing TLR4 and
MD-2 and the MyD88-dependent pathway *(118)*. The data on peptidoglcyan, a TLR2 lig-
and, in atherosclerosis also support this concept (*see* "Non-Pathogenic Microbes").
Finally, TLR3 and TLR9 are also expressed by mouse CD4+ T-cells, and their ligation
promotes survival of activated cells *(119,120)*, providing another mechanism promoting
adaptive immunity.

## RECIPROCAL INTERACTIONS BETWEEN INFLAMMATION AND LIPID METABOLISM

### *Foam Cell Formation*

Lipid metabolism and foam cell formation have been reviewed recently and excellently elsewhere *(2,13–15)*. Here, Figs. 1 and 4 and Table 3 are refered to, which point out some selected features. In the vessel wall, atherogenic apoB-containing lipoproteins interact directly with local proteoglycans leading to local retention *(121)*. CD36 and SR-A1/2 jointly are thought to mediate up to 90% of oxLDL uptake, but some other receptors may contribute as well (*see* Fig. 1) (Table 3). Lipoxygenases (LO) expressed by macrophages may contribute to oxidation of LDL (e.g., 12/15-LO as well as to formation of signaling lipid mediators (e.g., 5LO and leukotrienes), attracting macrophages. Indeed, genetic deficiency for 12/15-LO leads to reduced lesion formation in LDLR-deficient mice *(122)*, and partial deficiency of 5LO also dramatically limits lesion formation *(123)*. Expression of 5LO increases during atherogenesis, in monocytes, macrophages, and DC *(124)*. Interestingly, genetic epidemiological evidence supports that 5LO itself *(125)* and the 5LO-activating protein *(126)* are risk factors in atherosclerosis. Importantly, very recent and exciting data show that lipid metabolism and inflammation are reciprocally regulated, with a crucial role of the nuclear liver X receptors (LXR), the retinoid receptors, and peroxisome proliferator-activated receptor (PPAR)-γ. The legend to Fig. 4 discusses how engagement of these receptors crossregulates responses to ligation of the TLR by microbial and self-antigens.

### *Mechanisms Ascribed to oxLDL*

The potential mechanisms by which oxLDL influences atherosclerosis are numerous (reviewed in refs. *49,127,128*). These include: enhanced uptake of oxLDL by macrophages leading to foam cell formation; increase of expression of its own receptors on macrophages; induction of proinflammatory genes; chemotactic for monocytes and T-cells; immunogenicity leading to T-cells and antibodies specific for oxLDL; mitogenic as well as cytotoxic action, and induction of apoptosis; induction and activation of PPAR-γ.

There are intriguing but complex relations between oxLDL and specific autoantibodies. A murine IgM autoantibody (code EO6) generated from plasma cells in the spleen of an ApoE-deficient mouse recognizes a phosphorylcholine moiety on oxLDL. Surprisingly, the antigen recognition domain of this antibody turned out to be very similar to that of the highly conserved T15 natural antibody specifically recognizing phosphorylcholine. This led to the provocative hypothesis that recognition of phosphorylcholine on oxLDL, on apoptotic cells, and on pathogenic invaders alike is a mechanism used by natural "housekeeping" antibodies (e.g., T15), by newly formed autoantibodies (e.g., EO6) as well as by CRP. Hence, phosphorylcholine can be typified as a PAMP, also expressed by apoptotic host cells. Of note, this is not necessarily a monomeric ligand, but can be a clustered patch of molecules *(127)*. This PAMP-hypothesis is supported by successful decrease of atherosclerotic lesions on vaccination of LDLR-deficient mice with *Streptococcus pneumoniae (129)*. In some contrast with these exciting findings, in at least one experimental model, no evidence was found for clearance by autoantibody of mildly or heavily oxidized oxLDL *(130)*. However, specific antibody bound to oxLDL might still affect lesion formation.

## Functions of CRP and Relation to FcR and Complement Engagement

CRP is an acute phase protein synthesized by the liver, which acts as an innate immunity molecule by binding to phosphorylcholine present in microbial capsular polysaccharides, providing protection against pneumococcal infection. IL-6 is the main hepatic stimulus for CRP production. CRP is a potent activator of the classical complement pathway. Another function is the activation of IL-6 receptor shedding. CRP binds to macrophages and neutrophils by means of two of the Fc-γ receptors for IgG, CD32 (Fc-γ RIIa) being the low-affinity receptor and CD64 (Fc-γ R) being the high-affinity receptor *(131)*. CRP protects mice from LPS lethality by binding of both CD32 and CD64, hence increasing production of the anti-inflammatory cytokine IL-10 and downregulating proinflammatory IL-12 *(132)*.

As mentioned previously, CRP is a predictive marker for a range of vascular afflictions, including risk of myocardial infarction and stroke. Joint use of cholesterol and CRP measurements markedly improves predictive value, especially when LDL is low. Preventive measures including aspirin and statin treatment may be most beneficial at elevated CRP levels (lucidly reviewed by Blake and Ridker et al. *[4]*). Mechanisms by which CRP may contribute directly to lesion development remain to be fully elucidated, but most likely involve complement proteins and respective receptors as well as antibodies and Fc-receptors.

In a rat model, human CRP enhances coronary artery infarct size by approx 40% in a complement-dependent fashion *(133)*. A recent study demonstrated that CRP binds both oxLDL and apoptotic cells using a common ligand, which likely is phosphorylcholine. Hence, CRP may use this mechanism to assist in scavenging of oxLDL and apoptotic cells alike *(134)*.

## Lipid Metabolism and Infection

Cholesterol metabolism may directly impact at various points on the responsiveness of the immune system, such as predisposing the microvasculature to intense leukocyte-endothelial cell adhesion in response to inflammatory stimuli *(135)* or by increasing macrophage chemotaxis *(136)*. However, high-lipoprotein levels in plasma diminish systemic cytokine responses *(137)*, and impaired antibacterial immune responses were shown in genetically hypercholesterolemic ApoE-deficient mice *(138,139)*. Similarly, hypercholesterolemic mice lacking the LDL receptor are highly susceptible to disseminated *Candida albicans* infection *(140)*, indicating that in addition to local stimulatory effects in vascular inflammatory responses hypercholesterolemia may also exert negative effects on general immune responsiveness.

Although the role of hypercholesterolemia in the pathogenesis of atherosclerosis has been studied extensively in experimental mouse models, a thorough analysis of T-cell reactivity in these mice in response to a viral infection has only recently been described *(141)*. ApoE- and LDLR-deficient mice were infected with a hepatotropic strain of the lymphocytic choriomeningitis virus and MHC class I tetramers complexed with defined viral epitopes binding to their complementary T-cell receptor were used to follow activation and peripheral recruitment of virus-specific Cytotoxic T lymphocyte. In addition, antiviral T-cell effector function was followed by cytotoxicity and cytokine production assays. The results of this study indicate that hypercholesterolemia may substantially impair antiviral cellular immune responses leading to delayed viral clearance from the target organs. Hypercholesterolemia may thus disrupt the usually well-maintained pathogen–host equilibrium, ultimately leading to enhanced immunopathological disease.

These findings support the notion that altered immune-reactivity favors virus-induced vascular immunopathology *(142,143)*. Furthermore, mice with impaired IFN-γ responses are more susceptible to infection with murine CMV *(144)* or γ-herpesvirus 68 *(145)* and develop progressive chronic arterial inflammation. Similarly, *C. pneumoniae* preferentially infects predamaged atheromatous areas of the aorta in severely hypercholesterolemic ApoE- or LDLR-deficient mice, but only very rarely healthy aortas of normocholesterolemic C57BL/6 mice *(146)* or aortas of hypercholesterolemic mice before development of cholesterol-induced lesions *(147)*. It is therefore likely that the frequent association of *C. pneumoniae* and human CMV infection with atherosclerotic disease is due, at least in part, to altered immune-responsiveness and the subsequent impaired pathogen control. Importantly, herpesvirus infection *(142,148)* can further alter cholesterol metabolism. Thus, self-perpetuating immunopathological disease circuits may develop when chronic hypercholesterolemia-mediated immunosuppression impairs the usually well-balanced host–pathogen equilibrium.

The detrimental consequences of chronic T-cell-mediated inflammatory responses in the vascular wall can be demonstrated in a transgenic mouse model of inducible cardiovascular immunopathology. In SM-LacZ mice, the microbial β-galactosidase antigen is expressed exclusively in cardiomyocytes of the right heart and in arterial SMCs *(149)*. The transgene thus functions as a self-antigen mimicking a bacterial antigen that persists in the cardiovascular system. Interestingly, T-cells ignore the peripherally expressed antigen until the antigen is efficiently presented in secondary lymphoid organs. For example, immunization with DCs presenting α-galactosidase peptide elicits arteritis and myocarditis *(150)*. By crossing SM-LacZ mice onto the hypercholesterolemic apoE$^{-/-}$ background it was possible to determine the influence of hypercholesterolemia in the development of immune-mediated arterial inflammation and to evaluate the significance of immune-mediated arteritis in the chronological process of cholesterol-induced atherosclerosis. Hypercholesterolemia enhanced and perpetuated T-cell-mediated arterial inflammation and arterial inflammation significantly increased the susceptibility of the arterial wall to cholesterol-induced atherosclerosis *(150)*. Such mutual detrimental effects of vascular immunopathology and hypercholesterolemia have been observed in other experimental systems. For example, the number of IFN-γ-producing T-helper 1 cells infiltrating atherosclerotic lesions decreases under severe hypercholesterolemic conditions and the subsequent T-helper 1 to T-helper 2 switch results in the formation of IgG1 autoantibodies directed against oxidized LDL *(151)*. In addition, *C. pneumoniae* infection was shown to aggravate diet-induced atherosclerosis in normal C57BL/6 mice *(152)*. Overall, these data support the notion that the mutual perpetuation of pathogen- or autoimmunity-driven arterial inflammation and cholesterol-induced atherosclerosis may favor the vicious circle of chronic vascular injury.

### The Case of AAA vs Stenotic Atherosclerosis

AAA is an example of how the inflammation paradigm can be applied. Recent work *(153,154)* and references therein has modified the view that simple degenerative processes drive the aneurysm expansion by dissociating the normal lamellar organization of the aorta in AAA. Large numbers of inflammatory mononuclear cells are present, with activated CD4$^+$ T-cells and macrophages being the most abundant. There is local production of IFN-γ, TNF-α, and MMP-9, -2, -1, and -12. Based on data from animal studies as well as human postmortem material, the picture emerging is that infiltrating CD4$^+$ T-cells are the source of IFN-γ. This cytokine stimulates macrophages to produce MMP-9 and SMC

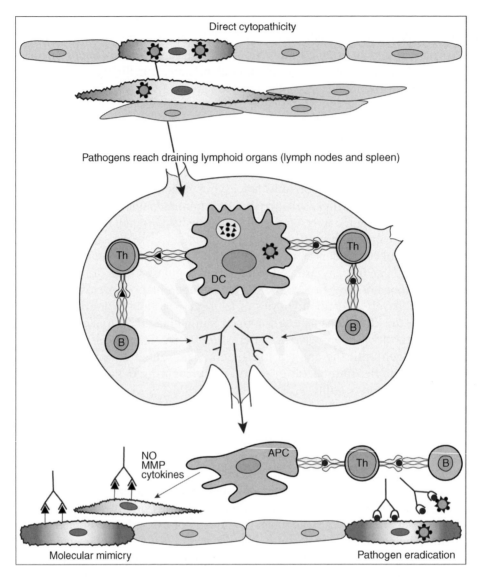

**Fig. 5.** Direct cytopathicity vs molecular mimicry as microbe effector mechanisms. This figure aims to clarify the complex issue of damage as a result of direct infection vs as a result of molecular mimicry (*see* also Table 8). The upper part shows direct cytopathic effects of infection. For activation of primary lymphocytes, the pathogen itself or its antigens need to reach the draining secondary lymphoid organs (middle part). DC activate lymphocytes by presenting individual antigens (filled circle, filled triangle) in the context of MHC. The desired effect is eradication of the pathogen by joint action of specific antibody (directed against "circle"-antigen) and T-cells (lower right hand side), cytokines and enzymes (e.g., NO, MMP). However, if a component of the pathogen bears structural resemblance ("triangle"-antigen on pathogen, and "triangle-stick"-antigen on host cells), crossreactive antibodies and T-cells may develop provoking tissue damage by molecular mimicry.

to produce MMP-2. In this way, the T-cells have a pivotal role in controlling composition of the extracellular matrix. The major contribution of IFN-γ is underscored by the finding that IFN-γ can induce arteriosclerotic changes in the absence of leukocytes, in a system where pig and human arteries are inserted into the aorta of immunodeficient mice *(155)*.

Interestingly, it has been argued that in AAA the immune response is mainly of a Th2 signature, with local expression of IL-4, -5, and IL-10, and paucity of IL-2 and IL-15 (Th1). Th2 cytokines induce a different pattern of matrix-degrading enzymes than Th1 cytokines. It was hence proposed that in this respect, AAA as an ectasia-inducing form of atherosclerosis is moleculary different from its diametrically opposed form of atherosclerosis, stenosis-producing plaques. It is of note that the prototypical Th1 cytokine IFN-γ is present in both forms.

## OPTIONS FOR INTERVENTION AND RESEARCH

Recent insight into inflammatory and immunological aspects of vascular disease spurs innovative experimental intervention. Unsurprisingly, there is no free lunch in anti-inflammatory therapy. Generic or targeted downregulation may affect protective immune responsiveness, whereas the chronic nature of cardiovascular disease would ask for continuous treatment. The clinical experience with therapeutic Mab against cytokines is not favorable (with the exception of TNF-α), which is perhaps easily explained by the redundant and pleiotropic action of this category of molecules. Chemokines and their receptors may offer a somewhat more specific target. As mentioned earlier, therapeutic Mab against adhesion molecules or CCR2 to prevent leukocyte migration into plaques are under active development, as are Mab blocking the interaction between costimulatory molecules, such as CD40 on APC and CD154 on activated T-cells. Exciting but challenging new immunological approaches are aimed at increasing activity of regulatory T-cells keeping inflammation in check, and induction of unresponsiveness in agressive T-cells by oral feeding of the relevant (auto)antigen or HSP *(156)*. The latter approach is hampered by the lack of positive identification of culprit (auto)antigens. Reduced exposure to a spectrum of pathogens (*see* Fig. 5) (Table 8) may be another approach, although the practicality of this is not *a priori* clear.

Success in antioxidative therapy based on insight into oxLDL function has been elusive: improved mechanistic insight into oxLDL function, better identification of risk groups likely to benefit from therapy, and selection of promising antioxidants are needed *(128)*. Drugs targeting LOs are also being evaluated. Finally, development of selective agonists and antagonists of TLR signaling pathways as well as PPAR/LXR (*see* Fig. 4) pathways are promising approaches, although the tight feedback and feedforward interconnections in lipid metabolism and inflammatory pathways may prove to be a major challenge *(157,158)*.

It is useful to distinguish between intervention that someday will be of clinical benefit to patients, and intervention which stimulates and potentially revolutionizes research. The latter is based on tools and technology available to interventional cardiologists, which are often stunningly advanced to the immunologist. Examples are the ever more sophisticated in vivo imaging techniques as well as intricate catheters (e.g., measuring micro temperature differences over the length of a plaque or allowing local delivery of agents) and stents (e.g., drug-eluting). These tools allow in vivo detection and manipulation of local inflammation, for instance, by delivery of therapeutic antibodies and intact infectious agents or microbial compounds engaging cellular receptors. Techniques to monitor plaque inflammation and activity in minimally invasive fashion in both man and animal models will prove invaluable. Scientific and technological close collaboration between "interventionists and inflammatists" will potentially bring about major advances.

## ACKNOWLEDGMENTS

The authors thank Tar van Os for artwork and Marcia Ijdo-Reintjes for secretarial assistance. Size constraints prohibited citation of all relevant primary literature. Instead it has been attempted to focus on authoritative reviews by experts in the field, providing useful general inroads for interested interventional cardiologists. This work was partly supported by grant 2001B077 from The Netherlands Heart Foundation, and by grant 32-63415.00 from the Swiss National Science Foundation to B.L.

## KEY POINTS ON IMMUNITY AND LIPIDS

- Primary (antigen inexperienced) lymphocytes are only effectively activated in the secondary lymphoid organs (spleen and lymph nodes).
- Secondary (antigen experienced) lymphocytes recirculate and are activated when properly exposed to their respective antigen by APC in affected organs.
- The normal flora at all mucosa, and notably in the gastrointestinal tract, contains abundant proinflammatory compounds, which may contribute to disease.
- Pathogen components can promote inflammation in the absence of replication.
- Pathogens can elicit inflammation at distal sites without a need for local replication in that site (echo effect).
- Fat tissue is an endocrine organ and its activity affects the immune system.
- Lipid metabolism and immune reactivity are not separated but closely intertwined.
- Hypercholesterolemia may disrupt the usually well-maintained pathogen-host equilibrium, ultimately leading to enhanced immunopathological disease.
- The mutual perpetuation of pathogen- or autoimmunity-driven arterial inflammation and cholesterol-induced atherosclerosis may favor the vicious circle of chronic vascular injury.

## KEY POINTS ON PLAQUE ASPECTS

- Plaque typing and plaque progression emphasize variation in composition.
- What explains plaque predilection sites?
- Shear stress affects plaque formation with high shear stress leading to increased particle retention time and uptake at plaque predilection sites.
- Vascular-associated lymphoid tissue occurs at predilection sites.
- Which factors in restenosis and intervention engage the immune system, for instance, tissue damage and repair releasing self-components binding to receptors?
- What are the factors determining culprit plaque (thrombus-forming, rupture prone) location and activity?

## KEY POINTS ON MAIN CELLULAR PLAYERS AND ANTIGENS INVOLVED IN ATHEROGENESIS

- Vessel wall: endothelium, SMC, fibroblasts, macrophages.
- Immune system: macrophages, CD4$^+$ T-cells. To a lesser extent: CD8$^+$ cytotoxic T-cells, B-cells (plasma cells).

- Candidate antigens in the plaque: oxLDL, HSP60, platelet β2 glycoprotein1b, pathogen components.
- T-cell activation can be antigen-independent, for example, stimulated by IL-15.

## ABBREVIATIONS

| | |
|---|---|
| AAA | abdominal artery aneurysm |
| APC | antigen-presenting cell |
| ApoE | apolipoprotein E |
| CCR | C-chemokine receptor |
| CXCR | C-X-C chemokine receptor |
| CD | cluster of differentiation |
| CLR | C-type lectin receptor |
| CRP | C-reactive protein |
| CTL | cytotoxic T lymphocyte |
| DC | dendritic cell |
| HDL | high-density lipoprotein |
| HLA | human leukocyte antigen (compare MHC) |
| HSP | heat shock protein 60 |
| ICAM | intercellular adhesion molecule |
| IFN | interferon |
| IL | interleukin |
| iNOS | inducible nitric oxide synthase |
| LDL | low-density lipoprotein |
| LO | lipoxygenase |
| LPS | lipopolysaccharide |
| LXR | liver X receptor |
| Mab | monoclonal antibody |
| MBL | mannose/mannan binding lectin |
| MHC | major histocompatibility complex (compare HLA) |
| MMP | matrix metalloproteinase |
| Nod | nucleotide-binding oligomerization domain |
| oxLDL | oxidized low-density lipoprotein |
| PAMP | pathogen associated molecular pattern |
| PPAR | peroxisome proliferator activated receptor |
| PRR | pattern recognition receptor |
| R | receptor |
| RXR | retinoid X receptor |
| RAG | recombinase activating gene |
| SMC | smooth muscle cell |
| SR | scavenger receptor |
| TGF | transforming growth factor |
| Th | T-helper |
| Treg | T-regulatory |
| TLR | Toll-like receptor |
| TNF | tumor necrosis factor |
| VCAM | vascular cellular adhesion molecule |
| VLDL | very low-density lipoprotein |

# REFERENCES

1. Wick G, Knoflach M, Xu Q. Autoimmune and inflammatory mechanisms in atherosclerosis. Annu Rev Immunol 2004;22:361–403.
2. Libby P. Inflammation in atherosclerosis. Nature 2002;420:868–874.
3. Feldmann M, Maini RN. Lasker Clinical Medical Research Award. TNF defined as a therapeutic target for rheumatoid arthritis and other autoimmune diseases. Nat Med 2003;9:1245–1250.
4. Blake GJ, Ridker PM. Novel clinical markers of vascular wall inflammation. Circ Res 2001;89: 763–771.
5. Janeway CA, Jr., Medzhitov R. Innate immune recognition. Annu Rev Immunol 2002;20:197–216.
6. Poltorak A, He X, Smirnova I, et al. Defective LPS signaling in C3H/HeJ and C57BL/10ScCr mice: mutations in Tlr4 gene. Science 1998;282:2085–2088.
7. Girardin SE, Philpott DJ. Mini-review: the role of peptidoglycan recognition in innate immunity. Eur J Immunol 2004;34:1777–1782.
8. Girardin SE, Hugot JP, Sansonetti PJ. Lessons from Nod2 studies: towards a link between Crohn's disease and bacterial sensing. Trends Immunol 2003;24:652–658.
9. de Boer OJ, Becker AE, van der Wal AC. T lymphocytes in atherogenesis-functional aspects and antigenic repertoire. Cardiovasc Res 2003;60:78–86.
10. Shevach EM. CD4+ CD25+ suppressor T-cells: more questions than answers. Nat Rev Immunol 2002;2:389–400.
11. Sakaguchi S. Naturally arising CD4+ regulatory t cells for immunologic self-tolerance and negative control of immune responses. Annu Rev Immunol 2004;22:531–562.
12. Vos Q, Lees A, Wu ZQ, Snapper CM, Mond JJ. B-cell activation by T-cell-independent type 2 antigens as an integral part of the humoral immune response to pathogenic microorganisms. Immunol Rev 2000;176:154–170.
13. Steinberg D. Atherogenesis in perspective: hypercholesterolemia and inflammation as partners in crime. Nat Med 2002;8:1211–1217.
14. Li AC, Glass CK. The macrophage foam cell as a target for therapeutic intervention. Nat Med 2002;8:1235–1242.
15. Repa JJ, Mangelsdorf DJ. The liver X receptor gene team: potential new players in atherosclerosis. Nat Med 2002;8:1243–1248.
16. Gordon S. Alternative activation of macrophages. Nat Rev Immunol 2003;3:23–35.
17. Duffield JS. The inflammatory macrophage: a story of Jekyll and Hyde. Clin Sci (Lond) 2003; 104:27–38.
18. Mosser DM. The many faces of macrophage activation. J Leukoc Biol 2003;73:209–212.
19. Mantovani A, Sozzani S, Locati M, Allavena P, Sica A. Macrophage polarization: tumor-associated macrophages as a paradigm for polarized M2 mononuclear phagocytes. Trends Immunol 2002; 23:549–555.
20. Boot RG, van Achterberg TA, van Aken BE, et al. Strong induction of members of the chitinase family of proteins in atherosclerosis: chitotriosidase and human cartilage gp-39 expressed in lesion macrophages. Arterioscler Thromb Vasc Biol 1999;19:687–694.
21. Boven LA, van Meurs M, Boot RG, et al. Gaucher cells demonstrate a distinct macrophage phenotype and resemble alternatively activated macrophages. Am J Clin Pathol 2004;122:359–369.
22. Furman MH, Ploegh HL. Lessons from viral manipulation of protein disposal pathways. J Clin Invest 2002;110:875–879.
23. Rescigno M, Urbano M, Valzasina B, et al. Dendritic cells express tight junction proteins and penetrate gut epithelial monolayers to sample bacteria. Nat Immunol 2001;2:361–367.
24. Macpherson AJ, Uhr T. Induction of protective IgA by intestinal dendritic cells carrying commensal bacteria. Science 2004;303:1662–1665.
25. Kraehenbuhl JP, Corbett M. Immunology. Keeping the gut microflora at bay. Science 2004;303: 1624–1625.
26. Shortman K, Liu YJ. Mouse and human dendritic cell subtypes. Nat Rev Immunol 2002;2:151–161.
27. Ardavin C. Origin, precursors and differentiation of mouse dendritic cells. Nat Rev Immunol 2003;3:582–590.
28. Lambrecht BN, Hammad H. Taking our breath away: dendritic cells in the pathogenesis of asthma. Nat Rev Immunol 2003;3:994–1003.
29. Aloisi F, Ria F, Adorini L. Regulation of T-cell responses by CNS antigen-presenting cells: different roles for microglia and astrocytes. Immunol Today 2000;21:141–147.
30. Figdor CG, de Vries IJ, Lesterhuis WJ, Melief CJ. Dendritic cell immunotherapy: mapping the way. Nat Med 2004;10:475–480.

31. Steinman RM, Hawiger D, Nussenzweig MC. Tolerogenic dendritic cells. Annu Rev Immunol 2003;21:685–711.

32. Boonstra A, Asselin-Paturel C, Gilliet M, et al. Flexibility of mouse classical and plasmacytoid-derived dendritic cells in directing T helper type 1 and 2 cell development: dependency on antigen dose and differential toll-like receptor ligation. J Exp Med 2003;197:101–109.

33. Eisenbarth SC, Piggott DA, Huleatt JW, Visintin I, Herrick CA, Bottomly K. Lipopolysaccharide-enhanced, toll-like receptor 4-dependent T helper cell type 2 responses to inhaled antigen. J Exp Med 2002;196:1645–1651.

34. Quezada SA, Jarvinen LZ, Lind EF, Noelle RJ. CD40/CD154 interactions at the interface of tolerance and immunity. Annu Rev Immunol 2004;22:307–328.

35. Laman JD, de Smet BJ, Schoneveld A, van Meurs M. CD40-CD40L interactions in atherosclerosis. Immunol Today 1997;18:272–277.

36. Mach F, Schonbeck U, Sukhova GK, et al. Functional CD40 ligand is expressed on human vascular endothelial cells, smooth muscle cells, and macrophages: implications for CD40-CD40 ligand signaling in atherosclerosis. Proc Natl Acad Sci USA 1997;94:1931–1936.

37. Lutgens E, Gorelik L, Daemen MJ, et al. Requirement for CD154 in the progression of atherosclerosis. Nat Med 1999;5:1313–1316.

38. Lutgens E, Cleutjens KB, Heeneman S, Koteliansky VE, Burkly LC, Daemen MJ. Both early and delayed anti-CD40L antibody treatment induces a stable plaque phenotype. Proc Natl Acad Sci USA 2000; 97:7464–7469.

39. Heeschen C, Dimmeler S, Hamm CW, et al. Soluble CD40 ligand in acute coronary syndromes. N Engl J Med 2003;348:1104–1111.

40. Phipps RP. Atherosclerosis: the emerging role of inflammation and the CD40-CD40 ligand system. Proc Natl Acad Sci USA 2000;97:6930–6932.

41. Lutgens E, Daemen MJ. CD40-CD40L interactions in atherosclerosis. Trends Cardiovasc Med 2002;12:27–32.

42. Gerritse K, Laman JD, Noelle RJ, et al. CD40-CD40 ligand interactions in experimental allergic encephalomyelitis and multiple sclerosis. Proc Natl Acad Sci USA 1996;93:2499–2504.

43. Laman JD, t Hart BA, Brok H, et al. Protection of marmoset monkeys against EAE by treatment with a murine antibody blocking CD40 (mu5D12). Eur J Immunol 2002;32:2218–2228.

44. Boon L, Brok HP, Bauer J, et al. Prevention of experimental autoimmune encephalomyelitis in the common marmoset (*Callithrix jacchus*) using a chimeric antagonist monoclonal antibody against human CD40 is associated with altered B-cell responses. J Immunol 2001;167:2942–2949.

45. Boon L, Laman JD, Ortiz-Buijsse A, et al. Preclinical assessment of anti-CD40 Mab 5D12 in cynomolgus monkeys. Toxicology 2002;174:53–65.

46. Rollins BJ. Chemokines and atherosclerosis: what Adam Smith has to say about vascular disease. J Clin Invest 2001;108:1269–1271.

47. Llodrá J, Angeli V, Liu J, Trogan E, Fisher EA, Randolph GJ. Emigration of monocyte-derived cells from atherosclerotic lesions characterizes regressive, but not progressive, plaques. Proc Natl Acad Sci USA 2004;101:11,779–11,784.

48. Ludewig B, Laman JD. The in and out of monocytes in atherosclerotic plaques: Balancing inflammation through migration. Proc Natl Acad Sci USA 2004;101:11,529–11,530.

49. Miller DH, Khan OA, Sheremata WA, et al. A controlled trial of natalizumab for relapsing multiple sclerosis. N Engl J Med 2003;348:15–23.

50. von der Thüsen JH, Kuiper J, van Berkel TJ, Biessen EA. Interleukins in atherosclerosis: molecular pathways and therapeutic potential. Pharmacol Rev 2003;55:133–166.

51. Matarese G, La Cava A. The intricate interface between immune system and metabolism. Trends Immunol 2004;25:193–200.

52. Van den Eertwegh AJ, Noelle RJ, Roy M, et al. In vivo CD40-gp39 interactions are essential for thymus-dependent humoral immunity. I. In vivo expression of CD40 ligand, cytokines, and antibody production delineates sites of cognate T-B-cell interactions. J Exp Med 1993;178:1555–1565.

53. Garside P, Ingulli E, Merica RR, Johnson JG, Noelle RJ, Jenkins MK. Visualization of specific B and T lymphocyte interactions in the lymph node. Science 1998;281:96–99.

54. Crivellato E, Vacca A, Ribatti D. Setting the stage: an anatomist's view of the immune system. Trends Immunol 2004;25:210–217.

55. Miller MJ, Wei SH, Cahalan MD, Parker I. Autonomous T-cell trafficking examined in vivo with intravital two-photon microscopy. Proc Natl Acad Sci USA 2003;100:2604–2609.

56. Cahalan MD, Parker I, Wei SH, Miller MJ. Real-time imaging of lymphocytes in vivo. Curr Opin Immunol 2003;15:372–377.

57. Silverman GJ, Carson DA. Roles of B-cells in rheumatoid arthritis. Arthritis Res Ther 2003;5(Suppl 4): S1–S6.

58. VanderLaan PA, Reardon CA, Getz GS. Site specificity of atherosclerosis: site-selective responses to atherosclerotic modulators. Arterioscler Thromb Vasc Biol 2004;24:12–22.

59. Faber BC, Heeneman S, Daemen MJ, Cleutjens KB. Genes potentially involved in plaque rupture. Curr Opin Lipidol 2002;13:545–552.

60. Naghavi M, Libby P, Falk E, et al. From vulnerable plaque to vulnerable patient: a call for new definitions and risk assessment strategies: Part II. Circulation 2003;108:1772–1778.

61. Naghavi M, Libby P, Falk E, et al. From vulnerable plaque to vulnerable patient: a call for new definitions and risk assessment strategies: Part I. Circulation 2003;108:1664–1672.

62. Millonig G, Schwentner C, Mueller P, Mayerl C, Wick G. The vascular-associated lymphoid tissue: a new site of local immunity. Curr Opin Lipidol 2001;12:547–553.

63. Bobryshev YV. Dendritic cells in atherosclerosis. In: Lotze MT, Thomson AW, eds. Dendritic Cells. Academic Press, London, UK, 2001, pp. 547–558.

64. de Winther MP, Hofker MH. New mouse models for lipoprotein metabolism and atherosclerosis. Curr Opin Lipidol 2002;13:191–197.

65. Allayee H, Ghazalpour A, Lusis AJ. Using mice to dissect genetic factors in atherosclerosis. Arterioscler Thromb Vasc Biol 2003;23:1501–1509.

66. Mestas J, Hughes CC. Of mice and not men: differences between mouse and human immunology. J Immunol 2004;172:2731–2738.

67. Binder CJ, Chang MK, Shaw PX, et al. Innate and acquired immunity in atherogenesis. Nat Med 2002;8:1218–1226.

68. Macpherson AJ, Harris NL. Interactions between commensal intestinal bacteria and the immune system. Nat Rev Immunol 2004;4:478–485.

69. Mallat Z, Besnard S, Duriez M, et al. Protective role of interleukin-10 in atherosclerosis. Circ Res 1999;85:e17–e24.

70. Laman JD, Schoneveld AH, Moll FL, van Meurs M, Pasterkamp G. Significance of peptidoglycan, a proinflammatory bacterial antigen in atherosclerotic arteries and its association with vulnerable plaques. Am J Cardiol 2002;90:119–123.

71. Nijhuis MM, Van Der Graaf Y, Melief MJ, et al. IgM antibody level against proinflammatory bacterial peptidoglycan is inversely correlated with extent of atherosclerotic disease. Atherosclerosis 2004;173:245–251.

72. Umetsu DT. Flu strikes the hygiene hypothesis. Nat Med 2004;10:232–234.

73. Yazdanbakhsh M, Kremsner PG, van Ree R. Allergy, parasites, and the hygiene hypothesis. Science 2002;296:490–494.

74. Strachan DP. Hay fever, hygiene, and household size. Bmj 1989;299:1259–1260.

75. Dahl ME, Dabbagh K, Liggitt D, Kim S, Lewis DB. Viral-induced T helper type 1 responses enhance allergic disease by effects on lung dendritic cells. Nat Immunol 2004;5:337–343.

76. Gibson FC, 3rd, Hong C, Chou HH, et al. Innate immune recognition of invasive bacteria accelerates atherosclerosis in apolipoprotein E-deficient mice. Circulation 2004;109:2801–2806.

77. Relman DA. The search for unrecognized pathogens. Science 1999;284:1308–1310.

78. Fabricant CG, Fabricant J, Litrenta MM, Minick CR. Virus-induced atherosclerosis. J Exp Med 1978;148:335–340.

79. Adam E, Melnick JL, Probtsfield JL, et al. High levels of cytomegalovirus antibody in patients requiring vascular surgery for atherosclerosis. Lancet 1987;2:291–293.

80. Zhou YF, Leon MB, Waclawiw MA, et al. Association between prior cytomegalovirus infection and the risk of restenosis after coronary atherectomy. N Engl J Med 1996;335:624–630.

81. Yonemitsu Y, Nakagawa K, Tanaka S, Mori R, Sugimachi K, Sueishi K. In situ detection of frequent and active infection of human cytomegalovirus in inflammatory abdominal aortic aneurysms: possible pathogenic role in sustained chronic inflammatory reaction. Lab Invest 1996;74:723–736.

82. Hendrix MG, Salimans MM, van Boven CP, Bruggeman CA. High prevalence of latently present cytomegalovirus in arterial walls of patients suffering from grade III atherosclerosis. Am J Pathol 1990;136:23–28.

83. Chiu B, Viira E, Tucker W, Fong IW. *Chlamydia pneumoniae*, cytomegalovirus, and herpes simplex virus in atherosclerosis of the carotid artery. Circulation 1997;96:2144–2148.

84. Jarvis MA, Nelson JA. Human cytomegalovirus persistence and latency in endothelial cells and macrophages. Curr Opin Microbiol 2002;5:403–407.

85. Speir E. Cytomegalovirus gene regulation by reactive oxygen species. Agents in atherosclerosis. Ann NY Acad Sci 2000;899:363–374.

86. Ameriso SF, Fridman EA, Leiguarda RC, Sevlever GE. Detection of Helicobacter pylori in human carotid atherosclerotic plaques. Stroke 2001;32:385–391.

87. Espinola-Klein C, Rupprecht HJ, Blankenberg S, et al. Impact of infectious burden on progression of carotid atherosclerosis. Stroke 2002;33:2581–2586.

88. Georges JL, Rupprecht HJ, Blankenberg S, et al. Impact of pathogen burden in patients with coronary artery disease in relation to systemic inflammation and variation in genes encoding cytokines. Am J Cardiol 2003;92:515–521.

89. Danesh J, Peto R. Risk factors for coronary heart disease and infection with Helicobacter pylori: meta-analysis of 18 studies. Bmj 1998;316:1130–1132.

90. Sriram S, Stratton CW, Yao S, et al. *Chlamydia pneumoniae* infection of the central nervous system in multiple sclerosis. Ann Neurol 1999;46:6–14.

91. Buljevac D, Verkooyen RP, Jacobs BC, et al. *Chlamydia pneumoniae* and the risk for exacerbation in multiple sclerosis patients. Ann Neurol 2003;54:828–831.

92. Balin BJ, Gerard HC, Arking EJ, et al. Identification and localization of *Chlamydia pneumoniae* in the Alzheimer's brain. Med Microbiol Immunol (Berl) 1998;187:23–42.

93. Gaydos CA, Summersgill JT, Sahney NN, Ramirez JA, Quinn TC. Replication of Chlamydia pneumoniae in vitro in human macrophages, endothelial cells, and aortic artery smooth muscle cells. Infect Immun 1996;64:1614–1620.

94. Maass M, Bartels C, Engel PM, Mamat U, Sievers HH. Endovascular presence of viable *Chlamydia pneumoniae* is a common phenomenon in coronary artery disease. J Am Coll Cardiol 1998;31:827–832.

95. Coombes BK, Mahony JB. *Chlamydia pneumoniae* infection of human endothelial cells induces proliferation of smooth muscle cells via an endothelial cell-derived soluble factor(s). Infect Immun 1999;67:2909–2915.

96. Saikku P, Leinonen M, Mattila K, et al. Serological evidence of an association of a novel Chlamydia, TWAR, with chronic coronary heart disease and acute myocardial infarction. Lancet 1988;2: 983–986.

97. Danesh J, Whincup P, Lewington S, et al. *Chlamydia pneumoniae* IgA titres and coronary heart disease; prospective study and meta-analysis. Eur Heart J 2002;23:371–375.

98. Danesh J, Whincup P, Walker M, et al. *Chlamydia pneumoniae* IgG titres and coronary heart disease: prospective study and meta-analysis. Bmj 2000;321:208–213.

99. Bartels C, Maass M, Bein G, et al. Association of serology with the endovascular presence of *Chlamydia pneumoniae* and cytomegalovirus in coronary artery and vein graft disease. Circulation 2000;101:137–141.

100. Smieja M, Mahony J, Petrich A, Boman J, Chernesky M. Association of circulating *Chlamydia pneumoniae* DNA with cardiovascular disease: a systematic review. BMC Infect Dis 2002;2:21.

101. Epstein SE, Zhu J, Burnett MS, Zhou YF, Vercellotti G, Hajjar D. Infection and atherosclerosis: potential roles of pathogen burden and molecular mimicry. Arterioscler Thromb Vasc Biol 2000;20:1417–1420.

102. Zhu J, Quyyumi AA, Norman JE, et al. Effects of total pathogen burden on coronary artery disease risk and C-reactive protein levels. Am J Cardiol 2000;85:140–146.

103. Prasad A, Zhu J, Halcox JP, Waclawiw MA, Epstein SE, Quyyumi AA. Predisposition to atherosclerosis by infections: role of endothelial dysfunction. Circulation 2002;106:184–190.

104. Zhu J, Nieto FJ, Horne BD, Anderson JL, Muhlestein JB, Epstein SE. Prospective study of pathogen burden and risk of myocardial infarction or death. Circulation 2001;103:45–51.

105. Rupprecht HJ, Blankenberg S, Bickel C, et al. Impact of viral and bacterial infectious burden on long-term prognosis in patients with coronary artery disease. Circulation 2001;104:25–31.

106. Kiechl S, Egger G, Mayr M, et al. Chronic infections and the risk of carotid atherosclerosis: prospective results from a large population study. Circulation 2001;103:1064–1070.

107. Mayr M, Kiechl S, Willeit J, Wick G, Xu Q. Infections, immunity, and atherosclerosis: associations of antibodies to *Chlamydia pneumoniae, Helicobacter pylori*, and cytomegalovirus with immune reactions to heat-shock protein 60 and carotid or femoral atherosclerosis. Circulation 2000;102: 833–839.

108. De Backer J, Mak R, De Bacquer D, et al. Parameters of inflammation and infection in a community based case-control study of coronary heart disease. Atherosclerosis 2002;160:457–463.

109. O'Connor S, Taylor C, Campbell LA, Epstein S, Libby P. Potential infectious etiologies of atherosclerosis: a multifactorial perspective. Emerg Infect Dis 2001;7:780–788.

110. Wright SD, Burton C, Hernandez M, et al. Infectious agents are not necessary for murine atherogenesis. J Exp Med 2000;191:1437–1442.

111. Kopp E, Medzhitov R. Recognition of microbial infection by Toll-like receptors. Curr Opin Immunol 2003;15:396–401.

112. Xu XH, Shah PK, Faure E, et al. Toll-like receptor-4 is expressed by macrophages in murine and human lipid-rich atherosclerotic plaques and upregulated by oxidized LDL. Circulation 2001;104:3103–3108.

113. Edfeldt K, Swedenborg J, Hansson GK, Yan ZQ. Expression of toll-like receptors in human atherosclerotic lesions: a possible pathway for plaque activation. Circulation 2002;105:1158–1161.

114. Kiechl S, Lorenz E, Reindl M, et al. Toll-like receptor 4 polymorphisms and atherogenesis. N Engl J Med 2002;347:185–192.

115. Erridge C, Stewart J, Poxton IR. Monocytes heterozygous for the Asp299Gly and Thr399Ile mutations in the Toll-like receptor 4 gene show no deficit in lipopolysaccharide signalling. J Exp Med 2003;197:1787–1791.

116. Vink A, Schoneveld AH, van der Meer JJ, et al. In vivo evidence for a role of toll-like receptor 4 in the development of intimal lesions. Circulation 2002;106:1985–1990.

117. Hollestelle SC, De Vries MR, Van Keulen JK, et al. Toll-like receptor 4 is involved in outward arterial remodeling. Circulation 2004;109:393–398.

118. Bulut Y, Faure E, Thomas L, et al. Chlamydial heat shock protein 60 activates macrophages and endothelial cells through Toll-like receptor 4 and MD2 in a MyD88-dependent pathway. J Immunol 2002;168:1435–1440.

119. Gelman AE, Zhang J, Choi Y, Turka LA. Toll-like receptor ligands directly promote activated CD4+ T-cell survival. J Immunol 2004;172:6065–6073.

120. Caramalho I, Lopes-Carvalho T, Ostler D, Zelenay S, Haury M, Demengeot J. Regulatory T-cells selectively express toll-like receptors and are activated by lipopolysaccharide. J Exp Med 2003;197:403–411.

121. Skalen K, Gustafsson M, Rydberg EK, et al. Subendothelial retention of atherogenic lipoproteins in early atherosclerosis. Nature 2002;417:750–754.

122. Cyrus T, Witztum JL, Rader DJ, et al. Disruption of the 12/15-lipoxygenase gene diminishes atherosclerosis in apo E-deficient mice. J Clin Invest 1999;103:1597–1604.

123. Mehrabian M, Allayee H, Wong J, et al. Identification of 5-lipoxygenase as a major gene contributing to atherosclerosis susceptibility in mice. Circ Res 2002;91:120–126.

124. Spanbroek R, Grabner R, Lotzer K, et al. Expanding expression of the 5-lipoxygenase pathway within the arterial wall during human atherogenesis. Proc Natl Acad Sci USA 2003;100:1238–1243.

125. Dwyer JH, Allayee H, Dwyer KM, et al. Arachidonate 5-lipoxygenase promoter genotype, dietary arachidonic acid, and atherosclerosis. N Engl J Med 2004;350:29–37.

126. Helgadottir A, Manolescu A, Thorleifsson G, et al. The gene encoding 5-lipoxygenase activating protein confers risk of myocardial infarction and stroke. Nat Genet 2004;36:233–239.

127. Hazen SL, Chisolm GM. Oxidized phosphatidylcholines: pattern recognition ligands for multiple pathways of the innate immune response. Proc Natl Acad Sci USA 2002;99:12,515–12,517.

128. Witztum JL, Steinberg D. The oxidative modification hypothesis of atherosclerosis: does it hold for humans? Trends Cardiovasc Med 2001;11:93–102.

129. Binder CJ, Horkko S, Dewan A, et al. Pneumococcal vaccination decreases atherosclerotic lesion formation: molecular mimicry between Streptococcus pneumoniae and oxidized LDL. Nat Med 2003;9:736–743.

130. Reardon CA, Miller ER, Blachowicz L, et al. Autoantibodies to OxLDL fail to alter the clearance of injected OxLDL in apolipoprotein E-deficient mice. J Lipid Res 2004;45:1347–1354.

131. Bharadwaj D, Stein MP, Volzer M, Mold C, Du Clos TW. The major receptor for C-reactive protein on leukocytes is fcgamma receptor II. J Exp Med 1999;190:585–590.

132. Mold C, Rodriguez W, Rodic-Polic B, Du Clos TW. C-reactive protein mediates protection from lipopolysaccharide through interactions with Fc gamma R. J Immunol 2002;169:7019–7025.

133. Griselli M, Herbert J, Hutchinson WL, et al. C-reactive protein and complement are important mediators of tissue damage in acute myocardial infarction. J Exp Med 1999;190:1733–1740.

134. Chang MK, Binder CJ, Torzewski M, Witztum JL. C-reactive protein binds to both oxidized LDL and apoptotic cells through recognition of a common ligand: Phosphorylcholine of oxidized phospholipids. Proc Natl Acad Sci USA 2002;99:13,043–13,048.

135. Henninger DD, Gerritsen ME, Granger DN. Low-density lipoprotein receptor knockout mice exhibit exaggerated microvascular responses to inflammatory stimuli. Circ Res 1997;81:274–281.

136. Navab M, Imes SS, Hama SY, et al. Monocyte transmigration induced by modification of low density lipoprotein in cocultures of human aortic wall cells is due to induction of monocyte chemotactic protein 1 synthesis and is abolished by high density lipoprotein. J Clin Invest 1991;88:2039–2046.

137. Netea MG, Demacker PN, Kullberg BJ, et al. Low-density lipoprotein receptor-deficient mice are protected against lethal endotoxemia and severe gram-negative infections. J Clin Invest 1996;97:1366–1372.

138. Roselaar SE, Daugherty A. Apolipoprotein E-deficient mice have impaired innate immune responses to Listeria monocytogenes in vivo. J Lipid Res 1998;39:1740–1743.

139. de Bont N, Netea MG, Demacker PN, et al. Apolipoprotein E knock-out mice are highly susceptible to endotoxemia and Klebsiella pneumoniae infection. J Lipid Res 1999;40:680–685.

140. Netea MG, Demacker PN, de Bont N, et al. Hyperlipoproteinemia enhances susceptibility to acute disseminated Candida albicans infection in low-density-lipoprotein-receptor-deficient mice. Infect Immun 1997;65:2663–2667.

141. Ludewig B, Jaggi M, Dumrese T, et al. Hypercholesterolemia exacerbates virus-induced immunopathologic liver disease via suppression of antiviral cytotoxic T-cell responses. J Immunol 2001;166:3369–3376.

142. Berencsi K, Endresz V, Klurfeld D, Kari L, Kritchevsky D, Gonczol E. Early atherosclerotic plaques in the aorta following cytomegalovirus infection of mice. Cell Adhes Commun 1998;5:39–47.

143. Persoons MC, Daemen MJ, Bruning JH, Bruggeman CA. Active cytomegalovirus infection of arterial smooth muscle cells in immunocompromised rats. A clue to herpesvirus-associated atherogenesis? Circ Res 1994;75:214–220.

144. Hamamdzic D, Harley RA, Hazen-Martin D, LeRoy EC. MCMV induces neointima in IFN-gammaR-/- mice: intimal cell apoptosis and persistent proliferation of myofibroblasts. BMC Musculoskelet Disord 2001;2:3.

145. Weck KE, Dal Canto AJ, Gould JD, et al. Murine gamma-herpesvirus 68 causes severe large-vessel arteritis in mice lacking interferon-gamma responsiveness: a new model for virus-induced vascular disease. Nat Med 1997;3:1346–1353.

146. Moazed TC, Kuo C, Grayston JT, Campbell LA. Murine models of *Chlamydia pneumoniae* infection and atherosclerosis. J Infect Dis 1997;175:883–890.

147. Hu H, Pierce GN, Zhong G. The atherogenic effects of chlamydia are dependent on serum cholesterol and specific to *Chlamydia pneumoniae*. J Clin Invest 1999;103:747–753.

148. Fabricant CG, Hajjar DP, Minick CR, Fabricant J. Herpesvirus infection enhances cholesterol and cholesteryl ester accumulation in cultured arterial smooth muscle cells. Am J Pathol 1981;105: 176–184.

149. Ludewig B, Ochsenbein AF, Odermatt B, Paulin D, Hengartner H, Zinkernagel RM. Immunotherapy with dendritic cells directed against tumor antigens shared with normal host cells results in severe autoimmune disease. J Exp Med 2000;191:795–804.

150. Ludewig B, Freigang S, Jaggi M, et al. Linking immune-mediated arterial inflammation and cholesterol-induced atherosclerosis in a transgenic mouse model. Proc Natl Acad Sci USA 2000;97:12,752–12,757.

151. Zhou X, Paulsson G, Stemme S, Hansson GK. Hypercholesterolemia is associated with a T helper (Th) 1/Th2 switch of the autoimmune response in atherosclerotic apo E-knockout mice. J Clin Invest 1998;101:1717–1725.

152. Blessing E, Campbell LA, Rosenfeld ME, Chough N, Kuo CC. *Chlamydia pneumoniae* infection accelerates hyperlipidemia induced atherosclerotic lesion development in C57BL/6J mice. Atherosclerosis 2001;158:13–17.

153. Xiong W, Zhao Y, Prall A, Greiner TC, Baxter BT. Key roles of CD4+ T-cells and IFN-gamma in the development of abdominal aortic aneurysms in a murine model. J Immunol 2004;172:2607–2612.

154. Schönbeck U, Sukhova GK, Gerdes N, Libby P. T(H)2 predominant immune responses prevail in human abdominal aortic aneurysm. Am J Pathol 2002;161:499–506.

155. Tellides G, Tereb DA, Kirkiles-Smith NC, et al. Interferon-gamma elicits arteriosclerosis in the absence of leukocytes. Nature 2000;403:207–211.

156. Maron R, Sukhova G, Faria AM, et al. Mucosal administration of heat shock protein-65 decreases atherosclerosis and inflammation in aortic arch of low-density lipoprotein receptor-deficient mice. Circulation 2002;106:1708–1715.

157. Ricote M, Valledor AF, Glass CK. Decoding transcriptional programs regulated by PPARs and LXRs in the macrophage: effects on lipid homeostasis, inflammation, and atherosclerosis. Arterioscler Thromb Vasc Biol 2004;24:230–239.

158. Lawrence T, Willoughby DA, Gilroy DW. Anti-inflammatory lipid mediators and insights into the resolution of inflammation. Nat Rev Immunol 2002; 2:787–795.

159. Castrillo A, Joseph SB, Vaidya SA, et al. Crosstalk between LXR and toll-like receptor signaling mediates bacterial and viral antagonism of cholesterol metabolism. Mol Cell 2003;12:805–816.

160. Janeway CA, P. T, M. W, Shlomchik MJ. Immunobiology, The immune system in health and disease. Garland, New York, USA, 2001, p. 732.

161. Yamamoto M, Takeda K, Akira S. TIR domain-containing adaptors define the specificity of TLR signaling. Mol Immunol 2004;40:861–868.

162. O'Neill LA. Immunology. After the toll rush. Science 2004;303:1481–1482.

163. Lucas AD, Greaves DR. Atherosclerosis: role of chemokines and macrophages. Expert Rev Mol Med 2001;2001:1–18.

164. Miller YI, Chang MK, Binder CJ, Shaw PX, Witztum JL. Oxidized low density lipoprotein and innate immune receptors. Curr Opin Lipidol 2003;14:437–445.
165. Young JL, Libby P, Schonbeck U. Cytokines in the pathogenesis of atherosclerosis. Thromb Haemost 2002;88:554–567.
166. Dansky HM, Charlton SA, Harper MM, Smith JD. T and B lymphocytes play a minor role in atherosclerotic plaque formation in the apolipoprotein E-deficient mouse. Proc Natl Acad Sci USA 1997;94:4642–4646.
167. Reardon CA, Blachowicz L, White T, et al. Effect of immune deficiency on lipoproteins and atherosclerosis in male apolipoprotein E-deficient mice. Arterioscler Thromb Vasc Biol 2001;21:1011–1016.
168. Daugherty A, Pure E, Delfel-Butteiger D, et al. The effects of total lymphocyte deficiency on the extent of atherosclerosis in apolipoprotein E-/- mice. J Clin Invest 1997;100:1575–1580.
169. Song L, Leung C, Schindler C. Lymphocytes are important in early atherosclerosis. J Clin Invest 2001;108:251–259.
170. Schönbeck U, Sukhova GK, Shimizu K, Mach F, Libby P. Inhibition of CD40 signaling limits evolution of established atherosclerosis in mice. Proc Natl Acad Sci USA 2000;97:7458–7463.
171. Gupta S, Pablo AM, Jiang X, Wang N, Tall AR, Schindler C. IFN-gamma potentiates atherosclerosis in ApoE knock-out mice. J Clin Invest 1997;99:2752–2761.
172. Whitman SC, Ravisankar P, Elam H, Daugherty A. Exogenous interferon-gamma enhances atherosclerosis in apolipoprotein E-/- mice. Am J Pathol 2000;157:1819–1824.
173. Pinderski LJ, Fischbein MP, Subbanagounder G, et al. Overexpression of interleukin-10 by activated T lymphocytes inhibits atherosclerosis in LDL receptor-deficient Mice by altering lymphocyte and macrophage phenotypes. Circ Res 2002;90:1064–1071.
174. Lee TS, Yen HC, Pan CC, Chau LY. The role of interleukin 12 in the development of atherosclerosis in ApoE-deficient mice. Arterioscler Thromb Vasc Biol 1999;19:734–742.
175. Whitman SC, Ravisankar P, Daugherty A. Interleukin-18 enhances atherosclerosis in apolipoprotein E(-/-) mice through release of interferon-gamma. Circ Res 2002;90:E34–E8.
176. Mallat Z, Gojova A, Marchiol-Fournigault C, et al. Inhibition of transforming growth factor-beta signaling accelerates atherosclerosis and induces an unstable plaque phenotype in mice. Circ Res 2001;89:930–934.
177. Lutgens E, Gijbels M, Smook M, et al. Transforming growth factor-beta mediates balance between inflammation and fibrosis during plaque progression. Arterioscler Thromb Vasc Biol 2002;22:975–982.
178. Nicoletti A, Kaveri S, Caligiuri G, Bariety J, Hansson GK. Immunoglobulin treatment reduces atherosclerosis in apo E knockout mice. J Clin Invest 1998;102:910–918.
179. Afek A, George J, Gilburd B, et al. Immunization of low-density lipoprotein receptor deficient (LDL-RD) mice with heat shock protein 65 (HSP-65) promotes early atherosclerosis. J Autoimmun 2000;14:115–121.
180. Freigang S, Horkko S, Miller E, Witztum JL, Palinski W. Immunization of LDL receptor-deficient mice with homologous malondialdehyde-modified and native LDL reduces progression of atherosclerosis by mechanisms other than induction of high titers of antibodies to oxidative neoepitopes. Arterioscler Thromb Vasc Biol 1998;18:1972–1982.
181. George J, Afek A, Gilburd B, et al. Hyperimmunization of apo-E-deficient mice with homologous malondialdehyde low-density lipoprotein suppresses early atherogenesis. Atherosclerosis 1998;138: 147–152.
182. Zhou X, Caligiuri G, Hamsten A, Lefvert AK, Hansson GK. LDL immunization induces T-cell-dependent antibody formation and protection against atherosclerosis. Arterioscler Thromb Vasc Biol 2001;21:108–114.
183. Buono C, Come CE, Witztum JL, et al. Influence of C3 deficiency on atherosclerosis. Circulation 2002;105:3025–3031.
184. Dollery CM, Owen CA, Sukhova GK, Krettek A, Shapiro SD, Libby P. Neutrophil elastase in human atherosclerotic plaques: production by macrophages. Circulation 2003;107:2829–2836.
185. Sukhova GK, Zhang Y, Pan JH, et al. Deficiency of cathepsin S reduces atherosclerosis in LDL receptor-deficient mice. J Clin Invest 2003;111:897–906.

# 7 Animal Restenosis Models

## From the Ideal Model to the Ideal Study

*Arturo G. Touchard, MD*
*and Robert S. Schwartz, MD*

## INTRODUCTION

Human coronary artery research is limited by an inability to control experiments and by the slowness of lesion development. Animal arterial injury models offer an opportunity for understanding restenosis mechanisms and for testing new treatments for safety and efficacy. In these models the pathophysiological aspects of disease can be simulated, variables can be controlled, and statistical data accrued in short time periods. The ideal animal restenosis model should have comparable human coronary anatomy, histology, and physiology. It should closely mimic human restenosis pathophysiology and reliably predict the outcome of human clinical trials. Other ideal characteristics include availability, inexpensive to acquire and maintain, and easy to handle. Many animal models have been used for restenosis studies. This variety comes because the ideal animal model does not exist. Each animal model has advantages and disadvantages. This chapter discusses the principal animal models described for restenosis studies, their characteristics, advantages, and disadvantages compared with humans, and the considerations necessary for proximity to and ideal animal model and study design.

## ANIMAL RESTENOSIS MODELS IN COMMON USE

Arterial restenosis in both humans and animals is a directed, reparative response after arterial insult. Similarly, all animal restenosis models are based on arterial injury. The arterial response to injury or the arterial healing induced by the injury will be the final cause of restenosis. There is no single arterial injury method that produces ideal

From: *Contemporary Cardiology: Essentials of Restenosis: For the Interventional Cardiologist*
Edited by: H. J. Duckers, E. G. Nabel, and P. W. Serruys © Humana Press Inc., Totowa, NJ

restenosis (repeatable, severe stenoses, similar to human physiology and histopathology, and so on). Several artery injuries have been developed, generally adapted to the animal model and their artery size. Common animals models used for restenosis studies include rodents (rats, mice, and rabbits), pigs, dogs, or primates. Frequent injury methods used in these models include mechanical injury overstretch artery with non-compliant angioplasty balloons inflated to high pressures, very compliant, low-pressure balloons for denudation injury *(1–3)*, wire loops *(4–8)*, or directional atherectomy, or injury induced by agents such chemical diet, electrical injury *(9)*, heat *(10)*, air desiccation *(11–13)*, irradiation *(14)*, or inducing severe inflammation with copper stents by foreign body implant *(15–18)*.

To enhance the lesion formation or for reproducing the human arterial angioplasty environment (such as atheroma presence), before or after the "principal" injury, other authors have developed complementary injurious methods. Animals can be placed on a high-fat high-cholesterol diet (chemical injury) or undergo other nondietary injury modes, alone or in tandem with the cholesterol diet. These create double or triple injury as models. It is unclear if such complementary injuries may positively or negatively affect final results of a study.

## *Rodents*

### RAT CAROTID ARTERY MODEL

Extensive studies on the response to vascular injury were performed in the rat carotid artery model years before angioplasty became known. These studies, based on denudation injury with a very compliant, low-pressure balloon, identified the intimal layer as a key site in the proliferative response. In this model, both carotid arteries are typically used in the same animal (Fig. 1). The rat carotid artery is injured either by air desiccation *(12,13)* or by balloon endothelial denudation *(1–3)*. A 2 French Fogarty balloon is advanced through an incision in the external carotid artery to the common carotid artery. The balloon is inflated and drawn through the artery (while inflated) for multiple passes, generally three or more times. The balloon is deflated and removed, and the external carotid artery is ligated.

### MOUSE ARTERIAL INJURY MODEL

The mouse arterial injury model came into use as a restenosis model owing to the widespread knowledge of the mouse genome and availability of powerful molecular biological methods in the mouse *(19,20)*. The small vessel size and their consequent manipulation have yielded several injury methods. They include a small guidewire rotated in the vessel *(4–6)*, transarterial electrical injury *(21,22)*, a nonconstricting hollow polyethylene tube place around the mouse carotid artery (in this technique the internal elastic lamina remains intact), or atherectomy.

### HYPERCHOLESTEROLEMIC RABBIT ILIAC MODEL

The rabbit atherosclerotic iliac restenosis model has been one of the most commonly used animal models. Although the restenotic lesions differ from human lesions, this model provides valuable insights for understanding the mechanism of repair after injury to an abnormal artery and for testing restenosis therapies *(23–31)*. Rabbit models are typically single-, double- ,or even triple-injury models: Usually a biochemical injury with hypercholesterolemic diets is followed by mechanical injury into both femoral arteries with a 3F Fogarty catheter (advanced and withdrawn five to six times to denude

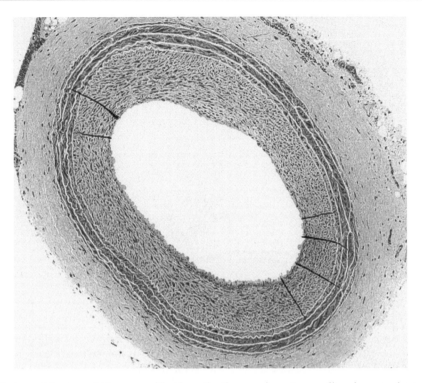

**Fig. 1.** Rat carotid artery. At low magnifications the three major artery wall regions can be seen. The inner layer is the intima, the outer layer (concentric white bands) is the adventitia. In between is the tunica media. Note the pink staining, corresponding to the elastic laminae in the tunica media, which is typical for the elastic arteries, such as the carotid artery. H&E staining. (Please *see* insert for color version.)

endothelium), or air desiccation. Four to six weeks after injury, both arteries are examined arteriographically for stenoses. If a significant lesion is found, an angioplasty (second mechanical injury) is performed under fluoroscopic guidance.

### Rabbit Ear Crush Injury Model

This is an interesting restenosis model, easy to perform, inexpensive, and can be produced rapidly in the ear arteries of New Zealand rabbits. Crush pressure is externally applied at two sites of the central ear artery of anesthetized hypercholesterolemic New Zealand rabbits. The rabbits are then maintained on a diet of 2.4% fat and 1% cholesterol. Area stenoses of roughly 40% of the original 0.5–1 mm diameter lumen develop, with neointimal thickening beginning at day 5.

## *Dog*

Dogs have been explored as an experimental model for restenosis mainly because of their size, cost, and ready availability. However, dogs have high fibrinolytic activity *(32)*, markedly different from the human coagulation system *(33)*. In addition, the canine vessel wall produces only a thin neointima when compared with other animal models *(34)* (Fig. 2). These considerations make the dog a poor model for restenosis.

## *Pig*

Lesions are created in porcine carotid or coronary arteries.

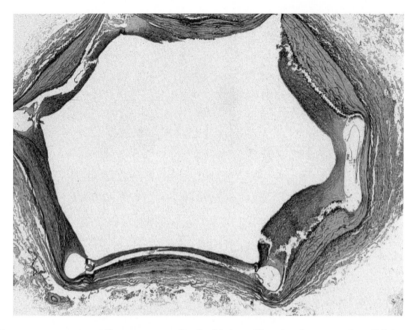

**Fig. 2.** Dog coronary artery after severe mechanical injury. Despite deep vessel wall injury partially extending to the external elastic lamina, the amount of neointima is minimal and clearly nonobstructive. Elastic van Giesson stain. (Please *see* insert for color version.)

### PORCINE CAROTID INJURY MODEL

The response of porcine carotid arteries to injury has been studied extensively *(35–37)*. In the porcine carotid injury model, denudation is usually achieved by advancing a 9 mm balloon catheter from the femoral artery into the common carotid artery. After inflation the balloon is drawn through the carotid three or four times, to cause endothelial denudation and occasionally deep arterial injury *(35,37–39)*.

### PORCINE CORONARY INJURY MODEL

The porcine heart and its coronary artery system have a size and anatomical structure very similar to that of humans (Fig. 3) *(18,40,41)*. The carotid arteries are typically used for arterial access in this model, although the femoral arteries may also be used without difficulty. Using the carotid rather than the femoral artery results in a lower occurrence of postoperative hematoma formation, which is frequently a problem in porcine femoral arteriotomies. Standard guide catheters and curves for human coronary angioplasty are used in both techniques for engagement of the left main or right coronary arteries, which is a great advantage of these models.

In this model, mechanical injury by oversizing the artery and endothelial denudation alone has proven successful. However, oversizing is a considerably stronger stimulus for smooth muscle cell proliferation than endothelial denudation alone. Oversizing the coronary artery can be achieved using a coronary angioplasty balloon *(42,43)* or oversized stent implantation *(44)*. This model produces a neointimal response virtually identical to human restenotic neointima in terms of cell size, cell density, and histopathological appearance *(34,41,45,46)*. Specimens from balloon-only injury typically show a single laceration of media, and specimens from oversized stent

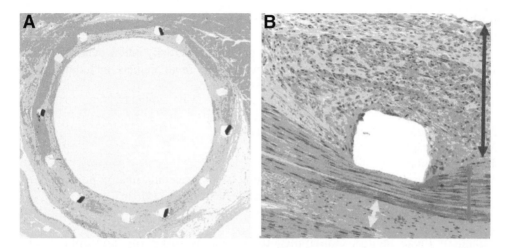

**Fig. 3.** Pig coronary artery **(A,B)**. Twenty eight days after mechanical injury (stent oversizing). This model produces a neointimal response (blue double head arrow) virtually identical to human restenotic neointima in terms of cell size, cell density, and histopathological appearance. Green double arrow: media. Yellow double arrow: adventitia. H&E staining. (Please *see* insert for color version.)

implantation show multiple injuries in the neighborhood of the stent wires, also very similar to human findings.

### Nonhuman Primates

Nonhuman primates bear phylogenetic resemblance to humans, a potentially singular advantage. The temporal sequence of proliferative response and thrombotic activity in coronary arteries is not well related to human restenosis and other animals. Their limited availability, legal restrictions, ethical concerns, and high cost, make this animal model impractical. Few studies using primate arteries to balloon catheter injury have thus been reported *(47–51)*.

### Transgenic Variants

A particularly powerful application of modern genetics to animal husbandry is the development of transgenic animals. Gene manipulation permits the selective deletion of one or more genes (knockout technology) or systemic gene transfer. This permits improved experimental controls and the observation of its effects at molecular, cellular, and histological levels. Rats and mice are the most advanced transgenic models. These animal models have well-defined genetic characterization; Transgenic and gene knockout animals are readily available.

### IS THERE A SPECIES-SPECIFIC ARTERIAL RESPONSE TO ARTERIAL INJURY?

A fundamental and universal survival mechanism is healing of the injured artery. However, all species have individualized molecular and cellular arterial healing mechanisms. Stenosis following injury differs immensely across species. Rats, mice, and porcine carotid injury models form hemodynamically significant stenoses only rarely. In hypercholesterolemic rabbits and porcine coronary arteries, macroscopic and hemodynamically significant stenoses may develop, but it does not occur systematically.

In general, six factors or phases, separated in time and partially interdependent, are common aspects in restenosis pathogenesis following injury in all animals, including humans:

1. Arterial damage (endothelial denudation, internal elastic lamina fracture, media injury, adventitial injury);
2. Platelet aggregation and Thrombus formation;
3. Elastic recoil;
4. Inflammation;
5. Smooth muscle cell migration, proliferation, and extracellular matrix production *(52)*, the principal responsible of the neointimal thickening *(53–56)*; and
6. Arterial remodeling.

Each of these factors contributes to restenosis following angioplasty alone *(57,58)*. However, following stent placement, endothelial damage, thrombosis, inflammation, and intimal hyperplasia appears to be the predominant pathology *(59,60)*. No single model appears to have all component processes identical to humans. Species-specific differences in arterial healing must be considered in study design and interpretation. Failure to account for these can cause confusion, potential data misinterpretation, or errors. Restenosis pathophysiology is described elsewhere in this book. The purpose of the present section is to highlight pathophysiological differences between species.

## *Arterial Damage and Injury Score*

All types of arterial injury begin with endothelial denudation, and progress to deeper injury. The degree and susceptibility to deeper injury exhibit species specificity. In the rat carotid model, injury typically shows endothelial denudation, remaining intact other arterial structures such the internal elastic lamina, media, and external elastic lamina (Fig. 1) *(61)*. This mild injury contrasts to deeper arterial injury usually observed in the rabbit iliac and porcine coronary arteries (Figs. 3 and 4), where internal elastic lamina and medial dissection is similar to the endothelial and medial damage following human percutaneous coronary intervention.

The type of injury may also induce different arterial injury degree even in the same animal. For example, arterial injury in rats is different, using a wire loop were only endothelial denudation is seen. This is compared with electric injury where wide necrosis zones from intima to adventitia can be seen. This different injury could stimulate different arterial healing phases in the same animal models.

Severity of mechanical injury across animal models might account for variability in neointimal hyperplasia. A porcine coronary injury score (Fig. 4) based on the integrity of the structural components of the vessel wall has resulted from such observations. This progressively relates superficial vessel wall damage (injury score of zero) to newly formed neointima that is very thin, as occurs with appropriately sized stenting. Stenoses develop progressively only when stent wires fracture the internal elastic lamina (score 1), or lacerate the media (score 2) or the external elastic lamina (score 3). It is unknown whether the elastin membranes influence the biomolecular aspects of neointima formation or if it can be regarded only as a marker for injury severity. There is evidence that the internal elastic membrane may function as a barrier for the diffusion of macromolecules from the lumen and as a base for the attachment of endothelial cells *(62)*. The injury score can be

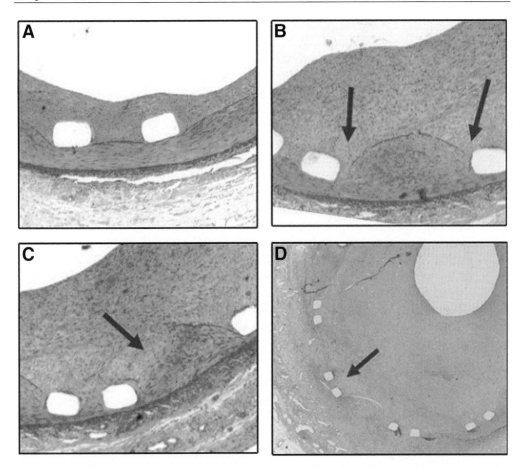

**Fig. 4.** Injury score in the porcine coronary artery. **(A)** Injury score of zero: Superficial vessel wall damage but internal elastic lamina is intact. **(B)** Score 1: stent wires have fractured the internal elastic lamina but media are intact. **(C)** Score 2: media are lacerated but external elastic lamina is intact. **(D)** Score 3: external elastic lamina is lacerated. (Please *see* insert for color version.)

used to compare studies and quantitate the response with potential therapies *(34,63,64)*. The peripheral arteries have been used similarly in examining the arterial response to injury *(65–67)*.

## Thrombus Formation: The Importance of the Thrombotic and Fibrinolytic Response

After arterial injury, the clotting and fibrinolytic mechanisms are activated. This response to vessel wall injury is substantially different across species *(32,33,41,68)*, and different amounts of mural thrombus can be seen depending the animal model used. In the rat carotid and canine models, significant fibrin-rich thrombus is rarely if ever found. Conversely, in the rabbit iliac and porcine model, macroscopic thrombus does occur and has been characterized in several reports. Primates have comparable fibrinolytic or hemostatic systems to humans. For example, baboons are prone to acute stent thrombosis within the first 3 d after the procedure, which is significantly different than the acute stent occlusion in pig arteries, which usually occurs within 6 h *(18,32,69)*.

Mural thrombus provides a scaf-fold for medial smooth muscle cell colonization. According to this concept, the amount of mural thrombus might govern the total neointimal burden.

This could explain, among other factors, why rat carotid and dog coronary arteries may not generate substantial neointimal volume (and macroscopic stenoses) in distinction to the rabbit and porcine models. Against this theory is that numerous anticoagulation trials have failed to impact restenosis, including warfarin, heparin, and direct thrombin inhibitors. However, whether these regimes eliminate local thrombus formation is unknown.

Differences in mural thrombus formation after angioplasty must be present in the design and interpretation of antithrombotic agents in various models. Animal models with higher tendency to thrombus formation (pigs, for example) can be more sensitive to antithrombotic agents than humans. It is thus possible that antithrombotic agents are effective for pigs but not for humans. Several examples exist in the literature, such prostacyclin *(70)*, aspirin *(71)*, and hirudin *(72–74)*, or low-molecular weight heparin *(75)*, where studies performed in pigs, show some efficacy of hemostatic interventions in the reduction of restenosis that failed in humans *(76–78)*. However, as discussed later, different end points in the animal studies may cause differences from human studies. As mural thrombus may provide a scaf-fold for medial smooth muscle cell colonization, the tendency to thrombus formation may be an explanation why some antiproliferative therapies demonstrate significant inhibition of neointimal hyperplasia in some animal models that do not translate to clinical trials. In summary, more or less thrombus formation must be present when choosing an animal model for antithrombotic therapy testing and in the extrapolation of the results in humans.

## *Inflammation*

Few studies document the role of inflammation in restenosis, although it is key. In addition, inflammation resolution is also important as it may produce a scar fibrosis, and resultant negative remodeling. In the rat carotid model of injury, there is remarkably little inflammatory response to injury. Hypercholesterolemic rabbits, porcine, and non-primate models show robust inflammatory reactions to injury (Fig. 5), with early mononuclear cell infiltration from the lumen into the thrombus *(68,79)*. In the porcine model inflammation is positively related to neointimal thickness *(80)*. Human studies of stented arteries also show acute inflammation early after implantation, especially when stenting is associated with medial injury or lipid core penetration *(81–83)*. Macrophage infiltration in atherectomy tissue and the activation status of blood mono-cytes correlate with an increased rate of restenosis *(84,85)*.

## *Smooth Muscle Cell Proliferation and Migration*

Although rat and mouse studies initiated the concept of proliferation, such proliferation and migration from media to intima, is considered a prominent feature in all animal models. Despite the observation that SMC neointima formation causes in-stent restenosis, the role of cell proliferation within the neointima remains controversial. It is uncertain if there is a species-specific cell proliferation and migration. Cell proliferation and migration in rats, mice, and pigs begin early after denudation (1 or 2 d) and proceed for the following 14–30 d (peaking in 2–3 wk) *(18,54,86)*. The Rabbit iliac model shows proliferation over the same period with peak at 8 d *(87)*. In nonhuman primates, proliferation is increased at 4 and 7 d but later declines to control rates *(50)*. Regardless of the fact that animal models show a hyperplastic response to injury, kinetics of cell proliferation in human vessels does not appear well defined. Human lesions show a comparative hypocellular response with abundant matrix.

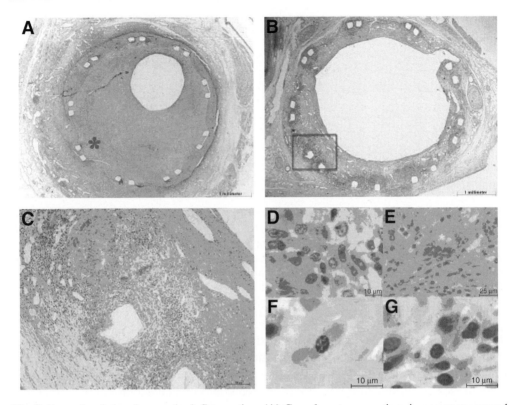

**Fig. 5.** Example of chronic vascular inflammation. **(A)** Granulomatous reactions in one artery around the penetrating struts (red asterisk). **(B)** Generalized granulomatous reaction in a stent venous section. **(C)** Magnified image (×100) of red square of B shows typical granulomatous reaction (*see* text). **(D)** Macrophages of Fig. C (×400). **(E)** Giant cell of Fig. C (yellow asterisk) (×200). **(F)** Plasma cells of Fig. C (×800). **(G)** Eosinophils of Fig. C (×800). and B × 20 Movat staining. C to G H&E staining. (Please *see* insert for color version.)

## *Elastic Recoil and Remodeling*

Acute elastic recoil immediately following balloon deflation and late vascular constriction (negative remodeling) *(88–91)* occur with PTCA alone, and are important aspects of restenosis pathophysiology in the present era. Coronary stents acting as a mechanical scaf-fold within the vessel, eliminating elastic recoil and vessel contracture. *(92,93)* Hypercholesterolemic rabbit *(94,95)*, porcine coronary artery *(96)*, and nonhuman primates *(97)* exhibit remodeling behavior in much the same fashion as man *(98)*. Mouse arteries tend to enlarge after angioplasty and appear naturally prone to positive remodeling *(21,99)*. Regardless that remodeling is lost in the stent era, animal models prone to positive or negative remodeling must be a consideration today as positive vascular remodeling occurs after bare-metal stent implantation *(92)*, after catheter-based radiation followed by conventional stent implantation *(93)* but not demonstrated, after drug-eluting stent implantation.

## DRUG STUDIES

Animal models have been used for testing new drugs, which will be tried in subsequently human clinical trials. Drug studies have two aims. First, they assess drug safety, and second, they assess the efficacy of the specific drug and reduce the restenosis rates.

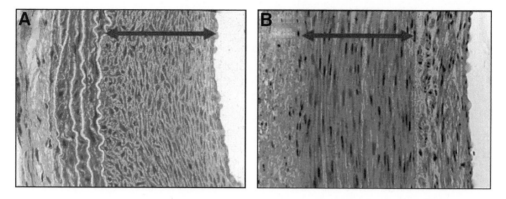

**Fig. 6.** Differences between elastic arteries and muscular arteries. **(A)** Rat carotid artery. The media (blue arrow) of elastic vessels is mostly elastin (large number of pink staining within the media), with proportionally fewer SMC (obscure structures). This is opposite to muscular arteries. **(B)** Porcine coronary artery as example of muscular arteries. Note that the media contain few elastin fibers and more SMC with their typical spindle form. The purpose of elastic conductance vessels is to convert the sudden systolic pressure impulse into potential energy. Muscular vessels design is to permit vessel diameter change in response to end-organ need for the muscular arteries. (Please *see* insert for color version.)

Recent examples of animals models assessing safety of new therapies are the porcine model prediction of acute and late stent thrombosis in brachytherapy *(100–102)* and inflammation from polymers of drug-eluting stents. Several studies show that many polymers induce an inflammatory response, which could induce neointima or thrombosis *(17,103–105)*, and may thus pose a concern for clinical stent application. They also show that among all polymers there are some, which may be more satisfactory *(105,106)*, showing minor inflammatory reactions to polymer-coated stents. These good results are compatible with those in humans.

The ideal experimental model to assess restenosis treatment would be one that reliably predicts the risks and outcome of human clinical trials. Although such an ideal model does not yet exist, experimental studies are ongoing. Many pharmacological agents, such as antiplatelet, anticoagulants, angiotensin-converting enzyme inhibitors, and antiproliferative drugs, have been tested successfully in animal models failed in human clinical trials. The marked disparity of results between animal model research and clinical trials has led to skepticism about the validity of animal models in restenosis research. The failure of animal studies to predict efficacy in preventing human restenosis is potentially attributable to two general factors. Species differences may in part be responsible, a factor not easily modified except with transgenic animals. Second, there are several modifiable factors, not taken into account, which are able to approach the current models to the ideal animal model.

### *Anatomically Different Arteries: Coronary vs Peripheral*

Coronary arteries are muscular vessels. Several studies use elastic arteries, despite the obvious differences (Fig. 6). The aorta, carotid, or iliac arteries are examples of elastic arteries. Several reasons exist for thinking that the type of artery may affect the studies positive predictive value. Elastic arteries stretch during angioplasty whereas muscular arteries are more likely to tear in response to balloon inflation. These characteristics may result in a higher degree of injury and subsequent stenosis for muscular arteries and perhaps explain why the rat carotid is resistant, showing typically only endothelial denudation with low-stenosis rates. Also, because neointimal hyperplasia in restenosis results from smooth muscle cell migration and proliferation, it is tempting to hypothesize that vessels containing proportionally more smooth muscle cells might respond more vigorously to arterial injury, affecting to the final stenosis.

Finally, it is possible that mechanisms responsible for restenosis in anatomically distinct vascular locations are different. Two different lineages of SMCs, responding differently to the same growth factors and cytokines have been identified in the media of large elastic arteries in the avian embryo (107,108). Also, different proliferative properties of SMC exist, analyzing human arterial and venous bypass vessels (109). In the same manner, it is likely that muscular and elastic arteries have different responses to injury. These differences suggest that the type of vessel chosen for instrumentation may significantly influence the outcome. For antirestenosis testing, coronary arteries are recommended. The role of other muscular arteries, such as brachial, radial, or femoral vessels, in animal models remains poorly defined.

### Clinical Relevance

An ideal response parameter between animal and humans does not yet exist. For efficacy assessment, animal model end points traditionally used quantitative measurements based on histopathological studies. Neointima area, neointima thickness, or residual lumen size are examples. They are measured precisely and compared across treatment groups using digital microscopic methods. Conversely, human clinical trials quantitative end points are based on angiographic measurements, where lumen diameter or percentage of luminal stenosis is measured by quantitative coronary analysis (QCA) or intravascular ultrasound (IVUS). Histopathological measurements by microscopy have higher sensitivity compared with angiography or IVUS. Neointimal thickness, for example, must be at least 0.36 mm to be detectable by angiography (110). Thus, in animal studies, when both treatment groups are compared, histological changes may be minimal, but can be statistically significant. This statistical significance may not translate to real life scenarios and might have little or no relevance, even if detectable by conventional methods like QCA or IVUS.

These end point differences are partially responsible for discrepant study results between animal and clinical studies, especially when the reduction in neointima formation is minimal. In addition to histopathological findings, it is recommended for efficacy assessment in animal studies that QCA or IVUS parameters. All parameters must be carefully analyzed together with the histological data. The small size of coronary arteries in many animal models, such as rat or mice makes certain models unsuitable for these purposes. A problem applying these techniques in assessing animal study efficacy is that with current animal models, repeatable significant stenoses cannot be achieved, so the statistical analysis does not have enough power. Currently, significant repeatable stenosis can be induced, producing severe injury. The penetration or rupture of the external elastic lamina is not useful for studying restenosis therapies, as it is such a severe injury it overwhelms the therapeutic modality, and the effect is lost to observation. Developing an animal model in which significant stenosis can be reproduced systematically for angiography and IVUS assessment is currently of paramount importance and remains under study.

### Small or Large Arteries?

Human studies assess binary angiographic stenosis (defined as stenosis diameter >50%). Artery size is important for restenosis angiographic evaluation. In small arteries (such as in mice, 0.4 mm diameter) a 50% angiographic restenosis is caused by microscopic neointimal thickening (as little as 100 μm). However, to produce the same 50% stenosis in human arteries (2.5–4 mm diameter), thickness more than 500 μm is required. To avoid misinterpretation with angiographic restenosis, arteries with size comparable with humans should be used.

## Drug Dosage and Timing Regimens

Other factors that may influence negative the predictive positive value of the animal studies are substantially for different drug-dose schedules from animal studies compared with human studies. Notable examples using different doses in animals than humans include the IECA *(111–113)*, colchicines *(114–116)*, or hirudin *(72,76)* studies. These drugs demonstrated reduced proliferative responses following angioplasty in animal models but not in clinical trials. In such studies up to 50 times higher drug doses were used in the animals compared with humans *(18)*. These differences raise the question of whether the negative results of the clinical trials were attributable to drug ineffectiveness species differences, or inadequate drug doses. It is possible but unlikely that the high doses used in animal models were comparable in efficacy if the same doses had been used in human trials.

Other example involves different drug timing. Hirudin studies demonstrated inhibition of neointimal formation by long-term (14 d), but not short-term administration (2 d) in pigs *(74)* and rats *(117)*. Human studies were carried out with only periprocedural drug administration, and negative human study results might be owing to inadequate duration of treatment rather than ineffectiveness of the drug *(74,78)*.

Animal studies should be performed more comparably with human studies. It is important to use the same doses (weight-adjusted doses) and identical drug timing. The time-course of the response and, therefore, the time required for an agent to be active may be very different in humans compared with animals. In general, the smaller the animal and the simpler the structure of the vessel wall, the faster the response to injury is completed. In contrast, successful therapy in humans may require chronic administration or a truly irreversible change in vessel wall cells rather than just a transient suppression or delay in cell proliferation.

## Arterial Injury Documentation

Clinical studies strongly support the concept of a relationship between vessel injury severity and restenosis risk. Larger initial lumen gains may lead to higher restenosis rates *(118,119)*. Animal models also show the same behavior, with a positive relationship between arterial injury (injury score) and neointimal thickness.

Vessel injury can be directly and semiquantitatively assessed in all models by histopathological assessment, a major advantage in animal models. Validating and analyzing the relation between arterial damage and neointimal formation for all present and future animal models and type of injuries are of paramount importance. If vessel injury is not accounted for as a covariate in studies, artifact-laden results may occur, because conclusions regarding differences in efficacy might result from differences in injury among the treated and control groups.

When mean injury scores and mean neointimal thickness for a histological section are compared (Fig. 7A), a highly significant linear regression results *(46,63,69)*. This linear regression yields a slope and a y-intercept (Fig. 7B). It has been shown that injury score regression slope appears relatively constant within a species (species-specific)

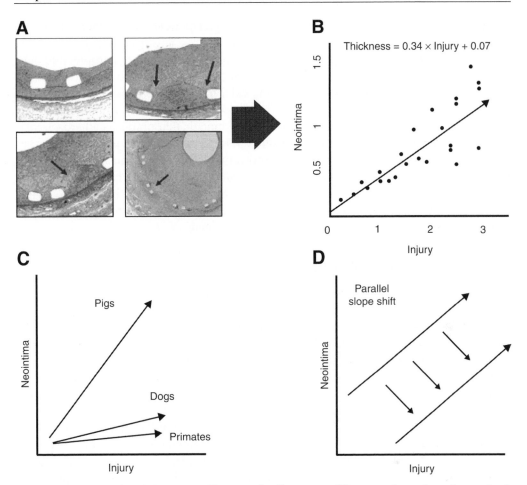

**Fig. 7.** Importance of the injury score. For more details *see* text. (Please *see* insert for color version.)

*(41)* (Fig. 7C). The linear regression evaluation has important implications. The regression slope can be used to estimate known and future animal models as a good model for restenosis efficacy testing. For example, the gentle slope of the dog or rat model with relatively little neointima in response to injury makes the dog a poor model for restenosis, whereas the steep slope of the pig model resembles the human response to angioplasty more closely and makes this model good to test restenosis therapies. The injury–neointimal thickness relationship of the baboon has a slope intermediate between dogs and pig model *(41,68,69)* (Fig. 7C). Linear regression can also be used for quantitative assessment of restenosis therapies, as restenosis therapies may affect the y-intercept, and for the same injury, they produce less neointimal thickness. This translates into a parallel linear regression (similar slope) but under the original (y intercept shifts downward) *(46,120)* (Fig. 7D).

## Unknowns in Models

The importance of several biological factors variability between species in restenosis or in the positive or negative predictive values are unknown. The impact of concomitant atherosclerosis in animal models is not well defined. Restenosis can be studied on either normal or previously injured arteries. The most commonly employed technique is the arterial injury over a normal coronary artery. The normal coronary artery of a young rat, rabbit, or pig differs distinctly from the atherosclerotic coronary artery of an older patient. Arteries of these animal models, even those of with hyperlipidemic diets (developing during a few weeks instead of decades as in humans), do not show densely fibrous and acellular plaques with ulceration, calcification, thrombosis, or hemorrhage into the vessel wall, all features of human restenosis. The impact of this atherosclerotic environment on restenosis and whether the use of models that produces atherosclerosis will have advantages over nonatherosclerotic models is also unknown.

Another consideration is the impact of protective molecules against atherosclerosis in restenoisis models such cholesteryl ester transferase or the high levels of HDL and low levels of LDL in mice. Cholesteryl ester transferase is present in humans, swine, and rabbits and is deficient in dogs and rodents. This enzyme explains in part the difficulty in inducing atheroma lesions in these latter animals *(121,122)*.

## CONCLUSIONS: THE IDEAL STUDY

Many "catastrophic" articles in the last decade have been written about the failure of animal models in predict results in human trials. These have generated distrust in the current animal models, but little true data exist about the true place for these models and their relation to humans. There is no doubt that animal models have significantly advanced the understanding of the mechanisms of restenosis formation and have served to improve the therapeutic options. For the moment, a single ideal global model does not exist, but promising research is ongoing in this area. At present, compromises in choosing an animal model are inevitable. A detailed species understanding for limitations and strength features must be considered for the specific purpose of the study (e.g., thrombosis vs migration), for the results interpretation and for human extrapolation. Taking in account all data commented in the present chapter, the "ideal model" should instead be considered of an "ideal study." A rational approach to the ideal study is important.

Arterial response to injury (pathogenesis) studies: Multiple animal models are valid. As this model serves to create hypothesis and subsequently new treatment strategies, minimal arterial changes may be sufficient. New hypothesis and treatment strategies should be confirmed in animal models that demonstrate good predictive values, such as the coronary porcine model. Safety studies: earlier comments about artery type, devices, dosage, and drug timing, animal pathophysiological differences must be considered. More close alignment with human stenting is strongly recommended. For this purpose, not all animal models would be valid.

Efficacy studies: The fundamental parameter besides safety studies is the amount of neointimal hyperplasia. Models with more neointima are typically the best models. It is of paramount importance to assess histological information along the same human end points, such as angiographic restenosis or IVUS. All results should be regularly reported and carefully evaluated. To date, considering all models, the porcine overstretch coronary artery appears closest to humans for global use as its coronary anatomy, physiology, and pathophysiology. In addition, it permits use of the same devices used in humans and produces the thickest neointima in response to injury.

Animal models will continue to provide more complete understanding of restenosis and to find the improved therapies for human restenosis. However, efforts for developing improved animal models must continue. New animal models, which are now under investigation may provide additional insight into new and important aspects of animal models that could predict the success of therapeutic interventions in animals and ultimately in humans.

## REFERENCES

1. Golden MA, Au YP, Kenagy RD, et al. Growth factor gene expression by intimal cells in healing polytetrafluoroethylene grafts. J Vasc Surg 1990;11:580–585.
2. Au YP, Kenagy RD, Clowes AW. Heparin selectively inhibits the transcription of tissue-type plasminogen activator in primate arterial smooth muscle cells during mitogenesis. J Biol Chem 1992;267:3438–3444.
3. Clowes AW, Clowes MM, Vergel SC, et al. The Renin-Angiotensin System and the Vascular Wall: From Experimental Models to Man: Heparin and Cilazapril Together Inhibit Injury-Induced Intimal Hyperplasia. Hypertension Suppl 1991;18:65–69.
4. Lindner V, Collins T. Expression of NF-kappa B and I kappa B-alpha by aortic endothelium in an arterial injury model. Am J Pathol 1996;148:427–438.
5. Lindner V, Reidy MA. Expression of VEGF receptors in arteries after endothelial injury and lack of increased endothelial regrowth in response to VEGF. Arterioscler Thromb Vasc Biol 1996;16:1399–1405.
6. Lindner V, Lappi DA, Baird A, et al. Original Contributions: Role of Basic Fibroblast Growth Factor in Vascular Lesion Formation. Circ Res 1991;68:106–113.
7. Reidy MA, Schwartz SM. Endothelial regeneration. III. Time course of intimal changes after small defined injury to rat aortic endothelium. Lab Invest 1981;44:301–308.
8. Walker LN, Ramsay MM, Bowyer DE. Endothelial healing following defined injury to rabbit aorta. Depth of injury and mode of repair. Atherosclerosis 1983;47:123–130.
9. Carmeliet P, Moons L, Stassen JM, et al. Vascular wound healing and neointima formation induced by perivascular electric injury in mice. Am J Pathol 1997;150:761–776.
10. Douek PC, Correa R, Neville R, et al. Dose-dependent smooth muscle cell proliferation induced by thermal injury with pulsed infrared lasers. Circulation 1992;86:1249–1256.
11. Fishman JA, Ryan GB, Karnovsky MJ. Endothelial regeneration in the rat carotid artery and the significance of endothelial denudation in the pathogenesis of myointimal thickening. Lab Invest 1975;32:339–351.
12. Sarembock IJ, Gertz SD, Thome LM, et al. Effectiveness of hirulog in reducing restenosis after balloon angioplasty of atherosclerotic femoral arteries in rabbits. J Vasc Res 1996;33:308–314.
13. Gellman J, Sigal SL, Chen Q, et al. The effect of tpa on restenosis following balloon angioplasty: a study in the atherosclerotic rabbit. J Am Coll Cardiol 1991;17:25A.
14. Fajardo LF, Berthrong M. Vascular lesions following radiation. Pathol Annu 1988;23:297–330.
15. Staab ME, Meeker DK, Edwards WD. et al. Reliable models of severe coronary stenosis in porcine coronary arteries: lesion induction by high temperature or copper stent. J Intervent Cardiol 1997;10:61–69.
16. Karas SP, Gravanis MB, Santoian EC, et al. Coronary intimal proliferation after balloon injury and stenting in swine: an animal model of restenosis. J Am Coll Cardiol 1992;20:467–474.
17. Murphy JG, Schwartz RS, Edwards WD, et al. Percutaneous polymeric stents in porcine coronary arteries. Initial experience with polyethylene terephthalate stents. Circulation 1992;86:1596–1604.
18. Schwartz RS. Animal models of human coronary restenosis. In: Topol EJ, ed. Textbook of interventional cardiology Saunders, Philadelphia, 1994, pp. 365–381.
19. Horiba M, Kadomatsu K, Nakamura E, et al. Neointima formation in a restenosis model is suppressed in midkine-deficient mice. J Clin Invest 2000;105:489–495.
20. Sata M, Maejima Y, Adachi F, et al. A mouse model of vascular injury that induces rapid onset of medial cell apoptosis followed by reproducible neointimal hyperplasia. J Mol Cell Cardiol 2000;32:2097–2104.
21. Carmeliet P, Moons L, Stassen JM, et al. Vascular wound healing and neointima formation induced by perivascular electric injury in mice. Am J Pathol 1997;150:761–776.
22. Carmeliet P, Collen D. Gene targeting and gene transfer studies of the plasminogen/plasmin system: implications in thrombosis, hemostasis, neointima formation, and atherosclerosis. FASEB J 1995;9:934–938.

23. Kalinowski M, Alfke H, Bergen S, et al. Comparative trial of local pharmacotherapy with L-arginine, r-hirudin, and molsidomine to reduce restenosis after balloon angioplasty of stenotic rabbit iliac arteries. Radiology 2001;219:716–723.

24. Nagae T, Aizawa K, Uchimura N, et al. Endovascular photodynamic therapy using mono-L-aspartyl-chlorin e6 to inhibit Intimal hyperplasia in balloon-injured rabbit arteries. Lasers Surg Med 2001; 28:381–388.

25. Kanamasa K, Otani N, Ishida N, et al. Suppression of cell proliferation by tissue plasminogen activator during the early phase after balloon injury minimizes intimal hyperplasia in hypercholesterolemic rabbits. J Cardiovasc Pharmacol 2001;37:155–162.

26. Zou J, Huang Y, Cao K, et al. Effect of resveratrol on intimal hyperplasia after endothelial denudation in an experimental rabbit model. Life Sci 2000;68:153–163.

27. Welt FG, Edelman ER, Simon DI, et al. Neutrophil, not macrophage, infiltration precedes neointimal thickening in balloon-injured arteries. Arterioscler Thromb Vasc Biol 2000;20:2553–2558.

28. Baumbach A, Oberhoff M, Bohnet A, et al. Efficacy of low-molecular-weight heparin delivery with the Dispatch catheter following balloon angioplasty in the rabbit iliac artery. Catheterization Cardiovasc Diag 1997;41:303–307.

29. Coats WD, Cheung DT, Han B, et al. Balloon angioplasty significantly increases collagen content but does not alter collagen subtype I/III ratios in the atherosclerotic rabbit iliac model. J Mol Cell Cardiol 1996;28:441–446.

30. Hansen DD, Auth DC, Vracko R, et al. Rotational atherectomy in atherosclerotic rabbit iliac arteries. Am Heart J 1988;115:160–165.

31. Jenkins RD, Sinclair IN, Leonard BM, et al. Laser balloon angioplasty versus balloon angioplasty in normal rabbit iliac arteries. Lasers Surg Med 1989;9:237–247.

32. Mason RG, Read MS. Some species differences in fibrinolysis and blood coagulation. J Biomed Mater Res 1971;5:121–128.

33. Kirschstein W, Simianer S, Dempfle CE, et al. Impaired fibrinolytic capacity and tissue plasminogen activator release in patients with restenosis after percutaneous transluminal coronary angioplasty (PTCA). Thromb Haemost 1989;62:772–775.

34. Schwartz RS, Edwards WD, Bailey KR, et al. Differential neointimal response to coronary artery injury in pigs and dogs. Implications for restenosis models. Arterioscler Thromb 1994;14: 395–400.

35. Fuster V, Badimon L, Badimon JJ, et al. The porcine model for the understanding of thrombogenesis and atherogenesis. Mayo Clin Proc 1991;66:818–831.

36. Steele P, Chesebro J, Stanson A, et al. Balloon angioplasty. Natural history of the pathophysiological response to injury in a pig model. Circ Res 1985;57:105–112.

37. Lam JYT, Chesebro JH, Steele PM, et al. Deep arterial injury during experimental angioplasty: Relationship to a positive Indium-111 labeled platelet scintigram, quantitative platelet deposition and mural thrombus. J Am Coll Cardiol 1986;8:1380–1386.

38. Worthley SG, Helft G, Fuster V, et al. Serial in vivo MRI documents arterial remodeling in experimental atherosclerosis. Circulation 2000;101:586–589.

39. Webster M, Chesebro J, Grill D, et al. The thrombotic and proliferative response to angioplasty in pigs after deep arterial injury: effect of intravenous thrombin inhibition with hirudin (abstr). Circulation 1991;84:II-580.

40. French JE, Jennings MA, Florey HW. Morphological studies on atherosclerosis in swine. Ann NY Acad Sci 1965;127:780–799.

41. Schwartz RS, Edwards WD, Huber KC, et al. Coronary restenosis: prospects for solution and new perspectives from a porcine model. Mayo Clin Proc 1993;68:54–62.

42. Heras M, Chesebro JH, Penny WJ, et al. Effects of thrombin inhibition on the development of acute platelet-thrombus deposition during angioplasty in pigs. Heparin versus recombinant hirudin, a specific thrombin inhibitor. Circulation 1989;79:657–65.

43. Schwartz RS, Murphy JG, Edwards WD, et al. Coronary artery restenosis and the "virginal membrane":smooth muscle cell proliferation and the intact internal elastic lamina. J Invest Cardiol 1991;3:3–8.

44. McKenna CJ, Burke SE, Opgenorth TJ, et al. Selective ET(A) receptor antagonism reduces neointimal hyperplasia in a porcine coronary stent model. Circulation 1998;97:2551–2556.

45. Schwartz RS, Murphy JG, Edwards WD, et al. Restenosis after balloon angioplasty. A practical proliferative model in porcine coronary arteries. Circulation 1990;82:2190–2200.

46. Schwartz RS, Huber KC, Murphy JG, et al. Restenosis and the proportional neointimal response to coronary artery injury: results in a porcine model. J Am Coll Cardiol 1992;19:267–274.

47. Geary RL, Adams MR, Benjamin ME, et al. Conjugated equine estrogens inhibit progression of atherosclerosis but have no effect on intimal hyperplasia or arterial remodeling induced by balloon catheter injury in monkeys. J Am Coll Cardiol 1998;31:1158–1164.

48. Hanson SR, Powell JS, Dodson T, et al. Effects of angiotensin converting enzyme inhibition with cilazapril on intimal hyperplasia in injured arteries and vascular grafts in the baboon. Hypertension 1991;18:II70–II76.

49. Geary RL, Koyama N, Wang TW, et al. Failure of heparin to inhibit intimal hyperplasia in injured baboon arteries. The role of heparin-sensitive and -insensitive pathways in the stimulation of smooth muscle cell migration and proliferation. Circulation 1995;91:2972–2981.

50. Geary RL, Williams JK, Golden D, et al. Time course of cellular proliferation, intimal hyperplasia, and remodeling following angioplasty in monkeys with established atherosclerosis. A nonhuman primate model of restenosis. Arterioscler Thromb Vasc Biol 1996;16:34–43.

51. Mondy JS, Williams JK, Adams MR, et al. Structural determinants of lumen narrowing after angioplasty in atherosclerotic nonhuman primates. J Vasc Surg 1997;26:875–883.

52. Clowes AW, Clowes MM, Fingerle J, et al. Kinetics of cellular proliferation after arterial injury. V. Role of acute distension in the induction of smooth muscle proliferation. Lab Invest 1989;60:360–364.

53. Hanke H, Strohschneider T, Oberhoff M, et al. Time course of smooth muscle cell proliferation in the intima and media of arteries following experimental angioplasty. Circ Res 1990;67:651–659.

54. Fingerle J, Johnson R, Clowes AW, et al. Role of platelets in smooth muscle cell proliferation and migration after vascular injury in rat carotid artery. Proc Natl Acad Sci USA 1989;86:8412–8416.

55. Casscells W. Migration of Smooth Muscle and Endothelial Cells: Critical Events in Restenosis. Circulation 1992;86:723–729.

56. Clowes A, Schwartz S. Significance of quiescent smooth muscle migration in the injured rat carotid artery. Circ Res 1985;56:139–145.

57. Landzberg BR, Frishman WH, Lerrick K. Pathophysiology and pharmacological approaches for prevention of coronary artery restenosis following coronary artery balloon angioplasty and related procedures. Prog Cardiovasc Dis 1997;39:361–398.

58. Currier JW, Faxon DP. Restenosis after percutaneous transluminal coronary angioplasty: have we been aiming at the wrong target? J Am Coll Cardiol 1995;25:516–520.

59. Braun-Dullaeus RC, Mann MJ, Dzau VJ. Cell cycle progression: new therapeutic target for vascular proliferative disease. Circulation 1998;98:82–89.

60. Gershlick AH, Baron J. Dealing with in-stent restenosis. Heart 1998;79:319–23.

61. Fingerle J, Au YP, Clowes AW, et al. Intimal lesion formation in rat carotid arteries after endothelial denudation in absence of medial injury. Arteriosclerosis 1990;10:1082–1087.

62. Sims FH. A comparison of structural features of the walls of coronary arteries from 10 different species. Pathology 1989;21:115–124.

63. Schwartz RS, Holder DJ, Holmes DR, et al. Neointimal thickening after severe coronary artery injury is limited by a short-term administration of a factor Xa inhibitor. Results in a porcine model. Circulation 1996;93:1542–1548.

64. Huber KC, Schwartz RS, Edwards WD, et al. Effects of angiotensin converting enzyme inhibition on neointimal proliferation in a porcine coronary injury model. Am Heart J 1993;125:695–701.

65. Kullo IJ, Simari RD, Schwartz RS. Vascular gene transfer : from bench to bedside. Arterioscler Thromb Vasc Biol 1999;19:196–207.

66. Simari RD. Gene Therapy for Restenosis. J Invasive Cardiol 1996;8:478–480.

67. Yang ZY, Simari RD, Perkins ND, et al. Role of the p21 cyclin-dependent kinase inhibitor in limiting intimal cell proliferation in response to arterial injury. Proc Natl Acad Sci USA 1996;93:7905–7910.

68. Schwartz RS, Holmes DR Jr., Topol EJ. The restenosis paradigm revisited: an alternative proposal for cellular mechanisms. J Am Coll Cardiol 1992;20:1284–1293.

69. Schwartz RS, Holmes DR. Pigs, dogs, baboons, and man: lessons for stenting from animal studies. J Intervent Cardiol 1994; 7:355–368.

70. Banning A, Brewer L, Wendt M, et al. Local delivery of platelets with encapsulated iloprost to balloon injured pig carotid arteries: effect on platelet deposition and neointima formation. Thromb Haemost 1997;77:190–196.

71. Clopath P. The effect of acetylsalicylic acid (ASA) on the development of atherosclerotic lesions in miniature swine. Br J Exp Pathol 1980;61:440–443.

72. Unterberg C, Sandrock D, Nebendahl K, et al. Reduced acute thrombus formation results in decreased neointimal proliferation after coronary angioplasty. J Am Coll Cardiol 1995;26:1747–1754.
73. Abendschein DR, Recchia D, Meng YY, et al. Inhibition of thrombin attenuates stenosis after arterial injury in minipigs. J Am Coll Cardiol 1996;28:1849–1855.
74. Gallo R, Padurean A, Toschi V, et al. Prolonged thrombin inhibition reduces restenosis after balloon angioplasty in porcine coronary arteries. Circulation 1998;97:581–588.
75. Buchwald AB, Unterberg C, Nebendahl K, et al. Low-molecular-weight heparin reduces neointimal proliferation after coronary stent implantation in hypercholesterolemic minipigs. Circulation 1992; 86:531–537.
76. Serruys PW, Herrman JP, Simon R, et al. A comparison of hirudin with heparin in the prevention of restenosis after coronary angioplasty. Helvetica Investigators. N Engl J Med 1995;333:757–763.
77. Bittl JA, Strony J, Brinker JA, et al. Treatment with bivalirudin (Hirulog) as compared with heparin during coronary angioplasty for unstable or postinfarction angina. Hirulog Angioplasty Study Investigators. N Engl J Med 1995;333:764–769.
78. Johnson GJ, Griggs TR, Badimon L. The utility of animal models in the preclinical study of inter- ventions to prevent human coronary artery restenosis: analysis and recommendations. On behalf of the Subcommittee on Animal, Cellular and Molecular Models of Thrombosis and Haemostasis of the Scientific and Standardization Committee of the International Society on Thrombosis and Haemostasis. Thromb Haemost 1999;81:835–843.
79. Aikawa M, Rabkin E, Okada Y, et al. Lipid lowering by diet reduces matrix metalloproteinase activ- ity and increases collagen content of rabbit atheroma: a potential mechanism of lesion stabilization. Circulation 1998;97:2433–2444.
80. Kornowski R, Hong MK, Tio FO, et al. In-stent restenosis: contributions of inflammatory responses and arterial injury to neointimal hyperplasia. J Am Coll Cardiol 1998;31:224–230.
81. Komatsu R, Ueda M, Naruko T, et al. Neointimal tissue response at sites of coronary stenting in humans: macroscopic, histological, and immunohistochemical analyses. Circulation 1998;98:224–233.
82. Farb A, Sangiorgi G, Carter AJ, et al. Pathology of acute and chronic coronary stenting in humans. Circulation 1999;99:44–52.
83. Grewe PH, Deneke T, Machraoui A, et al. Acute and chronic tissue response to coronary stent implan- tation: pathologic findings in human specimen. J Am Coll Cardiol 2000;35:157–163.
84. Moreno PR, Falk E, Palacios IF, et al. Macrophage infiltration in acute coronary syndromes. Implications for plaque rupture. Circulation 1994;90:775–778.
85. Pietersma A, Kofflard M, de Wit LE, et al. Late lumen loss after coronary angioplasty is associated with the activation status of circulating phagocytes before treatment. Circulation 1995;91: 1320–1325.
86. Zempo N, Koyama N, Kenagy RD, et al. Regulation of vascular smooth muscle cell migration and proliferation in vitro and in injured rat arteries by a synthetic matrix metalloproteinase inhibitor. Arterioscler Thromb Vasc Biol 1996;16:28–33.
87. Stadius ML, Gown AM, Kernoff R, et al. Cell proliferation after balloon injury of iliac arteries in the cholesterol-fed New Zealand White rabbit. Arterioscler Thromb 1994;14:727–733.
88. Lafont A, Guzman LA, Whitlow PL, et al. Restenosis after experimental angioplasty. Intimal, medial, and adventitial changes associated with constrictive remodeling. Circ Res 1995;76:996–1002.
89. Bauters C, Isner JM. The biology of restenosis. Prog Cardiovasc Dis 1997;40:107–116.
90. Mintz GS, Popma JJ, Hong MK, et al. Intravascular ultrasound to discern device-specific effects and mechanisms of restenosis. Am J Cardiol 1996;78:18–22.
91. Schwartz RS. Pathophysiology of restenosis: interaction of thrombosis, hyperplasia, and/or remodeling. Am J Cardiol 1998;81:14E–17E.
92. Shah VM, Mintz GS, Apple S, et al. Background incidence of late malapposition after bare-metal stent implantation. Circulation 2002;106:1753–1755.
93. Kay IP, Sabate M, Costa MA, et al. Positive geometric vascular remodeling is seen after catheter- based radiation followed by conventional stent implantation but not after radioactive stent implanta- tion. Circulation 2000;102:1434–1439.
94. Kakuta T, Usui M, Coats WD, Jr., et al. Arterial remodeling at the reference site after angioplasty in the atherosclerotic rabbit model. Arterioscler Thromb Vasc Biol 1998;18:47–51.
95. Kalef-Ezra J, Michalis LK, Malamou-Mitsi V, et al. External beam irradiation in angioplasted arteries of hypercholesterolemic rabbits. The dose and time effect. Cardiovasc Radiat Med 2002;3:20–25.

96. Waksman R, Rodriguez JC, Robinson KA, et al. Effect of intravascular irradiation on cell proliferation, apoptosis, and vascular remodeling after balloon overstretch injury of porcine coronary arteries. Circulation 1997;96:1944–1952.

97. Coats WD Jr., Currier JW, Faxon DP. Remodelling and restenosis: insights from animal studies. Semin Interv Cardiol 1997;2:153–158.

98. Schwartz RS, Topol EJ, Serruys PW, et al. Artery size, neointima, and remodeling: time for some standards. J Am Coll Cardiol 1998;32:2087–2094.

99. de Smet BJ, Pasterkamp G, van der Helm YJ, et al. The relation between de novo atherosclerosis remodeling and angioplasty-induced remodeling in an atherosclerotic Yucatan micropig model. Arterioscler Thromb Vasc Biol 1998;18:702–707.

100. Vodovotz Y, Waksman R, Kim WH, et al. Effects of intracoronary radiation on thrombosis after balloon overstretch injury in the porcine model. Circulation 1999;100:2527–2533.

101. Waksman R, Bhargava B, Mintz GS, et al. Late total occlusion after intracoronary brachytherapy for patients with in-stent restenosis. J Am Coll Cardiol 2000;36:65–68.

102. Waksman R. Late thrombosis after radiation. Sitting on a time bomb. Circulation 1999;100:780–782.

103. Dolmatch BL, Dong YH, Trerotola SO, et al. Tissue response to covered Wallstents. J Vasc Interv Radiol 1998;9:471–478.

104. De Scheerder IK, Wilczek KL, Verbeken EV, et al. Biocompatibility of polymer-coated oversized metallic stents implanted in normal porcine coronary arteries. Atherosclerosis 1995;114:105–114.

105. van der Giessen WJ, Lincoff AM, Schwartz RS, et al. Marked inflammatory sequelae to implantation of biodegradable and nonbiodegradable polymers in porcine coronary arteries. Circulation 1996;94:1690–1697.

106. Satler LF, Mintz G. Promises, promises: the covered stent. Catheter Cardiovasc Interv 2000;50:89.

107. Topouzis S, Majesky MW. Smooth muscle lineage diversity in the chick embryo. Two types of aortic smooth muscle cell differ in growth and receptor-mediated transcriptional responses to transforming growth factor-beta. Dev Biol 1996;178:430–445.

108. Majesky MW, Dong XR, Topouzis S. Smooth muscle cell diversity and the extracellular matrix in a rat model of restenosis. P R Health Sci J 1996;15:187–191.

109. Yang Z, Oemar BS, Carrel T, et al. Different proliferative properties of smooth muscle cells of human arterial and venous bypass vessels: role of PDGF receptors, mitogen-activated protein kinase, and cyclin-dependent kinase inhibitors. Circulation 1998;97:181–187.

110. Strauss BH, Juilliere Y, Rensing BJ, et al. Edge detection versus densitometry for assessing coronary stenting quantitatively. Am J Cardiol 1991;67:484–490.

111. Pratt RE, Dzau VJ. Pharmacological strategies to prevent restenosis: lessons learned from blockade of the renin-angiotensin system. Circulation 1996;93:848–852.

112. Hermans WR, Foley DP, Rensing BJ, et al. Morphologic changes during follow-up after successful percutaneous transluminal coronary balloon angioplasty: quantitative angiographic analysis in 778 lesions—further evidence for the restenosis paradox. MERCATOR Study Group (Multicenter European Research trial with Cilazapril after Angioplasty to prevent Transluminal Coronary Obstruction and Restenosis). Am Heart J 1994;127:483–494.

113. Faxon DP. Effect of high dose angiotensin-converting enzyme inhibition on restenosis: final results of the MARCATOR Study, a multicenter, double-blind, placebo-controlled trial of cilazapril. The Multicenter American Research Trial With Cilazapril After Angioplasty to Prevent Transluminal Coronary Obstruction and Restenosis (MARCATOR) Study Group. J Am Coll Cardiol 1995;25:362–369.

114. O'Keefe JH, Jr., McCallister BD, Bateman TM, et al. Ineffectiveness of colchicine for the prevention of restenosis after coronary angioplasty. J Am Coll Cardiol 1992;19:1597–1600.

115. Freed M, Safian RD, O'Neill WW, et al. Combination of lovastatin, enalapril, and colchicine does not prevent restenosis after percutaneous transluminal coronary angioplasty. Am J Cardiol 1995;76:1185–1188.

116. Tanaka K, Honda M, Kuramochi T, et al. Prominent inhibitory effects of tranilast on migration and proliferation of and collagen synthesis by vascular smooth muscle cells. Atherosclerosis 1994;107:179–185.

117. Gerdes C, Faber-Steinfeld V, Yalkinoglu O, et al. Comparison of the effects of the thrombin inhibitor r-hirudin in four animal models of neointima formation after arterial injury. Arterioscler Thromb Vasc Biol 1996;16:1306–1311.

118. Beatt KJ, Serruys PW, Luijten HE, et al. Restenosis after coronary angioplasty: the paradox of increased lumen diameter and restenosis. J Am Coll Cardiol 1992;19:258–266.
119. Roubin GS, Douglas JS, Jr., King SB, 3rd, et al. Influence of balloon size on initial success, acute complications, and restenosis after percutaneous transluminal coronary angioplasty. A prospective randomized study. Circulation 1988;78:557–565.
120. Ramee SR, White CJ. Percutaneous coronary angioscopy. In: Topol EJ ed. Textbook of interventional cardiology Saunders, Philadelphia, 1994, pp. 1122–1135.
121. Tall AR. Plasma lipid transfer proteins. J Lipid Res 1986;27:361–367.
122. Narayanaswamy M, Wright KC, Kandarpa K. Animal models for atherosclerosis, restenosis, and endovascular graft research. J Vasc Interv Radiol 2000;11:5–17.

# II  GENETIC BASIS OF RESTENOSIS

# 8

# The Genomics of Restenosis

*Thomas W. Johnson,* Bsc, MBBS, MRCP
*and Karl R. Karsch,* MD

## INTRODUCTION

Interventional cardiology took off in 1977, with the development of percutaneous coronary balloon angioplasty *(1)*. Despite immediate success in regaining vessel patency, long-term results were undermined by luminal loss secondary to the vessel injury induced by the balloon *(2,3)*. A decade later a new technique involving stent deployment had been designed to overcome vessel recoil *(4)*, initially, considered the major contributor to the loss of lumen diameter. Rather than ridding interventional cardiology of restenosis, a purely iatrogenic process, stents have shifted the focus of attention toward the phenomenon of intimal hyperplasia *(5)*.

Now, a further 10 yr on and great excitement has been generated by the discovery of sirolimus' and paclitaxel's capacity to inhibit the intimal response encountered following the deployment of intracoronary stents *(6,7)*. A sceptic might speculate that in 10-yr time the focus will have shifted again, and further novel therapies will be in production targeting the latest culprit of restenosis unmasked by today's technology. However, major changes in molecular biology technology have occurred in the last decade giving us new insight into pathophysiological mechanisms and thus offering us novel methods of diagnosis and therapy *(8)*. It is quite obvious that the phenomenon of restenosis is secondary to a complex interaction between extrinsic factors of predisposition (e.g., diabetes, small vessels, long lesions, and so on) and a multiplicity of genes.

Without an idea of the hierarchy of communication, between genes and the extrinsic factors, attempts at halting the process can only be governed by best guess, thus

From: *Contemporary Cardiology: Essentials of Restenosis: For the Interventional Cardiologist*
Edited by: H. J. Duckers, E. G. Nabel, and P. W. Serruys © Humana Press Inc., Totowa, NJ

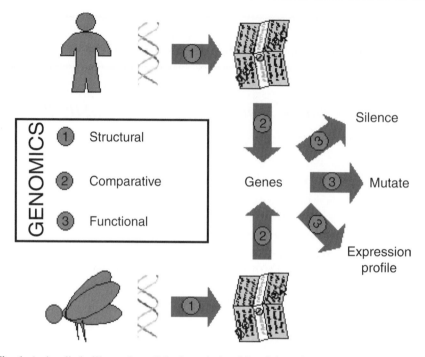

**Fig. 1.** A simplistic illustration of the interrlationship of the subspecialities of genomics.

diminishing any likelihood of abolishing restenosis. The advent of genomics has changed this, allowing investigators to observe gene function and to interrogate disease mechanisms at the molecular level. Consequently, the next decade will be an exciting time of new discovery. The purpose of this chapter is to introduce the new technologies available within the field of genomics and to relate this to how they might impact on the understanding and therapy of restenosis.

## AN INTRODUCTION TO GENOMICS

Following its proposal in the 1980s, the human genome project has accelerated exponentially. The first major landmark came in June 2000 with the release of a "first draft" of the genome, by which time "Genomics," the scientific discipline of mapping, sequencing and analyzing genomes, was well established. Three years on and more than 100 organisms have had their genomes completely sequenced (*see* list www.ncbi. nlm.nih.gov/entrez/query.fcgi?db=Genome), completion of the final draft of the human genome was announced in April 2003. Numerous subspecialities have evolved within this relatively immature field; structural, comparative, and functional genomics, and all are reliant on highly advanced computational analysis, which itself has evolved into the subspeciality of Bioinformatics *(9)*. Figure 1 graphically demonstrates the interrelationship between the subspecialties of genomics.

In brief, structural genomics *(10)* represents the sequencing of the genome and ultimately will culminate in the construction of genetic, physical, and transcript maps of organisms. Mapping of genes using tandem-repeat polymorphisms allows comparison of the human genome against the genomes of model organisms and other vertebrates— comparative genomics. Comparison with model organism genomes, for example, the fruit fly (*Drosophila melanogaster*) or nematode worm (*Caenorhabditis elegans*), both with well-characterized genomes, can aid the interrogation of distant, yet related human genes with unknown function.

Additionally, comparison of the human genome with those from other vertebrates and mammals demonstrates the highly conserved nature of many genes. Subsequently, the gene map from one species can be used to reveal the location of a target gene in a related species. Furthermore, comparison of nontranscriptional domains can highlight important sequences, conserved in many species, attributed with roles in the regulation of gene expression. Functional genomics relies on the data gathered from structural and comparative analysis of the genome; it focuses on gaining an understanding of the function of genes and gene products.

Therefore, genomics—the interrogation of the genome—potentially allows the linking of gene expression with biological behavior. The shift in emphasis from studying single genes to assessing the whole genome simultaneously has led to the creation of vast databases of information, allowing collaboration in the generation of gene structure, the mapping of genes within the genome, assessment in gene functionality, and the postulation of the interrelations of "clusters" of genes. Linking of gene expression to biological behavior requires more than just an explicit understanding of the genome, as ultimately it is the gene products that act as effectors. The mere presence of a gene does not reflect functionality therefore much energy has been invested in the assessment of both the transcriptome, *transcriptomics*, and the eventual pool of effector proteins, *proteomics*.

"Transcriptomics" falls within the auspices of functional genomics and is covered within this review, however the vast discipline of proteomics is now established as a research field in its own right, the proteomics of restenosis is covered separately within this book. The combination of genomics, transcript profiling, and proteomics will give insight into the mechanisms of disease, allow identification of diagnostic and prognostic markers and highlight suitable targets for therapy. These disciplines remain relative newcomers to the field of molecular biology and consequently the associated technology and the understanding of the principles underpinning these processes are rapidly advancing—new molecular biology techniques, reliant on the colossal processing power of computers, have allowed the profiling of 100–1000s of genes/transcripts concurrently and therefore opened up this exciting field of science to widespread application.

## GENOMIC TOOLS

The tools available for genomic and transcriptomic study have been revolutionized since the first suggestions of sequencing the human genome in the 1980s.

### Sequencing Tools

As the relative importance of genomic study and the suggested uses of genomic information escalated so too did commercial interest. The creation of the first commercial genomics company, Celera Genomics, in 1998, potentially jeopardized the international, and cooperative approach taken by the human genome project. Instead, commercial competition galvanized the public sector and resulted in a boost in public spending and triggered an unprecedented acceleration in the production of raw sequence. Until 1998 approx 6% of the human genome had been sequenced within 3 yr 90% was complete. Sequencing is still achieved using methods first described by Sanger in the 1970s *(11)*.

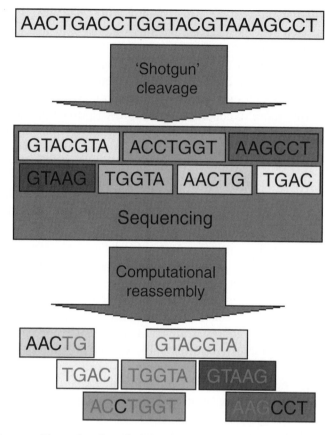

**Fig. 2.** A flow diagram, illustrating the principle of "shot-gun" cleavage, used to facilitate genomic sequencing.

The genome's size prevents analysis in its entirety; therefore it is broken into smaller pieces for sequencing. Genome fragments of about 150 kB are inserted into bacterial artificial chromosomes for cloning. The clones are then further fragmented or "shotgunned" to produce manageable segments of DNA for sequencing, i.e., about 1500 base pairs (bps). Repeated shotgun fragmentation of the clones allows piecing together of the entire clone following sequencing (*see* Fig. 2).

### Sequence Polymorphisms and Association Studies

Following completion of the sequencing of the human genome, mapping of genes onto chromosomes has been facilitated by detection of sequence polymorphisms (polymorphic DNA markers) *(12)*. The presence of polymorphic DNA markers located throughout the human genome has facilitated the mapping of genes onto other individuals and species genomes. Rare Mendelian disorders, attributable to single gene defects can be highlighted by careful analysis of short-tandem repeat polymorphisms located close to the target gene in unison with detection of disease phenotype, thus permitting identification of causative mutations.

However, restenosis like atherosclerosis and hypertension is a complex disorder involving the interaction of several genes, and consequently harder to decipher. Single nucleotide polymorphisms (SNPs), frequently occurring inherited sequence polymorphisms (about every 300–500 bp) might possibly reveal genetic associations with more complex diseases. It has been postulated that a subset of SNPs contribute to the genetic risk of complex disorders *(13)*. Genes of relevance to a particular disorder can be sequenced and the SNPs present within the region noted—SNP association study. Comparison of the same chromosomal region in numerous individuals demonstrates patterns of SNP distribution—individuals with similar clustering of SNPs share the same haplotype. Haplotypes represent descendence from a common ancestral chromosome. For example, it is possible that a particular haplotype is more likely to associate with in-stent restenosis, thus detection would be a useful marker of risk and thus facilitate extra measures of precaution.

## *Gene Function Assessment*

The combination of new high-throughput technologies and a complete draft of the human genome enable investigators to interrogate gene function in two ways. Either, through manipulation of a specific gene, by mutation or altered expression, to assess the effect on phenotype, or, the genetic profile of various phenotypes can be compared to reveal genes involved in characterizing the phenotype *(14)*. The tools available to assess function either through gene manipulation or profiling of phenotypes have advanced rapidly since the first suggestion of sequencing the human genome in the 1980s. The fundamental techniques for functional genomics are described in the following subheadings.

### PHENOTYPE GENERATION BY MUTATION/GENE MANIPULATION

Chemical Mutagenesis remains an important method of elucidating gene function. By its nature it is obviously limited to animal models, commonly the zebra fish, a vertebrate, and the mouse, a mammal. Commonly, males are exposed to a mutagen that induces mutations at high frequency throughout the genome, before mating with a wild-type female. The first generation progeny are then phenotypically assessed for dominant mutations, this may include simple observation, morphological analysis, biochemical tests, and genetic sequencing. Homozygotes for mutations can be generated by mating first-generation males with wild-type females and then with the female progeny of this cross. *See* Fig. 3, taken from Rubin and Tall's review entitled "Perspectives for vascular genomics" *(12)*.

### RNA Interference Technology

A new technique of RNA interference (RNAi) allows silencing of individual genes by post-transcriptional disruption of gene function. Loss of all messenger RNA (mRNA) produced by a gene effectively silences it, a project is underway to produce human cell lines each with a silenced gene, the first phase has focused on approx 8000 genes but the intention is to have a library of cell lines for all 30,000 + genes within the genome by mid-2004. An obvious drive for this new technique is the ability to silence genes required for the proliferation of cancerous cell lines. Restenosis has often been likened to a mitotic process and current best therapy utilizes antimitotic agents, therefore RNAi technology may be of use in cell lines obtained from restenotic tissue samples. However, it is well known that only limited information can be gleaned from isolated cell lines and consequently RNAi technology cannot give a complete answer.

The disadvantage of mutational methods for functional gene assessment is the reliance on the investigator to select an individual gene of interest. As mentioned earlier, the complex, and as yet not fully understood, nature of restenosis in addition to the existence of more than 30,000 genes within the human genome makes gene selection

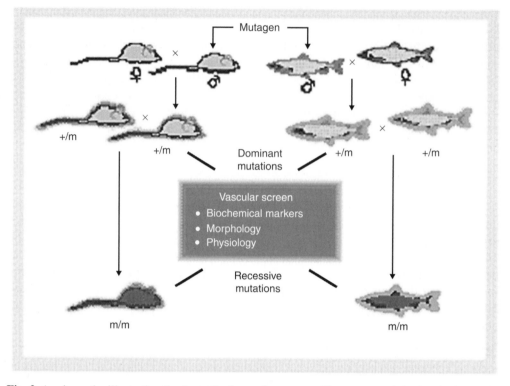

**Fig. 3.** A schematic, illustrating the theoretical use of genome-wide mutagenesis in the elucidation of gene function.

more of a lottery than a scientific process. If the understanding of the disease process was complete, then a definitive therapy would be rapidly achievable. However, these techniques have arrived before the full understanding of the complex process of in-stent restenosis, consequently investigators have utilized the technology to assess their favored targets. It is possible that a cure for restenosis might be found using these technologies alone but the chance is slim.

The emergence of high-throughput technologies capable of gene, transcript or protein profiling enable assessment of phenotype at a molecular level, offering up the opportunity to define mechanisms of disease process, markers of risk, disease progression or regression, and most importantly specific targets for therapy and possibly cure. Therefore, the use of mutational models, RNAi silencing, "knockout" models and vector-driven gene over- and under-expression would be best used in confirming effect detected by these more widespread assessments of the entire genetic milieu within its environment.

## RELATIONSHIP OF PHENOTYPE WITH GENE EXPRESSION

The genome varies very little between cells, however, levels of gene transcription within cells are sensitive to multiple intrinsic and extrinsic factors, thus study of the transcriptome acts as a good meter of gene expression. Transcriptomics, a component of functional genomics allows investigation of the complex interrelationships between genes and facilitates the generation of expression profiles for various phenotypes that can be compared with revealed putative mechanisms of physiological and pathological functions.

Differential display and subtractive hybridization, both well-established techniques in molecular biology can be utilized to assess expression *(15)*, however, they have

been superseded by newer high-throughput technologies facilitating rapid, reproducible, and widespread comparison of gene expression, for example, complementary
DNA (cDNA) and oligonucleotide microarray systems, and serial analysis of gene
expression (SAGE) *(16)*.

## Microarrays

Microarrays *(15,17,18)* require the selection of a known library of genes for profiling. Fragments of double-stranded cDNA or shorter single-stranded oligonucleotide
sequences are spotted onto a solid support, usually glass, silicon, or nylon, using pins
or an ink-jet printer. Advancing technology has allowed increasingly dense array production, currently more than 20,000 sequences can be displayed per array, and in the
near future it is possible that the entire genome will be displayed on a single chip.
Microarray analysis requires labeling of RNA extracted from sample tissue with a fluorescent or radioactive probe. If the quantity of RNA extracted from the test tissue is
limited then polymerase chain reaction (PCR) amplification is permitted, however, it
can potentially distort subsequent profile analysis.

Following labeling of the test RNA/cDNA, the sample is hybridized to the microarray—complementary sequences bind to the solid support whereas nonmatching
sequences are washed off (*see* Fig. 4). An expression profile can be assessed by the use
of two individual probes for test and control RNA extracts and subsequent comparison
of fluorescence between the two samples. Therefore, genes can be assessed as overexpressed, repressed, or equivalent.

## Serial Analysis of Gene Expression

SAGE *(15,19,20)* requires no previous knowledge of genetic sequence, and is therefore capable of detecting novel genes. An initial PCR amplification step allows the
analysis of small samples (50–500 ng of mRNA or 5–50 μg of total RNA). SAGE relies
on the ability to identify mRNA transcripts by a unique short oligonucleotide sequence
located close to its 3′ poly-A tail, *see* Fig. 5.

Briefly, mRNA is purified from total cellular RNA by passage through solid phase
oligo(dT) magnetic beads. Subsequently, cDNA is synthesized from the mRNA and
digested with a restriction enzyme, the resulting 3′-most fragments (anchored to the dT
beads) are then ligated with two different linkers containing PCR primer sites. The
linkers possess a recognition site for a type IIS restriction enzyme, which cuts 10-bp 3′
from the anchoring enzyme recognition site, thus producing unique oligonucleotide
sequences for each mRNA transcript. The 10-bp tags or SAGE tags, bound to linkers
are then ligated to form "ditags" and PCR amplified.

Subsequently, the linkers are cleaved and the ditags are then serially ligated into
concatemers, cloned, and sequenced using an automated sequencer. Software allows
identification of sequences and measurement of their relative frequency. Obviously,
SAGE is limited by the accuracy of sequencing; misplacement of a single base will
result in a loss of data. Equally, any variations in "ditag" amplification between linker
sets will affect any data relating to frequency of expression.

Although a 10-bp sequence tag should theoretically give rise to more than one million
different sequence combinations and thus be adequate to discriminate between the
approx 35,000 genes within the human genome, not all genes within the unannotated
genome can be detected. Therefore a modification that extends the length of the SAGE
tag has been introduced to overcome this problem—"LongSAGE." LongSAGE utilizes
a type IIS restriction enzyme capable of cleaving cDNA 17-bp 3′ of the anchoring

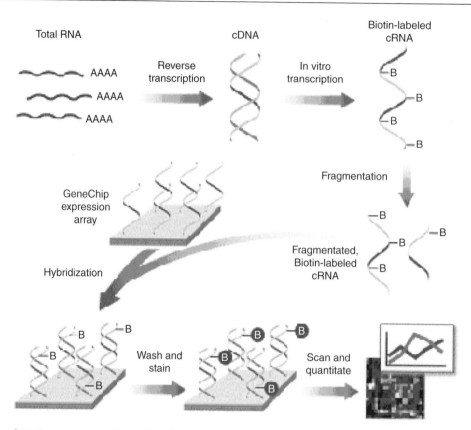

**Fig. 4.** A flow diagram, illustrating the processes involved in microarray systems. Sample RNA is labeled with a biotin probe (B) before hybridization to the microarray, which carries thousands of known nucleic acid probes. The quantity of label associated with each probe location on the array permits the study of gene expression.

site—these lengthened tags heighten sensitivity and consequently enable matching to the unannotated genome.

Currently, only sample availability and the ethical issues surrounding tissue retention limit profiling of genes, transcripts, and proteins. As the technology advances sample size is becoming less of an issue, it is now possible to profile genetic material from a single cell! Thus, phenotypes can be defined at a molecular level using profiles derived from human tissue, the major limitation now lies with the vast quantity of data generated by such high-throughput techniques, therefore much time is being spent advancing computational power—bioinformatics has become a separate field within molecular biological science *(9)*, and will not be covered within this review.

## APPLICATION OF GENOMICS TO RESTENOSIS

Hundreds of studies have been undertaken in an attempt to find methods to suppress the response to experimental vascular injury, most commonly by balloon over-stretch injury to rodent, rabbit, or pig arteries *(21–23)*. Although many have succeeded in the suppression of an injury response in animal models, very few have translated into viable clinical therapies. This discrepancy highlights the existence of fundamental differences between animal models and clinical reality *(24)*. First, there is great

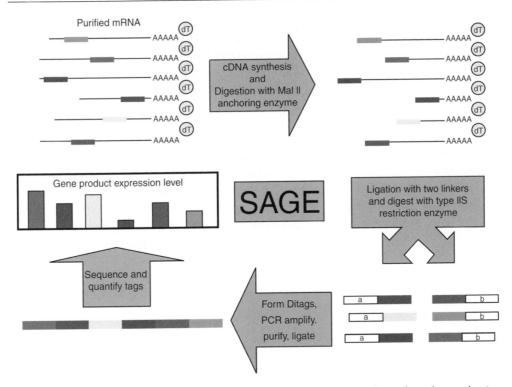

**Fig. 5.** A schematic representation of the SAGE protocol. (Please *see* insert for color version.)

disparity between the use of therapies in juvenile animals, undergoing injury of healthy arteries, against application in an aged human population with severely diseased vessels. Second, the injury induced in small animals varies markedly from that elicited in humans, i.e., endothelial denudation rather than extensive endothelial and medial disruption. Use of swine and nonhuman primates combined with coronary overstretch injury has reduced the gap between animal models and reality; however, size, cost, and ethical issues prevent their widespread use. Genomics offers new uses for such animal models and potentially may refine and reduce the scientific communities reliance on nonhuman experimentation. Rather than being the "test bed" for best guess therapy, genomic interrogation of the human restenotic process may provide specific targets for treatment; these can then be tested in well-established animal models of restenosis before human trailing.

Genomics offers enumerable avenues of new biomedical research, however, within the field of restenosis most work, to-date, has concentrated on the development of risk markers, through assessment of SNP and haplotype associations within populations susceptible to in-stent restenosis and the probing for genes involved in the restenotic process, using methods of profiling gene and transcript expression, from which platform further exploration of target genes or clusters of genes can be undertaken.

## EXISTING DATA WITHIN THE FIELD OF RESTENOSIS GENOMICS

Unlike other cardiovascular pathologies, a small animal genetic model of restenosis cannot be readily produced. As previously discussed, great disparity exists between the nature of injury caused by balloon inflation in small animal and human arteries, and expense, and ethics prevent large-scale experimentation in large animal/nonhuman primate models. Therefore, early investigation of restenosis at the genomic level has concentrated on finding who is the most susceptible and which genes are responsible in those individuals with restenosis. Gene profiling of tissue extracted from restenotic lesions has generated vast amounts of data and offered up numerous targets for therapy, this is discussed at length in the Chapter 9.

Much interest has been shown in attempting to highlight individuals at risk of restenosis before percutaneous coronary intervention. Numerous haplotype and SNP association studies have been performed, only a few associations have been found. Such studies require the investigator to select a gene of interest and assess the effect of known polymorphisms on phenotype. To date, positive associations include homozygosity for the *T*-allele of the PvuII polymorphism of the α-estrogen receptor in women *(25)*, a 6A6A metalloproteinase-3 genotype (only with balloon angioplasty) *(26)*, E-selectin Ser128Arg genotype *(27)*, and angiotensin converting enzyme gene DD genotype *(28)*. However, negative associations include 677C/T and 1298A/C polymorphisms of methylenetetrahydrofolate reductase gene *(29)*, a polymorphic marker of the gene encoding interleukin-1 receptor antagonist *(30)*, and gene polymorphisms of tumor necrosis factor-α, lymphotoxin-α, and interleukin-10 *(31)*.

## FUTURE DIRECTIONS

Genomics potentially holds the key to the appropriate targeting of therapy at a molecular/genetic level. Cardiovascular genomics remains in its infancy, moreover, restenosis genomics is "embryonic"—in September 2003 only a handful of papers addressing in-stent restenosis genomics could be found on an extensive PubMed search. As SNP and haplotype association studies continue, increasingly sensitive screening tools will be developed enabling interventional cardiologists to tailor intervention to the individual not just the lesion type. The emergence of microarray technology capable of screening the entire human genome will allow the temporal genetic profiling of the restenotic process to be realized. Subsequently, genes implicated in the process can be interrogated with regards their function and pathological role, thus developing the understanding of restenosis. In parallel with the advancing understanding of the pathological process, new targets for therapeutic intervention will arise. Rather than seeking a cure for restenosis, genomics may offer a method of prevention. However, amidst the excitement surrounding genomics and its potential, it must be remembered that assessment of the genome only reveals part of the story, it must not be considered on its own but instead in combination with analysis of the transcriptome and proteome. Gene expression and gene function cannot be used as direct surrogates of transcript or protein function.

## SUMMARY

- SNP association studies in large cohorts of patients undergoing percutaneous coronary intervention, combined with phenotype may lead to the detection of markers of risk.
- High-throughput technologies have enabled investigators to interrogate restenotic gene expression without previous knowledge of the genes involved and despite small sample sizes.
- Expression profiling can highlight genes of importance in the restenotic process.

- Comparison genomics has an important role in deriving function for unknown genes through mapping onto model genomes or those of related species.
- Genomics must be assessed in combination with information from the transcriptome and proteome otherwise it is meaningless.

# GLOSSARY

## Genome

The complete "library" of genetic information for an individual, containing more than three billion bp, distributed across 22 autosomal chromosomes (1–22) and two sex chromosomes (X and Y). The genome contains, in encrypted form (>30,000 genes), all the information required to create that individual.

## Transcriptome

Despite almost all cells containing the required information to translate its DNA into mRNA transcripts for all human genes, mRNA production varies between cells and differing environments. Gene expression, i.e., mRNA transcription from DNA is controlled by transcriptional factors present within the nucleus, which interact with regulatory regions bordering the coding regions genes (nontranscriptional domains). Therefore, assessment of mRNA production from specific cell types in defined conditions results in the creation of a transcriptome.

## Proteome

The mere presence of mRNA cannot predict the resulting pool of proteins. The mRNA transcribed from DNA needs modification before translation into protein, it contains coding sequences (exons), flanked by irrelevant sequences (introns). Splicing (removal of introns to join exons) can vary and thus result in the production of different protein products. Therefore, the proteome refers to the effective protein produced from a defined transcriptome.

## Genotype

Generally refers to the complement of genes carried by an individual. Every individual carries two copies of each gene, one inherited from their father and the other from their mother. Variations in genes exist (alleles) and these can be defined through interrogation of the genes sequence. Homozygosity relates to the carriage of two identical genes whereas heterozygosity refers to the presence of two variants of a single gene.

## Phenotype

Variations in genes (alleles) and gene expression result in observable differences between individuals and can predispose to disease. The phenotype is defined as the observed characteristics of an individual. In part, the phenotype can be predicted by an individuals genotype.

## Polymorphisms

Comparison of a single gene between two individuals will reveal variations in nucleotide sequence, these can impact dramatically on protein formation if located within coding regions of the gene. Sequence changes within the noncoding (intron) regions are less likely to result in changes to protein production. Frequently occurring variations in nucleotide sequence are called *polymorphisms*, alleles with a frequency of less than 1% or sequence changes directly related to disease are known as *mutations (32)*. Nucleotide sequence variations can be single or multiple.

## *Haplotype*

Haplotype refers to patterns/clusters of polymorphisms within a gene sequence, detected in subsets of a population. It is a direct consequence of descendence from a common ancestral chromosome.

## REFERENCES

1. Gruntzig AR, Senning A, Siegenthaler WE. Nonoperative dilatation of coronary-artery stenosis: percutaneous transluminal coronary angioplasty. N Engl J Med 1979;301(2):61–68.
2. Essed CE, Van den Brand M, Becker AE. Transluminal coronary angioplasty and early restenosis. Fibrocellular occlusion after wall laceration. Br Heart J 1983;49(4):393–396.
3. Zarins CK, Lu CT, Gewertz BL, Lyon RT, Rush DS, Glagov S. Arterial disruption and remodeling following balloon dilatation. Surgery 1982;92(6):1086–1095.
4. Sigwart U, Puel J, Mirkovitch V, Joffre F, Kappenberger L. Intravascular stents to prevent occlusion and restenosis after transluminal angioplasty. N Engl J Med 1987;316(12):701–706.
5. Karas SP, Gravanis MB, Santoian EC, Robinson KA, Anderberg KA, King SB 3rd. Coronary intimal proliferation after balloon injury and stenting in swine: an animal model of restenosis. J Am Coll Cardiol 1992;20(2):467–474.
6. Suzuki T, Kopia G, Hayashi S, et al. Stent-based delivery of sirolimus reduces neointimal formation in a porcine coronary model. Circulation 2001;104(10):1188–1193.
7. Sousa JE, Costa MA, Abizaid A, et al. Lack of Neointimal Proliferation After Implantation of Sirolimus-Coated Stents in Human Coronary Arteries : A Quantitative Coronary Angiography and Three-Dimensional Intravascular Ultrasound Study. Circulation 2001;103(2):192–195.
8. Savill J. Molecular genetic approaches to understanding disease. BMJ 1997;314(7074):126–129.
9. Winslow RL, Boguski MS. Genome informatics: current status and future prospects. Circ Res 2003;92(9):953–961.
10. Burley SK. An overview of structural genomics. Nat Struct Biol 2000;7(Suppl):932–934.
11. Sanger F, Coulson AR. A rapid method for determining sequences in DNA by primed synthesis with DNA polymerase. J Mol Biol 1975;94(3):441–448.
12. Rubin EM, Tall A. Perspectives for vascular genomics. Nature 2000;407(6801):265–269.
13. Risch N, Merikangas K. The future of genetic studies of complex human diseases. Science 1996;273(5281):1516–1517.
14. Yaspo ML. Taking a functional genomics approach in molecular medicine. Trends Mol Med 2001;7(11):494–501.
15. Henriksen PA, Kotelevtsev Y. Application of gene expression profiling to cardiovascular disease. Cardiovasc Res 2002;54(1):16–24.
16. Velculescu VE, Zhang L, Vogelstein B, Kinzler KW. Serial analysis of gene expression. Science 1995;270(5235):484–487.
17. Cook SA, Rosenzweig A. DNA Microarrays: Implications for Cardiovascular Medicine. Circ Res 2002;91(7):559–564.
18. Moldovan L, Moldovan NI. Trends in genomic analysis of the cardiovascular system. Arch Pathol Lab Med 2002;126(3):310–316.
19. Patino WD, Mian OY, Hwang PM. Serial Analysis of Gene Expression: Technical Considerations and Applications to Cardiovascular Biology. Circ Res 2002;91(7):565–569.
20. Green CD, Simons JF, Taillon BE, Lewin DA. Open systems: panoramic views of gene expression. J Immunol Methods 2001;250(1–2):67–79.
21. Schwartz RS. Animal models of human coronary restenosis. In: Topol EJ, ed. Textbook of Interventional Cardiology. W.B. Saunders, Philadelphia, PA, 1994, pp. 365–381.
22. Kantor B, Ashai K, Holmes DR Jr, Schwartz RS. The experimental animal models for assessing treatment of restenosis. Cardiovasc Radiation Med 1999;1(1):48–54.
23. Ferns GA, Avades TY. The mechanisms of coronary restenosis: insights from experimental models. Int J Exp Pathol 2000;81(2):63–88.

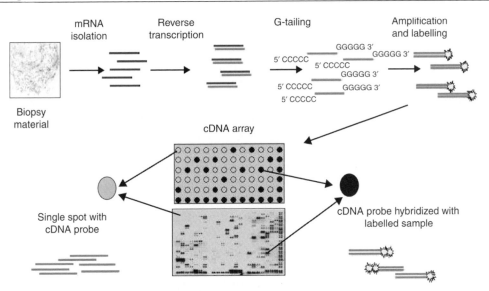

**Fig. 1.** Protocol for PCR-based gene-expression profiling. The basic goal of the protocol is to introduce two binding sites of the PCR primers into all transcripts allowing alike amplification of each transcript. The first primer-binding site consists in a flanking region that lies at the 5′-end of the random cDNA synthesis primer, the second primer-binding site is introduced trough a tailing step. After lysis of frozen tissue, mRNA is isolated and reverse transcribed. Subsequent to the tailing reaction, cDNA was amplified and labeled with digoxigenin by PCR. Denatured, labeled probes are hybridized to cDNA arrays and filter bound probes are detected by chemiluminescence.

intensity by a factor of 2.5 at a descriptive $p$ value $\leq 0.05$) to more complex statistical methods for cluster identification *(4)*.

There are numerous modifications of this technique, which share the essential steps of the experimental setup, but are different in many details of mRNA preparation and amplification as well as array technololgy. The latest generation of arrays, such as the Affymetrix™ (Santa Clara, CA) arrays, are miniaturized and can assay more than 60,000 oligonucleotides on one chip.

## ELUCIDATION OF MECHANISMS OF RESTENOSIS

Restenosis is the most important limitation of percutaneous angioplasty procedures. Although stent implantation reduces the risk of restenosis compared with other percutaneous treatment modalities, angiographic restenosis rates continue to range around 30% *(5,6)*. More than 90% of the late lumen loss after stent implantation is caused by neointima formation *(7)*. Neointima formation is considered an arterial healing response, which is initiated by dedifferentiation of vascular smooth muscle cells (SMCs), followed by emigration and proliferation with subsequent elaboration of abundant extracellular matrix *(8–10)*. The current knowledge is mainly based on

1. Histological analysis of vessel tissue from patients that have passed away;
2. Animal models in general;
3. The use of specifically designed "knockout mice;" and
4. In vitro experiments, for example, with cell cultures.

Therefore, gene-expression analyses of SMCs cultured under pathophysiological conditions or of animal or human samples from neointima after vascular injury were needed.

## IN VITRO EXPERIMENTS

In vitro, mechanical stress leads to responses in SMCs that are similar to those after balloon injury *(11)*. The first study that analyzed the molecular response of SMCs to mechanical stress systematically by gene-expression profiling using cDNA arrays was reported by Feng et al. *(11)*. This group investigated the expression of 5000 genes with putative relevance to neointima formation. They found that only three transcripts were induced more than 2.5-fold: cyclooxygenase-1, tenascin-C, and plasminogen activator inhibitor-1. Downregulated genes were P-selectin ligand, interleukin (IL)-1β, matrix metalloproteinase-1, and thrombomodulin *(11)*. Schaub et al. *(12)* demonstrated that induction of apoptosis by Fas/FADD-activation mediates a specific mRNA expression program of inflammatory genes in SMCs. This included upregulation of IL-8, monocyte chemolactic protein-1, plasminogen activator inhibitor type 2, IL-6 growth-regulated protein-1, and IL-1a. The inflammatory responses increased the recruitment of macrophages to the site of vessel injury in a rat model *(12)*.

## ANIMAL EXPERIMENTS

In a systematic approach, Geary et al. *(13)*, analyzed the gene-expression pattern of neointimal SMCs 4 wk after aortic grafting in cynomolgus monkeys. They compared these expression patterns with those of SMCs from healthy aorta and vena cava *(13)*. Thereby, the authors were able to characterize gene expression events associated with neointima formation and to provide the basis for novel hypotheses. Only 13 genes were upregulated in neointimal SMCs compared with aortic SMCs, whereas 134 genes were downregulated. For example, specific collagen subtypes, like collagen-I, -III, -VI, and -V and other matrix genes like versican were upregulated in neointimal SMCs emphasizing the pivotal role of extracellular matrix synthesis in the pathogenesis of neointima formation *(13)*.

## STUDIES IN PATIENTS

Despite abundant animal data, molecular mechanisms of neointima formation had been investigated on only a limited basis in patients. Therefore, the authors sought to establish a method for profiling gene expression in human in-stent neointima *(2)*. As an initial step, the authors were able to demonstrate that gene-expression patterns of human neointima retrieved by helix-cutter atherectomy can be reliably analyzed by cDNA array technology. The expression of 2435 genes in atherectomy specimens and blood cells of patients with in-stent restenosis, normal coronary artery specimens, and cultured human SMCs were investigated *(1)*. The tissue retrieved from in-stent restenosis by helix-cutter atherectomy exhibited known gene-expression patterns of neointima, such as the upregulation of cyclooxygenase-1 or the downregulation of desmin *(2)*. Additionally, previously unknown gene expression events of neointima, including downregulation of mammary-derived growth inhibitor and upregulation of FK506 binding protein 12 were discovered. Of the 223 differentially expressed genes, 37 genes indicated activation of interferon (IFN)-γ signaling in neointimal SMCs *(1)*. In cultured SMCs, IFN-γ inhibited apoptosis. Genetic disruption of IFN-γ signaling in a mouse model of restenosis significantly reduced the vascular proliferative response. Therefore, the data suggest an important role of IFN-γ in the control of neointima proliferation *(1)*.

Zhang et al. *(14)* analyzed differential gene expression in cultured SMCs explanted from neointima from human in-stent restenosis and compared it with the gene-expression pattern of cultured SMCs from aorta and coronary artery from patients undergoing renal or cardiac transplantation. They identified 32 genes that were upregulated in SMCs from human neointima. Consistent with the authors gene-expression analysis of human neointima from in-stent restenosis *(2)*, they also described upregulation of thrombospondin-1.

## THERAPEUTIC DEVELOPMENT

Gene-expression profiling in conjunction with current knowledge of pathophysiological role of the genes analyzed may help identify novel therapeutic targets. For example, thrombospondin-1 that was found to be upregulated in human neointima is involved in SMC proliferation and migration *(15)*. Accordingly, blockade of thrombosponsin-1 by specific antibodies reduced neointima formation in balloon-injured rat carotid arteries by decreasing the number of proliferating SMCs *(16)*. Thus, the consistent results from the independent gene-expression analyses provide a rationale to test antibody blockade of thrombospondin-1 in humans.

Another example of this paradigm are the findings regarding upregulation of FKBP12 in human neointima *(2)*. FKBP12 is the receptor for sirolimus, which in animal models reduced neointima formation. By the same time, the authors found upregulation of FKBP12 in human neointima by gene-expression profiling, the first clinical study showed that sirolimus-coated stents dramatically decrease the risk of in-stent restenosis in patients without increasing the risk of other major adverse cardiac events *(17,18)*. Additionally, it has been recently shown that sirolimus treatment with a high oral loading dose regimen before coronary intervention resulted in a significant reduction of restenosis after placement of bare stents. In this study, the plasma concentration of sirolimus on the day of the procedure correlated inversely with the late lumen loss at follow-up *(19)*.

In several animal models of restenosis after angioplasty, it has been shown that sirolimus inhibits the proliferative response causing neointima formation by enhancement of the level of $p27^{KIP1}$ protein and activation of retinoblastoma protein (pRb) *(8,20)*. Nevertheless, this pathway does not appear to be the only mechanism involved in the beneficial action of sirolimus. Sirolimus also inhibits neointima formation in $p27^{KIP1}$-knockout mice through $p27^{KIP1}$-independent mechanisms *(21)*.

Sirolimus, an immunosuppressive, binds to cytosolic FKBP-12 and this complex inhibits the protein kinase mammalian target of rapomycin (mTOR) *(22)*. The mTOR kinase is essential for viability and regulates translation initiation and cell-cycle progression by altering the phosphorylation state of downstream targets like the p70 S6 kinase (p70S6K) *(23)*. In T lymphocytes, inhibition of mTOR by sirolimus leads to dephosphorylation and thereby inactivation of p70S6K and to hypophosphorylation and thereby activation of pRb *(24)*. The p70S6K is an important regulator of cell-cycle progression in response to mitogens that play pivotal roles in neointima formation, like placelet-derived growth factor and angiotensin *(25,26)*.

In the gene-expression analysis of human neointima from in-stent restenosis study, the authors showed that p70S6K-II and FKBP-12 were upregulated in cells from human in-stent neointima *(1)*. However, a systematic analysis of the effect of sirolimus on neointima formation in vivo has not been carried out yet. Therefore, the authors investigate the regulation of mammalian target of rapomycin kinase and the effect of sirolimus on p70S6K, pRb activity, and on global gene-expression patterns in coronary artery SMCs

*(27)*. mTOR was nuclear translocated and phosphorylated in coronary artery smooth muscle cells (CASMCs) and T cells from human neointima from the coronary in-stent restenosis indicative for an activation of mTOR during neointima formation in humans.

Comparative gene-expression analysis of CASMCs treated with sirolimus revealed downregulation of the transcription factor E2F-1, a key regulator of $G_1$/S-phase entry, and of various pRb/E2F-1-regulated genes. In addition, changes in the expression of genes associated with replication, apoptosis, and inflammation were found. Furthermore, sirolimus decreased the gene expression of endothelial monocyte-activating polypeptide (EMAP)-II. This decrease of EMAP-II expression was reflected in a reduced adhesiveness of CASMCs for monocytic cells. Addition of EMAP-II counteracted the antiadhesive effect of sirolimus. Therefore, EMAP-II may include a mechanism of sirolimus-mediated reduction of the proinflammatory activation of CASMCs *(27)*.

The effects of sirolimus on the downregulation of genes involved in cell-cycle progression, apoptosis, proliferation, and extracellular matrix formation in CASMCs provide further insight into how sirolimus reduces CASMC proliferation. The data suggest an additional antiadhesive and thereby anti-inflammatory effect of sirolimus: by inhibiting the expression of the monocyte chemoattractant EMAP-II, sirolimus leads to a decrease in CASMC adhesiveness and thereby may block the early recruitment of inflammatory cells to the injured arteries. This effect may further reduce the vascular proliferative response in humans.

## PERSPECTIVES

Major progress has been made in the availability of technologies to analyze global gene-expression patterns in clinical samples *(28)*. Although gene-expression profiling can provide important information about molecular mechanisms of disease, such as neointima formation, one has to be aware of the pitfalls and limitations of these analyses. Gene-expression profiling represents an effective and powerful tool to generate hypotheses of potential pathophysiological relevance and to identify novel therapeutic targets. On the other hand, a careful validation and verification of the gene-expression data is essential. Therefore, the new approach of gene-expression profiling cannot replace conventional methods such as validation by Northern or Western blotting or proof of concept in experimental animals, such as knockout or transgenic mice. Nevertheless, increased availability of this technology will bring into light some of the thus far ill-understood features of cardiovascular disease and will help identify new, potentially more individualized therapeutic options.

## REFERENCES

1. Zohlnhöfer D, Richter T, Neumann F, et al. Transcriptome analysis reveals a role of interferon-gamma in human neointima formation. Mol Cell 2001b;7:1059–1069.
2. Zohlnhöfer D, Klein CA, Richter T, et al. Gene expression profiling of human stent-induced neointima by cDNA array analysis of microscopic specimens retrieved by helix cutter atherectomy: Detection of FK506-binding protein 12 upregulation. Circulation 2001a;103:1396–1402.
3. Klein CA, Seidl S, Petat-Dutter K, et al. Combined transcriptome and genome analysis of single micrometastatic cells. Nat Biotechnol 2002;20:387–392.
4. Ramoni MF, Paola Sebastiani P, Isaac S, Kohane IS. Cluster analysis of gene expression dynamics. Proc Natl Acad Sci USA 2002;99:9121–9126.
5. Serruys PW, de Jaegere P, Kiemeneij F, et al. A comparison of balloon-expandable-stent implantation with balloon angioplasty in patients with coronary artery disease. Benestent Study Group. N Engl J Med 1994;331:489–495.

6. Fischman DL, Leon MB, Baim DS, et al. A randomized comparison of coronary-stent placement and balloon angioplasty in the treatment of coronary artery disease. Stent Restenosis Study Investigators. N Engl J Med 1994;331:496–501.

7. Mintz GS, Popma JJ, Hong MK, et al. Intravascular ultrasound to discern device-specific effects and mechanisms of restenosis. Am J Cardiol 1996;78:18–22.

8. Poon M, Badimon JJ, Fuster V. Overcoming restenosis with sirolimus: from alphabet soup to clinical reality. Lancet 2002;359:619–622.

9. Geary RL, Nikkari ST, Wagner WD, Williams JK, Adams MR, Dean RH. Wound healing: a paradigm for lumen narrowing after arterial reconstruction. J Vasc Surg 1998;27:96–106.

10. Schwartz RS. Pathophysiology of restenosis: interaction of thrombosis, hyperplasia, and/or remodeling. Am J Cardiol 1998;81:14E–17E.

11. Feng Y, Yang JH, Huang H, et al. Transcriptional profile of mechanically induced genes in human vascular smooth muscle cells. Circ Res 1999;85:1118–1123.

12. Schaub FJ, Han DK, Liles WC, et al. Fas/FADD-mediated activation of a specific program of inflammatory gene expression in vascular smooth muscle cells. Nat Med 2000;6:790–796.

13. Geary RL, Wong JM, Rossini A, Schwartz SM, Adams LD. Expression profiling identifies 147 genes contributing to a unique primate neointimal smooth muscle cell phenotype. Arterioscler Thromb Vasc Biol 2002;22:2010–2016.

14. Zhang QJ, Goddard M, Shanahan C, Shapiro L, Bennett M. Differential gene expression in vascular smooth muscle cells in primary atherosclerosis and in stent stenosis in humans. Arterioscler Thromb Vasc Biol 2002;22:2030–2036.

15. Scott-Burden T, Resink TJ, Baur U, Burgin M, Buhler FR. Activation of S6 kinase in cultured vascular smooth muscle cells by submitogenic levels of thrombospondin. Biochem Biophys Res Commun 1988a;150:278–286.

16. Chen D, Asahara T, Krasinski K, et al. Antibody blockade of thrombospondin accelerates reendothelialization and reduces neointima formation in balloon-injured rat carotid artery. Circulation 1999;100:849–854.

17. Sousa JE, Costa MA, Abizaid A, et al. Lack of Neointimal Proliferation After Implantation of Sirolimus-Coated Stents in Human Coronary Arteries : A Quantitative Coronary Angiography and Three-Dimensional Intravascular Ultrasound Study. Circulation 2001;103:192–195.

18. Marx SO, Marks AR. Bench to bedside: the development of sirolimus and its application to stent restenosis. Circulation 2001;104:852–855.

19. Hausleiter J, Kastrati A, Mehilli J, et al. Randomized, double-blind, placebo-controlled trial of oral sirolimus for restenosis prevention in patients with in-stent restenosis: the Oral Sirolimus to Inhibit Recurrent In-stent Stenosis (OSIRIS) trial. Circulation 2004;110:790–795.

20. Gallo R, Padurean A, Jayaraman T, et al. Inhibition of intimal thickening after balloon angioplasty in porcine coronary arteries by targeting regulators of the cell cycle. Circulation 1999;99:2164–2170.

21. Roque M, Reis ED, Cordon-Cardo C, et al. Effect of p27 deficiency and sirolimus on intimal hyperplasia: in vivo and in vitro studies using a p27 knockout mouse model. Lab Invest 2001;81:895–903.

22. Gingras AC, Raught B, Sonenberg N. Regulation of translation initiation by FRAP/mTOR. Genes Dev 2001;15:807–826.

23. Raught B, Gingras AC, Sonenberg N. The target of sirolimus (TOR) proteins. Proc Natl Acad Sci USA 2001;98:7037–7044.

24. Brennan P, Babbage JW, Thomas G, Cantrell D. p70(s6k) integrates phosphatidylinositol 3-kinase and sirolimus-regulated signals for E2F regulation in T lymphocytes. Mol Cell Biol 1999;19:4729–4738.

25. Pearson RB, Thomas G. Regulation of p70s6k/p85s6k and its role in the cell cycle. Prog Cell Cycle Res 1995;1(21–32):21–32.

26. Scott-Burden T, Resink TJ, Baur U, Burgin M, Buhler FR. Amiloride sensitive activation of S6 kinase by angiotensin II in cultured vascular smooth muscle cells. Biochem Biophys Res Commun 1988b;151:583–589.

27. Zohlnhöfer D, Nührenberg TG, Neumann FJ, et al. Sirolimus effects transcriptional programs in smooth muscle cells controlling proliferative and inflammatory properties. Mol Pharmacol 2004;65:880–889.

28. Napoli C, Lerman LO, Sica V, Lerman A, Tajana G, de Nigris F. Microarray analysis: a novel research tool for cardiovascular scientists and physicians. Heart 2003;89:597–604.

# 10 Proteomics and Restenosis

*Santhi K. Ganesh, MD*
*and Elizabeth G. Nabel, MD*

## CONTENTS

## INTRODUCTION

The human genome sequence is now known. With the completion of the human genome project, focus has shifted to the immense task of understanding the function of genes and their roles in disease processes. The proteome is defined as the complement of proteins expressed by the genome. The ultimate expression of the genome is the proteome. As proteins are the actual molecular workhorses that carry out gene function within cells, proteomic studies are functional genomic investigations. Investigation at the protein level is directly reflective of cellular function and alterations in disease states. Proteome analysis provides highly detailed information because protein expression and function is regulated through multiple mechanisms, including post-translational modification, compartmentalization, protein–protein interactions, varying degradation patterns. Novel advances in protein–analysis technologies have yielded powerful analytic tools that can now be applied to biomedical research. The methods used in proteomics are based on pairing of these tools with the human genome sequence. These methods allow profiling of proteins and determination of protein modifications for the purposes of defining disease mechanisms and biomarker discovery. Several specific proteins have known roles in vascular injury responses, many of which have been directly implicated in the development of restenosis. As functional genomics pushes the current thinking past individual gene function in disease processes, proteomics will be used to precisely define molecular functions and the interconnections between functional gene networks and pathways. Furthermore, the definition of protein-level interactions is expected to highlight novel disease mechanisms and provide further insight into altered cellular function in cardiovascular diseases.

From: *Contemporary Cardiology: Essentials of Restenosis: For the Interventional Cardiologist*
Edited by: H. J. Duckers, E. G. Nabel, and P. W. Serruys © Humana Press Inc., Totowa, NJ

# PROTEOMICS

## Background

Several reasons exist for focusing on protein analysis. Expression profiles of mRNA within a cell do not necessarily reflect the amount of active protein within the cell. Although amino acid sequence of a protein can be inferred from DNA sequence, the gene sequence does not describe alternative splice variants or post-translational modifications that may be essential for any given protein's function and activity. Furthermore, the genome sequence is static and does not adequately reflect dynamic cellular processes, and even mRNA expression provides only one level of information regarding the ultimate expression and function of a gene. The overall concept of proteomics and the rationale for its study are straightforward. However, investigation of the proteome presents significant technical challenges. The proteome is incrementally complex compared with the study of DNA or mRNA because proteins are made of 20 amino acids, as opposed to four nucleotides. Protein sequencing strategies are available, but these are not nearly as high-throughput as DNA sequencing or mRNA hybridization for identification. The dynamic range of protein abundance is larger, up to $10^9$ in the case of plasma *(1)* (Fig. 1). The study of low-abundance proteins is hampered by the lack of amplification methods. Additionally, the diversity of functional regulation of proteins can additionally make analysis more complex. Protein function is regulated through a variety of mechanisms, including alternative splicing of transcripts, contranslational and post-translational modification, compartmentalization within cells, protein–protein interactions and varying degradation patterns. Examination of protein–protein interactions alone demonstrates a high-degree of complexity *(2)* (Fig. 2). However, significant technical advances in proteomic instrumentation makes study of the proteome possible. As proteomics aims to identify proteins as well as define the cellular and biochemical functions of identified proteins under various conditions, proteomics investigations are more complex but are accordingly highly revealing. Proper study design and informed application of the available technologies are essential to getting the most from any proteomics study *(3)*. Using clearly defined experimental approaches, the knowledge that can now be obtained using proteomics is beyond what has been possible in the past and is leading to new understanding of cellular function and disease pathophysiology.

Examples of successful proteomic applications in cardiovascular research include the determination of downstream effectors of protein kinase C signaling during myocardial preconditioning and functional regulators of apoptosis in vascular smooth muscle cells *(4,5)*. Functional post-translational modifications of contractile proteins in myocardial tissue have been defined and suggest mechanisms for myocardial preconditioning and stunning *(6–8)*. As proteomic technologies develop and applications in cardiovascular research broaden, significant understanding of disease mechanisms, prediction of responses to pharmacological therapies and biomarker discovery will be possible *(9)*.

## Clinical Proteomics

Clinical proteomics is a new field of applied proteomics, primarily used in the context of biomarker determination. Beyond the identification and characterization of individual protein biomarkers, newer proteomics tools, such as mass spectrometry (MS), have shown early promise for novel biomarker assessments. One such example is the use of surface enhanced laser desporption-ionziation time-of-flight MS for diagnostic proteomics, in which the mass spectrum resulting from analysis of complex body

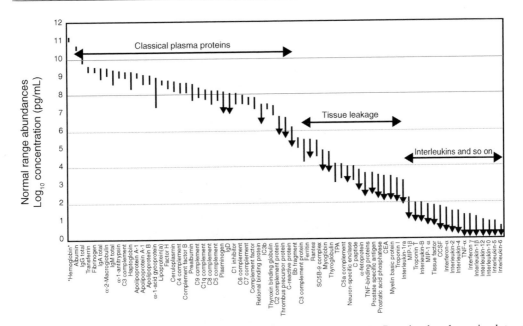

**Fig. 1.** Dynamic range of 70 proteins in the human plasma proteome *(1)*. Protein abundance is plotted on a log scale and spans over eleven orders of magnitude. Classical plasma proteins are clustered on the left. Proteins expressed in states of tissue leakage, such as enzymes and troponins, are clustered in the center. Cytokines, which are known to be of relatively low abundance in plasma, are clustered on the right. Reproduced with permission *(1)*.

fluids, such as serum, is used as a biomarker for disease in itself. That is, the spectral signals serve as a biomarker, regardless of not knowing individual protein identities that make up the mass spectral signals. In surface enhanced laser desporption-ionziation technology, the sample is subjected to interaction with a specialized surface, on which proteins are captured by the process of adsorption, electrostatic interaction or affinity chromatography on a solid-phase chip surface *(10)*.

The proteins are then ionized and detected, using laser desorption/ionization. From this, a mass spectrum is reported. Analysis of multiple spectra is achieved using advanced computational methods to determine spectral patterns distinctive of disease states. The strength of this approach lies in the ability to simultaneously assay many proteins in a complex mixture. In this manner, proteomic diagnostics is potentially an effective method to evaluate groups of proteins in unison for biomarker purposes. The use of sets of proteins as opposed to a single protein marker is expected to enhance the sensitivity and specificity for disease-state identification. This approach has been successfully applied in pilot studies in the field of cancer diagnostics. Validation in larger Food and Drug Administration-sponsored trials is currently ongoing *(11–14)*. The application of this type of pattern recognition approach is just beginning in the field of cardiovascular research and has significant potential to aid in the prediction or diagnosis of the occurrence of specific vascular injury responses.

## METHODS

### *Proteomics Tools*

The tools used in proteomics are based on well-established analytic methods that have been recently adapted for use in proteomic investigations. Publication of the draft

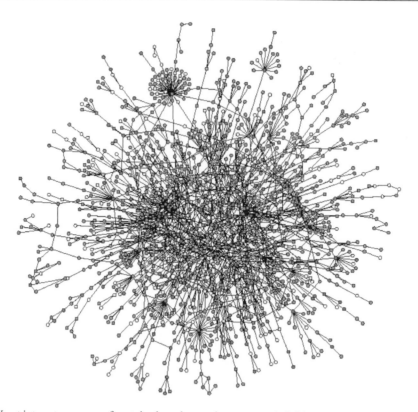

**Fig. 2.** Yeast interactome map of proteins based on early yeast two-hybrid measurements in *Saccaromyces cerevisiae (2)*. A high degree of interconnectedness has been observed in maps of protein–protein interactions, illustrating the complexity of the proteome. Reproduced with permission *(2)*.

human genome sequence resulted in an explosion of proteomic databases and tools with which to identify proteins based on sequence data. In combination, these two advances have enabled proteomic approaches in biomedical research. The key steps in proteomics are the separation of complex mixtures of proteins and the identification of proteins using MS. The typical workflow of a proteomic investigation starts with separation of a complex protein sample, such as that derived from a tissue or cells. Two-dimensional gel electrophoresis (2DGE) and liquid chromatography are two well-established protein separation strategies and have been scaled to high-throughput applications with use of robotics and automated multidimensional separation strategies. Once proteins are separated, individual protein spots, in the case of gels or fractions and in the case of chromatographic separation are digested with an enzyme, such as trypsin, which will cleave at predictable locations within a protein. This results in peptide fragments that have a predictable mass.

The peptides are then analyzed with MS to determine mass and matched against a database created from an in silico translation of the genome sequence, considering the enzyme used to cleave proteins (Fig. 3). Mass-based matches made in this manner are often sufficient to unambiguously identify a protein. In the case where the protein identity is still not clearly determined, possibly owing to post-translational or other modifications that may alter the exact mass of a peptide, tandem MS can be performed. In this method, peptides are broken into sequential ions, from which direct amino acid

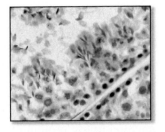

Exact proteins from tissue or cells

  Separate proteins

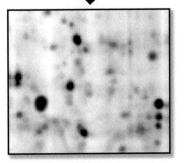

Two-dimensional gel

Enzymatic cleavage of individual protein spots

Analyze peptides with mass spectrometry

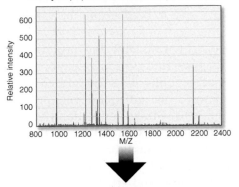

Match peptide masses against translated
genome database with in silco digestion results

Identify proteins

**Fig. 3.** Typical proteomic workflow for peptide mass fingerprinting. Proteins are isolated from the cells or tissue of interest and separated. In this example, two-dimensional gel electrophoresis is the separation method. Individual protein spots are then cut out of the gel, enzymatically digested into peptides of which mass is determined using mass spectrometry. Reproduced with permission *(42)*.

sequence is determined. This method can provide unequivocal protein identification as well as additional information, such as the existence of a specific post-translation modification at a specific amino acid. These proteomic findings must then be interpreted in the context of known or predicted biological function. Adaptations of these techniques for higher throughput and more sophisticated proteome investigations are an area of rapid technological development. Although gene expression profiling more commonly refers to transcript analyses, methods to quantify as well as identify proteins offer the tantalizing potential to use protein expression as a new gene expression method *(15)*.

## *Interpretation of Proteomics Data*

Proteomic data analysis requires similar considerations as in the interpretation of microarrays, with special attention to reproducibility and the statistical issue of multiple hypothesis testing. Reproducibility of assays, such as 2DGE can be problematic, and meaningful comparisons between two samples may be challenging. One weakness of all proteomic techniques is the limited detection of low-abundance proteins. This is a problem common to any large-scale analysis and is seen in transcript profiling studies as well. However, the wide dynamic range of protein abundance presents a larger challenge in proteomics. Coverage of the proteome is additionally complicated by the various properties of proteins. Hydrophobicity, extreme charge states or isoelectric mobility, location within membranes, and the presence of certain post-translational modifications can diminish the ability to detect and identify certain proteins. New fluorescent dye systems for 2DGE now allow for the analysis of two samples on one gel, providing a robust means for controlling for technical factors during the 2DGE. Additionally, these fluorescent dyes have improved sensitivity over standard protein-detection methods. Other advances in automation, microfluidics and nanotechnology are expected to significantly assist the widespread application of proteomics technology as well. Finally, any findings of a proteomic study, much like a microarray transcript profiling study, must be followed by functional validation of the specific findings. This is a necessary step to both ensure the validity and functional significance of any findings.

Combined investigations of transcript and protein expression show special promise for determining gene function because cross-validation can be performed across both sets of genomic data. Integrated global quantitative analyses of biological information from multiple levels provide detailed insight into the operation of a system *(16)*. Modeling of detailed cell signaling and other pathways is assisted, and further examination of the model can then be performed to understand the properties of the system. This approach has been applied in experimental systems of yeast, where galactose utilization has been analyzed under various conditions and after various perturbations, such as gene inactivation, investigations were performed to determine mRNA expression, protein expression, protein–protein interactions, and protein–DNA interactions. This investigation yielded a detailed map of galactose utilization pathways, regulatory networks, and relationship to other biochemical pathways *(16)*. These types of integrated approaches hold promise in functional genomic investigations as a systems biology approach to understanding the human genome as well and hold particular promise for understanding the perturbations in systems that cause disease.

## PROTEOMICS IN RESTENOSIS

The application of proteomics to understand vascular injury responses will shed light on vascular homeostatic and disease mechanisms that lead to restenosis. Several distinct proteins are already known to have important roles in potentiating inflammatory and proliferative mechanisms. Examples are 12-lipoxygenase products, transforming growth factor-β, leukocyte β 2-integrins, M-cerebral spinal fluid, vascular cell adhesion molecule-1, tumor necrosis factor-α, Interleukin-8, Interferon-γ and the nuclear factor-κB pathways *(17–30)*. Several of these proteins that have well-understood inflammatory functions are additionally known to be mitogenic signals, triggering the exit of vascular smooth muscle cells from $G_0/G_1$ and entry into the cell cycle. Several specific genes in cell-cycle regulatory pathways also have defined roles in the development of restenosis. Proteomics offers the advantage of being able to fill in such functional pathways, by both demonstrating protein expression and defining the state of individual proteins *(31)*. For example, phosphorylation of specific cell cycle proteins, such as p27Kip1, is known to regulate its stability and function *(32)*. Proteomics is the only approach that can adequately address the question of what post-translational modifications to proteins occur on a global basis after vascular injury, and what may be the functional consequences of these.

Another example of the importance of understanding post-translational modification of proteins is the discovery of the role of advanced glycosylation end products (AGE) after arterial injury. In the setting of arterial injury, AGE formation and deposition is stimulated *(33)*. AGE bind to a multiligand receptor (RAGE) and trigger augmentation of processes known to be central in neointimal lesion development, including inflammatory responses, cellular migration and proliferation *(34)*. RAGE is a multiligand member of the immunoglobulin superfamily of cell surface molecules, interacts with distinct molecules implicated in homeostasis, development, and inflammation, and certain diseases, such as diabetes. RAGE is expressed at low levels in adult tissues in homeostasis, but highly upregulated at sites of vascular pathology *(35–37)*. The glycosylated proteins that are ligands to RAGE are the product of extensive post-translational modification that are thought to play a significant role in the vasculopathy observed in diabetics. Binding of RAGE by a ligand triggers activation of key cell signaling pathways, such as p21 (ras), MAP kinases, NF-κB, and cdc42/rac, thereby reprogramming cellular properties *(38–40)*. Furthermore, in this study, RAGE expression was demonstrated to modulate the expression of genes known to have important roles in vascular homeostasis, such as tenascin C, an extracellular matrix protein with antiadhesive effects, and MMP12, an enzyme capable of degrading arterial elastin. Blockade of RAGE-dependent cellular activation suppressed transcripts for these genes and diminished neointimal hyperplasia. Because post-translational modification of proteins is understood to be an acute response mechanism, proteomic applications in this type of investigation would clarify acute responses. Downstream targets of activated cell signaling pathways can also be filled in using a global approach. In the example provided, further understanding of the importance of AGE and related protein modifications in the mechanism restenosis may also help to explain clinical observations, such as the finding that restenosis is more prevalent among diabetics *(41)*.

## SUMMARY

The development of proteomics offers exciting and novel approaches to examine disease processes at a molecular level. Proteomics is already beginning to unravel many of the complexities of gene function in homeostatic as well as pathological conditions. The application of proteomics to understanding responses to vascular injury and the development of restenosis will be highly enhanced by the technological advances that continue to be made in this field. As proteomics technology continues to improve, it will be possible in the near future to obtain a more comprehensive picture of the pathological vascular injury responses that culminate in the development of restenosis.

# REFERENCES

1. Anderson NL, Anderson NG. The human plasma proteome: history, character, and diagnostic prospects. Mol Cell Proteomics 2002;1:845–867.
2. Hasty J, McMillen D, Collins JJ. Engineered gene circuits. Nature 2002;420:224–230.
3. Arrell DK, Neverova I, Van Eyk JE. Cardiovascular proteomics: evolution and potential. Circ Res 2001;88:763–773.
4. Ping P, Zhang J, Pierce WM Jr, Bolli R. Functional proteomic analysis of protein kinase C epsilon signaling complexes in the normal heart and during cardioprotection. Circ Res 2001;88:59–62.
5. Taurin S, Seyrantepe V, Orlov SN, et al. Proteome analysis and functional expression identify mortalin as an antiapoptotic gene induced by elevation of [Na+]i/[K+]i ratio in cultured vascular smooth muscle cells. Circ Res 2002;91:915–922.
6. Arrell DK, Neverova I, Fraser H, Marban E, Van Eyk JE. Proteomic analysis of pharmacologically preconditioned cardiomyocytes reveals novel phosphorylation of myosin light chain 1. Circ Res 2001;89:480–487.
7. Foster DB, Noguchi T, VanBuren P, Murphy AM, Van Eyk JE. C-terminal truncation of cardiac troponin I causes divergent effects on ATPase and force: implications for the pathophysiology of myocardial stunning. Circ Res 2003;93:917–924.
8. Buscemi N, Foster DB, Neverova I, Van Eyk JE. p21-activated kinase increases the calcium sensitivity of rat triton-skinned cardiac muscle fiber bundles via a mechanism potentially involving novel phosphorylation of troponin I. Circ Res. 2002;91:509–516.
9. Patterson SD, Aebersold RH. Proteomics: the first decade and beyond. Nat Genet 2003;33:311–323.
10. Issaq HJ, Conrads TP, Prieto DA, Tirumalai R, Veenstra TD. SELDI-TOF MS for diagnostic proteomics. Anal Chem 2003;75:148A–155A.
11. Petricoin EF, Ardekani AM, Hitt BA, et al. Use of proteomic patterns in serum to identify ovarian cancer. Lancet 2002;359:572–577.
12. Adam BL, Qu Y, Davis JW, et al. Serum protein fingerprinting coupled with a pattern-matching algorithm distinguishes prostate cancer from benign prostate hyperplasia and healthy men. Cancer Res 2002;62:3609–3614.
13. Yanagisawa K, Shyr Y, Xu BJ, et al. Proteomic patterns of tumour subsets in non-small-cell lung cancer. Lancet 2003;362:433–439.
14. Pusch W, Flocco MT, Leung SM, Thiele H, Kostrzewa M. Mass spectrometry-based clinical proteomics. Pharmacogenomics 2003;4:463–476.
15. Pasa-Tolic L, Lipton MS, Masselon CD, et al. Gene expression profiling using advanced mass spectrometric approaches. J Mass Spectrom 2002;37:1185–1198.
16. Ideker T, Thorsson V, Ranish JA, et al. Integrated genomic and proteomic analyses of a systematically perturbed metabolic network. Science 2001;292:929–934.
17. Hayashi S, Watanabe N, Nakazawa K, et al. Roles of P-selectin in inflammation, neointimal formation, and vascular remodeling in balloon-injured rat carotid arteries. Circulation 2000;102:1710–1717.
18. Kumar A, Hoover JL, Simmons CA, Lindner V, Shebuski RJ. Remodeling and neointimal formation in the carotid artery of normal and P-selectin-deficient mice. Circulation 1997;96:4333–4342.
19. Gu JL, Pei H, Thomas L, et al. Ribozyme-mediated inhibition of rat leukocyte-type 12-lipoxygenase prevents intimal hyperplasia in balloon-injured rat carotid arteries. Circulation 2001;103:1446–1452.
20. Smith JD, Bryant SR, Couper LL, et al. Soluble transforming growth factor-beta type II receptor inhibits negative remodeling, fibroblast transdifferentiation, and intimal lesion formation but not endothelial growth. Circ Res 1999;84:1212–1222.
21. Ward MR, Agrotis A, Kanellakis P, Hall J, Jennings G, Bobik A. Tranilast prevents activation of transforming growth factor-beta system, leukocyte accumulation, and neointimal growth in porcine coronary arteries after stenting. Arterioscler Thromb Vasc Biol 2002;22:940–948.

22. Horvath C, Welt FG, Nedelman M, Rao P, Rogers C. Targeting CCR2 or CD18 inhibits experimental in-stent restenosis in primates: inhibitory potential depends on type of injury and leukocytes targeted. Circ Res 2002;90:488–494.

23. Simon DI, Dhen Z, Seifert P, Edelman ER, Ballantyne CM, Rogers C. Decreased neointimal formation in Mac-1(–/–) mice reveals a role for inflammation in vascular repair after angioplasty. J Clin Invest 2000;105:293–300.

24. Hojo Y, Ikeda U, Katsuki T, et al. Chemokine expression in coronary circulation after coronary angioplasty as a prognostic factor for restenosis. Atherosclerosis 2001;156:165–170.

25. Zohlnhofer D, Richter T, Neumann F, et al. Transcriptome analysis reveals a role of interferon-gamma in human neointima formation. Mol Cell 2001;7:1059–1069.

26. Libby P, Ganz P. Restenosis revisited—new targets, new therapies. N Engl J Med 1997;337:418–419.

27. Collins T, Read MA, Neish AS, Whitley MZ, Thanos D, Maniatis T. Transcriptional regulation of endothelial cell adhesion molecules: NF-kappa B and cytokine-inducible enhancers. Faseb J 1995;9:899–909.

28. Shi C, Zhang X, Chen Z, Robinson MK, Simon DI. Leukocyte integrin Mac-1 recruits toll/interleukin-1 receptor superfamily signaling intermediates to modulate NF-kappaB activity. Circ Res 2001; 89(10):859–865.

29. Bourcier T, Sukhova G, Libby P. The nuclear factor kappa-B signaling pathway participates in dysregulation of vascular smooth muscle cells in vitro and in human atherosclerosis. J Biol Chem 1997; 272(25):15,817–15,824.

30. Breuss JM, Cejna M, Bergmeister H, Kadl A, Baumgartl G, Steurer S, et al. Activation of nuclear factor-kappa B significantly contributes to lumen loss in a rabbit iliac artery balloon angioplasty model. Circulation 2002;105(5):633–638.

31. Elia AE, Cantley LC, Yaffe MB. Proteomic screen finds pSer/pThr-binding domain localizing Plk1 to mitotic substrates. Science 2003;299(5610):1228–1231.

32. Boehm M, Yoshimoto T, Crook MF, Nallamshetty S, True A, Nabel GJ, et al. A growth factor-dependent nuclear kinase phosphorylates p27(Kip1) and regulates cell cycle progression. EMBO J 2002;21(13):3390–3401.

33. Schmidt AM, Hasu M, Popov D, Zhang JH, Chen J, Yan SD, et al. Receptor for advanced glycation end products (AGEs) has a central role in vessel wall interactions and gene activation in response to circulating AGE proteins. Proc Natl Acad Sci USA 1994;91(19): 8807–8811.

34. Sakaguchi T, Yan SF, Yan SD, Belov D, Rong LL, Sousa M, et al. Central role of RAGE-dependent neointimal expansion in arterial restenosis. J Clin Invest 2003;111(7):959–972.

35. Park L, Raman KG, Lee KJ, Lu Y, Ferran LJ, Jr., Chow WS, et al. Suppression of accelerated diabetic atherosclerosis by the soluble receptor for advanced glycation endproducts. Nat Med 1998;4(9): 1025–1031.

36. Bucciarelli LG, Wendt T, Qu W, Lu Y, Lalla E, Rong LL, et al. RAGE blockade stabilizes established atherosclerosis in diabetic apolipoprotein E-null mice. Circulation 2002;106(22):2827–2835.

37. Wendt T, Bucciarelli L, Qu W, Lu Y, Yan SF, Stern DM, et al. Receptor for advanced glycation endproducts (RAGE) and vascular inflammation: insights into the pathogenesis of macrovascular complications in diabetes. Curr Atheroscler Rep 2002;4(3):228–237.

38. Taguchi A, Blood DC, del Toro G, Canet A, Lee DC, Qu W, et al. Blockade of RAGE-amphoterin signalling suppresses tumour growth and metastases. Nature 2000;405(6784):354–360.

39. Hofmann MA, Drury S, Fu C, Qu W, Taguchi A, Lu Y, et al. RAGE mediates a novel proinflammatory axis: a central cell surface receptor for S100/calgranulin polypeptides. Cell 1999;97(7):889–901.

40. Schmidt AM, Yan SD, Brett J, Mora R, Nowygrod R, Stern D. Regulation of human mononuclear phagocyte migration by cell surface-binding proteins for advanced glycation endproducts. J Clin Invest 1993;91(5):2155–2168.

41. Mathew V, Gersh BJ, Williams BA, Laskey WK, Willerson JT, Tilbury RT, et al. Outcomes in patients with diabetes mellitus undergoing percutaneous coronary intervention in the current era: a report from the Prevention of REStenosis with Tranilast and its Outcomes (PRESTO) trial. Circulation 2004;109(4):476–480.

42. Ganesh SK, Nabel EG. Genomics and Gene Transfer. In: Fuster V, Topol E, Nabel E (eds). *Atherosclerosis and Coronary Artery Disease,* Lippincott Williams Wilkens, Philadelphia, 2004, pp. 647–661.

# 11 Contribution of Circulating Progenitor Cells to Vascular Repair and Lesion Formation

*Masataka Sata, MD, PhD*
*and Kenneth Walsh, PhD*

## CONTENTS

## INTRODUCTION

The accumulation of smooth muscle cells (SMCs) plays a principal role in atherogenesis, postangioplasty restenosis, and transplantation-associated vasculopathy. Therefore, much effort has been expended in targeting the migration and proliferation of medial SMCs to prevent occlusive vascular remodeling. Recent findings have suggested that bone marrow-derived precursors can also give rise to vascular cells that contribute to repair, remodeling, and lesion formation. This article overviews recent findings on circulating vascular progenitor cells and describes potential therapeutic strategies that target these cells.

## CONTRIBUTION OF SMCS TO VASCULAR LESIONS

Exuberant accumulation of SMCs plays a principal role in the pathogenesis of vascular diseases (1–4). In atherosclerotic plaques, SMC proliferate and synthesize extracellular matrix, contributing to lesion mass. Percutaneous coronary interventions (PCIs) have been widely adopted for the treatment of coronary atherosclerosis. However, a significant fraction of these procedures fail as a result of postangioplasty restenosis (5). Although the increasing use of new devices for dilatation of stenosed arteries has lowered the incidence of acute complications, restenosis still limits the long-term outcome of percutaneous interventions (6).

From: *Contemporary Cardiology: Essentials of Restenosis: For the Interventional Cardiologist*
Edited by: H. J. Duckers, E. G. Nabel, and P. W. Serruys © Humana Press Inc., Totowa, NJ

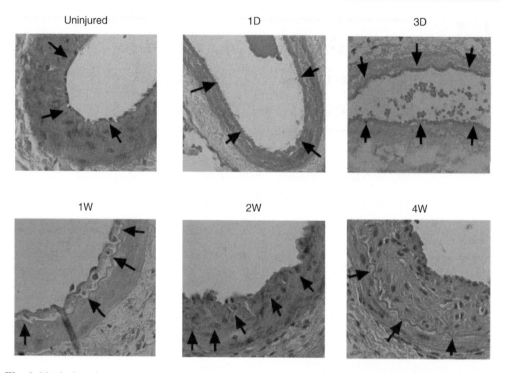

**Fig. 1.** Neointima formation in the absence of medial cells. A large wire was inserted into the femoral artery of C57BL/6J mice. The injured arteries were harvested at the indicated time-points. At 1, 3, and 7 d after the injury, the media contained few cells. At 1 wk, thin neointimal formation was observed on the luminal side of the internal elastic lamina. The neointimal hyperplasia continued to grow for 3 or 4 wk after which lesion formation did not advance further. Arrows indicate internal elastic lamina. Reproduced with permission from Elsevier Science. (Please *see* insert for color version.)

Furthermore, SMC hyperplasia is a major cause of postcoronary bypass surgery occlusion *(7,8)* and graft vasculopathy after transplantation *(9)*. Therefore, much effort has been devoted to understand the molecular pathways that regulate SMC behavior.

## Sources of SMCs in Lesions

It has been hypothesized that dedifferentiated SMC migrate from the media to the subendothelial space, where they proliferate and contribute to atherogenesis *(2)*. Similarly, it has been assumed that all of the neointimal cells in postangioplasty restenosis and graft vasculopathy are derived from adjacent medial SMCs *(3)*. Thus, numerous pharmacological and gene therapies have been focused on targeting medial SMCs *(10–21)*. However, there are several observations that challenge the simple model of SMC migration from the media to the intimal lesion.

1. Very few articles have documented SMC migration across the internal elastic lamina from the tunica media into the subendothelial layer. On the other hand, many studies have shown that blood cells attach to the luminal side of the injured artery before the development of neointimal hyperplasia *(22,23)*.
2. It has been observed that neointima can rapidly form in the absence of medial cells, which can be killed by severe injury (Fig. 1) *(22)*. In this study, it was also noted that neointimal cells were negative for SMC markers and appeared to be hematopoietic at 1 wk postinjury.

3. Many studies have reported that SMC hyperplasia can be prevented by blocking chemokines or adhesion molecules *(24,25)*, which play a crucial role in recruiting blood cells but have little or no effect on the migration and proliferation of SMC *(24)*.
4. Neointimal SMC express a number of hematopoietic lineage markers, including FK506-binding protein 12, interferon regulatory factor, and proinflammatory proteins *(26,27)*.

Collectively, these findings suggest that some of the neointimal SMC may be derived from blood cells rather than medial cells. Direct evidence in support of this hypothesis was recently provided in several models of vascular diseases *(28–31)*.

## CONTRIBUTION OF BONE MARROW CELLS TO VASCULAR LESIONS

In addition to the conventional assumption that damaged vessels are repaired by adjacent parenchymal cells, an accumulating body of evidence indicates that somatic stem cells are mobilized to participate in vascular repair and regeneration. These studies suggest that bone marrow is an additional source of vascular cells that contribute pathological remodeling in postangioplasty restenosis, transplant-associated arteriosclerosis, and hyperlipidemia-induced atherosclerosis.

### *Transplant-Associated Arteriosclerosis*

The contribution of bone marrow cells to vascular lesions was first investigated in graft vasculopathy, a robust form of atherosclerosis which rapidly develops in transplanted organs *(9,30)*. In this study, heterotopic cardiac transplantation was performed between wild-type mice and ROSA26 mice *(28,29)*, which express LacZ ubiquitously (LacZ-mice) *(32,33)*. Four weeks after transplantation, allografts were harvested and stained with X-gal (5-bromo-4-chloro-3-indolyl β-D-galactopyranoside) (Fig. 2).

The lumens of large epicardial coronary arteries and their smaller branches and arterioles were narrowed because of concentric neointimal hyperplasia. The majority of the neointima was made up of recipient cells expressing LacZ *(28,29)*. It was also observed that some of the medial SMC, as well as endothelial cells (ECs), had been replaced by recipient cells. Immunofluorescence studies revealed that LacZ-positive cells in the neointima expressed various markers for SMC, including myosin heavy chain, calponin, h-caldesmon, and α-smooth muscle actin (α-SMA) *(29)*. Conversely, when LacZ-positive hearts were transplanted into wild-type mice, LacZ-negative neointima developed on the LacZ-positive coronary arteries.

Furthermore, *in situ* hybridization of the allografts from female to male mice revealed that most of the neointimal cells corresponded to cells from the recipients *(28)*. These results indicated that the majority of the neointimal cells derived from the recipient cells, but not from the medial cells of donor origin. Consistent with these observations, others independently reported that recipient cells are a major source of graft vasculopathy in aortic transplantation models *(34–39)*. Moreover, it was reported that most of the neointimal cells and ECs were derived from recipients in human transplant-associated arteriosclerosis after renal transplantation *(40,41)*.

To identify the potential source of recipient cells that contribute to allograft vasculopathy, bone marrow transplantation (BMT) was performed from LacZ mice to wild-type mice (BMTLacZ → wild mice). After 4–8 wk, wild-type hearts were transplanted into the BMTLacZ → wild mice. Four weeks after cardiac transplantation, most of the neointimal cells were found to be LacZ-positive. Similarly, when wild-type hearts were transplanted into wild-type mice whose bone marrow had been reconstituted with that

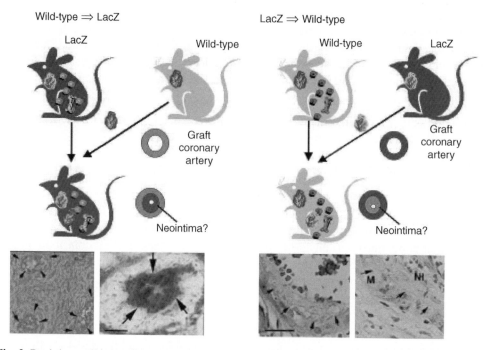

**Fig. 2.** Recipient cells contribute to graft-vasculopathy. When wild-type hearts were transplanted into LacZ mice, 90% of neointima cells were LacZ-positive and thus originating from the recipient (left; bar = 50 μm). Conversely, LacZ-negative recipient cells formed neointima on the LacZ-positive coronary arteries after cardiac transplantation from LacZ-mice to wild-type mice (right; bar = 25 μm). Arrows in histological panels indicate internal lamina. Reproduced with permission from Nature Publishing Company. (Please *see* insert for color version.)

of transgenic mice that express green fluorescent protein (GFP) mice (bone marrow of transgenic GFP [BMTGFP] → wild mice) *(29)*, it was observed that GFP-positive cells accumulated on the luminal side of the graft coronary arteries. Immunofluorescence analysis revealed that some of the GFP-positive cells in graft vasculopathy expressed α-SMA. These results indicate that recipient bone marrow cells may substantially contribute to neointimal formation in transplanted grafts.

## Contribution of Bone Marrow Cells to Vascular Remodeling After Mechanical Injury

Bone marrow cells can also contribute to the pathogenesis of lesion formation after mechanical vascular injury (Fig. 3) *(29–31)*. For these experiments, the bone marrow of wild-type mice were replaced with that of LacZ-mice (BMTLacZ → wild mice). It was found that transplanted LacZ bone marrow cells had settled in bone marrow, spleen, and thymus, whereas no LacZ-positive cell was detected in uninjured femoral arteries of BMTLacZ → wild mice. Four to eight weeks after BMT, a large wire was inserted into the femoral artery of BMTLacZ → wild mice, leading to complete endothelial denudation and marked enlargement of the lumen (Fig. 1) *(22,42,43)*. The cellularity of the medial layer decreased as a result of acute onset of SMC apoptosis *(44)*. One week after the injury, the artery remained dilated, and X-gal staining revealed that LacZ-positive cells attached to the luminal side of the injured vessels. LacZ-positive cells did not express markers for SMC (α-SMA) or ECs (CD31).

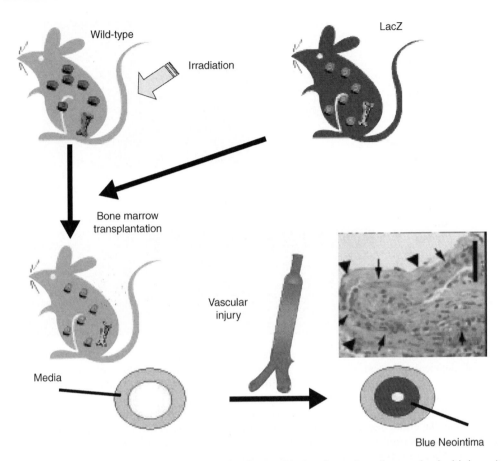

**Fig. 3.** Contribution of bone marrow cells to healing and lesion formation after mechanical injury. A large wire was inserted into the femoral artery of wild-type mice whose bone marrow had been reconstituted with that of LacZ mice. At 4 wk, neointima formation was observed. About 60% of neointima cells and 40% of media cells were LacZ-positive, and thus derived from the bone marrow. Arrows and arrowheads in histological panel indicate internal and external elastic lamina, respectively. Scale bar = 50 μm. Reproduced with permission from Nature Publishing Company. (Please *see* insert for color version.)

At later time-points the dilated lumen gradually narrowed as result of neointimal hyperplasia *(29,31)*. Immunofluorescence double-staining of lesions at these time-points documented that some bone marrow-derived LacZ-positive cells in the neointimal lesions expressed α-SMA or CD31 *(31)*. These results indicate that bone marrow cells may give rise to vascular cells, following mechanical endovascular injury.

### *Bone Marrow-Derived SMC-Like Cells in Atherosclerotic Plaques*

To evaluate the potential source of SMC observed in atherosclerotic plaques *(4)*, the bone marrow of 8-wk-old ApoE$^{-/-}$ mice was replaced with that of GFP-mice (BMT-GFP → ApoE$^{-/-}$ mice) or ROSA26-mice (BMTLacZ → ApoE$^{-/-}$ mice) *(29)*. The recipient mice were fed a western-type diet for 8 wk, starting at 4 wk after BMT *(45)*, and marker-positive cells accumulated in atherosclerotic plaques developing in the aorta of BMTGFP → ApoE$^{-/-}$ mice (Fig. 4). These bone marrow-derived cells expressed a smooth muscle cell marker (α-SMA). Furthermore, an immunogold-labeling for LacZ

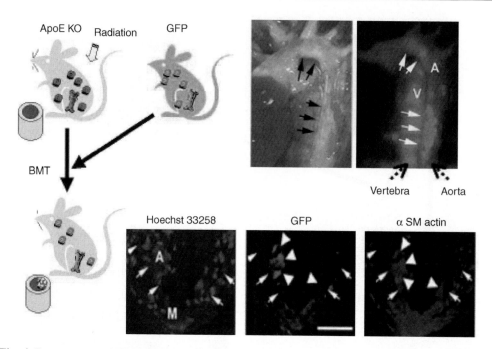

**Fig. 4.** Bone marrow-derived SMC in atherosclerotic plaques. BMT was performed from GFP-mice to ApoE-deficient mice, and animals were maintained on a Western diet. The aortas of BMTGFP → ApoE$^{-/-}$ mice were observed under a xenon fiberoptic light source. Arrows indicate atherosclerotic plaques. A, aorta; V, vertebra. Cross-sections of the aorta of BMTGFP → ApoE$^{-/-}$ mice were stained with Cy3-conjugated anti-α smooth muscle actin antibody (red) and Hoechst 33258 (blue). Arrows indicate internal elastic lamina. Arrowheads indicate GFP-positive cells (green) expressing α-SMA (red) in atherosclerotic lesions. Scale bar = 50 μm. Reproduced with permission from Nature Publishing Company. (Please *see* insert for color version.)

identified bone marrow-derived SMC-like cells with a "synthetic" phenotype appearance. Therefore, these results suggest that some of the SMC-like cells observed in hyperlipidemia-induced atherosclerotic plaques may originate from bone marrow.

### *Injury-Dependent Recruitment of Progenitor Cells*

Numerous reports have demonstrated that neointimal cells are heterogeneous and that SMC in vascular lesions are made up of cells of diverse origin *(31,46,47)*. It has been shown that the cellular constituents of a lesion differ depending on the type of vascular injury *(31)*. A recent study compared three types of mechanical injury in the same mouse model whose bone marrow had been reconstituted with that of GFP- or LacZ-mice (Fig. 5) *(31)*. After wire-mediated endovascular injury, a significant number of the neointimal and medial cells were derived from bone marrow. In contrast, marker-positive cells were seldom detected in the lesion induced by perivascular cuff replacement, and only a few bone marrow-derived cells in the neointima following ligation of the common carotid artery.

These findings suggest that the mode of injury is crucial for the recruitment of bone marrow-derived cells to tissue remodeling and that bone marrow cells substantially contribute to lesion formation only when arteries are subjected to severe injuries *(31)*. Therefore, circulating progenitors would be predicted to only contribute to vascular remodeling in humans when arteries are subjected to severe injuries, such as percutaneous

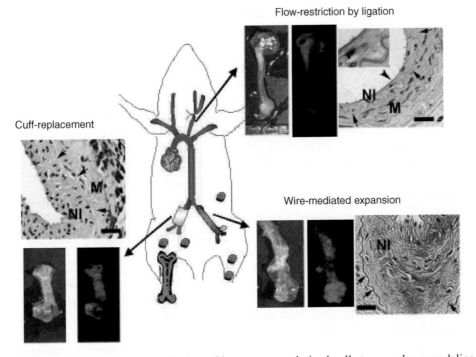

**Fig. 5.** Marked diversity in the contribution of bone marrow-derived cells to vascular remodeling. Three distinct types of mechanical injuries were induced in the same mouse whose bone marrow had been reconstituted with that of GFP⁻ or LacZ⁻ mice. Endovascular injury was induced by inserting a large wire into the left femoral artery (wire-mediated expansion). Perivascular injury was induced by placing a polyethylene tube around the right femoral artery of the same mouse (Cuff-replacement). Flow-restriction vascular injury was induced by ligating the left common carotid artery (flow-restriction by ligation). The injured arteries of BMTLacZ → ApoE⁻/⁻ mice were harvested at 4 wk and observed with a GFP-lighting system and a cooled charge-coupled device camera (macroscopic panels). Scale bar = 1 mm. In BMTLacZ → Wild mice, the injured arteries were stained with X-gal to detect LacZ. Paraffin-embedded sections were rehydrated and stained with hematoxylin. Arrows indicate the internal elastic lamina. Arrowheads indicate LacZ⁺ cells (histological panels). Scale bar = 20 μm. Reproduced with permission from Lippincott Williams & Wilkins. (Please *see* insert for color version.)

coronary intervention, transplantation, and plaque rupture *(29–31,42,43,48)*. Consistent with this notion, an analysis of sex-mismatched bone marrow transplant subjects revealed that the recruitment of bone marrow-derived SMC is more extensive in diseased compared with undiseased segments *(49)*.

### *Fractions of Bone Marrow Cells That Contribute to Vascular Remodeling*

Pluripotent cells in bone marrow are classified as hematopoietic stem cells (HSCs) *(50)* and mesenchymal stem cells *(51)*. Although it was assumed that HSCs give rise only to blood cells of hematopoietic lineage, recent reports suggest that they may have the broader potential to differentiate into various cell types, including epithelial cells *(52)*, hepatocytes *(53,54)*, and cardiomyocytes *(55,56)*. To identify the bone marrow cells that have the potential to generate vascular cells, a HSC-enriched fraction (c-Kit⁺, Sca-1⁺, Lin⁻) was isolated from the bone marrow of LacZ-mice by fluorescence-activated cell sorting *(29)* and 3000 cells were injected into lethally irradiated wild-type mice. Four weeks after bone marrow reconstitution, the femoral arteries of recipient mice were mechanically injured with a large wire *(22)*. At 4 wk after the injury, the neointima and the media contained many LacZ-positive cells *(29)*, some of which expressed α-SMA. LacZ-positive cells were also found to contribute to endothelial regeneration *(29)*. These findings suggest that the c-Kit$^+$, Sca-1$^+$, Lin$^-$ fraction of bone marrow cells may have the potential to differentiate into either SMC or ECs that participate in vascular remodeling. In contrast, Wagers et al. extensively analyzed organs of wild-type mice whose bone marrow had been reconstituted with a single HSC. The authors concluded that transdifferentiation of HSCs into other lineages is an extremely rare event *(57)*. The apparent discrepancy between these two studies could derive from the analysis of noninjured vs injured tissues or from the possibility that other cell types in the c-Kit$^+$, Sca-1$^+$, Lin$^-$ fraction contribute to the lesion. However, a recent study on ischemic myocardium failed to detect the contribution of hematopoietic cells to cardiac, smooth, or endothelial phenotype *(58)*. Thus, we investigated the vascular lesion induced by wire after the bone marrow was reconstituted by a single HSC *(59)*. Although a single HSC showed an appreciable level of hematopoietic engraftment activity, very few cells in the lesion were derived from a single HSC. Our result suggests that it is a rare property for a highly purified HSC to transdifferentiate into vascular cells, whereas the KSL fraction of bone marrow cells contained a distinct population that could substantially contribute to lesion formation. Although the KSL fraction is considered to be enriched in HSCs *(50)*, mesenchymal stem cells or multipotent cells that are more primitive than HSCs could be included in this fraction. It is plausible that those non-hematopoietic cells in the KSL fraction might be responsible for the KSL-derived endothelial-like cells or smooth muscle-like cells observed in the vascular lesion *(29)*.

### *Cell Fusion as a Possible Mechanism of Bone Marrow Contribution to Vascular Repair*

Many animal experiments have indicated that adult stem cells can transdifferentiate into other lineages *(52,60,61)*. Similar conclusions have also been reported in gender-mismatched human BMT studies *(52,54)*. On the other hand, recent articles suggest that adult stem cells can adopt a tissue-specific phenotype by cell fusion in vitro *(62,63)* and in vivo *(64,65)*, rather than by transdifferentiation. It is possible that cell fusion can account for, at least in part, the accumulation of bone marrow-derived SMC-like cells in vascular lesions *(30)*. Consistent with this notion, previous reports documented polyploidization of vascular SMC in response to mechanical and humoral stimuli *(66)*. However, spontaneous cell fusion between recipient and donor-derived cells appears to be a rare event when examined in a murine model of cardiac transplantation *(67)*.

## THERAPEUTIC STRATEGIES TARGETING CIRCULATING VASCULAR PROGENITOR CELLS

Much effort has been devoted to targeting the migration and proliferation of medial SMC to prevent vascular lesions *(68)*. Recent findings indicate that bone marrow-derived smooth muscle progenitor cells might represent an additional target for treatment to prevent vascular diseases (Fig. 6) *(30)*. Consistent with this notion is the observation that transient myelosuppression can inhibit SMC hyperplasia in balloon-injured coronary arteries *(69)*. Similar effects can be obtained through inhibition of chemokine *(24)* or adhesion molecule *(25)*, which may play a crucial role

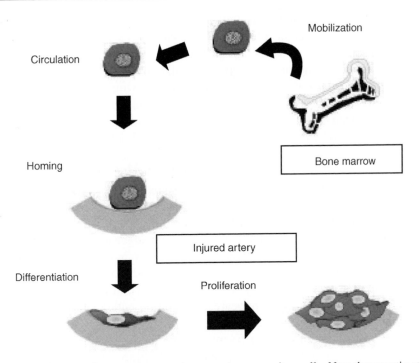

**Fig. 6.** Therapeutic strategies targeting putative vascular progenitor cells. New therapeutic strategies for vascular diseases may involve targeting the mobilization, circulation, homing, differentiation, or proliferation of bone marrow-derived vascular progenitor cells.

in recruitment and homing of putative smooth muscle progenitors. Recently, the sirolimus-eluting stent has emerged as a promising strategy to inhibit post-PCI restenosis *(70,71)*. Because sirolimus is an immunosuppressive drug, it is plausible that it functions to inhibit bone marrow-derived vascular precursor cells when delivered locally to the site of vascular injury. We reported sirolimus potently inhibits differentiation of human vascular progenitor cells *(72)*. The potent inhibitory effects of sirolimus on circulating smooth muscle progenitor cells may, at least in part, mediate the clinical efficacy of SES. Sirolimus potentially also may affect re-endothelialization after stent implantation, causing late thrombosis after interruption of anti-platelet therapy.

### Gene Therapy Through Targeting Circulating Progenitors

It may be possible to develop gene therapies to vascular diseases that target vascular progenitor cells. One potential approach could involve the Fas/Fas ligand (FasL) system *(73,74)*. Fas is a death receptor that transmits an apoptosis-inducing signaling when activated by its ligand, FasL *(75,76)*. Studies have shown that ectopic or augmented expression of FasL may have utility for treating vascular diseases *(77–79)*. FasL induces apoptosis in Fas-bearing vascular SMC *(77)*, whereas ECs are refractory to FasL overexpression *(77,80,81)*. Thus, the local delivery of FasL to sites of balloon injury is predicted to reduce SMC number by inducing apoptotic cell death, although this treatment would not inhibit the beneficial process of re-endothelialization at this same site *(77,82)*.

Moreover, local delivery of FasL is predicted to kill bone marrow-derived progenitors as well as inflammatory cells at these lesions because these cells express Fas *(79,80)*. Consistent with this notion, it was reported that ECs could be genetically modified to overexpress functional, cell-surface FasL by adenovirus-mediated gene transfer in vitro or by transgenic approaches in vivo without undergoing self-destruction *(82,83)*. In a rodent model of transplant graft vasculopathy, endothelial overexpression of FasL attenuated homing of hematopoietic cells at 1 wk post-transplantation *(78)*. These vessels also displayed reduced neointima formation at 1 and 2 mo post-transplantation. Thus, it is conceivable that endothelial cell-specific overexpression of FasL inhibits transplant arteriosclerosis by preventing accumulation of smooth muscle-like progenitors, with little effect in endothelial cell-like progenitors.

### *Implications for Regenerative Medicine*

There is increasing enthusiasm for the use of somatic stem cells for "cell transplantation therapy" and "tissue engineering" *(84)*. However, given the pluripotency of adult stem cells, they may potentially differentiate into unfavorable cell-types. In fact, similarities between stem cells and cancer cells have been suggested *(85,86)*, and studies in animal models have shown somatic stem cells participate in pathological remodeling in remote organs *(28,29,87)*. Thus, attention should be paid to potential adverse effects as well as beneficial aspects caused by the transplanted stem cells in the clinic. In this regard, a recent clinical trial with myocardial infarction patients has shown that granulocyte colony-stimulating factor mobilization of stem cells and subsequent infusion of such cells improved cardiac performance and angiogenesis *(88)*. However, this improvement was associated with an unexpectedly high rate of in-stent restenosis, which led to the premature termination of the trial.

## CONCLUSIONS

In summary, findings indicate that bone marrow cells contribute not only to the healing process of injured organs, but also to pathological vascular remodeling. These findings may provide the basis for the development of new therapeutic strategies for vascular diseases that involve targeting the mobilization, homing, differentiation, and proliferation of bone marrow-derived vascular progenitor cells. Therefore, further experiments that dissect molecular mechanisms by which progenitors are recruited and differentiate at the site of injury are warranted.

## REFERENCES

1. Ross R. Atherosclerosis-An inflammatory disease. N Eng J Med 1999;340:115–126.
2. Ross R. Rous-Whipple Award Lecture. Atherosclerosis: a defense mechanism gone awry. Am J Pathol 1993;143:987–1002.
3. Ross R. Genetically modified mice as models of transplant atherosclerosis. Nat Med 1996;2:527–528.
4. Ross R. The pathogenesis of atherosclerosis: a perspective for the 1990s. Nature 1993;362:801–809.
5. Nobuyoshi M, Kimura T, Nosaka H, et al. Restenosis after successful percutaneous transluminal coronary angioplasty: serial angiographic follow-up of 229 patients. J Am Coll Cardiol 1988;12:616–623.
6. Kearney M, Pieczek A, Haley L, et al. Histopathology of in-stent restenosis in patients with peripheral artery disease. Circulation 1997;95:1998–2002.
7. Callow AD. Molecular biology of graft occlusion. Curr Opin Cardiol 1995;10:569–576.
8. Sarjeant JM, Rabinovitch M. Understanding and treating vein graft atherosclerosis. Cardiovasc Pathol 2002;11:263–271.
9. Billingham ME. Cardiac transplant atherosclerosis. Transplant Proc 1987;19:19–25.
10. Clausell N, Milossi S, Sett S, Rabinovitch M. In vivo blockade of tumor necrosis factor-$\alpha$ in cholesterol-fed rabbits after cardiac transplant inhibits acute coronary artery neointimal formation. Circulation 1994;89:2768–2779.

11. Chang MW, Barr E, Lu MM, Barton K, Leiden JM. Adenovirus-mediated over-expression of the cyclin/cyclin-dependent kinase inhibitor, p21 inhibits vascular smooth muscle cell proliferation and neointima formation in the rat carotid artery model of balloon angioplasty. J Clin Invest 1995;96:2260–2268.

12. Smith RC, Wills KN, Antelman D, et al. Adenoviral constructs encoding phosphorylation-competent full-length and truncated forms of the human retinoblastoma protein inhibit myocyte proliferation and neointima formation. Circulation 1997;96:1899–1905.

13. Pollman MJ, Hall JL, Mann MJ, Zhang L, Gibbons GH. Inhibition of neointimal cell bcl-x expression induces apoptosis and regression of vascular disease. Nature Med 1998;4:222–227.

14. Chen D, Krasinski K, Chen D, et al. Down-regulation of cyclin-dependent kinase activity and cyclin A promoter activity in vascular smooth muscle cells by p27 (KIP-1), an inhibitor of neointima formation in the rat carotid artery. J Clin Invest 1997;99:2334–2341.

15. George SJ, Johnson JL, Angelini GD, Newby AC, Baker AH. Adenovirus-mediated gene transfer of the human TIMP-1 gene inhibits smooth muscle cell migration and neointimal formation in human saphenous veins. Hum Gene Ther 1998;9:867–877.

16. George SJ, Angelini GD, Capogrossi MC, Baker AH. Wild-type p53 gene transfer inhibits neointima formation in human saphenous vein by modulation of smooth muscle cell migration and induction of apoptosis. Gene Ther 2001;8:668–676.

17. Izawa A, Suzuki J, Takahashi W, Amano J, Isobe M. Tranilast inhibits cardiac allograft vasculopathy in association with p21(Waf1/Cip1) expression on neointimal cells in murine cardiac transplantation model. Arterioscler Thromb Vasc Biol 2001;21:1172–1178.

18. Rebsamen MC, Sun J, Norman AW, Liao JK. 1alpha,25-dihydroxyvitamin D3 induces vascular smooth muscle cell migration via activation of phosphatidylinositol 3-kinase. Circ Res 2002;91:17–24.

19. Ohno T, Gordon D, San H, et al. Gene therapy for vascular smooth muscle cell proliferation after arterial injury. Science 1994;265:781–784.

20. Yang Z, Simari R, Perkins N, et al. Role of the p21cyclin-dependent kinase inhibitor in limiting intimal cell proliferation in response to arterial injury. Proc Natl Acad Sci USA 1996;93:7905–7910.

21. Chang MW, Barr E, Seltzer J, et al. Cytostatic gene therapy for vascular proliferative disorders with a constitutively active form of the retinoblastoma gene product. Science 1995;267:518–522.

22. Sata M, Maejima Y, Adachi F, et al. A mouse model of vascular injury that induces rapid onset of medial cell apoptosis followed by reproducible neointimal hyperplasia. J Mol Cell Cardiol 2000;32:2097–2104.

23. Feldman LJ, Mazighi M, Scheuble A, et al. Differential expression of matrix metalloproteinases after stent implantation and balloon angioplasty in the hypercholesterolemic rabbit. Circulation 2001;103:3117–3122.

24. Furukawa Y, Matsumori A, Ohashi N, et al. Anti-monocyte chemoattractant protein-1/monocyte chemotactic and activating factor antibody inhibits neointimal hyperplasia in injured rat carotid arteries. Circ Res 1999;84:306–314.

25. Hayashi S, Watanabe N, Nakazawa K, et al. Roles of P-selectin in inflammation, neointimal formation, and vascular remodeling in balloon-injured rat carotid arteries. Circulation 2000;102:1710–1717.

26. Zohlnhofer D, Klein CA, Richter T, et al. Gene expression profiling of human stent-induced neointima by cDNA array analysis of microscopic specimens retrieved by helix cutter atherectomy: detection of FK506-binding protein 12 upregulation. Circulation 2001;103:1396–1402.

27. Zohlnhofer D, Richter T, Neumann FJ, et al. Transcriptome analysis reveals a role of interferon-gamma in human neointima formation. Mol Cell 2001;7:1059–1069.

28. Saiura A, Sata M, Hirata Y, Nagai R, Makuuchi M. Circulating smooth muscle progenitor cells contribute to atherosclerosis. Nat Med 2001;7:382–383.

29. Sata M, Saiura A, Kunisato A, et al. Hematopoietic stem cells differentiate into vascular cells that participate in the pathogenesis of atherosclerosis. Nat Med 2002;8:403–409.

30. Sata M. Circulating vascular progenitor cells contribute to vascular repair, remodeling, and lesion formation. Trends Cardiovasc Med 2003;13:249–253.

31. Tanaka K, Sata M, Hirata Y, Nagai R. Diverse contribution of bone marrow cells to neointimal hyperplasia after mechanical vascular injuries. Circ Res 2003;93:783–790.

32. Friedrich G, Soriano P. Promoter traps in embryonic stem cells: a genetic screen to identify and mutate developmental genes in mice. Genes Dev 1991;5:1513–1523.

33. Zambrowicz BP, Imamoto A, Fiering S, Herzenberg LA, Kerr WG, Soriano P. Disruption of overlapping transcripts in the ROSA βgeo 26 gene trap strain leads to widespread expression of β-galactosidase in mouse embryos and hematopoietic cells. Proc Natl Acad Sci USA 1997;94: 3789–3794.

34. Shimizu K, Sugiyama S, Aikawa M, et al. Host bone-marrow cells are a source of donor intimal smooth- muscle-like cells in murine aortic transplant arteriopathy. Nat Med 2001;7:738–741.
35. Hillebrands JL, Klatter FA, van Den Hurk BM, Popa ER, Nieuwenhuis P, Rozing J. Origin of neointimal endothelium and alpha-actin-positive smooth muscle cells in transplant arteriosclerosis. J Clin Invest 2001;107:1411–1422.
36. Hu Y, Davison F, Ludewig B, et al. Smooth muscle cells in transplant atherosclerotic lesions are originated from recipients, but not bone marrow progenitor cells. Circulation 2002;106:1834–1839.
37. Hillebrands JL, Klatter FA, Rozing J. Origin of vascular smooth muscle cells and the role of circulating stem cells in transplant arteriosclerosis. Arterioscler Thromb Vasc Biol 2003;23:380–387.
38. Hillebrands JL, Klatter FA, van Dijk WD, Rozing J. Bone marrow does not contribute substantially to endothelial-cell replacement in transplant arteriosclerosis. Nat Med 2002;8:194–195.
39. Hillebrands J, vdH BM, Klatter FA, Popa ER, Nieuwenhuis P, Rozing J. Recipient origin of neointimal vascular smooth muscle cells in cardiac allografts with transplant arteriosclerosis. J Heart Lung Transplant 2000;19:1183–1192.
40. Grimm PC, Nickerson P, Jeffery J, et al. Neointimal and tubulointerstitial infiltration by recipient mesenchymal cells in chronic renal-allograft rejection. N Engl J Med 2001;345:93–97.
41. Lagaaij EL, Cramer-Knijnenburg GF, van Kemenade FJ, van Es LA, Bruijn JA, van Krieken JH. Endothelial cell chimerism after renal transplantation and vascular rejection. Lancet 2001;357:33–37.
42. Sata M, Sugiura S, Yoshizumi M, Ouchi Y, Hirata Y, Nagai R. Acute and chronic smooth muscle cell apoptosis after mechanical vascular injury can occur independently of the Fas-death pathway. Arterioscler Thromb Vasc Biol 2001;21:1733–1737.
43. Sata M, Tanaka K, Ishizaka N, Hirata Y, Nagai R. Absence of p53 Leads to Accelerated Neointimal Hyperplasia After Vascular Injury. Arterioscler Thromb Vasc Biol 2003;23:1548–1552.
44. Perlman H, Maillard L, Krasinski K, Walsh K. Evidence for the rapid onset of apoptosis in medial smooth muscle cells following balloon injury. Circulation 1997;95:981–987.
45. Plump AS, Smith JD, Hayek T, et al. Severe hypercholesterolemia and atherosclerosis in apolipoprotein E-deficient mice created by homologous recombination in ES cells. Cell 1992;71:343–353.
46. Li S, Fan YS, Chow LH, et al. Innate diversity of adult human arterial smooth muscle cells: cloning of distinct subtypes from the internal thoracic artery. Circ Res 2001;89:517–525.
47. Zalewski A, Shi Y, Johnson AG. Diverse origin of intimal cells: smooth muscle cells, myofibroblasts, fibroblasts, and beyond? Circ Res 2002;91:652–655.
48. Kaushal S, Amiel GE, Guleserian KJ, et al. Functional small-diameter neovessels created using endothelial progenitor cells expanded ex vivo. Nat Med 2001;7:1035–1040.
49. Caplice NM, Bunch TJ, Stalboerger PG, et al. Smooth muscle cells in human coronary atherosclerosis can originate from cells administered at marrow transplantation. Proc Natl Acad Sci USA 2003;100:4754–4759.
50. Osawa M, Hanada K, Hamada H, Nakauchi H. Long-term lymphohematopoietic reconstitution by a single CD34-low/negative hematopoietic stem cell. Science 1996;273:242–245.
51. Prockop DJ. Marrow stromal cells as stem cells for nonhematopoietic tissues. Science 1997;276:71–74.
52. Krause DS, Theise ND, Collector MI, et al. Multi-organ, multi-lineage engraftment by a single bone marrow-derived stem cell. Cell 2001;105:369–377.
53. Alison MR, Poulsom R, Jeffery R, et al. Hepatocytes from non-hepatic adult stem cells. Nature 2000;406:257.
54. Lagasse E, Connors H, Al-Dhalimy M, et al. Purified hematopoietic stem cells can differentiate into hepatocytes in vivo. Nat Med 2000;6:1229–1234.
55. Orlic D, Kajstura J, Chimenti S, et al. Bone marrow cells regenerate infracted myocardium. Nature 2001;410:701–705.
56. Orlic D, Kajstura J, Chimenti S, et al. Mobilized bone marrow cells repair the infracted heart, improving function and survival. Proc Natl Acad Sci USA 2001;98:10,344–10,349.
57. Wagers AJ, Sherwood RI, Christensen JL, Weissman IL. Little evidence for developmental plasticity of adult hematopoietic stem cells. Science 2002;297:2256–2259.
58. Balsam LB, Wagers AJ, Christensen JL, Kofidis T, Weissman IL, Robbins RC. Haematopoietic stem cells adopt mature haematopoietic fates in ischaemic myocardium. Nature 2004;428:607–608.
59. Sahara M, Sata M, Matsuzaki Y, et al. Comparison of various bone marrow fractions in the ability to participate in vascular remodeling after mechanical injury. Stem Cells 2005;23:874–878.
60. Korbling M, Estrov Z. Adult stem cells for tissue repair — a new therapeutic concept? N Engl J Med 2003;349:570–582.
61. LaBarge MA, Blau HM. Biological progression from adult bone marrow to mononucleate muscle stem cell to multinucleate muscle fiber in response to injury. Cell 2002;111:589–601.

atherosclerosis. In contrast; however, to the slow progression of atherosclerosis, VSMC hyperplasia often develops rapidly and occurs during the first 2 wk after vascular injury *(9)*. The initial event is an acute alteration of the endothelial cell homeostasis inflicted by the vascular injury. Endothelial cell denudation and upregulation of adhesion molecules in the remaining endothelial cells result in an acute inflammatory response characterized by early attachment of neutrophils and monocytes to the injured vessel lumen. Chemokines and growth factors released from inflammatory cells as well as from endothelial cells and VSMCs lead to further invasion of inflammatory cells, such as neutrophils, monocytes, and T-cells, from the adventitia toward the injured area *(10)*. Release of metalloproteases degrades extracellular matrix components, which loosens medial VSMCs from their surrounding connecting tissue *(11)*. This enables the VSMC to proliferate on stimulation by growth factors like platelet-derived growth factor, basic fibroblast growth factor, insulin-like growth factor-1, and transforming growth factor-β *(12–17)*. Subsequently, medial VSMCs migrate toward the intima of the injured area, complete several additional rounds of cell division before they finally form the neointima. This process is necessary to re-establish the vessel integrity after vascular injury and requires a fine balance between induction of proliferation and inhibition of proliferation. Unbalanced arterial wound repair results either in an accelerated neointima formation and restenosis or in an incomplete wound repair with prothrombotic tendencies. This balance is achieved by a fine tuned interaction between the different cell compartments. Bone marrow transplantation (BMT) experiments utilizing mice models with genetic defects in cellular function of inflammatory cells have demonstrated the important role of inflammatory cells in arterial wound repair. BMT from a mouse model with increased inflammatory responses into wild-type mice accelerated the neointima formation after mechanical injury. In addition, T-cell depletion decreases the neointima formation in a mouse model of accelerated neointima formation. This is quite surprising, as T-cells represent only a small percentage of all inflammatory cells found within the vascular lesion. These findings suggest a dominate role of inflammatory cells in arterial wound repair. However, reciprocal BMT with normal BM into a mouse model with a proliferative phenotype also resulted in an accelerated neointimal formation *(10)*. This implies that there is not one cell type that regulates the arterial wound repair program. The orchestration of several different cell compartments is necessary to restore the vessel integrity after vascular injury. The concept gets even more complex with the discovery of circulating and local stem cells, which may play an important role in the regenerative process after vascular injury or in the development of atherosclerosis.

## STEM CELLS

Although local smooth muscle cell (SMC) and endothelial cells will proliferate in response to injury or stimulus there is now increasing evidence that stem and progenitor cells may participate in the repair processes of blood vessels. These stem/progenitor cells may be derived from local cells residing within the vessel itself or be circulating in the blood. Traditionally, postnatal neovascularization was believed to occur through the proliferation and migration of local endothelial cells, which would rapidly recover an injured/denuded area of a vessel or sprout into new vessels *(18)*. Endothelial progenitor cells were first described by Asahara et al in 1997 *(19)* and are a fraction of circulating hematopoietic progenitor cells, which express the hematopoietic stem cell markers CD133/ CD34 and various endothelial markers (VE-cadherin, CD31, von Willebrand factor, VEGFR2, Tie2, CD146) (20). These cells can incorporate into sites of neo angiogenesis where they adopt an endothelial-like phenotype. There is also evidence that endothelial-like cells may also originate from circulating myelo-monocytic cells but these cells may have a reduced angiogenic potential and not be true endothelial progenitor cells (20). Numerous studies have shown that these bone marrow/ blood-derived cells can participate in neo-angiogensis at sites of vascular injury or ischemia, not only in animal models but also in clinical studies (21). For example, patients implanted with left-ventricular assist devices were fond to have CD34+ VEGFR2+ bone marrow-derived cells, lining the artificial surface of these devices (22).

Although there have been fewer studies on smooth muscle progenitor cells, it appears that there are progenitor cells that exist circulating in blood and also locally in some blood vessels. Mouse hematopoietic stem cells can differentiate into SMCs and under certain circumstances can contribute to postangioplasty restenosis, graft vasculopathy, and atherosclerosis (23). Although human data at present are limited, it appears that cells with a VSMC phenotype can be cultured from blood (24), and in patients who have received BM transplants, donor-derived neointimal cells were found within vascular lesions at necroscopy (25).

Although most recent research has focused on circulating BM-derived cells there is also evidence that there may well be local tissue stem cells that may be important for producing endothelial and SMCs. In mice there have been found to be pluripotent stem cells in tissues, such as skeletal and cardiac muscle, which have the ability to differentiate into endothelium as well as other cell types (26–28). It has also been demonstrated that the adventitia of some blood vessels in the mouse harbor vascular progenitor cells capable of differentiating into SMCs (29). The biological significance of these local stem cells is not yet clear.

The frequency of circulating EPCs within the blood is extremely low although levels rise after mobilization from the bone marrow under appropriate stimuli. Mobilization of stem cells from their niche within the bone marrow is determined by the local environment, which is contributed to by fibroblasts, osteoblasts, and endothelial cells as well as local and systemic cytokines. Mobilization of EPCs has been found to be increased by a number of cytokines, such as vascular endothelial growth factor (VEGF), erythropoetin, granulocyte colony-stimulating factor, stromal cell-derived factor-1, and also by the use of statins and by exercise, trauma, and surgery (21). Physiologically, ischemia is believed to be the predominant signal to induce EPC mobilization from the bone marrow. It is speculated that stem cells reside in a nonproliferative state. Under appropriate stimuli, such as VEGF or placental growth factor, EPCs are mobilized. VEGF induces the production of matrix metalloproteinose (MMP)-9 within the BM, which causes an increase in soluble Kit ligand (stem cell factor). Soluble Kit ligand results in increased cycling of quiescent stem and progenitor cells and enhanced translocation to a vascular niche that is conductive to stem-cell proliferation, differentiation, and mobilization to the peripheral circulation (30). Angiogenic cytokine-mediated MMP-9 activation is a crucial checkpoint in controlling the cell turnover and hence mobilization of EPCs. Some evidence also points to the role of the cell cycle inhibitors p21[Cip1] (31) and p27[Kip1] (10) as being important in controlling the proliferation and mobilization of EPC and BM-derived SMCs although there is clearly more work to be done to understand the proliferation, migration, homing, and differentiation of these cells.

Recent evidence indicates that EPCs/BM-derived cells are also important in the pathogenesis of atherosclerosis. Patients with established coronary artery disease have decreased numbers of circulating EPCs *(32)* but so do patients with risk factors for atherosclerosis, such as smoking, diabetes or hypercholesterolemia *(33)*. EPC numbers also correlate with markers of vascular function. Although the exact reason for a decrease in EPCs under these circumstances is not known, it has been speculated that depletion of EPCs may itself be a risk factor for vascular disease and that EPCs may play an important role in blood vessel regeneration. Certainly, in animal models there is good evidence that EPCs take part in repair of injured or damaged blood vessels. The reduction of EPCs seen in atherosclerosis may be a result of depletion of the bone marrow stem cell pool or owing to reduced mobilization, impaired homing or a failure of differentiation.

In addition, EPCs and BM-derived cells are also incorporated into atheroma and neointima. Genetically marked BM-derived cells can integrate into neoimtima and atheroma *(23,34)*.

It is quite likely that there is a fine balance between re-endotheliazation of an injured blood vessel, which may be beneficial and excessive cellular infiltration, which may lead to restenosis after angioplasty or plaque instability in atherosclerosis.

The full clinical and biological relevance of stem and progenitor cells is not yet established. There is considerable interest in further dissecting the biology of these progenitors, and investigating their role as potential targets for therapeutic agents.

## CELL CYCLE

The proliferation of local vascular cells and reactive BM-derived cells are important determinants in the pathology of vascular diseases. The biological program that controls these cells is the cell cycle *(35)*. The cell cycle receives inputs from the surrounding environment of the cell and the nutrition/energy and DNA status from inside the cell. The output of the cell cycle determines the fate of the cell. This can be proliferation or senescence, differentiation or dedifferentiation, apoptosis or even migration. This paragraph focuses on the molecular mechanism of cell cycle control and its impact on vascular disease. Cell cycle progression occurs in a defined sequential manner, which leads to the historical definition of the different cell cycle phases. Most cells of a developed organism are in a quiescent stage called $G_0$. On mitogenic stimulation the cell enters the cell cycle at the $G_1$ phase. Progression through $G_1$ phase is associated with an increase in protein and RNA synthesis in anticipation of DNA replication in S-phase. The transition from the $G_1$ to S-phase is crucial for cell cycle progression. As long as the cell is in $G_1$ phase it is sensitive to mitogenic stimulation and mitogen withdrawn would stop the cell cycle progression and cell duplication. As soon as the cell enters S-phase, it is committed to continue the cell cycle progression independent of mitogen stimulation. Before starting S-phase, cells have to ensure that the environmental conditions are appropriate for cell division. Several molecular networks, receiving the appropriate signals govern the transition from $G_1$ to S-phase. This transition is called the check point or restriction point. S-phase entry is associated with the initiation of DNA replication, which occurs at multiple defined sites on the chromosomes. The whole genome is duplicated only once and with high accuracy. Any mistake in copying the DNA needs to be detected and repaired. This takes place during the $G_2$-phase of the cell cycle. After duplicating its contents, the cell is faced with the challenge of distributing the cellular contents equally between two daughter cells. This is achieved during mitosis, which begins with the condensation of chromosomes and the formation of a

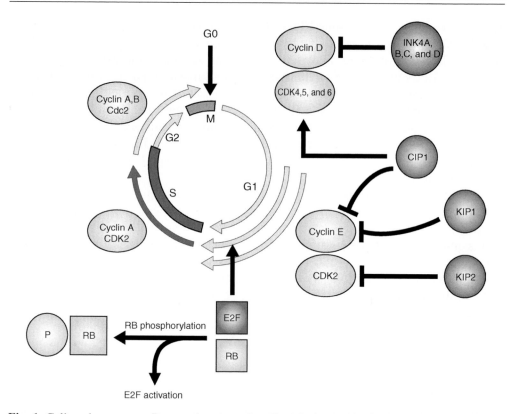

**Fig. 1.** Cell cycle program. Progression through cell cycle is cooperatively regulated by cyclin-dependent kinases, the activities of which are controlled by the cyclin-dependent kinases inhibitors. The cyclin-dependent kinases inhibitors have been assigned to two families on the basis of their structure: the INK4 proteins (INK4A–INK4D) and the CIP/KIP proteins (CIP1, KIP1, and KIP2). E2F, transcription factor E2F; P, phosphate group; RB, retinoblastoma tumor-suppressor protein. Adapted from ref. *93.*

mitotic spindle. The spindle microtubules attach to the two sister chromatids of each chromosome through kinetochores, and the nuclear envelop breaks down. After each spindle is aligned correctly with its chromatids, the sister chromatids are pulled apart. Following separation of the replicated genomes, the chromosomes decondense and the nuclear envelop is reformed. Finally, the formation of the two daughter cells is completed by the partitioning of the cytoplasm in a process called cytokinesis. The proper execution of mitosis is controlled by several check points to ensure precise separation of the sister chromatids and equal distribution of genetic information into the two daughter cells.

The central regulatory protein complexes involved in the cell cycle are the cyclins and their catalytic subunits the cyclin-dependent kinases (CDKs) *(36–38).* The various members of this family have distinct functions in different phases of the cell cycle (Fig. 1). After mitogen stimulation and cell cycle entry from $G_0$ into $G_1$, the first cyclins to be expressed are the D-cyclins (D1/2/3) with their catalytic units CDK4/5/6. These cyclins serve as mitogen sensors transmitting the mitogenic signal toward the nucleus of the cell. However, complete deletions of all D/CDK complexes in a knock out mice model does not affect cell cycle control in the majority of cells during development, indicating that D-cyclins are not the only modulators of cell cycle progression and other signal pathways exist to transfer the mitogenic signal toward the cell cycle machinery in the nucleus *(39)*.

Cyclin D is assembled with the catalytic unit, CDK, in the cytoplasm and translocated to the nucleus where it phosphorylates the retinoblastoma protein (Rb) and the other related pocket proteins p107 and p130. Rb is the central protein complex containing several transcription factors and cofactors necessary for S-phase entry *(40)*. On phosphorylation by cyclin D/CDK2, Rb allows the activation of the E2F family of transcription factors. These proteins are necessary for the induction of the first wave of proteins required for $G_1$/S-phase progression. Among them is cyclin E with its catalytic subunit CDK2. Cyclin E/CDK2 complex is essential and required for cell cycle progression. Together with cyclin D/CDK it hyperphosphorylate Rb and the other pocket proteins, which is necessary for the full activation of the S-phase transcriptional program. The activity of the cyclin/CDK complex is tightly regulated by several mechanisms. The most important regulators of the cyclin/CDK kinase activity are the cyclin-dependent kinase inhibitor (CKI) INK4 and Cip/Kip protein families *(41)*. The INK4 family is named after its ability to inhibit CDK4. It consists of p15[INK4B] *(42)*, p16[INK4A] *(43)*, p18[INK4C] and p19[INK4D] *(44)*. They bind to monomeric CDK4 and CDK6 at the same region as cyclin D and inhibit the formation of the active cyclin D/CDK complex. The second family of CKIs called Cip/Kip contains p21[Cip1] *(45–48)*, p27[Kip1] *(49–51)*, and p57[Kip2] *(52,53)*. They strongly inhibit the CDK2-containing complex by blocking the kinase catalytic core and therefore the substrate access. The regulation of CDK activity by CKI during $G_1$-S progression is complex and contains several positive and negative feedback mechanisms. The progression through $G_1$ into S-phase entry is the only phase of the cell cycle sensitive to mitogenic stimulation. The $G_1$/S-phase regulatory network between cyclin/CDK complexes and CKI is fundamentally important for the regulation of cell proliferation in vascular disease and is explained in more detail (Fig. 2).

The initial event after mitogenic stimulation is assembly of the cyclin D and CDK complex in the cytoplasm. This requires the factors Cip/Kip CKI p21[Cip1] and p27[Kip1] *(54,55)*. Although this seems counterproductive p21[Cip1] and p27[Kip1] do not inhibit the in vivo activity of the cyclin D/CDK complex. Together with the complex they are translocated to the nucleus where they prevent the premature activation of the cyclin E/CDK2 complex. Nuclear cyclin D/CDK has two major functions. First, it phosphorylates Rb and other pocket proteins *(56)*, second, it titrates p27[Kip1] away from cyclin E/CDK2, without been inhibited by the CKI. Free cyclin E/CDK2 complexes phosphorylate cyclinE/CDK2 bound p27[Kip1], which leads to rapid degradation of p27[Kip1] by the 26S proteasome *(57–59)*. The cyclin E/CDK2 complexes are now fully activated. p27[Kip1] is not only phosphorylated by cyclin E/CDK2. Early in $G_1$ progression p27[Kip1] is phosphorylated by KIS at serine 10, which initiates nuclear export of p27[Kip1] *(10)*. This decreases nuclear p27[Kip1] and supports $G_1$-S phase progression *(60,61)*. In the cytoplasm serine 10 phosphorylated p27[Kip1] can be degraded or it binds through its carboxy terminal domain to RhoA and interferes with RhoA activation by guanine-nucleotide-exchange factors. By interfering with RhoA activation, p27[Kip1] inhibits or promotes cell migration, depending on the cell type *(62,63)*. This might represent an important link how cell-cycle controlling factors can switch the fate of a cell from a proliferative to a migratory phenotype. Distinct from the Cip/Kip CKI, high expression of the INK4 CKI blocks formation of the active cyclin D/CDK complex. By doing so, the Cip/Kip CKIs are no longer sequestered by the cyclin

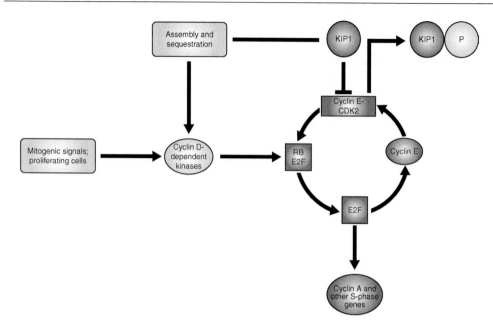

**Fig. 2.** Regulation of $G_1$/S transition. Mitogenic signals promote the assembly of cyclin D, cyclin-dependent kinases (CDKs) and CIP/KIP proteins into a complex. Sequestration of CIP/KIP proteins lowers the inhibitory threshold and facilitates activation of cyclin E/CDK2 complexes. The cyclin D/CDK and cyclin E/CDK complexes contribute sequentially to phosphorylation of the retinoblastoma tumor suppressor protein (RB), which cancels RB repression of E2F-family members, and promotes entry into S-phase. CIP, CDK-inhibitory protein; E2F, transcription factor E2F; KIP, CDK-inhibitory protein; P, phosphate group. Adapted from ref. *93.*

D/CDK complex and are available to inhibit the cyclin E/CDK2 complex. Hence, upregulation of Ink4 CKI directly blocks cyclin D/CDK activity and indirectly inhibits Cyclin E/CDK2 activity through the Cip/Kip CKIs.

The entrance of the cell into S-phase is accompanied with an increase of cyclin A/CDK2. Both cyclin E/CDK2 and cyclin A/CDK2 activities are necessary for the initiation of DNA replication and the completion of DNA replication only once in each cycle *(64–66)*. In addition cyclin A/CDK2 promotes the transcription of histones and other genes involved in the replication process *(67,68)*. After proceeding through S- and $G_2$-phase the cell enters the M-phase of the cell cycle. The dramatic morphological changes occurring in M-phase are under the control of Cdk1 (Cdc2) in association with cyclin A and Cyclin B. Cyclin B rises late in S-phase and remains high throughout $G_2$ and M-phase *(69)*. The morphological changes are closely associated with the activity of the cyclin B/Cdk1 complex and structural proteins like nuclear lamins, nucleolar proteins, centrosomal proteins, and Eg5 (a kinesin-related motor) have all been described as substrates *(70)*. The different stages in M-phase are characterized by a rapid and coordinated destruction of cyclin A and cyclin B *(71)*. Ubiquitin-mediated degradation is the main pathway for ridding cells of cell cycle proteins that have executed their function. This mechanism makes sure that cell cycle progression is unidirectional and does not reoccur inappropriately. Cyclin A and B are marked for destruction by the anaphase promoting complex, for $G_1$ cyclins the Skp-Cullin F box complex controls their timely degradation *(72)*. In summary, the cell cycle is a complex regulatory network controlling precisely each step for cell duplication. The cyclin/CDKs complexes together with their modifiers are the central regulators receiving mitogenic signals and controlling the progression through the cell-cycle clock.

## CELL CYCLE REGULATION AND VSMC HYPERPLASIA

Normally, VSMCs in the media of normal arteries are quiescent in $G_0$ phase of the cell cycle. After vascular injury VSMCs are stimulated to divide by mitogens. After several rounds of cell division cell proliferation ceases when arterial wound is complete. The CKIs have distinct temporal and spatial patterns of expression in normal, injured, and diseased arteries in vivo. $p27^{Kip1}$ is constitutively expressed in VSMCs of normal arteries, but is rapidly downregulated after vascular injury during mitogen-induced VSMC proliferation *(73)*. VSMCs synthesize collagen and other extracellular matrix molecules that signal back in autocrine and paracrine feedback loops to cause upregulation of $p27^{Kip1}$ and downregulation of cyclin E/CDK2 *(74)*. $p27^{Kip1}$ expression persists within intimal VSMCs after the wound is completely healed. In contrast, $p21^{Cip1}$ protein is not observed in VSMCs of normal arteries, but is upregulated along with $p27^{Kip1}$ in the later phases of arterial wound repair. $p16^{INK4}$ expression is low in normal and injured arteries. These patterns of protein expression are observed in several animal models of vascular disease including mice, rats, and pigs *(75,76)*. In human coronary arteries, $p27^{Kip1}$ is expressed within medial and intimal VSMCs of normal and atherosclerotic arteries, including the VSMCs of new blood vessels within the atherosclerotic plaque. $p21^{Cip1}$ is present only in advanced atherosclerotic lesions, and $p16^{INK4}$ is not detectable in normal or diseased human arteries *(77)*. These distinct temporal and spatial patterns of expression suggest that the CIP/KIP CKIs regulate $G_1$/S-phase progression in vascular cells and promote favorable vascular remodeling. Gene transfer and gene deletion experiments have confirmed these observational studies. $p27^{Kip1}$ or $p21^{Cip1}$ expression in VSMCs in vitro causes $G_1$ arrest by inhibition of CDK2 activity. Gene transfer of vectors that encode $p27^{Kip1}$ or $p21^{Cip1}$ into balloon injured arteries produces a significant reduction of VSMCs proliferation and neointimal-lesion formation. Deletion of $p27^{Kip1}$ and $p21^{Cip1}$ genes in mice accelerates cellular proliferation resulting in excessive neo intimal growth and impaired arterial wound repair *(10)*.

The CKI proteins also regulate VSMC migration through $p27^{Kip1}$. VSMC migration in vitro is inhibited by treatment of cells with rapamycin *(78)*. Rapamycin is a macrolide antibiotic, which prevents growth factor-dependent downregulation of $p27^{Kip1}$ through inhibition of the serine/threonine kinase $p70^{S6}$ *(79)*. Rapamycin also inhibits VSMC migration from wild-type mice but not from $p27^{-/-}$ mice, suggesting a $p27^{Kip1}$-dependent mechanism *(80)*.

The biology of vascular repair is characterized by discrete phases. Coincident with VSMC migration and proliferation, macrophages, neutrophils, and T-lymphocytes infiltrate the intima creating an acute inflammatory response. The degree of inflammatory response is dependent on the activation of inflammatory cells, such as macrophages and T-cells. $p27^{Kip1}$ plays a central role not only in the activation of these cells types but also in regulating the pool size of inflammatory cells in the BM. The inflammatory phase is followed by a synthetic phase in which VSMCs synthesize extracellular matrix proteins, including transforming growth factor-β. Polymerized type 1 collagen fibrils, a mature form of collagen, increase $p27^{Kip1}$ protein levels through integrin signaling and inhibition of $p70^{S6}$ kinase. In contrast, monomeric collagen, present following matrix degradation during vascular injury, induces VSMC proliferation through downregulation of p27$^{Kip1}$ *(74)*. Thus, extracellular matrix protein signaling leads to changes in CKI expression and VSMC proliferation.

## MOLECULAR TARGETS FOR VASCULAR THERAPIES

Recent therapies for vascular proliferative diseases have focused on targeting the cell cycle. Restenosis and in-stent restenosis have been treated in animal models by the overexpression of the CKIs p27$^{Kip1}$ and p21$^{Cip1}$ using adenoviral gene transfer. These studies, which demonstrate proof of principle for the rationale of cell cycle inhibition, coupled with advances in-stent technology have provided the platform for a new class of therapeutic devices and agents. Novel stents have been coated with drugs that inhibit VSMC proliferation and migration. Currently, sirolimus (rapamycin)-eluting stents and polymer-based paclitaxel-eluting stents have proven effective at preventing restenosis in large randomized controlled clinical trials.

Rapamycin is a natural fermentation product of *Streptomyces hygroscopicus*. It was discovered in 1964 in a soil sample from Rapa Nui (Easter Island) by a Canadian medical research expedition *(81)*. Although it has antifungal properties, it was not developed as an antibiotic owing to its potent immunosuppressive effects. Subsequent molecular and cellular studies have elucidated its properties. Rapamycin binds the cytosolic receptor FKBP12, leading to inhibition of the protein kinase TOR (target of rapamycin), elevation of p27$^{Kip1}$ and G$_1$ arrest. Rapamycin blocks G$_1$-S phase transition and proliferation of T-cell lymphocytes by upregulating p27$^{Kip1}$ *(79)*. Recently, these observations have been extended to VSMCs *(82,83)*. In addition to its antiproliferative properties, rapamycin inhibits VSMC migration. Rapamycin-coated stents have been approved for clinical use first in Europe and recently in the United States. Two large randomized, double-blinded, multicenter trials in Europe (RAVEL) and United States (SIRIUS) demonstrated significant improvements in angiographic and clinical outcomes compared with bare metal stents in patients with de novo lesions in native coronary arteries *(84,85)*.

Paclitaxel is an equally promising approach that is also undergoing clinical testing. This agent is a derivative of diterpenoid that was isolated from the bark of a yew tree, *Taxus brevifolia (86)*. Paclitaxel induces tubulin polymerization, which results in unstable microtubules *(87)*. Microtubules are an essential component of the mitotic spindle and are required for cell division and maintaining cell shape. They are also required for other cellular functions including motility, anchorage and intracellular signal transduction. Paclitaxel and other antimicrotubule drugs have a principal role in the treatment of certain malignancies, and more recently; this agent has been shown to inhibit VSMC migration and proliferation *(88)*. The drug inhibits intimal hyperplasia in animal models of restenosis *(89)*, and the results of randomized, double-blinded, multicenter clinical trials (TAXUS, ELUTES, and ASPECT) indicate comparable efficacy in preventing restenosis into rapamycin *(90–92)*.

## REFERENCES

1. Libby P. Inflammation in atherosclerosis. Nature 2002;420:868–874.
2. Ross R. Atherosclerosis is an inflammatory disease. Am Heart J 1999;138:S419–S420.
3. Glass CK, Witztum JL. Atherosclerosis. the road ahead. Cell 2001;104:503–516.

4. Nakashima Y, Chen YX, Kinukawa N, Sueishi K. Distributions of diffuse intimal thickening in human arteries: preferential expression in atherosclerosis-prone arteries from an early age. Virchows Arch 2002;441:279–288.

5. Li H, Cybulsky MI, Gimbrone MA Jr., Libby P. An atherogenic diet rapidly induces VCAM-1, a cytokine-regulatable mononuclear leukocyte adhesion molecule, in rabbit aortic endothelium. Arterioscler Thromb 1993;13:197–204.

6. Qiao JH, Tripathi J, Mishra NK, et al. Role of macrophage colony-stimulating factor in atherosclerosis: studies of osteopetrotic mice. Am J Pathol 1997;150:1687–1699.

7. Lee RT, Libby P. The unstable atheroma. Arterioscler Thromb Vasc Biol 1997;17:1859–1867.

8. Clowes AW, Schwartz SM. Significance of quiescent smooth muscle migration in the injured rat carotid artery. Circ Res 1985;56:139–145.

9. Clowes AW, Reidy MA, Clowes MM. Kinetics of cellular proliferation after arterial injury. I. Smooth muscle growth in the absence of endothelium. Lab Invest 1983;49:327–333.

10. Boehm M, Olive M, True AL, et al. Bone marrow-derived immune cells regulate vascular disease through a p27(Kip1)-dependent mechanism. J Clin Invest 2004;114:419–426.

11. Margolin L, Fishbein I, Banai S, et al. Metalloproteinase inhibitor attenuates neointima formation and constrictive remodeling after angioplasty in rats: augmentative effect of alpha(v)beta(3) receptor blockade. Atherosclerosis 2002;163:269–277.

12. Ferns GA, Raines EW, Sprugel KH, Motani AS, Reidy MA, Ross R. Inhibition of neointimal smooth muscle accumulation after angioplasty by an antibody to PDGF. Science 1991;253:1129–1132.

13. Jawien A, Bowen-Pope DF, Lindner V, Schwartz SM, Clowes AW. Platelet-derived growth factor promotes smooth muscle migration and intimal thickening in a rat model of balloon angioplasty. J Clin Invest 1992;89:507–511.

14. Majesky MW, Lindner V, Twardzik DR, Schwartz SM, Reidy MA. Production of transforming growth factor beta 1 during repair of arterial injury. J Clin Invest 1991;88:904–910.

15. Nabel EG, Yang ZY, Plautz G, et al. Recombinant fibroblast growth factor-1 promotes intimal hyperplasia and angiogenesis in arteries in vivo. Nature 1993;362:844–846.

16. Nabel EG, Yang Z, Liptay S, et al. Recombinant platelet-derived growth factor B gene expression in porcine arteries induce intimal hyperplasia in vivo. J Clin Invest 1993;91:1822–1829.

17. Grant MB, Wargovich TJ, Ellis EA, Caballero S, Mansour M, Pepine CJ. Localization of insulin-like growth factor I and inhibition of coronary smooth muscle cell growth by somatostatin analogues in human coronary smooth muscle cells. A potential treatment for restenosis? Circulation 1994;89:1511–1517.

18. Folkman J. Seminars in Medicine of the Beth Israel Hospital, Boston. Clinical applications of research on angiogenesis. N Engl J Med 1995;333:1757–1763.

19. Asahara T, Murohara T, Sullivan A, et al. Isolation of Putative Progenitor Endothelial Cells for Angiogenesis. Science 1997;275:964–966.

20. Rafii S, Lyden D. Therapeutic stem and progenitor cell transplantation for organ vascularization and regeneration. Nat Med 2003;9:702–712.

21. Urbich C, Dimmeler S. Endothelial progenitor cells: characterization and role in vascular biology. Circ Res 2004;95:343–353.

22. Peichev M, Naiyer AJ, Pereira D, et al. Expression of VEGFR-2 and AC133 by circulating human CD34(+) cells identifies a population of functional endothelial precursors. Blood 2000;95:952–958.

23. Sata M, Saiura A, Kunisato A, et al. Hematopoietic stem cells differentiate into vascular cells that participate in the pathogenesis of atherosclerosis. Nat Med 2002;8:403–409.

24. Simper D, Stalboerger PG, Panetta CJ, Wang S, Caplice NM. Smooth Muscle Progenitor Cells in Human Blood. Circulation 2002;106:1199–1204.

25. Caplice NM, Bunch TJ, Stalboerger PG, et al. Smooth muscle cells in human coronary atherosclerosis can originate from cells administered at marrow transplantation. Proc Natl Acad Sci USA 2003;100:4754–4759.

26. Majka SM, Jackson KA, Kienstra KA, Majesky MW, Goodell MA, Hirschi KK. Distinct progenitor populations in skeletal muscle are bone marrow derived and exhibit different cell fates during vascular regeneration. J Clin Invest 2003;111:71–79.

27. Jiang Y, Vaessen B, Lenvik T, Blackstad M, Reyes M, Verfaillie CM. Multipotent progenitor cells can be isolated from postnatal murine bone marrow, muscle, and brain. Exp Hematol 2002;30:896–904.

28. Beltrami AP, Barlucchi L, Torella D, et al. Adult cardiac stem cells are multipotent and support myocardial regeneration. Cell 2003;114:763–776.

29. Hu Y, Zhang Z, Torsney E, et al. Abundant progenitor cells in the adventitia contribute to atherosclerosis of vein grafts in ApoE-deficient mice. J Clin Invest 2004;113:1258–1265.

30. Rabbany SY, Heissig B, Hattori K, Rafii S. Molecular pathways regulating mobilization of marrow-derived stem cells for tissue revascularization. Trends Mol Med 2003;9:109–117.

31. Bruhl T, Heeschen C, Aicher A, et al. p21Cip1 levels differentially regulate turnover of mature endothelial cells, endothelial progenitor cells, and in vivo neovascularization. Circ Res 2004;94: 686–692.

32. Vasa M, Fichtlscherer S, Aicher A, et al. Number and migratory activity of circulating endothelial progenitor cells inversely correlate with risk factors for coronary artery disease. Circ Res 2001;89:E1–E7.

33. Hill JM, Zalos G, Halcox JP, et al. Circulating endothelial progenitor cells, vascular function, and cardiovascular risk. N Engl J Med 2003;348:593–600.

34. Luttun A, Tjwa M, Moons L, et al. Revascularization of ischemic tissues by PlGF treatment, and inhibition of tumor angiogenesis, arthritis and atherosclerosis by anti-Flt1. Nat Med 2002;8:831–840.

35. Nurse P. A Long Twentieth Century of the Cell Cycle and Beyond. Cell 2000;100:71–78.

36. Murray AW. Recycling the Cell Cycle: Cyclins Revisited. Cell 2004;116:221–234.

37. Evans T, Rosenthal ET, Youngblom J, Distel D, Hunt T. Cyclin: a protein specified by maternal mRNA in sea urchin eggs that is destroyed at each cleavage division. Cell 1983;33:389–396.

38. Lee MG, Nurse P. Complementation used to clone a human homologue of the fission yeast cell cycle control gene cdc2. Nature 1987;327:31–35.

39. Malumbres M, Sotillo R, Santamaria D, et al. Mammalian Cells Cycle without the D-Type Cyclin-Dependent Kinases Cdk4 and Cdk6. Cell 2004;118:493–504.

40. Harbour JW, Dean DC. The Rb/E2F pathway: expanding roles and emerging paradigms. Genes Dev 2000;14:2393–2409.

41. Sherr CJ, Roberts JM. CDK inhibitors: positive and negative regulators of G1-phase progression. Genes Dev 1999;13:1501–1512.

42. Hannon GJ, Beach D. p15INK4B is a potential effector of TGF-beta-induced cell cycle arrest. Nature 1994;371:257–261.

43. Serrano M, Hannon GJ, Beach D. A new regulatory motif in cell-cycle control causing specific inhibition of cyclin D/CDK4. Nature 1993;366:704–707.

44. Hirai H, Roussel MF, Kato JY, Ashmun RA, Sherr CJ. Novel INK4 proteins, p19 and p18, are specific inhibitors of the cyclin D-dependent kinases CDK4 and CDK6. Mol Cell Biol 1995;15:2672–2681.

45. Gu Y, Turck CW, Morgan DO. Inhibition of CDK2 activity in vivo by an associated 20K regulatory subunit. Nature 1993;366:707–710.

46. Harper JW, Adami GR, Wei N, Keyomarsi K, Elledge SJ. The p21 Cdk-interacting protein Cip1 is a potent inhibitor of G1 cyclin-dependent kinases. Cell 1993;75:805–816.

47. el-Deiry WS, Tokino T, Velculescu VE, et al. WAF1, a potential mediator of p53 tumor suppression. Cell 1993;75:817–825.

48. Xiong Y, Hannon GJ, Zhang H, Casso D, Kobayashi R, Beach D. p21 is a universal inhibitor of cyclin kinases. Nature 1993;366:701–704.

49. Polyak K, Kato JY, Solomon MJ, et al. p27Kip1, a cyclin-Cdk inhibitor, links transforming growth factor-beta and contact inhibition to cell cycle arrest. Genes Dev 1994;8:9–22.

50. Polyak K, Lee MH, Erdjument-Bromage H, et al. Cloning of p27Kip1, a cyclin-dependent kinase inhibitor and a potential mediator of extracellular antimitogenic signals. Cell 1994;78:59–66.

51. Toyoshima H, Hunter T. p27, a novel inhibitor of G1 cyclin-Cdk protein kinase activity, is related to p21. Cell 1994;78:67–74.

52. Lee MH, Reynisdottir I, Massague J. Cloning of p57KIP2, a cyclin-dependent kinase inhibitor with unique domain structure and tissue distribution. Genes Dev 1995;9:639–649.

53. Matsuoka S, Edwards MC, Bai C, et al. p57KIP2, a structurally distinct member of the p21CIP1 Cdk inhibitor family, is a candidate tumor suppressor gene. Genes Dev 1995;9:650–662.

54. LaBaer J, Garrett MD, Stevenson LF, et al. New functional activities for the p21 family of CDK inhibitors. Genes Dev 1997;11:847–862.

55. Cheng M, Olivier P, Diehl JA, et al. The p21(Cip1) and p27(Kip1) CDK 'inhibitors' are essential activators of cyclin D-dependent kinases in murine fibroblasts. Embo J 1999;18:1571–1583.

56. Ewen ME, Sluss HK, Sherr CJ, Matsushime H, Kato J, Livingston DM. Functional interactions of the retinoblastoma protein with mammalian D-type cyclins. Cell 1993;73:487–497.

57. Pagano M, Tam SW, Theodoras AM, et al. Role of the ubiquitin-proteasome pathway in regulating abundance of the cyclin-dependent kinase inhibitor p27. Science 1995;269:682–685.

58. Sheaff RJ, Groudine M, Gordon M, Roberts JM, Clurman BE. Cyclin E-CDK2 is a regulator of p27Kip1. Genes Dev 1997;11:1464–1478.

59. Vlach J, Hennecke S, Amati B. Phosphorylation-dependent degradation of the cyclin-dependent kinase inhibitor p27. Embo J 1997;16:5334–5344.

60. Rodier G, Montagnoli A, Di Marcotullio L, et al. p27 cytoplasmic localization is regulated by phosphorylation on Ser10 and is not a prerequisite for its proteolysis. Embo J 2001;20:6672–6682.

61. Ishida N, Hara T, Kamura T, Yoshida M, Nakayama K, Nakayama KI. Phosphorylation of p27Kip1 on serine 10 is required for its binding to CRM1 and nuclear export. J Biol Chem 2002;277: 14,355–14,358.

62. Besson A, Gurian-West M, Schmidt A, Hall A, Roberts JM. p27Kip1 modulates cell migration through the regulation of RhoA activation. Genes Dev 2004;18:862–876.

63. McAllister SS, Becker-Hapak M, Pintucci G, Pagano M, Dowdy SF. Novel p27(kip1) C-terminal scatter domain mediates Rac-dependent cell migration independent of cell cycle arrest functions. Mol Cell Biol 2003;23:216–228.

64. Pagano M, Pepperkok R, Verde F, Ansorge W, Draetta G. Cyclin A is required at two points in the human cell cycle. Embo J 1992;11:961–971.

65. Girard F, Strausfeld U, Fernandez A, Lamb NJ. Cyclin A is required for the onset of DNA replication in mammalian fibroblasts. Cell 1991;67:1169–1179.

66. Ohtsubo M, Theodoras AM, Schumacher J, Roberts JM, Pagano M. Human cyclin E, a nuclear protein essential for the G1-to-S phase transition. Mol Cell Biol 1995;15:2612–2624.

67. Obaya AJ, Sedivy JM. Regulation of cyclin-Cdk activity in mammalian cells. Cell Mol Life Sci 2002;59:126–142.

68. Bell SP. The origin recognition complex: from simple origins to complex functions. Genes Dev 2002;16:659–672.

69. Gautier J, Minshull J, Lohka M, Glotzer M, Hunt T, Maller JL. Cyclin is a component of maturation-promoting factor from *Xenopus*. Cell 1990;60:487–494.

70. Musacchio A, Hardwick KG. The spindle checkpoint: structural insights into dynamic signalling. Nat Rev Mol Cell Biol 2002;3:731–741.

71. Amon A, Irniger S, Nasmyth K. Closing the cell cycle circle in yeast: G2 cyclin proteolysis initiated at mitosis persists until the activation of G1 cyclins in the next cycle. Cell 1994;77:1037–1050.

72. Harper JW, Burton JL, Solomon MJ. The anaphase-promoting complex: it's not just for mitosis any more. Genes Dev 2002;16:2179–2206.

73. Tanner FC, Yang ZY, Duckers E, Gordon D, Nabel GJ, Nabel EG. Expression of cyclin-dependent kinase inhibitors in vascular disease. Circ Res 1998;82:396–403.

74. Koyama H, Raines EW, Bornfeldt KE, Roberts JM, Ross R. Fibrillar collagen inhibits arterial smooth muscle proliferation through regulation of Cdk2 inhibitors. Cell 1996;87:1069–1078.

75. Yang ZY, Simari RD, Perkins ND, et al. Role of the p21 cyclin-dependent kinase inhibitor in limiting intimal cell proliferation in response to arterial injury. Proc Natl Acad Sci USA 1996;93:7905–7910.

76. Chen D, Krasinski K, Sylvester A, Chen J, Nisen PD, Andres V. Downregulation of cyclin-dependent kinase 2 activity and cyclin A promoter activity in vascular smooth muscle cells by p27(KIP1), an inhibitor of neointima formation in the rat carotid artery. J Clin Invest 1997;99:2334–2341.

77. Tanner FC, Boehm M, Akyurek LM, et al. Differential effects of the cyclin-dependent kinase inhibitors p27(Kip1), p21(Cip1), and p16(Ink4) on vascular smooth muscle cell proliferation. Circulation 2000;101:2022–2025.

78. Poon M, Marx SO, Gallo R, Badimon JJ, Taubman MB, Marks AR. Rapamycin inhibits vascular smooth muscle cell migration. J Clin Invest 1996;98:2277–2283.

79. Nourse J, Firpo E, Flanagan WM, et al. Interleukin-2-mediated elimination of the p27Kip1 cyclin-dependent kinase inhibitor prevented by rapamycin. Nature 1994;372:570–573.

80. Sun J, Marx SO, Chen HJ, Poon M, Marks AR, Rabbani LE. Role for p27(Kip1) in Vascular Smooth Muscle Cell Migration. Circulation 2001;103:2967–2972.

81. Vezina C, Kudelski A, Sehgal SN. Rapamycin (AY-22,989), a new antifungal antibiotic. I. Taxonomy of the producing streptomycete and isolation of the active principle. J Antibiot (Tokyo) 1975; 28:721–726.

82. Marx SO, Marks AR. Bench to bedside: the development of rapamycin and its application to stent restenosis. Circulation 2001;104:852–855.

83. Marx SO, Jayaraman T, Go LO, Marks AR. Rapamycin-FKBP inhibits cell cycle regulators of proliferation in vascular smooth muscle cells. Circ Res 1995;76:412–417.

84. Morice MC, Serruys PW, Sousa JE, et al. A randomized comparison of a sirolimus-eluting stent with a standard stent for coronary revascularization. N Engl J Med 2002;346:1773–1780.

85. Moses JW, Leon MB, Popma JJ, et al. Sirolimus-eluting stents versus standard stents in patients with stenosis in a native coronary artery. N Engl J Med 2003;349:1315–1323.

86. Wani MC, Taylor HL, Wall ME, Coggon P, McPhail AT. Plant antitumor agents. VI. The isolation and structure of taxol, a novel antileukemic and antitumor agent from *Taxus brevifolia*. J Am Chem Soc 1971;93:2325–2327.

87. Schiff PB, Horwitz SB. Taxol stabilizes microtubules in mouse fibroblast cells. Proc Natl Acad Sci USA 1980;77:1561–1565.

88. Sollott SJ, Cheng L, Pauly RR, et al. Taxol inhibits neointimal smooth muscle cell accumulation after angioplasty in the rat. J Clin Invest 1995;95:1869–1876.

89. Heldman AW, Cheng L, Jenkins GM, et al. Paclitaxel stent coating inhibits neointimal hyperplasia at 4 weeks in a porcine model of coronary restenosis. Circulation 2001;103:2289–2295.

90. Gershlick A, De Scheerder I, Chevalier B, et al. Inhibition of restenosis with a paclitaxel-eluting, polymer-free coronary stent: the European evaLUation of pacliTaxel Eluting Stent (ELUTES) trial. Circulation 2004;109:487–493.

91. Colombo A, Drzewiecki J, Banning A, et al. Randomized study to assess the effectiveness of slow- and moderate-release polymer-based paclitaxel-eluting stents for coronary artery lesions. Circulation 2003;108:788–794.

92. Park SJ, Shim WH, Ho DS, et al. A paclitaxel-eluting stent for the prevention of coronary restenosis. N Engl J Med 2003;348:1537–1545.

93. Nabel EG. CDKs and CKIs: molecular targets for tissue remodelling. Nat Rev Drug Discov 2002; 1:587–598.

# 13 Arterial Remodeling

*Gerard Pasterkamp, PhD,*
*Bradley H. Strauss, MD, PhD,*
*and Dominique de Kleijn, PhD*

## CONTENTS

## INTRODUCTION

Arterial remodeling is recognized as an important determinant in most vascular pathology in which narrowing of the lumen is the predominant feature. Not only expansive remodeling, for example, enlargement, but also constrictive remodeling, for example, shrinkage, is observed in arterial occlusive disease *(1–5)*. Expansive remodeling prevents and constrictive remodeling accelerates narrowing of the lumen *(1–5)*. Also in restenosis after balloon angioplasty, in both experimental research *(6–8)* as well as in humans *(9)*, constrictive remodeling is the most important determinant of luminal renarrowing *(10)*.

The descriptive observations on the existence of the different remodeling modes and their relation with luminal (re)narrowing has changed the perception on the mechanisms of arterial occlusive disease. Not just plaque formation or intimal hyperplasia, but the response to intima and plaque formation predominantly determines the degree of luminal narrowing *(10)*. The mechanisms of arterial constrictive remodeling are not fully understood. Latest research point to an important role for matrix (collagen) turnover orchestrated by inflammatory processes and protease activity.

## ARTERIAL REMODELING AFTER ANGIOPLASTY

The process of restenosis following balloon injury is divided in three phases *(11)*.

1. Endothelial denudation and subsequent platelet adhesion and aggregation and activation of coagulation cascade.

From: *Contemporary Cardiology: Essentials of Restenosis: For the Interventional Cardiologist*
Edited by: H. J. Duckers, E. G. Nabel, and P. W. Serruys © Humana Press Inc., Totowa, NJ

2. The proliferative phase, consists of medial smooth muscle cell (SMC) and fibroblast proliferation and migration toward the arterial lumen with the formation of neointima. This phase is stimulated by several growth factors, mainly platelet-derived growth factor, and fibroblast growth factor.
3. The synthesis and accumulation of extracellular matrix (ECM) that enhances intimal formation and induces constrictive remodeling.

For a long time, restenosis after balloon injury was considered to be the cause of intimal hyperplasia. However, constrictive remodeling is now recognized as the major factor in restenosis after angioplasty and atherectomy in humans (12,13) as had been suggested earlier in experimental animals (6,7). Angiographic restenosis is predominantly found to be the result of inward remodeling, with moderate plaque growth. In one human study, the decrease in vessel size accounted for 66% of the late lumen area loss (12). Moreover, Luo et al. (14) reported that 83% of the late loss after balloon angioplasty might be attributed to a decrease in vessel size. An unique study in humans was performed by Kimura et al. (13), who performed serial intravascular studies at 24 h, 1, and 6 mo after balloon angioplasty or coronary atherectomy to evaluate the time-course of geometric remodeling. They reported that geometric remodeling after coronary angioplasty was a biphasic phenomenon: after 24 h and 1 mo the artery enlarges and that inward remodeling occurs predominantly between 1 and 6 mo after the procedure, thus distinguishing it from early elastic recoil (13). This longitudinal study pointed out that constrictive remodeling is clearly distinguished from early elastic recoil (13).

Nowadays, in most centers, stents are used in more than 80% of procedures, as they provide both a more reliable immediate result and improved restenosis rates compared with regular balloon angioplasty. Although, the stent will prevent inward remodeling of the arterial wall, expansive remodeling is still possible. In that case enlargement of the arterial size does not affect lumen size but will result in intimal hyperplasia outside the stent struts.

### *Arterial Remodeling and Stenting*

Constrictive remodeling after balloon angioplasty is prevented by stenting (15). Neointima formation is the only determinant of lumen loss after stenting. However, intimal hyperplasia behind the stent struts may result in outward remodeling. Kay et al. (16) assessed the extent of expansive remodeling after stenting with radioactive stents and stenting with subsequent catheter-based irradiation. Catheter-based irradiation resulted in an increase in vessel area behind the stent compared with radioactive and nonradioactive stenting. In addition, constrictive remodeling was observed at the stent edges in the radioactive stenting group but not in the catheter-based radioactive stenting group. Thus, different patterns of remodeling exist between conventional, radioactive, and catheter-based radiotherapy with stenting. The authors (16) concluded that users of irradiation need to be alerted to the deleterious remodeling seen at the stent edges after higher dose radioactive stent implantation and behind the stents after catheter-based radiation and stenting.

More recently, the same research group investigated changes in vessel area dimensions by catheter-based β-irradiation following stenting or balloon angioplasty in humans. They observed expansive remodeling in the β-irradiated arteries in both the stented as well as in the balloon dilated arteries that accommodated tissue growth. The conclusion was quite provocative stating that after β-irradiation, stenting may not play an important role in the prevention of constrictive remodeling *(17)*. Another study from Rotterdam demonstrated that γ-irradiation following balloon angioplasty of peripheral arteries also resulted in enhanced expansive remodeling *(18)*.

Thus, it is generally accepted that stenting prevents constrictive remodeling and subsequent luminal narrowing. However, expansion of the arterial size by atherosclerotic plaque formation is still possible in in-stented arteries.

## ARTERIAL REMODELING AND ECM TURNOVER

Collagen fibers represent the major component of the ECM in many tissues including the arteries. Vascular collagen plays a key role in the maintenance of tissue integrity, and together with elastin, in the control of vessel wall elasticity. Collagen turnover encompasses biosynthesis, crosslinking and breakdown of fibers. In general, the rate of collagen turnover in normal blood vessels is very slow *(19,20)*. Data generated from in vitro and in vivo studies, have shown that under certain pathological circumstances, such us neointima appearance following vascular injury and plaque formation, the collagen turnover is altered. It has been reported that changes in collagen content might directly influence the mode of arterial remodeling following injury *(21)*.

Quantitative studies of collagen synthesis and content determination after experimental balloon injury have shown that collagen accumulation occurs over a much longer time frame than cell proliferation. Collagen synthesis continued at high rates for at least the first 4 wk after balloon angioplasty, whereas total collagen content continued to increase for up to 12 wk *(22)*. Other studies have shown increased collagen mRNA expression during the first week after arterial injury followed by collagen accumulation during the first month *(23)*. Other matrix proteins such as elastin also showed a gradual increase in deposition in the arterial wall over several months *(24)*. The collagen accumulation after stenting is even more dramatic and an almost twofold increase in collagen content at 10 wk compared with balloon angioplasty alone is noted *(25)* and this collagen accumulation is present in both the intimal and adventitial layers of the vessel wall.

The analysis of human restenosis specimens have confirmed the prominent role of ECM accumulation after arterial injury was first observed in animal models *(26,27)*. Recently Chung et al. *(28)* have also shown that the cellularity of the neointimal lesion after arterial stenting in humans is quite low after the first 3 mo. Neointima was hypercellular in the early weeks after stenting, but became hypocellular with prominent cell loss with passage of time *(28)*.

Most arterial collagen is observed in the adventitial layer. Adventitial thickening is commonly observed in animal models following arterial balloon injury *(29)*. Moreover, adventitial collagen content is found to be associated with the degree of constrictive remodeling following angioplasty *(21,30)*. Inhibition of matrix metalloprotease activity resulted in less collagen accumulation in the adventitia and also in less constrictive remodeling, which would support the role of adventitial collagen accumulation in constrictive remodeling following angioplasty. The mechanisms of increased collagen accumulation after arterial injury are still being investigated and not fully understood. The paradoxical effect of matrix metalloprotease inhibitors, which surprisingly inhibit adventitial collagen accumulation, has already been mentioned. More recently, also a role for angiotensin II type 1 receptor *(31)* and transforming growth factor-β *(32)* have been suggested.

In rabbit arteries, collagen content is significantly lower in restenotic vs non-restenotic vessel after balloon angioplasty *(33)*, which is difficult to reconcile with a presumed increased adventitial collagen content in constrictive remodeling *(8)*. Thus, controversial reports exist on the relation between adventitial thickness, collagen content, and the mode of arterial remodeling after balloon angioplasty. Probably not the deposit of total collagen but the maturation with subsequent conformational changes and crosslinking of collagen are an important determinant of geometrical changes within the arterial wall. After synthesis and release, cleavage of the collagen propeptides occurs, followed by self-assembly into collagen fibrils. The final enzymatic modification in the collagen fibril formation is the formation of intra- and intermolecular crosslinks by lysyl oxidase *(34,35)*.

Lysyl oxidase is a copper-dependent enzyme that initiates the crosslinking of collagen and elastin fibers to form insoluble collagen fibers. Lysyl oxidase expression is increased during various biological processes that are characterized by extensive ECM remodeling and crosslinking of collagen molecules that will eventually result in scar contraction and fibrosis *(36)*. Increased lysyl oxidase activity has been implicated in the pathogenesis of atherosclerosis *(37)*, whereas inhibition of arterial remodeling can be achieved by lysyl oxidase inhibition *(38)*. Although lysyl oxidase is a key molecule in the collagen fiber maturation pathway, in vivo expression of lysyl oxidase after balloon injury has not been studied in relation to other members of collagen fiber maturation pathway and arterial remodeling.

Recently, a rabbit balloon injury model to study temporal changes in arterial lysyl oxidase and collagen I expression, collagen fiber content, and collagen crosslinking was used. The authors demonstrate that following arterial injury, collagen crosslinking first decreases probably because of collagen accumulation, followed by crosslinking of the new collagen fibers and constrictive remodeling of the artery. The results suggested that not collagen synthesis but subsequent collagen crosslinking might be a critical process in lumen stenosis following arterial injury *(39)* (Smeets et al., unpublished observation).

## ARTERIAL REMODELING AND PROTEASE ACTIVITY

Matrix metalloproteases (MMPs) degrade the collageneous fibrous cap and thereby destabilize the atherosclerotic plaque. MMP-1 degrades collagen into gelatins, which facilitate SMC migration *(40)*. Thus, blocking of MMP activity might impair the ability of SMCs to migrate and subsequently form an intimal layer. Indeed, MMPs are upregulated following balloon angioplasty and after blood flow cessation *(41,42)*. Recently, the authors studied the effect of the MMP-inhibitors batimastat and marimastat on late lumen loss after balloon angioplasty in the pig. In the atherosclerotic pig, batimastat reduced late lumen loss by 50%, which was completely attributed to impaired constrictive remodeling *(43)*. In the nonatherosclerotic pig, marimastat completely abolished constrictive remodeling resulting in reduction of late lumen loss of more than 50% *(44)*. Intimal hyperplasia was not influenced by MMP-inhibition. These experimental studies show that breakdown of the ECM is a prerequisite for an artery to shrink in response to balloon angioplasty. However, one has to keep in mind that proteases are also obligatory for the maturation of procollagen: propeptides are cleaved by bone morphogenetic protein-1 and a furin like protease *(45)*. As nonspecific MMP-inhibitors are tested, it should be studied whether the effect of MMP-inhibition in experimental studies is attributed to the suppression of matrix breakdown, collagen maturation, or both.

However, there are some divergent reports. Cherr et al. *(46)* used RO113-2908, another nonspecific MMP inhibitor, without effect on intimal hyperplasia in an atherosclerotic primate stent model. Administration of batimastat and marimastat in a micropig model also showed no effect on intimal hyperplasia *(47,48)* after balloon angioplasty, but lack of benefit in these studies may be explained by the catch up phenomenon *(49)* resulting from the brief duration of drug administration. Rat models of carotid balloon injury with GM6001 have shown an inhibitory effect on cell migration and intimal hyperplasia at 1 and 2 wk, but a catch-up phenomenon by 4 wk *(49)*.

So far the role of collagen turnover is been considered as the major matrix constituent. Also a role for elastin degradation by MMPs has been considered as a potential mechanism to inhibit restenosis following arterial injury. Recently, MMP3 polymorphism has found to be associated with the incidence of restenosis *(50)*. Elastase inhibitors have also been shown to reduce intimal hyperplasia after balloon injury. The group has reported a 43% reduction in intimal area with overexpression of the serine protease inhibitor, elafin, in a rabbit carotid injury model *(51)*. Elafin has also been shown to be effective in preventing intimal hyperplasia in other models of vascular injury such as transplant arteriopathy and vein-graft degeneration *(52,53)*.

## ARTERIAL REMODELING: A ROLE FOR IMMUNITY?

In atherosclerotic disease it is well recognized that a strong relation exists between the mode of arterial remodeling and the presence of inflammatory cells. Expansive remodeling and aneurysm formation have been associated with the presence of inflammatory cells, whereas constrictively remodeled lesions mostly appear to have a stable, noninflammatory phenotype *(54,55)*. In animal models it has been demonstrated that the presence of macrophages are associated with the expansive remodeling response *(56)*. Perivascular inflammation is also commonly observed following balloon angioplasty *(57)*. Literature on the role of inflammatory cells in constrictive remodeling following angioplasty hides contradictions. Costa et al. *(58)* showed that an inverse relation exists between late lumen loss following coronary intervention, and the presence of CD *(66)*, which is a marker for neutrophil activation. This report would suggest a beneficial effect of neutrophil activation in the remodeling response *(58)*.

Next to atherosclerotic remodeling and remodeling following angioplasty, much research has been performed on the remodeling process following alterations in blood flow. This well-controlled research may also provide insight into the potential role of ligands and receptors that are recognized for their role in the innate immunity. Biomechanical effects of increased blood flow on the vascular wall are of primary importance for collateral vessel growth *(59)*. It is still unclear how the vascular wall senses these biomechanical effects but the endothelium plays an important role in its response *(60)*. Flow changes can upregulate activation of MMPs *(61)*, considered to be important for remodeling in general *(48,62,63)*.

Endothelial cells sense shear stress and various patterns of flow resulting in regulating the expression of intracellular-adhesion molecule 1, vascular-adhesion molecule 1 *(64)*, monocyte-chemoattractant molecule 1 *(65)*, and MMP-9 *(66)*. All these molecules can contribute to monocyte–arterial wall interactions important in the remodeling of the wall. The role of monocytes in stimulating arteriogenesis is still unclear, but it has been suggested that their production of growth factors might play a role *(67)*. Infusion of monocyte chemotactic protein-1 *(67)* as well as of a bolus of lipopolysacharide (LPS), which activates monocytes *(68)*, stimulated arterial conductance after femoral artery occlusion in the rabbit. This not only supports the role of monocytes in arteriogenesis, but also suggest a role for the Toll-like receptor (Tlr)4, which is the receptor for LPS, in arterial remodeling.

### *Arterial Remodeling and Tlr4*

Tlr4 is the receptor for exogenous LPS *(69)*, endogenous heat shock protein (Hsp)60 *(70)*, and the extra domain A of fibronectin *(71)* present in alternatively spliced fibronectin also known as cellular fibronectin. Tlr4 expression has recently been described in atherosclerotic arteries in endothelial cells, macrophages *(72,73)*, and advential fibroblasts *(74)*. Moreover, Tlr4 polymorphism is associated with carotid intima thickness in humans *(75)*. Recently, Boekholdt et al. *(76)* found that Tlr4 polymorphism modify the efficacy of statin therapy and the risk of cardiovascular events. This points again to a potential contribution of Tlr4 to cardiovascular disease although the exact mechanistic role of Tlr4 remains obscure.

Using a mouse femoral cuff model, it was recently demonstrated that Tlr4 is involved in neointima formation *(74)*. Although the role of Tlr4 remains unknown, it has been shown that Tlr4 activation results in the in vitro production of cytokines and MMP-9 *(71)*, a protease associated with structural changes of the arterial wall involving cell migration and collagen (matrix) breakdown *(77)*.

In the mouse, femoral artery cuff model Tlr4 activation by LPS-stimulated plaque formation and subsequent expansive arterial remodeling in the atherosclerotic ApoE3 (Leiden) transgenic mouse and in the wild-type mice. However, in the Tlr4-deficient mice, no compensatory expansive arterial remodeling was observed in response to neointima formation *(78)*. In another model, ligation of one of the common carotid arteries in wild-type mice resulted in expansive remodeling without neointima formation in the contralateral carotid artery. This effect was associated with an increase in Tlr4 expression and extra domain A and Hsp60 mRNA levels.

In contrast, expansive remodeling was not observed following a similar carotid ligation procedure in the Tlr4-deficient mice *(78)*. It was determined that in the Tlr4-deficient mouse, collagen-density increased significantly in the contralateral, whereas it did not change in the wild-type mouse. These results suggest that accumulation of collagen prevented the expansive remodeling and that Tlr4 is an important cellular receptor affecting the collagen turnover. It is suggested that regulation of Tlr4 and its endogenous ligands, extra domain A, and Hsp60, are potential novel targets available for therapeutic control of arterial remodeling.

## ARTERIAL REMODELING: INTERVENTIONS

Animal and clinical research has been performed to study the effect of chemical and molecular compounds that potentially inhibit the constrictive remodeling response following coronary angioplasty. Some of them will be briefly discussed here.

### *The Endothelium as a Therapeutic Target*

In restenotic arterial remodeling the possibility of a regulating role for shear stress is currently being explored. Recently, Krams et al. *(79)* locally quantified shear stress in three dimensional vessel reconstructions after balloon angioplasty in the Yucatan micropig. They reported that the level of decrement in shear stress predicted the loss of vessel area during follow-up after balloon angioplasty. This observation is somewhat surprising because by balloon angioplasty the shear registrating cell (endothelium) is removed and after reendothelization is initially dysfunctional *(80)*. The local shear stress as determined after angioplasty was found to be more predictive than the acute luminal gain. Supportive for the role of shear stress in the remodeling response is the observation that low flow upregulates MMP-2 after balloon injury *(81)*.

Constrictive remodeling has been prevented successfully by inhibiting oxidative stress *(82,83)*. In humans, the antioxidant probucol has proven to exert its antirestenotic effects by improving expansive remodeling after angioplasty *(83)*. However, in contrast with other serial intravascular ultrasound studies, in this clinical study, constrictive remodeling was not a predominant feature in the control group who did not receive probucol. Thus, it could not be concluded that constrictive remodeling was prevented by probucol, although it did enhance the expansive remodeling response. Theoretically, this positive effect of probucol can be explained by preventing endothelial dysfunction, low-density lipoprotein oxidation, or MMP activation.

Endothelial function is impaired after balloon angioplasty *(80)* and can be restored by local delivery of the nitric oxide (NO) precursor L-arginine *(84)*. In addition, angiographic improvement of the lumen is observed late (>6 mo) after balloon angioplasty *(85)*, possibly because of the temporary absence of the endothelial function. Conflicting reports exist on the effect of L-arginine administration on postangioplasty remodeling *(86,87)*. In the pig, adenovirus-mediated transfer of human endothelial NO-synthase, reduced the late lumen loss after balloon angioplasty by both reduction of neointima and enlargement of the vessel area *(88)*. Reduction of luminal narrowing and constrictive remodeling following balloon angioplasty was also observed in pigs when intrapericardial nitric oxide levels were augmented *(89)*. Also supporting the role of NO in arterial remodeling is the observation that physical training induces endothelial nitric oxide synthase expression and reduces constrictive remodeling following balloon angioplasty in rats *(90)*.

### The Matrix as a Therapeutic Target

Changes in arterial wall structure occurs in all types and modes of arterial remodeling. In restenotic *(91)* and flow-induced remodeling *(92)* structural matrix changes occur late in the remodeling process. It is likely to assume that the vascular wall uses common pathways to initiate and maintain the different types of remodeling although mechanical triggers may differ. For collagen breakdown, it is reported that in *de novo* atherosclerotic remodeling, in postangioplasty remodeling as well as in flow-related remodeling matrix metalloproteinases (MMP) play an important role *(63,93)*. MMP inhibition studies support this postulation *(63,93)*. Next to collagen breakdown, also synthesis and maturation of collagen are appropriate targets to intervene in the arterial remodeling process. Synthesis can be affected by using an inhibitor of collagen synthesis *(94)* but also the maturation process of collagen might be an appropriate target by, for instance, interfering in collagen crosslinking *(38)*. Other potential sites of application are bone morphogenetic protein-1 and a furin-like proprotein convertase that are responsible for the N- and C-terminal cleavage of collagen-1 during maturation *(45)*.

### The Coagulation Pathway as a Therapeutic Target

Tissue factor is a low-molecular weight glycoprotein that initiates the extrinsic clotting cascade. Tissue factor pathway inhibitor is a natural inhibitor of the tissue factor initiated coagulation. Two animal studies have been performed in which the effect of tissue factor pathway inhibitor *(TFPI)* gene delivery was investigated *(95,96)*. Both studies revealed an improvement of luminal diameter following intervention by *TFPI* gene delivery. This gain in lumen area could be attributed to a decrease in neointima formation. However, the study performed in rabbits also showed a significant inhibitory effect on constrictive remodeling *(95)*.

## *Radiation and Phototherapy*

Ionizing radiation has been shown to reduce vascular lesion formation after balloon injury and stenting *(97)*. In the pig coronary artery, irradiation also resulted in a larger vessel perimeter *(98)*. Thus, brachytherapy might have a beneficial effect on both intimal hyperplasia and on constrictive remodeling after balloon angioplasty. Suggested potential mechanisms by which irradiation might influence arterial remodeling are impairment of macrophage population *(99)*.

In an iliac rabbit model, van Leeuwen et al. *(100)* observed significantly less constrictive remodeling when saline flush was performed during excimer laser angioplasty. This effect may be attributed to the direct irradiation of the arterial wall during saline flush or the impaired response to injury. Another type of radiation by long wavelength ultraviolet light and psoralen as adjuvant (psoralen ultraviolet radiation A) augmented the loss of vessel area after balloon angioplasty *(101)*. More recently, ultraviolet B-activated psoralen also was found to reduce luminal narrowing by constrictive remodeling following balloon angioplasty in rabbits *(102)*. In another study aminolaevulinic acid was used as an adjuvant in combination with photodynamic therapy to successfully block constrictive remodeling following balloon injury in a rabbit model *(103)*. The latter study revealed that this photodynamic therapy was associated with cellular depletion and elimination of cholinergic innervations.

## ARTERIAL REMODELING: CONCLUSIONS

Arterial remodeling is a major determinant of obstructive cardiovascular disease. Compared with plaque/neointima formation, the mechanisms of the different remodeling modes have been relatively unexplored. Recently, several investigators have reported successful blocking of the constrictive remodeling response after balloon injury. With rapidly accumulating knowledge of the mechanisms of arterial remodeling, potential targets for intervention are being identified that have great potential for future therapeutic strategies in the treatment of obstructive arterial disease. Whether this therapeutic window will also open for stenotic culprit lesions merits careful consideration. With the increasing potency of the drug-eluding stents, it is questionable whether pharmaceutical approaches will improve the outcomes of the mechanical stent.

## REFERENCES

1. Pasterkamp G, Wensing PJW, Post MJ, Hillen B, Mali WPTM, Borst C. Paradoxical arterial wall shrinkage contributes to luminal narrowing of human atherosclerotic femoral arteries. Circulation 1995;91:1444–1449.
2. Pasterkamp G, Borst C, Post MJ, et al. Atherosclerotic arterial remodeling in the superficial femoral artery: individual variation in local compensatory enlargement response. Circulation 1996;93:1818–1825.
3. Nishioka T, Luo H, Eigler NL, Berglund H, Kim CJ, Siegel RJ. Contribution of inadequate compensatory enlargement to development of human coronary artery stenosis: an in vivo intravascular ultrasound study. J Am Coll Cardiol 1996;27:1571–1576.
4. Mintz GS, Kent KM, Pichard AD, Satler LF, Popma JJ, Leon MB. Contribution of inadequate arterial remodeling to the development of focal coronary artery stenoses: an intravascular ultrasound study. Circulation 1997;95:1791–1798.

5. Pasterkamp G, Schoneveld AH, van Wolferen WA, et al. The impact of atherosclerotic arterial remodeling on percentage luminal stenosis varies widely within the arterial system: a post mortem study. Arterioscler Thromb Vasc Biol 1997;17:3057–3063.

6. Post MJ, Borst C, Kuntz RE. The relative importance of arterial remodeling compared with intimal hyperplasia in lumen renarrowing after balloon angioplasty. Circulation 1994;89:2816–2821.

7. Kakuta T, Currier JW, Haudenschild CC, Ryan TJ, Faxon DP. Differences in compensatory vessel enlargement, not intimal formation, account for restenosis after angioplasty in the hypercholesterolemic rabbit model. Circulation 1994;89:2809–2815.

8. Lafont A, Guzman LA, Whitlow RL, Goormastic M, Fredrick J, Chisolm GM. Restenosis after experimental angioplasty: intimal, medial, and adventitial changes associated with constrictive remodeling. Circulation Res 1995;76:996–1002.

9. Mintz GS, Popma JJ, Pichard AD, et al. Arterial remodeling after coronary angioplasty. A serial intravascular ultrasound study. Circulation 1996;94:35–43.

10. Pasterkamp G, Fitzgerald PF, de Kleijn DP. Atherosclerotic expansive remodeled plaques: a wolf in sheep's clothing. J Vasc Res 2002;39:514–523.

11. Faxon DP, Coats W, Currier J. Remodeling of the coronary artery after vascular injury. Prog Cardiovasc Dis 1997;40:129–140.

12. Mintz GS, Popma JJ, Pichard AD, et al. Arterial remodeling after coronary angioplasty. A serial intravascular ultrasound study. Circulation 1996;94:35–43.

13. Kimura T, Kaburagi S, Tamura T, et al. Remodeling of human coronary arteries undergoing coronary angioplasty or atherectomy. Circulation 1997;96:475–483.

14. Luo H, Nishioka T, Eigler NL, et al. Coronary artery restenosis after balloon angioplasty in humans is associated with circumferential coronary constriction. Atheroscler Thromb Vasc Biol 1996;16:1393–1398.

15. Post MJ, de Smet BJGL, ven der Helm Y, Borst C, Kuntz R. Arterial remodeling after balloon angioplasty or stenting in an atherosclerotic model. Circulation 1997;96:996–1003.

16. Kay IP, Sabaté M, Costa MA, et al. Positive geometric remodeling is seen after catheter-based irradiation followed by conventional stent implantation, but not after radioactive stent implantation. Circulation 2000;102:1484–1489.

17. Kozuma K, Costa MA, van der Giessen WJ, et al. Intitial observation regarding changes in vessel dimensions after balloon angioplasty and stenting followed by catheter-based beta-radiation. Is stenting necessary in the setting of catheter-based radiotherapy? Eur Heart J 2002;23:641–649.

18. Hagenaars T, A Po IF, van Sambeek MR, et al. Gamma radiation induces positive vascular remodeling after balloon angioplasty: a prospective, randomized intravascular ultrasound scan study. J Vasc Surg 2002;36:318–324.

19. Janicki JS, Brower GL, Henegar JR, Wang L. Ventricular remodeling in heart failure: the role of myocardial collagen. Adv Exp Med Biol 1995;382:239–245.

20. Tanaka S, Koyama H, Ichii T, et al. Fibrillar collagen regulation of plasminogen activator inhibitor-1 is involved in altered smooth muscle cell migration. Arterioscler Thromb Vasc Biol 2002;22:1573–1578.

21. Sierevogel MJ, Velema E, van der Meer FJ, et al. Matrix metalloproteinase inhibition reduces adventitial thickening and collagen accumulation following balloon dilation. Cardiovasc Res 2002;55:864–869.

22. Strauss BH, Robinson R, Batchelor WB, et al. In vivo collagen turnover following experimental balloon angioplasty injury and the role of matrix metalloproteinases. Circ Res 1996;79:541–550.

23. Karim MA, Miller DD, Farrar MA, et al. Histomorphometric and biochemical correlates of arterial procollagen gene expression during vascular repair after experimental angioplasty. Circulation 1995;91:2049–2057.

24. Strauss BH, Chisholm RJ, Keeley FW, Gotlieb AI, Logan RA, Armstrong PW. Extracellular matrix remodeling after balloon angioplasty injury in a rabbit model of restenosis. Circ Res 1994;75:650–658.

25. Li C, Cantor W, Nili N, et al. Arterial repair after stenting and the effects of GM6001, a matrix metalloproteinase inhibitor. J Am Coll Cardiol 2002;39:1852–1858.

26. Strauss BH, Umans VA, van Suylen RJ, et al. Directional atherectomy for treatment of restenosis within coronary stents: clinical, angiographic and histologic results. J Am Coll Cardiol 1992;20:1465–1473.

27. Farb A, Sangiorgi G, Carter AJ, et al. Pathology of acute and chronic coronary stenting in humans. Circulation 1999;99:44–52.

28. Chung IM, Gold HK, Schwartz SM, Ikari Y, Reidy MA, Wight TN. Enhanced extracellular matrix accumulation in restenosis of coronary arteries after stent deployment. J Am Coll Cardiol 2002; 40:2072–2081.

29. Andersen HR, Maeng M, Thorwest M, Falk E. Remodeling rather than neointimal formation explains luminal narrowing after deep vessel wall injury: insights from a porcine coronary (re)stenosis model. Circulation 1996;93:1716–1724.

30. Lafont A, Durand E, Samuel JL, et al. Endothelial dysfunction and collagen accumulation: two independent factors for restenosis and constrictive remodeling after experimental angioplasty. Circulation 1999;100:1109–1115.

31. Eto H, Biro S, Miyata M, et al. Angiotensin II type I receptor participates in extracellular matrix production in the late stage of remodeling after vascular injury. Cardiovasc Res 2003;59:200–211.

32. Ryan ST, Koteliansky VE, Gotwals PJ, Lindner V. Transforming growth factor-beta-dependent events in vascular remodeling following arterial injury. J Vasc Res 2003;40:37–46.

33. Coats WD, Whittaker P, Cheung DT, Currier JW, Han B, Faxon DP. Collagen content is significantly lower in restenotic versus nonrestenotic vessels after balloon angioplasty in the atherosclerotic rabbit model. Circulation 1997;95:1293–1300.

34. Smith-Mungo LI, Kagan HM. Lysyl oxidase: properties, regulation and multiple functions in biology. Matrix Biol 1998;16:387–398.

35. Csiszar K. Lysyl oxidases: a novel multifunctional amine oxidase family. Prog Nucleic Acid Res Mol Biol 2001;70:1–32.

36. Kagan HM. Intra- and extracellular enzymes of collagen biosynthesis as biological and chemical targets in the control of fibrosis. Acta Trop 2000;77:147–152.

37. Kagan HM, Raghavan J, Hollander W. Changes in aortic lysyl oxidase activity in diet-induced atherosclerosis in the rabbit. Arteriosclerosis 1981;1:287–291.

38. Spears JR, Zhan H, Khurana S, Karvonen RL, Reiser KM. Modulation by beta-aminopropionitrile of vessel luminal narrowing and structural abnormalities in arterial wall collagen in a rabbit model of conventional balloon angioplasty versus laser balloon angioplasty. J Clin Invest 1994;93:1543–1553.

39. Smeets MB, Sierevogel MJ, Perree J, Voorbij HAM, Pasterkamp G, de Kleijn DPV. Collagen accumulation in the adventitia precedes constrictive remodeling after balloon dilation. Submitted unpublished observation.

40. Kuzuya M, Kanda S, Sasaki T, et al. Deficiency of gelatinase a suppresses smooth muscle cell invasion and development of experimental hyperplasia. Circulation 2003;108:1375–1381.

41. Godin D, Ivan E, Johnson C, Magid R, Galis ZS. Remodeling of carotid artery is associated with increased expression of matrix metalloproteinases in mouse blood flow cessation model. Circulation 2000;102:2861–2666.

42. Bassiouny HS, Song RH, Hong XF, Singh A, Kocharyan H, Glagov S. Flow regulation of 72-kD collagenase IV (MMP-2) after experimental arterial injury. Circulation 1998;98:157–163.

43. de Smet BJGL, Robertus JL, Rebel JMJ, van der Helm YJM, Borst C, Post MJ. Metalloproteinase inhibition reduces constrictive arterial remodeling following balloon angioplasty: a study in the atherosclerotic yucatan micropig. J Am Coll Cardiol 1999;33:88A.

44. Sierevogel MJ, Pasterkamp G, Velema E, de Kleijn DPV, de Smet BJGL, Borst C. MMP inhibition following balloon angioplasty inhibits constrictive remodeling in favour of expansive enlargement: an intravascular ultrasound study. Eur Heart J 1999;20:S367.

45. Imamura Y, Steiglitz BM, Greenspan DS. Bone morphogenetic protein-1 processes the NH2-terminal propeptide, and a furin-like proprotein convertase processes the COOH-terminal propeptide of pro-alpha1(V) collagen. J Biol Chem 1998;273(42):27,511–27,517.

46. Cherr GS, Motew SJ, Travis JA, et al. Metalloproteinase inhibition and the response to angioplasty and stenting in atherosclerotic primates. Arterioscler Thromb Vasc Biol 2002;22:161–166.

47. Sierevogel MJ, Pasterkamp G, Velema E, et al. Oral matrix metalloproteinase inhibition and arterial remodeling after balloon dilation : an intravascular ultrasound study in the pig. Circulation 2001;103:302–307.

48. de Smet BJ, de Kleijn D, Hanemaaijer R, et al. Metalloproteinase inhibition reduces constrictive arterial remodeling after balloon angioplasty: a study in the atherosclerotic Yucatan micropig. Circulation 2000;101:2962–2067.

49. Bendeck MP, Irvin C, Reidy MA. Inhibition of matrix metalloproteinase activity inhibits smooth muscle cell migration but not neointimal thickening after arterial injury. Circ Res 1996;78:38–43.

50. Humphries S, Bauters C, Meirhaeghe A, Luong L, Bertrand M, Amouyel P. The 5A6A polymorphism in the promotor of the stromelysin-1 (MMP3) gene as a risk factor for restenosis. Eur Heart J 2002;23:721–725.
51. Barolet AW, Nili N, Cheema A, et al. Arterial elastase activity after balloon angioplasty and effects of elafin, an elastase inhibitor. Arterioscler Thromb Vasc Biol 2001;21:1269–1274.
52. O'Blenes SB, Zaidi SH, Cheah AY, McIntyre B, Kaneda Y, Rabinovitch M. Gene transfer of the serine elastase inhibitor elafin protects against vein graft degeneration. Circulation 2000;102:III289–III295.
53. Cowan B, Baron O, Crack J, Coulber C, Wilson GJ, Rabinovitch M. Elafin, a serine elastase inhibitor, attenuates post-cardiac transplant coronary arteriopathy and reduces myocardial necrosis in rabbits afer heterotopic cardiac transplantation. J Clin Invest 1996;97:2452–2468.
54. Pasterkamp G, Schoneveld AH, van der Wal AC, et al. Relation of arterial geometry to luminal narrowing and histological markers for plaque vulnerability: the remodeling paradox. J Am Coll Cardiol 1998;32:655–662.
55. Pasterkamp G, Schoneveld AH, Hijnen DJ, et al. Atherosclerotic arterial remodeling and the localization of macrophages and matrix metalloproteases 1, 2 and 9 in the human coronary artery. Atherosclerosis 2000;150:245–253.
56. Ivan E, Khatri JJ, Johnson C, et al. Expansive arterial remodeling is associated with increased neointimal macrophage foam cell content: the murine model of macrophage-rich carotid artery lesions. Circulation 2002;105:2686–2691.
57. Okamoto E, Couse T, De Leon H, et al. Perivascular inflammation after balloon angioplasty of porcine coronary arteries. Circulation 2001;104:2228–2235.
58. Costa MA, de Wit LE, de Valk V, et al. Indirect evidence for a role of subpopulation of activated neutrophils in the remodeling process after percutaneous coronary intervention. Eur Heart J 2001;22:580–586.
59. Carmeliet P. Angiogenesis in health and disease. Nat Med 2003;9:653–660.
60. Langille BL, O'Donnell F. Reductions in arterial diameter produced by chronic decreases in blood flow are endothelium-dependent. Science 1986;231:405–407.
61. de Kleijn DP, Sluijter JP, Smit J, et al. Furin and membrane type-1 metalloproteinase mRNA levels and activation of metalloproteinase-2 are associated with arterial remodeling. FEBS Lett 2001;501:37–41.
62. Galis ZS, Khatri JJ. Matrix metalloproteinases in vascular remodeling and atherogenesis: the good,the bad, and the ugly. Circulation Res 2002;90:251–262.
63. Abbruzzese TA, Guzman RJ, Martin RL, Yee C, Zarins CK, Dalman RL. Matrix metalloproteinase inhibition limits arterial enlargements in a rodent arteriovenous fistula model. Surgery 1998;124:328–34, discussion 334–335.
64. Walpola PL, Gotlieb AI, Cybulsky MI, Langille BL. Expression of ICAM-1 and VCAM-1 and monocyte adherence in arteries exposed to altered shear stress. Arterioscler Thromb Vasc Biol 1995;15:2–10. Erratum in: Arterioscler Thromb Vasc Biol 1995;15:429.
65. Shyy JY, Lin MC, Han J, Lu Y, Petrime M, Chien S. The cis-acting phorbol ester "12-O-tetradecanoylphorbol 13-acetate"-responsive element is involved in shear stress-induced monocyte chemotactic protein 1 gene expression. Proc Natl Acad Sci USA 1995;92:8069–8073.
66. Magid R, Murphy TJ, Galis ZS. Expression of matrix metalloproteinase-9 in endothelial cells is differentially regulated by shear stress: role of c-Myc. J Biol Chem 2003;278:32,994–32,999.
67. Ito WD, Arras M, Winkler B, Scholz D, Schaper J, Schaper W. Monocyte chemotactic protein-1 increases collateral and peripheral conductance after femoral artery occlusion. Circ Res 1997;80:829–837.
68. Arras M, Ito WD, Scholz D, Winkler B, Schaper J, Schaper W. Monocyte activation in angiogenesis and collateral growth in the rabbit hindlimb. J Clin Invest 1998;101:40–50.
69. Poltorak A, He X, Smirnova I, et al. Defective LPS signaling in C3H/HeJ and C57BL/10ScCr mice: mutations in Tlr4 gene. Science 1998;282:2085–2088.
70. Ohashi K, Burkart V, Flohe S, Kolb H. Cutting edge: heat shock protein 60 is a putative endogenous ligand of the toll-like receptor-4 complex. J Immunol 2000;164:558–561.
71. Okamura Y, Watari M, Jerud ES, et al. The extra domain A of fibronectin activates Toll-like receptor 4. J Biol Chem 2001;276:10,229–10,233.
72. Xu XH, Shah PK, Faure E, et al. Toll-like receptor-4 is expressed by macrophages in murine and human lipid-rich atherosclerotic plaques and upregulated by oxidized LDL. Circulation 2001;104:3103–3108.

73. Edfeldt K, Swedenborg J, Hansson GK, Yan ZQ. Expression of toll-like receptors in human atherosclerotic lesions: a possible pathway for plaque activation. Circulation 2002;105:1158–1161.
74. Vink A, Schoneveld AH, van der Meer JJ, et al. In vivo evidence for a role of toll-like receptor 4 in the development of intimal lesions. Circulation 2002;106:1985–1990.
75. Kiechl S, Lorenz E, Reindl M, et al. Toll-like receptor 4 polymorphisms and atherogenesis. N Engl J Med 2002;347:185–192.
76. Boekholdt SM, Agema WR, Peters RJ, et al. Variants of toll-like receptor 4 modify the efficacy of statin therapy and the risk of cardiovascular events. Circulation 2003;107:2416–2421.
77. Galis ZS, Johnson C, Godin D, et al. Targeted disruption of the matrix metalloproteinase-9 gene impairs smooth muscle cell migration and geometrical arterial remodeling. Circ Res 2002;91:852–859.
78. Hollestelle SCG, de Vries M, van Keulen JK, Schoneveld AH, van Middelaar BJ, Pasterkamp G, Quax PHA, de Kleijn DPV. Toll-like receptor 4 is involved in outward arterial remodeling. Circulation 2004;109:393–398.
79. Krams R, Wentzel JJ, Oomen JAF, et al. Shear stress in atherosclerosis, and vascular remodeling. Semin Intervent Cardiol 1998;3:39–44.
80. Weidinger FF, McLenachan JM, Cybulsky MI, et al. Persistent dysfunction of regenerated endothelium after balloon angioplasty of rabbit iliac artery. Circulation 1990;81:1667–1679.
81. Bassiouny HS, Song RH, Hong XF, Singh A, Kocharyan H, Glagov S. Flow regulation of 72-kD collagenase IV (MMP-2) after experimental arterial injury. Circulation 1998;98:157–163.
82. Nunes GL, Sgoutas DS, Redden RA, et al. Combination of vitamins C and E alters the response to coronary balloon injury in the pig. Arterioscl Thromb Vasc Biol 1995;15:156–165.
83. Côté G, Tardif JC, Lesperance J, et al. Effects of probucol on vascular remodeling after coronary angioplasty. Circulation 1999;99:3035.
84. Schwarzacher SP, Lim TT, Wang B, et al. Local intramural delivery of L-arginine enhances nitric oxide generation and inhibits lesion formation after balloon angioplasty. Circulation 1997;95:1863–1869.
85. Ormiston JA, Stewart FM, Roche AH, Webber BJ, Whitlock RM, Webster MW. Late regression of the dilated site after coronary angioplasty: a 5 year quantitative angiographic study. Circulation 1997;96:468–474.
86. Bosmans JM, Vrints CJ, Kockx MM, Bult H, Cromheeke KMC, Herman AG. Continuous perivascular L-Arginine delivery increases total vessel area and reduces neointimal thickening after experimental balloon dilation. Arterioscl Thromb Vasc Biol 1999;19:767–776.
87. Le Tourneau T, van Belle E, Corseaux D, et al. Role of nitric oxide in restenosis after experimental balloon angioplasty in the hypercholesterolemic rabbit: effects on neointimal hyperplasia and vascular remodeling. J Am Coll Cardiol 1999;33:876–882.
88. Varenne O, Pislaru S, Gillijns H, et al. Local adenovirus-mediated transfer of human endothelial nitric oxide synthase reduces luminal narrowing after coronary angioplasty in pigs. Circulation 1998;98:919–926.
89. Baek SH, Hrabie JA, Keefer LK, Hou D, Fineberg N, Rhoades R, March KL. Augmentation of intrapericardial nitric oxide level by a prolonged-release nitric oxide donor reduces luminal narrowing after porcine coronary angioplasty. Circulation 2002;105:2779–2784.
90. Indolfi C, Torella D, Coppola C, et al. Physical training increases eNOS vascular expression and activity and reduces restenosis after balloon angioplasty or arterial stenting in rats. Circ Res 2002;91:1190–1197.
91. de Smet BJGL, Pasterkamp G, van der Helm YJ, Borst C, Post MJ. The relation between *de novo* atherosclerotic remodeling and angioplasty-induced remodeling in an atherosclerotic yucatan micropig model. Arterioscler Thromb Vasc Biol 1998;188:702–707.
92. Langille BL, O'Donnell F. Reductions in arterial diameter produced by chronic decreases in blood flow are endothelium-dependent. Science 1986;231:405–407.
93. de Smet BJGL, Robertus JL, Rebel JMJ, van der Helm YJM, Borst C, Post MJ. Metalloproteinase inhibition reduces constrictive arterial remodeling following balloon angioplasty: a study in the atherosclerotic yucatan micropig. J Am Coll Cardiol 1999;33:88A.
94. Choi ET, Callow AD, Sehgal NL, Brown DM, Ryan US. Halofuginone, a specific collagen type I inhibitor, reduces anastomotic intimal hyperplasia. Arch Surg 1995;130(3):257–261.
95. Yin X, Yutani C, Ikeda Y, et al. Tissue factor pathway inhibitor gene delivery using HVJ-AVE liposomes markedly reduces restenosis in atherosclerotic arteries. Cardiovasc Res 2002;56:454–463.
96. Singh R, Pan S, Mueske CS, et al. Role for tissue factor pathway in murine model of vascular remodeling. Circ Res 2001;89:71–76.

97. Mazur W, Ali MN, Khan M, et al. High dose rate intracoronary radiation for inhibition of neointimal formation in the stented and balloon injured porcine models of restenosis: angiographic, morphometric and histopathologic analyses. Int J Radiat Oncol Biol Phys 1996;36:777–788.

98. Waksman R, Rodriguez JC, Robinson KA, et al. Effect of intravascular irradiation on cell proliferation, apoptosis, and vascular remodeling after balloon overstretch injury of porcine coronary arteries. Circulation 1997;96:1944–1952.

99. Rubin P, Williams JP, Riggs PN, et al. Cellular and molecular mechanisms of radiation inhibition of restenosis. part I: role of the macrophage and platelet-derived growth factor. Int J Radiat Oncol Biol Phys 1998;40:929–941.

100. Van Leeuwen TG, Velema E, Pasterkamp G, Post MJ, Borst C. Saline flush during excimer laser angioplasty: short and long term effects in the rabbit femoral artery. Lasers Surg Med 1998;23:128–140.

101. Perree J, van Leeuwen TG, Velema E, Borst C. Psoralen and long wavelength ultraviolet radiation as an adjuvant therapy for prevention of intimal hyperplasia and constrictive remodeling after balloon angioplasty. Lasers Surg Med 1998;23:281–290.

102. Perree J, van Leeuwen TG, Velema E, Smeets M, de Kleijn D, Borst C. UVB-activated psoralen reduces luminal narrowing after balloon dilation because of inhibition of constrictive remodeling. Photochem Photobiol 2002;75:68–75.

103. Gabeler EE, van Hilligersberg R, Statius van Eps RG, Sluiter W, Mulder P, van Urk H. Endovascular photodynamic therapy with animoleavulinic acid prevents balloon induced hyperplasia and constrictive remodeling. Eur J Endovasc Surg 2002;24:322–331.

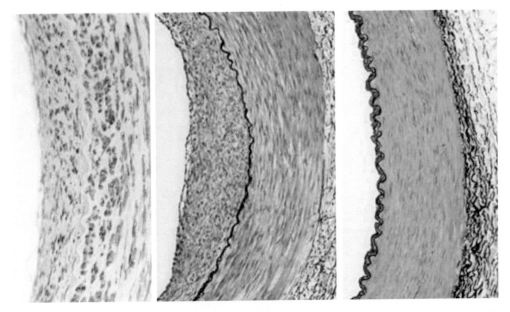

**Color Plate 1.** Response to injury, normal artery wall. (Fig. 1B, Chapter 2; *see* complete caption on p. 11.)

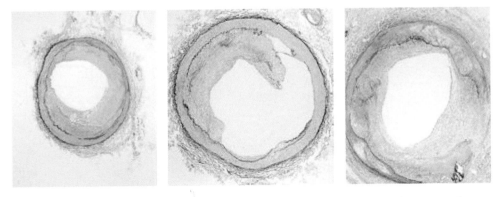

**Color Plate 2.** Response to injury, atherosclerotic artery wall. (Fig. 2, Chapter 2; *see* complete caption on p. 12.)

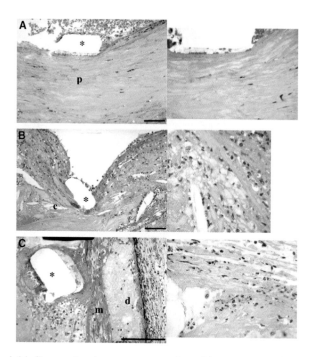

**Color Plate 3.** Arterial inflammation in coronary arteries with stents placed less than or equal to 3 d antemortem. (Fig. 1, Chapter 4; *see* complete caption on p. 49.)

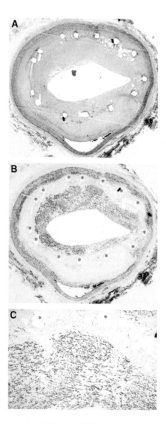

**Color Plate 4.** In-stent restenosis. (Fig. 4, Chapter 4; *see* complete caption on p. 52.)

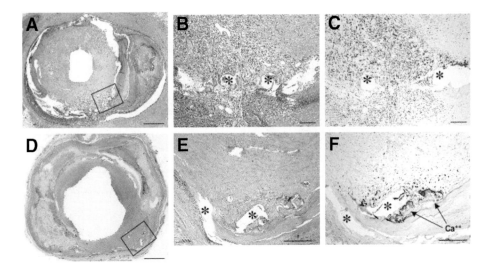

**Color Plate 5.** Neointimal macrophages and neointimal growth. (Fig. 5, Chapter 4; *see* complete caption on p. 54.)

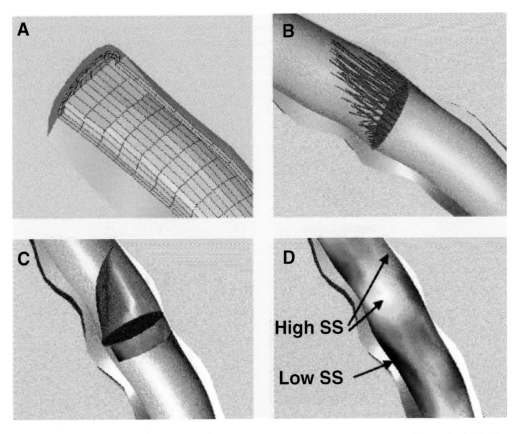

**Color Plate 6. (A)** After lumen meshing, computational flow dynamics allows **(B)** detailed velocity determination at any cross-section. From this **(C)** the local velocity profile and wall WSS (colored band) are derived. Ultimately, **(D)** WSS is calculated at any location of the lumen wall as shown in color-code. (Fig. 3, Chapter 5; *see* complete caption on p. 63.)

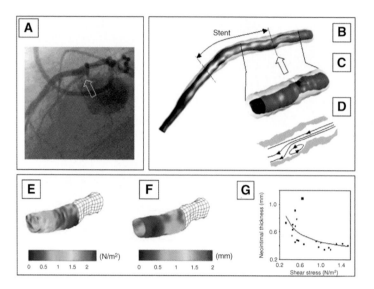

**Color Plate 7. (A)** Lateral angiographic view of the left anterior descending coronary artery after stent placement. Open arrow indicates location of step-up. **(B)** 3D (ANGUS) reconstruction of the coronary artery shown in A, clearly showing the step-up phenomenon at the proximal edge of the stent (open arrow). **(C)** Segment in which detailed analysis of the temporal WSS variations is performed. **(D)** Cartoon showing the existence of a region with retrograde velocities and flow separation. **(E)** Averaged WSS over the cardiac cycle color-coded at the surface of the stented region of the 3D reconstruction. **(F)** Neointimal thickness color-coded at the lumen surface of the stented region. **(G)** In-stent average neointimal thickness per cross-section vs the WSS averaged over the cardiac cycle and per cross-section showing a nonlinear inverse relationship (NIH = $0.3 + 0.2 \times \text{WSS}^{-1}$[mm]; $r^2 = 0.34$, $p < 0.01$). (Fig. 7, Chapter 5; *see* caption on p. 73.)

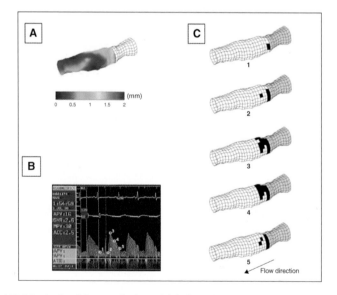

**Color Plate 8. (A)** Neointimal hyperplasia, which is color-coded at the 3-dimensionally reconstructed lumen at baseline. The perspective view of Figure 8A and 8C differs from Fig. 7. **(B)** Doppler measurements used for the time-dependent flow calculations. **(C)** At 5 time-points during the cardiac cycle, locations (black) in the stent experience retrograde axial velocities. (Fig. 8, Chapter 5; *see* complete caption on p. 74.)

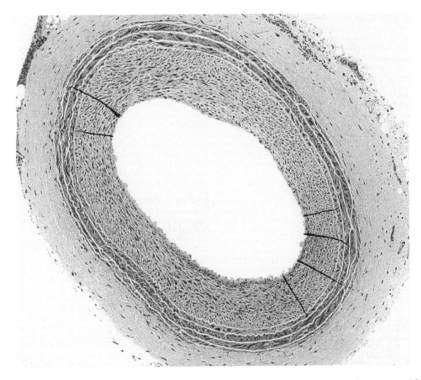

**Color Plate 9.** Rat carotid artery. (Fig. 1, Chapter 7; *see* complete caption on p. 133.)

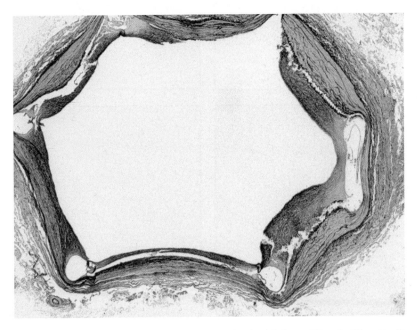

**Color Plate 10.** Dog coronary artery after severe mechanical injury. (Fig. 2, Chapter 7; *see* complete caption on p. 134.)

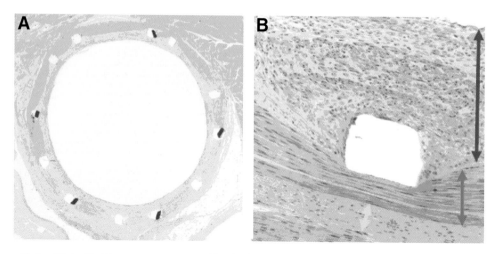

**Color Plate 11.** Pig coronary artery. (Fig. 3, Chapter 7; *see* complete caption on p. 135.)

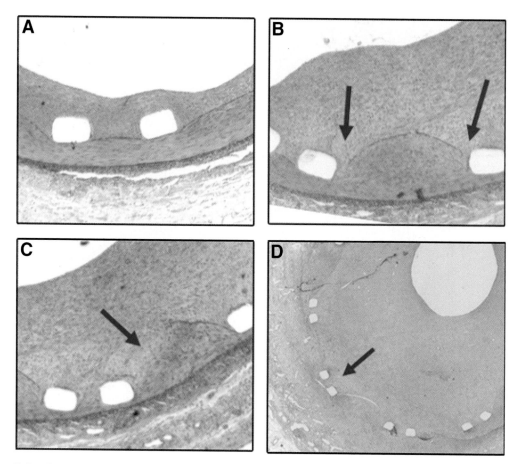

**Color Plate 12.** Injury score in the porcine coronary artery. (Fig. 4, Chapter 7; *see* complete caption on p. 137.)

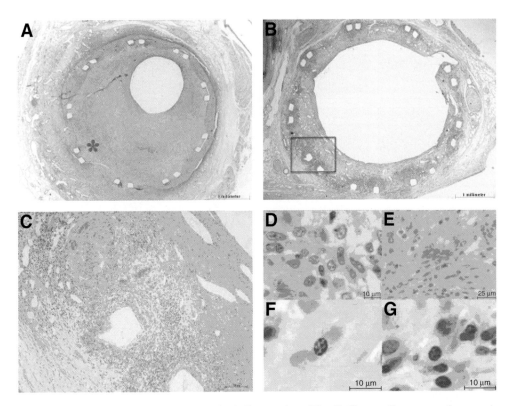

**Color Plate 13.** Example of chronic vascular inflammation. (Fig. 5, Chapter 7; *see* complete caption on p. 139.)

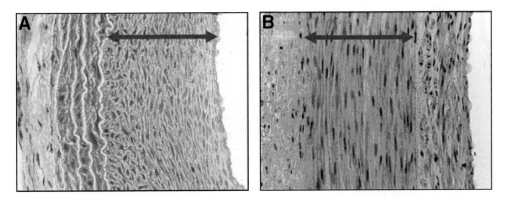

**Color Plate 14.** Differences between elastic arteries and muscular arteries. (Fig. 6, Chapter 7; *see* complete caption on p. 140.)

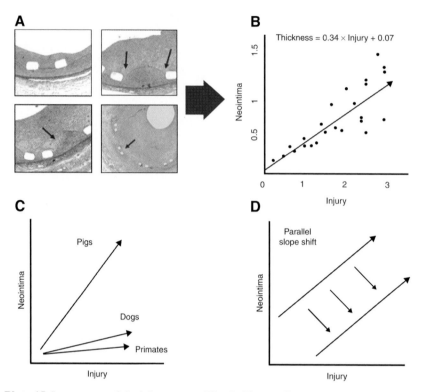

**Color Plate 15.** Importance of the injury score. (Fig. 7, Chapter 7; *see* complete caption on p. 143.)

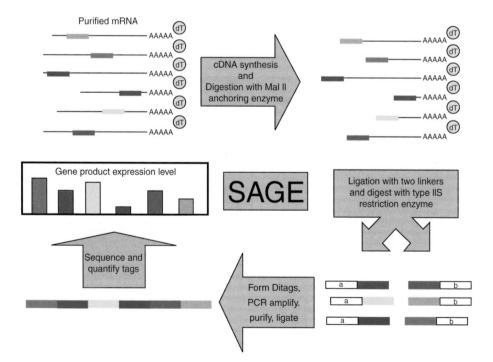

**Color Plate 16.** A schematic representation of the SAGE protocol. (Fig. 5, Chapter 8; *see* caption on p. 161.)

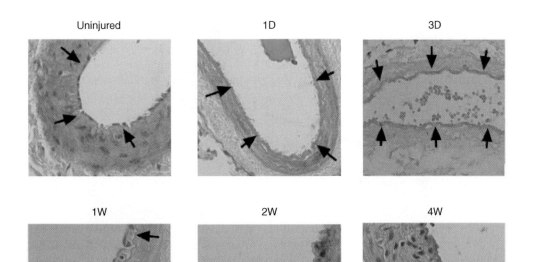

**Color Plate 17.** Neointima formation in the absence of medial cells. (Fig. 1, Chapter 11; *see* complete caption on p. 186.)

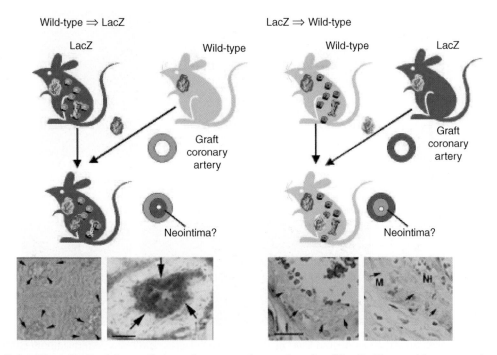

**Color Plate 18.** Recipient cells contribute to graft-vasculopathy. (Fig. 2, Chapter 11; *see* complete caption on p. 188.)

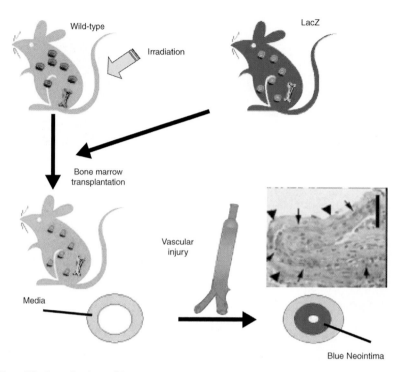

**Color Plate 19.** Contribution of bone marrow cells to healing and lesion formation after mechanical injury. (Fig. 3, Chapter 11; *see* complete caption on p. 189.)

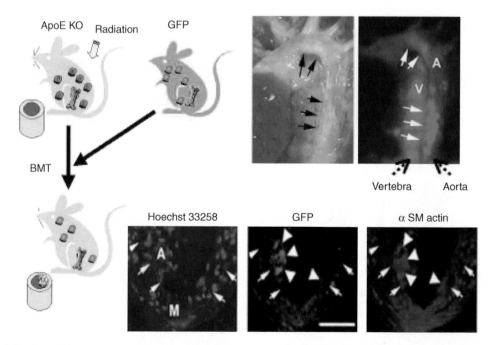

**Color Plate 20.** Bone marrow-derived SMC in atherosclerotic plaques. BMT was performed from GFP-mice to ApoE-deficient mice, and animals were maintained on a Western diet. (Fig. 4, Chapter 11; *see* complete caption on p. 190.)

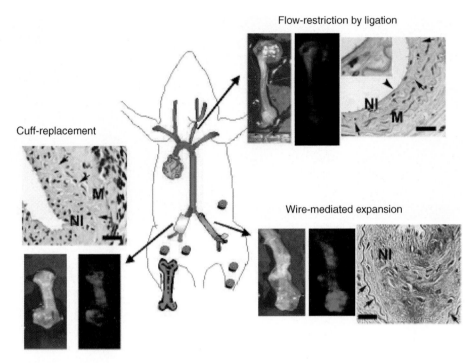

**Color Plate 21.** Marked diversity in the contribution of bone marrow-derived cells to vascular remodeling. (Fig. 5, Chapter 11; *see* complete caption on p. 191.)

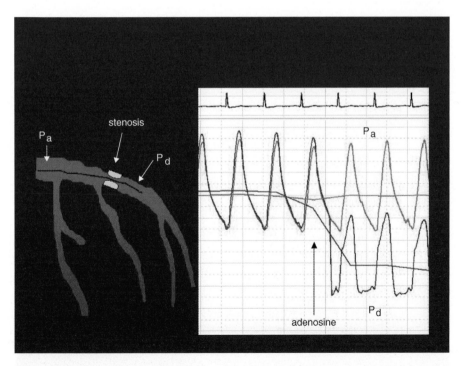

**Color Plate 22.** Fractional flow reserve can be derived easily by means of a 0.014-in. pressure guide wire, which is placed distally to a stenosis of questionable hemodynamic relevance. (Fig. 1, Chapter 15; *see* complete caption on p. 249.)

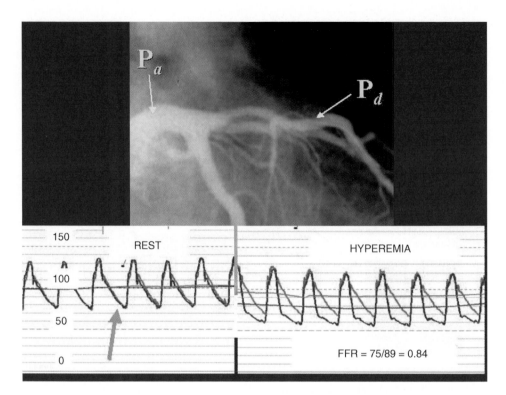

**Color Plate 23.** A 50-yr-old man was scheduled for control angiography. (Fig. 3, Chapter 15; *see* complete caption on p. 253.)

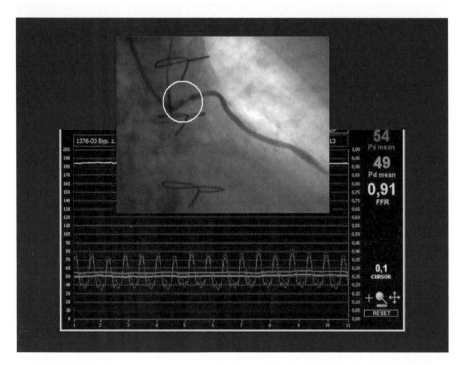

**Color Plate 24.** Angiogram of a venous graft to a small obtuse marginal branch, which was treated with stent implantation (bare metal stent) 8 mo ago. (Fig. 4, Chapter 15; *see* complete caption on p. 254.)

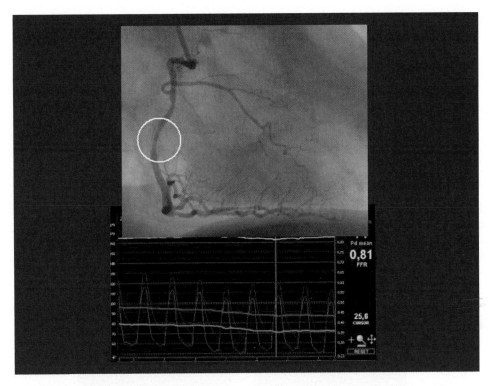

**Color Plate 25.** A 58-yr-old male was scheduled for PCI of the LAD. (Fig. 5, Chapter 15; *see* complete caption on p. 255.)

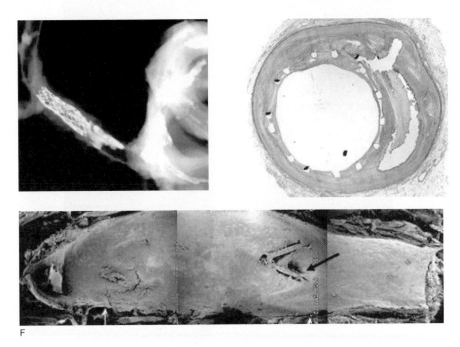

**Color Plate 26.** Widely patent sirolimus-eluting stent in the right coronary artery (left upper panel). Light microscopic section demonstrated a thin healed intimal hyperplasia (right, upper panel). (Fig. 2, Chapter 22; *see* complete caption on p. 358.)

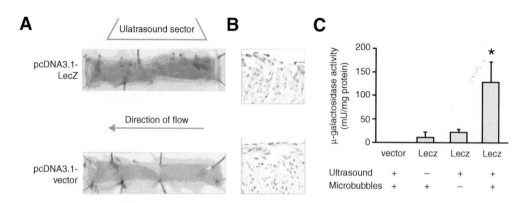

**Color Plate 27.** Ultrasound-induced disruption of DNA3.1-*LacZ*-coated microbubbles improves gene delivery. (Fig. 2, Chapter 24; *see* complete caption on p. 386.)

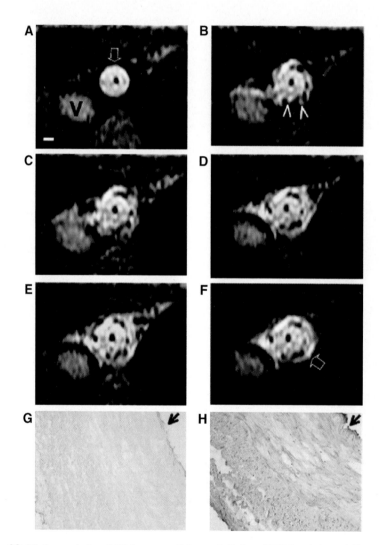

**Color Plate 28.** High-resolution MR images of the gadolinium/GFP lentivirus delivery in the iliac artery of a pig. (Fig. 3, Chapter 24; *see* complete caption on p. 388.)

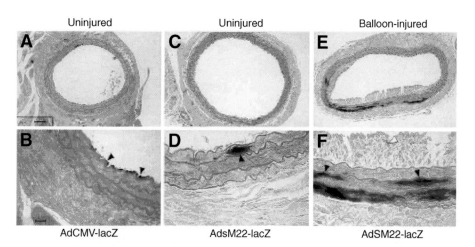

Uninjured       Uninjured       Balloon-injured

AdCMV-lacZ       AdsM22-lacZ       AdSM22-lacZ

**Color Plate 29.** *lacZ*-transgene expression in uninjured and balloon-injured rat carotid arteries infected with *AdSM22-lacZ* and *AdCMV-lacZ*. (Fig. 4, Chapter 24; *see* complete caption on p. 390.)

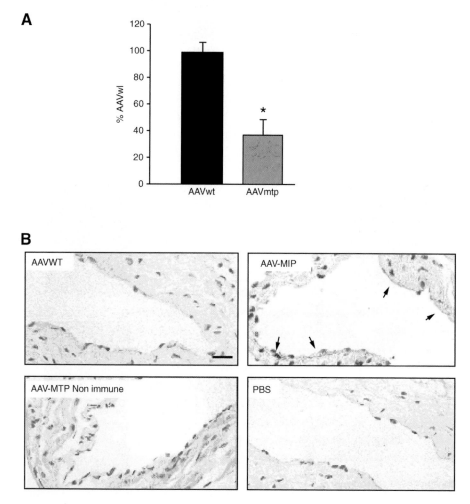

**Color Plate 30.** AAV expressing targeting peptide (MTP) decreases liver uptake and increases systemic vascular targeting in vivo. (Fig. 6, Chapter 24; *see* complete caption on p. 393.)

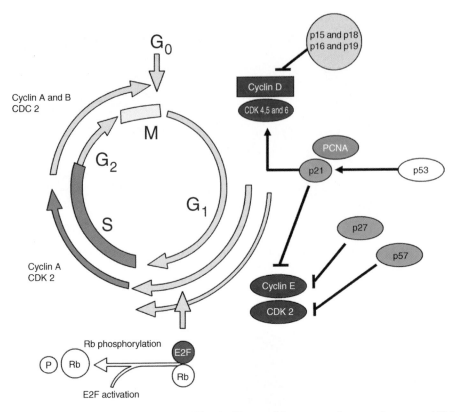

**Color Plate 31.** Cell cycle pathways. (Fig. 1, Chapter 26; *see* complete caption on p. 410.)

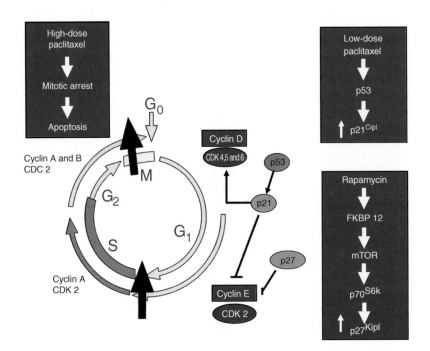

**Color Plate 32.** Structure of sirolimus (left) and paclitaxel, along with their effects on the biology of the vasculature. (Fig. 3, Chapter 26; *see* caption on p. 415.)

# 14    The Role of eNOS in Vascular Diseases

*Alexey Kuroedov, MD,*
*Francesco Cosentino, MD, PhD,*
*Felix C. Tanner, MD, and Thomas F. Lüscher, MD*

## CONTENTS

THREE ISOFORMS OF NOS
SYNTHESIS OF NO
REGULATION OF NO PRODUCTION
MEASUREMENT OF NO PRODUCTION
MECHANISMS OF DECREASED NO BIOAVAILABILITY
ROLE OF NO IN PATHOGENESIS OF VASCULAR DISEASES
KEY NOTES
REFERENCES

## THREE ISOFORMS OF NOS

The demonstration in 1980 of the phenomenon of endothelium-dependent relaxations and of the release of endothelium-derived relaxing factor (EDRF) led to a search for the chemical identity of this factor. In the next few years, EDRF was shown to be an extremely labile molecule and some of its properties were described. Eventually, it was shown that vascular endothelial cells release nitric oxide (NO) and that this compound accounted for the vasodilatory and platelet inhibitory effects of EDRF *(1)*. The only source of NO in the body is enzyme NO synthase (NOS). Up to now three isoforms of NOS have been described. Two isoforms are constitutively expressed, although their expression may be modulated: nNOS (or NOSI) is expressed in neurons, and eNOS (or NOSIII) is expressed in endothelial cells, cardiac myocytes, and blood platelets. The expression of third isoform (NOSII) is not constitutive but is induced by various cytokines and bacterial products; that is why NOSII also is defined as inducible NOS (iNOS) *(2)*. Accordingly, being overexpressed on stimulation with cytokines or lipopolysaccharide iNOS generates 100–1000-fold more NO than its constitutive counterparts whose roles are involved in physiological regulation *(3)*. The function of NO in the cardiovascular system has been investigated very intensively during the past two

From: *Contemporary Cardiology: Essentials of Restenosis: For the Interventional Cardiologist*
Edited by: H. J. Duckers, E. G. Nabel, and P. W. Serruys © Humana Press Inc., Totowa, NJ

decades. The bewildering array of publications about the NO gives us no chance to discuss the role of all three NOS isoforms in pathogenesis of vascular diseases within one chapter. Taking into consideration the fact that eNOS is apparently the most crucial one the chapter has been limited to the discussion of only this isoform.

## SYNTHESIS OF NO

The human NOSIII mRNA is encoded by 26 exons spanning 21–22 kb of genomic DNA. The gene is present as a single copy in the haploid human genome. The human NOSIII gene has been assigned to the 7q35-7q36 region of chromosome 7 *(4)*.

NO is synthesized from L-arginine through a five electron oxidation step through the formation of the intermediate $N^G$-hydroxy-L-arginine *(5)*. The substrates for NOS-mediated NO production are the amino acid L-arginine, molecular oxygen, and NADPH. Cofactors that are required for NO generation are tetrahydrobiopterin ($BH_4$), flavin adenine dinucleotide, and flavin mononucleotide. Furthermore, the enzyme contains binding sites for heme and calmodulin. After the binding of calcium-loaded calmodulin to eNOS between COOH-terminal reductase and $NH_2$-terminal oxygenase domain of eNOS, electrons are donated by NADPH in the reductase domain, which are subsequently shuttled through the calmodulin-binding domain toward the heme-containing eNOS oxygenase domain, which in turn may result in the formation of the enzyme products citrulline and NO *(2,6)*. eNOS also contains a motif involved in the binding of zinc. Each eNOS dimmer contains one zinc ion, which plays a role in stabilization of the dimeric molecule *(7)*. eNOS contains a myristoyl group that is covalently attached to the glycine residue at its $NH_2$ terminus. Myristoylation targets eNOS in the Golgi complex, where it is palmitoylated *(8)*. eNOS palmitoylated on two cysteine residues near the $NH_2$ terminus (cystein-15 and -26). This modification is reversible, requiring eNOS myristoylation, which stabilizes the association of eNOS with the membrane, and is required for a proper localization of eNOS *(9)*.

## REGULATION OF NO PRODUCTION

Simulation of endothelium with hormones that induce a rise in intracellular calcium levels, such as bradykinin, estradiol, serotonin, vascular endothelial growth factor (VEGF), and histamine leads to increased NO production by eNOS. $Ca^{2+}$ release from intracellular stores and $[Ca^{2+}]_i$ from extracellular space promote the binding of calmodulin to eNOS *(2)*.

Calmodulin binding to the calmodulin-binding motif is thought to displace an adjacent autoinhibitory loop on eNOS, thus facilitating the electron transfer from NADPH to the reductase domain flavins or from the flavins to the oxygenase domain heme iron, resulting in increased NO production. Thr-495 is constitutively phosphorylated in all of the endothelial cells investigated today and is a negative regulatory site. That is, phosphorylation is associated with a decrease in enzyme activity. The link between phosphorylation and NO production can be explained by interference with the binding of calmodulin to the calmodulin-binding domain. In endothelial cells stimulated with a $Ca^{2+}$-elevating agonist, substantially more calmodulin binds to eNOS when Thr-495 is dephosphorylated. The constitutively active kinase that phosphorylate eNOS Thr-495 is most probably protein kinase C; a finding that could account for the fact that protein kinase C inhibitors and the downregulation of PKC markedly increase endothelial NO production *(10–12)*.

Physiological regulation of eNOS activity may be better understood in regard to its specific intracellular localization. The functional pool of endothelial eNOS is assigned to caveolae. Caveolae are small (70–90 nm in diameter), invaginated foldings of the plasmalemmal membrane that are distinctively enriched in cholesterol and glycosphingolipids, and structurally maintained by oligomerized caveolins that also serve as scaffolds for the assembly of multiprotein signaling complexes within these specialized membrane compartments *(13)*. Caveolae are involved in signal transduction by ensuring the compartmenting of signaling molecules, such as G protein and tyrosine kinase-associated receptors, as well as eNOS. Interaction of eNOS with caveolin-1 occurs through the caveolin-1 scaffolding domain (N-terminal residues 81–101) and results in the inhibition of the enzyme. The equilibrium between eNOS bound to caveolin and caveolin-free eNOS determines the basal component of eNOS-dependent NO release in endothelial cells. This interaction may be required to protect the cell from undesired, potentially cytotoxic, or nonphysiological burst of NO in response to small fluctuations in intracellular calcium. In the presence of increased $Ca^{2+}$, calmodulin binds not only to eNOS but also to caveolin that in turn promotes the dissociation of eNOS from caveolin *(14)*. eNOS activation by hemodynamic shear stress as well as by isometric vessel contraction is independent of calcium *(15)*. Shear stress-induced eNOS activation is regulated by a potassium channel, which might act as a mechanochemical transducer within the plasma membrane of the endothelial cell *(16)*.

Phosphorylation of Ser-1177 in molecule eNOS by Akt has been proposed to be crucial in calcium-independent upregulation of eNOS activity. Accumulating data about time-relationships between Ser-1177 phosphorylation and agonist induced NO synthesis led to conclusions about involvement of Ser-1177 in autoinhibition of eNOS activity. In basal conditions, eNOS is kept inactive also by interaction with Hsp 90. This ubiquitous 90 kDA, heat-shock protein is expressed at high levels (accounting for up to 1–2% of total cellular protein content) in the cytosol (even in unstressed conditions) *(17)*. It functions as a chaperone for the proper folding of specific protein substrates, including many signal transduction molecules (e.g., nonreceptor tyrosine kinases, transcription factors, and eNOS, among others) *(18)*. Hsp 90 is associated with eNOS in resting endothelial cells and, on stimulation with VEGF, oestrogen, histamine, shear stress, and statins, the association between the two proteins is increased, resulting in enhanced NO production *(19)*. Thus, Hsp 90-dependent repression of eNOS activity is attributable to the $Ca^{2+}$-dependent and $Ca^{2+}$-independent pathways. It is important to note that, the protein kinase Akt, the kinase involved in activating the phosphorylation of eNOSon serine 1177, is another client protein for hsp90 and binds to a sequence of hsp90 that does not overlap with those involved in the binding of eNOS. Therefore, hsp90 was recently proposed as an adaptor between Akt and its substrate, eNOS *(17)*.

Fluid flow across the endothelium, also referred to as shear stress, upregulates eNOS expression *(20)*. eNOS promoter also contains other putative *cis*-elements, including Sp1 and GATA motifs, a sterol regulatory element, estrogen–responsive elements, a nuclear factor-1 element, a cAMP-responsive element, and activator proteins-1 and -2 binding sites *(21,22)*. eNOS expression is also up regulated by cyclic strain, estrogen, VEGF, insulin, basic fibroblast growth factor, epidermal growth factor, and transforming growth factor (TGF)-β *(2)*. NO has been shown to be involved in a negative-feedback regulatory mechanism and decreases eNOS expression through a cGMP-mediated process *(23)*.

# MEASUREMENT OF NO PRODUCTION

Basically two main approaches to study the role of eNOS in cardiovascular diseases have been used by different groups. First, the pharmacological inhibition of NO or genetic manipulation (eNOS knockout and eNOS transgenic mice) made possible the conclusion of involvement of eNOS with high specificity. Second, direct measurement of NO production in all kinds of laboratory models of vascular diseases as well as in patients gave integral information about activity of eNOS *(24)*. Technical problem the researchers always faced is the short lifetime of NO.

An indirect measurement of eNOS activity by assessment of endothelium-dependent vasodilation rather gives integral information about endothelial function than specifically about L-arginine/NOS-pathway. The contribution of NO to endothelium-dependent relaxation, for example, is best estimated by determining the inhibitory effects of inhibitors of eNOS, scavengers of NO in the extracellular space (oxyhemoglobine), and inhibitors of soluble guanylate cyclase. However, the contribution of NO may be underestimated using these inhibitors. Indeed, the conventional concentrations of NOS inhibitors may not totally prevent the formation of NO. Similarly, inhibitors of soluble guanylate cyclase obviously only prevent the effects of NO owing to activation of that enzyme, and thus mediated by cGMP, although NO may affect other cellular events. Finally, the inhibitors used may have pharmacological actions not related to the L-arginine-NO pathway *(25)*.

Because NO is a free radical, the spin trapping of NO or NO-related intermediates appear to be simple and straightforward. Pronai et al. *(26)* in their initial study used two different spin-traps: 3,5-dibromo-4-nitrosobenzenesulfonate (DBNBS) and 2-methyl-2-nitrosopropane (MNP). Activation of platelets with a low concentration of collagen and in the presence of DBNBS or MNP has yielded several EPR-detectable spin adducts. DBNBS and MNP spin adducts have been generated during platelet activation in the presence of $Ca^{2+}$ and of a cytosol-depleted L-arginine preparation from washed platelets to which L-arginine was subsequently added. The formation of these DBNBS and MNP spin adducts has been abolished by the eNOS inhibitor $N^{\omega}$-methyl-L-arginine, suggesting that these originated from a product of NOS. Diethyl-dithiocarbamate chelating ferrous ion is also successfully used during EPR detection of NO as a precursor of spin traps for the quantification of released NO both in vitro and in vivo. This method is based on the high-affinity of water insoluble iron–dithiocarbamate complexes toward NO. The nitrosyl iron–dithiocarbamate complex is formed with characteristic triplet EPR spectrum *(27)*. Malinski et al. *(28)* developed a porphyrinic based microsensor for NO detection in a single cell. This sensor combines the electrocatalytic properties of conductive polymeric porphyrins and the selectivity of Naflon film, which excludes nitrite, a major interferential. This sensor is sensitive enough to monitor changes in NO concentrations in a biological system with a response time of less than 10 ms.

# MECHANISMS OF DECREASED NO BIOAVAILABILITY

All known risk factors (hyperglycemia, hyperlipidemia, and hyperhomocysteinemia) as well as all know ischemic events (stable angina, acute coronary syndromes, and peripheral occlusive diseases) are associated with increased oxidative stress. Accumulated data demonstrates a clear link between the rise in reactive oxygen species (ROS) production and decreased NO availability in vascular tissue. Several molecular mechanisms can be involved.

In 1990, Beckman and associates first found that the reaction of NO with superoxide could take place under physiological conditions and lead to the formation of peroxynitrite ($ONOO^-$). This not only results in the fall of NO availability but also has much worse consequences. $ONOO^-$ oxidizes sulfhydryls, can nitrate, and hydroxilate aromatic rings, and also oxidize lipids, proteins, and DNA. The reactions of $ONOO^-$ are greatly facilitated by the presence of metal-iron centers or heme-thiolate clusters *(29,30)*.

Interestingly, there is now evidence that small amounts of $ONOO^-$ may be generated during aggregation of normal platelets. Thus, it is likely that under physiological conditions $ONOO^-$, when generated by platelets, is rapidly detoxified and converted to NO donors following reactions with platelet membrane thiols. The oxidizing stress could decrease the efficiency of this regulating mechanism *(29,31)*. Under certain conditions, NOS may generate superoxide instead of NO, a process called NOS uncoupling (i.e., uncoupling of NADPH oxidation and NO synthesis) *(32)*. The ability of NOS to produce superoxide was first demonstrated in neuronal NOS and then extended to eNOS. The switch from the normal state to the uncoupled state is mainly determined through the amounts of available L-arginine and $BH_4$. When there is an abundance of both factors, eNOS produces NO. When the concentration of one of these factors (L-arginine and $BH_4$) is relatively low, eNOS generates superoxide *(2)*.

In turn, increased production of ROS results in a decrease of the intracellular $BH_4$ pool. With elevated oxidative stress, the oxidation of $BH_4$ is enhanced and vascular tissue levels of 7,8-dihydrobiopterin is increased. Only the completely reduced (tetrahydro) form of biopterin supports NOS coupling of NADPH oxidation to NO synthesis. It has been proposed that in addition to the absolute availability of $BH_4$, the ratio of $BH_4$/7,8-dihydrobiopterin to the ratio of reduced and oxidized biopterin, is important for determining the rates of NO production vs uncoupled superoxide formation from eNOS. Partially oxidized analogs of $BH_4$ potentially compete with $BH_4$ for eNOS binding and enhanced rates of superoxide formation from eNOS, even in the presence of saturating L-arginine concentration *(33)*.

Therefore, oxidative stress causes "uncoupling" of eNOS not only by decreasing $BH_4$ levels but also by increasing the ratio of $BH_4$/7,8-dihydrobiopterin. Increased $BH_2$ levels potentially compete with $BH_4$ for eNOS binding and worsen eNOS uncoupling. Recently, a mouse model of $BH_4$ deficiency has been developed by use of the sperm mutagen N-ethyl-N'-nitrosourea *(34)*. The hyperphenylalaninemic mouse mutant (hph-1) displays 90% deficiency in GTP cyclohydrolase I activity, the enzyme catalyzing the first committed step in $BH_4$ synthesis. This enzyme deficiency results in reduced tissue $BH_4$ concentrations compared with concentrations in the wild-type mice of the same strain.

Another mechanism that may implicate to eNOS inhibition in conditions of oxidative stress is accumulation of its endogenous inhibitors *(35)*. The endogenous inhibitors of eNOS are asymmetric dimethylarginine (ADMA) and N-monomethylarginine (NMA). As it is the predominant species (plasma levels of ADMA are 10-fold greater than those of NMA), further discussion will focus on ADMA. This molecule is an arginine analog that competes with L-arginine for NOS *(36)*. Dimethylarginine dimethylaminohydrolase (DDAH) metabolizes the methylarginines ADMA and NMA to citrulline and methylamines *(37)*. Inhibition of ADMA degradation leads to its accumulation and adverse effects on the vasculature. DDAH is exquisitely sensitive to oxidative stress. The vulnerability of DDAH to oxidative attack is likely conferred by the sulfhydryl groups that are critical for its activity. The sulfhydryl group of Cys-249 can also be nitrosylated in a reversible reaction with NO that also inhibits DDAH activity.

The nitrosylation of DDAH and subsequent inhibition of ADMA metabolism may represent a physiological form of negative feedback on NOS activity. Transgenic mice overexpressing human DDAH have reduced plasma ADMA levels. This genetically induced reduction in plasma ADMA levels is associated with increased NOS activity in the skeletal muscle and heart, as well as in the doubling of urinary nitrogen oxides. Not surprisingly, the increase in NOS activity is associated with a 10% decline in systemic resistance and systolic arterial pressure *(34,38)*.

## ROLE OF NO IN PATHOGENESIS OF VASCULAR DISEASES

### *Arterial Hypertension*

The vasculature is in a constant state of active dilation mediated by NO. Endothelial cells continuously release small amounts of NO, producing a basal level of vascular smooth muscle relaxation through stimulation of guanilate cyclase in smooth muscle cells. Guanylate cyclase belongs to the family of heterodimeric heme proteins and catalyzes the formation of cGMP, which is utilized as an intracellular amplifier and secondary messenger in a large range of physiological responses *(39,40)*. NO binds to the heme moiety of guanylate cyclase, disrupting the planar form of the heme iron. The resulting conformational change activates the enzyme *(41)*. Its product cGMP modulates the function of protein kinases, phosphodiesterases, ion channels, and other physiologically important targets. Vascular smooth muscle relaxation is mediated by a cGMP-dependent protein kinase that phosphorylates and activates a calcium-sensitive potassium channel *(39)*. In addition, cGMP acts as an endogenous inhibitor of the phosphodiesterase, which are responsible for breakdown of cAMP.

Both in vitro and in vivo studies have demonstrated that basal and stimulated production of NO in endothelial cells plays a key role in the regulation of vascular tone *(42–44)*. L-Arginine analogs, such as $N^G$-monomethyl-L-arginine (L-NMMA), $N^G$-nitro-L-arginine-methyl ester (L-NAME), and $N^G$-nitro-L-arginine, cause endothelium-dependent contractions in a number of isolated vessels. The inhibitory effect of these compounds is prevented by L-arginine *(1)*. Intravenous injections of L-NMMA into anaesthetized rabbits resulted in an immediate and substantial rise in blood pressure, which could be reversed by L-arginine. The blood pressure-elevating and vasoconstrictive effects of L-NMMA have now been demonstrated in a number of species, including man. These inhibitors have no intrinsic constrictor activity on vascular smooth muscle; their activity is entirely endothelium-dependent and results from the inhibition of endogenous vasodilatation. A highly reproducible model of chronic hypertension in animals owing to treatment with L-NMMA, is the clear evidence that resistant vessels in basal condition in healthy organism are under permanent control by NO. A High level of arterial pressure has been demonstrated in eNOS deficient mice. Vice versa, animals overexpressing human eNOS are hypotensive *(1)*.

Furthermore, a renal mechanism for regulation of blood pressure involves eNOS. NO modulates the constrictor actions on the afferent arteriole *(2,45,46)*. NO is also a crucial modulator of renal medullary blood flow, allowing pressure natriuresis *(2,47)*. NO production and inactivation might be heterogeneously affected in different forms of hypertension. Indeed, in Dahl salt-sensitive rats, endothelium-dependent relaxations are impaired, but no release of vasoconstrictor prostanoids can be demonstrated *(48)*.

It was reported that $H_2O_2$ formed through eNOS becomes a mediator of endothelium-dependent relaxations in intact coronary arteries depleted of $BH_4$ *(49)*.

Whereas $O_2^-$ is a potent mediator of endothelium-dependent contraction, $H_2O_2$ is a potent vasodilator. In this work, confirmation that eNOS rather than other sources produced most of the $O_2^-$ in prehypertensive SHR came from experiments showing $O_2^-$ release after treatment with a NO agonist, as well as its inhibition with known cNOS inhibitors. The rapid accumulation of $O_2^-$ concentration in the presence of A23187 suggests that production of $O_2^-$ is calcium-dependent like the production of NO by eNOS. Furthermore, as with NO production, $O_2^-$ production can be inhibited by L-arginine analogs, such as L-NMMA and L-NAME. It was observed that the sum of the $O_2^-$ produced by all noncNOS sources, without A23187 (basal release), accounts for only 25–30% of the total $O_2^-$ produced after stimulation by A23187. Therefore, it can be assumed that the remaining 70–75% is associated with calcium-dependent eNOS *(50)*.

## *Atherosclerosis*

Atherosclerosis accounts for a half of morbidity and mortality in Western countries. An impairment of endothelium-dependent relaxations is present in atherosclerotic vessels even before vascular structural changes occur and represent the reduced eNOS-derived NO bioavailability. Blair et al. *(51,52)* reported that endothelial cell exposure to oxidized low-density lipoprotein (LDL), which results in caveolar cholesterol depletion, rapidly caused the translocation of both eNOS and caveolin from caveolae, thereby leading to a marked decline in acetylcholine-induced eNOS activation.

eNOS expression is upregulated by low concentrations of oxidized LDL or its major atherogenic phospholipids—lysophosphatidylcholine *(53)*. An increased eNOS expression by lysophosphatidylcholine and moderate amounts of oxidized LDL may implicate an endothelial antiatherosclerotic defense mechanism at the early stages of lesion formation. Sp1 has been shown to be involved in lysophosphatidylcholine—induced eNOS upregulation. High concentrations of oxidized LDL lower eNOS expression *(2,54)*. Measurements of NO release with a porphyrinic microsensor in atherosclerotic human carotid arteries and normal mammary arteries obtained during surgery, have revealed reduced NO production in atherosclerotic segments that were accompanied by marked reduction of immuno-reactive eNOS in luminal endothelial cells *(55)*.

Chronic treatment with L-arginine, a substrate for NOS, inhibits atherosclerotic lesion formation in animal models of atherosclerosis, such as diet-induced atherosclerosis models of rabbits, and LDL-receptor knockout mice *(56)*. On the contrary, NOS inhibitors like L-NAME significantly accelerate atherosclerotic lesion development, suggesting that inhibition of endogenous NO synthesis facilitates the progression of atherosclerosis *(33,57)*. The interaction between lipids and eNOS seems to be the most crucial step in the pathogenesis of the vascular lesion formation. Experiments on mice with normal lipid level did not demonstrate clear involvement of the L-arginine/eNOS-pathway in remodeling of big vessels that are the usual target of atherosclerosis *(58)*. In wild-type mice, long-term treatment with L-NAME caused significant medial thickening and perivascular fibrosis in coronary microvessels but not in large coronary arteries. Importantly, in eNOS-deficient mice, treatment with L-NAME also caused an extent of medial thickening and perivascular fibrosis in coronary microvessels that was comparable with that in wild-type mice.

Knowles et al *(59)* first demonstrated that a genetic lack of eNOS resulted in enhanced atherosclerosis. Kuhlencordt et al. *(60)* also reported that eNOS deficiency promoted atherosclerosis in Apo E/eNOS double-knockout mice. In contrast, Shi et al.

*(61)* reported the paradoxical reduction of atherosclerotic lesion size in high-cholesterol diet-induced atherosclerosis in eNOS-double-knockout (eNOS-ko) mice compared with wild-type mice. They fed mice a "high-cholesterol diet" (15% fat, 1.25% cholesterol, and 0.5% sodium cholate for 12 wk) and then examined the lesion size in the aortic sinus. They found that eNOS-ko mice had much smaller aortic sinus lesions than did wild-type mice. L-NAME reduced LDL oxidation by endothelial cells from wild-type mice but not from eNOS-ko mice. Based on these findings they speculated that eNOS may contribute to the oxidation of LDL under the circumstance of hypercholesterolemia, and that the absence of eNOS-mediated LDL oxidation may lead to the reduction of atherosclerotic lesion formation in eNOS-ko mice *(33)*.

Ozaki M et al. *(62,63)* have crossed eNOS-transgenic mice (eNOS-Tg) with apo E-ko mice and fed them a "high-cholesterol diet." Paradoxically, after 8 wk on a high-cholesterol diet, the atherosclerotic lesion areas in the aortic sinus were increased by more than twofold in apoE-ko/eNOS-Tg mice compared with apoE-ko mice. Also, aortic tree lesion areas were approx 50% larger in apoE-ko/eNOS-Tg mice after 12 wk on a high-cholesterol diet. In apoE-ko they found the presence of eNOS dysfunction, demonstrated by lower NO production relative to eNOS protein levels and enhanced super oxide production in the endothelium. They found decreased vascular BH4 levels and increased 7,8-dihydrobiopterin levels in apoE-ko/eNOS-Tg *(33,64)*.

In contrast, van Haperen et al. *(65)* also crossbred apoE-ko mice with another line of eNOS transgenic mice that they created, and reported that atherosclerotic lesion size was reduced by eNOS overexpression. Regarding the mechanisms, they cited reductions in blood pressure and plasma cholesterol levels. In their study, eNOS overexpression was associated with 20- to 25-mmHg reduction in mean blood pressure and a 15% decrease in plasma cholesterol levels.

Kawashima and Yokoyama *(33)*, who scrupulously analyzed the protocols of all the aforementioned studies have explained the discrepancy in results of different groups by an apparent difference in the balance between NO and superoxide production from the endothelium, owing to the differences in the chows applied. The increase of plasma cholesterol levels achieved by the "Western-type" diet used in van Harpen was much more modest compared with that achieved by feeding a "high-cholesterol" diet in all studies performed by research group of Yokoyama.

The endothelial cytoskeletal network usually maintains the shape of the endothelial cell, which is essential for the relative impermeability of the endothelial lining of the vessel wall. Increased endothelial permeability is a characteristic sign of atherosclerotic vessels. Interestingly, NO is important for stability of the endothelial cytoskeleton and therefore has a role in the relative impermeability of the endothelium *(66)*. In contrast, under certain conditions (e.g., hypoxia) and dependent on the vascular bed, endothelial permeability is enhanced as a result of VEGF-induced increases in NO levels *(2,67)*. Thus, hyperlipidemia through decrease of NO availability can directly affect endothelial permeability, which can result in accumulation of plasma proteins in subendothelial space.

On the other hand, NO decreases NF-kB activity through stabilization of its inhibitory subunit, IkBα. Prevention of NF-kB activation results in an abolishment of cytokine-induced adhesion molecules expression. Thus, surface expression of vascular cell adhesion molecule-1, intercellular adhesion molecule-1, and P-selectin are important triggers of atherosclerotic lesions, and in condition of decreased NO availability will be dramatically increased *(68)*.

## *Diabetes Mellitus*

The relation between diabetes and premature cardiovascular disease is well established *(69)*. Atherosclerosis and microangiopathy are the principal causes of morbidity and mortality in patients with diabetes mellitus *(70)*. Atherosclerosis occurs earlier in diabetics than in nondiabetics and is more severe and diffuse. Several studies have shown impairment of endothelium-dependent relaxations to various receptor-mediated vasodilators in different vascular beds from diabetic animals *(71–73)*. It has been suggested that, in diabetes, oxidative stress plays a key role in the pathogenesis of vascular complications. Accelerated flux of glucose through glycolysis and feeding of pyruvate to the tricarbonic acid cycle overloads mitochondria, causing excessive generation of free radicals *(74)*. Nishikawa et al. *(75)* have determined that the source of free radicals in endothelial cells incubated in high glucose transports glycolysis-derived pyruvate in mitochondria at the level of complex II (succinate:ubiquinone oxidoreductase), one of the four inner membrane-associated complexes central to oxidative phosphorylation.

Another mechanism whereby high glucose can stimulate oxidative stress is the autoxidation of glucose in the presence of transition metals as well as the generation of ROS during the process of glycation *(76,77)*. Indeed the development from Schiff base to Amadori to advanced glycation end products is accompanied by ROS-generating reactions at various steps *(78)*.

Activation of PKC by glucose has been implicated in the regulation and activation of membrane-associated NAD(P)H-dependent oxidases and subsequent production of superoxide anion. Indeed, the activity of NAD(P)H oxidase and level of its protein are increased in internal mammary arteries and saphenous veins of patients with diabetes *(79)*. The authors found a marked increase in the NAD(P)H oxidase subunit p22phox expression in human aortic endothelial cells incubated with high glucose.

Paradoxically, it was demonstrated that in human aortic endothelial cells, high glucose increases eNOS expression. However, up regulation of eNOS is associated with increased superoxide anion production, suggesting that NO is inactivated by $O2^-$ *(80)*.

It was demonstrated that high glucose, through PKC induces oxidative stress and up regulation of COX-2. Glucose-induced COX-2 upregulation is associated with a shift in the balance of vasodilatory (6-keto-PGF1$\alpha$) and vasoconstricting (TXB2) eicosanoids produced by the endothelial cells in favour of the latter. Prostaglandin H2 is the common precursor for prostaglandins, thronboxane, and PGI2. PGI2 is synthesized from prostaglandin H2 by a specific enzyme, PGIS. Exposure to high glucose increased PGIS protein expression. However, increased formation of NO/O2-reaction product was associated with tyrosine nitration of PGIS. Tyrosine nitration is a mechanism of selective inactivation of PGIS by peroxynitrite. The authors ruled out that COX-2 is a source of ROS. Indeed, targeting COX-2 by indomethacin, a nonselective inhibitor, did not affect glucose-induced ROS generation *(81)*.

## *Chronic Ischemia*

Pharmacological administration of L-arginine to patients suffering from coronary artery disease and peripheral arterial obstructive disease alleviated the symptoms of arterial insufficiency *(29)*. Mainly through regulation of vascular diameter eNOS can ensure an adequate blood support of the tissues. Nevertheless, the antiaggregant effect of NO on platelets should not be underestimated. Blood platelets play a pivotal role in the quality of tissue perfusion. A failure to maintain blood in its fluid state leads to thrombosis.

During 1990–1993, Moncada, Palmer, and Radomski provided detailed biochemical and pharmacological characteristics of platelet NOS and measured the release of NO from stimulated platelets using a selective porphyrinic micro sensor *(82,83,84).* NO inhibits the activation cascade of mediators generated by all known pathways of platelet aggregation, including matrix metalloproteinase-2-dependent platelet aggregation, and some pathways of platelet adhesion to subendothelium *(29).*

Bypass graft disease of the vessels used for correction of ischemic myocardium is also tightly related with eNOS function. Both the internal mammary artery and the saphenous vein are used to construct coronary-artery bypass grafts. It was demonstrated that the release of NO differs in venous and arterial grafts. The authors studied endothelium-dependent relaxation in internal mammary arteries, internal mammary veins, and saphenous veins obtained from patients undergoing coronary bypass surgery. Acetylcholine ($10^{-8}$ to $10^{-4}$ $M$), thrombin (1 U per milliliter), and adenosine diphosphate ($10^{-7}$ to $10^{-4}$ $M$) evoked potent endothelium-dependent relaxation in the mammary artery but weak response in the saphenous vein. In the mammary artery, relaxation was greatest in response to acetylcholine ($86 \pm 4\%$ reduction in norepinephrine-induced tension), followed by thrombin ($44 \pm 7\%$) and adenosine diphosphate ($39 \pm 8\%$). In the saphenous and mammary veins, relaxation was less than 25%. Relaxation was unaffected by indomethacin but was inhibited by methylene blue and hemoglobin, which suggests that NO was the mediator. Endothelium-independent relaxation in response to sodium nitroprusside was similar in arteries and veins *(85).*

In mammary arteries, histamine ($10^{-8}$ to $3 \pm 10^{-6}$ $M$) induced relaxations in rings with ($70 \pm 5\%$), but not without endothelium. The response was inhibited by methylene blue or hemoglobin, but not meclofenamate, therefore NO was delineated as the mediator. Because chlorpheniramine but not cimetidine inhibited the response, NO was released by the H1-histaminergic receptor. In contrast, in saphenous veins histamine caused only weak or absent endothelium-dependent relaxation, but contractions were enhanced in rings with endothelium. Serotonin did not induce endothelium-dependent relaxations, but contractions were markedly greater in veins compared with arteries. The endothelium inhibited the maximal contraction to serotonin in arteries but not in veins. Thus, NO protects against contractions induced by histamine and serotonine in the mammary artery but not in the saphenous vein. This may be important for improved graft function and patency of the artery compared with that of the vein *(86).*

### Ischemia-Reperfusion

A common problem in patients undergoing reperfusion after myocardial infarction is myocardial perfusion-function mismatch. A significant number of patients have persistent ventricular dysfunction despite restoration of flow to the optimal level in epicardial vessels. This dysfunction, owing to myocardial stunning or hibernation, was shown to be associated with poor intramural microcirculatory flow. The underlying mechanism appears to be vascular dysfunction at the microcirculatory level *(87).*

Vascular injury after reperfusion begins very early with an endothelial triggering phase followed by a neutrophil amplification phase. Within 2.5–5 min of reperfusion the endothelium becomes dysfunctional and NO formation decreases. Within 20 min, leucocyte adhesiveness increases, leucocytes adhere to endothelium, and neutrophils migrate across the endothelium into reperfused tissue. The activated neutrophils release cytotoxic and chemotactic substances, such as cytokines, proteases, leukotrienes, and ROS *(87,88).*

Mice with eNOS deletion showed increased necrosis after ischemia-reperfusion and increased expression of P-selectin *(89)*. Several studies have shown that eNOS-derived NO is cardioprotective during ischemia-reperfusion and decreased infarction size *(90–92)*. In the dog model, NOS inhibition with L-NNA worsened stunning after ischemia-reperfusion *(87)*. eNOS-ko mice also lost the benefit from preconditioning with repetitive ischemic cycles *(90)*. Study of Sumeray et al. *(91)* in eNOS-ko mice showed an increased infarct size attributable to a permanent decrease in coronary flow, confirming the protective vasodilatory properties of NO. By contrast, with the shortest ischemic time (16 min) at constant coronary flow and pacing showed an improved functional inotropic, lusitropic, and metabolic (phosphocreatine and ATP) recovery, suggesting a detrimental effect of NO in ischemia-reperfusion, at least in isolated hearts under these experimental conditions *(93)*. Also, in isolated rabbit hearts with ischemia-reperfusion L-NAME induces cardio protection *(87)*. In isolated rat hearts perfused with polymorphonuclear neutrophils containing perfusate, L-NAME increases cardiac dysfunction during ischemia-reperfusion and an NO donor improved function. The NOS inhibitor L-NNA worsened hypoperfusion in the dog model with coronary stenosis.

Furthermore, endogenous NO produced by additional NOS isoform induction may exert cardioprotective effects. Accordingly, eNOS-ko mice in the study by Kanno et al. *(94)* showed a compensatory induction of iNOS after 30 min of ischemia, which resulted in improved function attributed to cardioprotective iNOS-derived NO production.

Experimental evidence suggests that after ischemia-reperfusion, early and severe endothelial dysfunction is largely because of the production of ROS arising from endothelial cell xanthine oxidase activity. During ischemia ATP is degraded to hypoxanthine, and xanthine dehydrogenase is converted to xanthine oxidase, and on reperfusion, xanthine oxidase converts hypoxanthine to uric acid and produces ROS.

The phenomenon of "ischemic preconditioning" has been recognized for almost two decades. In experimental animals and humans, a brief period of ischemia has been shown to protect the heart from more prolonged episodes of ischemia, and reduced the degree of impaired ventricular function or subsequent damage. Ischemic preconditioning is classified into two distinct components: the classic early preconditioning and the delayed or late preconditioning, each with its own biological mechanism of adaptation. A substantial body of evidence now supports a critical role for constitutive NOS in the early triggering of the induction of a iNOS *(95)*. This in turn, ensures a sustained production of cardio protective NO. Specifically, enhanced NO production by iNOS, moderately and specifically overexpressed in myocytes is essential to mediate the antistunning and anti-infarct action of late preconditioning elicited by five different stimuli (ischemia, adenosine A1 agonists, opioid δ1 agonists, endotoxine derivates, and exercise), suggesting that the upregulation of this enzyme is a central mechanism whereby the myocardium protects itself from ischemia *(17,96,97)*. The molecular and functional aspects of ischemia-induced late preconditioning that can be reproduced by the administration of NO donors in lieu of ischemia in experimental animals and more recently in patients, indicates that NO is also sufficient to induce late preconditioning *(17)*.

## *Promotion of Angiogenesis*

NO is an endothelial survival factor, inhibiting apoptosis and increases endothelial cell proliferation. Furthermore, NO enhances endothelial migration *(35)*. Human umbilical venous endothelial cells in a three-dimensional gel elaborate NO and form capillary-like structures when stimulated by bFGF or VEGF. The capillary tube formation induced by these growth factors is abolished by the NOS antagonist L-NAME. Similarly, inhibition of NOS ablates the angiogenic effects of substance P or TGF-β in vitro. In the rabbit cornea model of angiogenesis, VEGF-induced angiogenesis is blocked by L-NAME. The angiogenic response to hindlimb ischemia is impaired in eNOS-deficient mice, an effect that cannot be reversed by VEGF *(35)*.

Sonveaux et al. *(98)* used mice deficient for the caveolin-1 gene (Cav−/−) to examine the impact of caveolae suppression in a model of adaptive angiogenesis obtained after femoral artery resection. Evaluation of the ischemic tissue perfusion and histochemical analysis revealed that contrary to Cav+/+ mice, Cav−/− mice failed to recover a functional vasculature and actually lost part of the ligated limbs, thereby recapitulating the effects of the NOS inhibitor L-NAME administrated to operated Cav+/+ mice. They also isolated endothelial cells from Cav−/− aorta and showed that on VEGF stimulation, NO production and endothelial tube formation were dramatically abrogated when compared with Cav+/+ endothelial cells. The Ser-1177 eNOS phosphorylation, the 495 dephosphorylation, and also the ERK phosphorylation were similarly altered in VEGF-treated Cav−/− endothelial cells.

## Prevention of Restenosis

Prevention of restenosis and major cardiac events after percutaneous coronary intervention is of enormous public health importance. Enormous high rate of smooth muscle cells proliferation is a culprit event that leads to restenosis formation. NO donors inhibit VSMC proliferation, and the overexpression of NOS in the rat carotid artery reduces neointima formation after balloon dilatation *(99)*.

Cell-cycle progression is mediated by cycline-dependent kinases (cdk). Progression in G1 phase and entry into S phase are related to the activity of cdk2 in cycline E and later with cycline A complexes. Cycline E expression increases during G1 and peaks at G1-to-S transition; it enters into complexes with cdk2 throughout this time period. Cycline A expression late in G1 is important for G1-to-S transition, because the inhibition of cycline A kinase prevents S phase entry. The cdk activity is also affected by cyclin-dependent kinase inhibitors (cki). Both p21 and p27 are cki that interfere with cyclin E and cyclin A kinase activity. p21 is present in cdk complexes of proliferating cells during all phases of the cycle; the conversion of active into inactive complexes is achieved through alteration of the ratio of p21 to cdk *(100)*. p27 levels are high in growth factor-deprived cells and decline in response to growth factor stimulation; mitogens are the main factor regulating the p27 level. Consistent with these observations in cultured cells, the vascular p27 level in vivo is inversely related to the degree of proliferation after balloon dilatation and thus permits proliferation in the presence of mitogens, whereas p21 is induced during the phase of declining proliferation and contributes to rendering the vessel quiescent *(101)*.

The study of the molecular mechanism of antiproliferate effect of NO has revealed that NO inhibits VSMC proliferation by inducing G1 phase arrest owing to specific alterations in cell-cycle regulation. The NO donor DETANO inhibited vascular smooth muscle cells proliferation in a concentration-dependent manner. The effect of NO on proliferation was related to G1 arrest, mediated by complete inhibition of cdk2 kinase activity owing to a lower level of both cdk2 and cyclin A as well as by a higher level of p21 protein. The signal transduction processes that underlie this effect remain unknown, although neither cGMP nor cAMP seems to be involved *(102)*.

From the other side, impairment of vascular wound healing (decreased endothelization) is another predictor of restenosis-formation after percutaneous balloon angioplasty. Apoptosis or programmed cell death is an essential mechanism to maintain the adequate rate of endothelization of injured vessels. Local releasing factors like cytokines and autacoids are the main regulators of apoptotic rate in endothelium. Recently, Dimmeler at al described a detailed mechanism for how NO counteracts the proapoptotic effects of cytokines *(103)*. According to their finding the activation of interleukin-1β-converting enzyme (ICE)-like and cysteine protease protein (CPP)-32-like cysteine proteases are required to mediate TNFα-induced apoptosis of HUVEC. Endothelial-derived NO as well as exogenous NO donors in their study inhibited TNFα-induced cysteine protease activation. Inhibition of CPP-32 enzyme activity was owing to specific S-nitrosylation of cystein 163, a functionally essential amino acid conserved among ICE/CPP-32-like proteases *(103)*.

## KEY NOTES

1. The only source of NO in the body is enzyme NOS. Two isoforms (endothelial NOS and neural NOS) are constitutively expressed, although their expression may be modulated. The expression of iNOS is not constitutive but is induced by various cytokines and bacterial products.

2. NO is protective for the vessels only if its production is optimal. Increased NO production could be even more detrimental for the vessels because of peroxynitrite formation.

3. Oxidative stress, independent on the source of free radicals, appears to be a universal molecular trigger for eNOS dysfunction. On the other hand, "uncoupled" eNOS becomes itself the significant source of superoxide.

4. Three important molecular mechanisms of eNOS dysfunction during oxidative stress are known: quenching of NO by superoxide with subsequent peroxynitrite formation; oxidation of $BH_4$; and accumulation of endogenous inhibitors of eNOS—asymmetric ADMA owing to inhibition of redox-sensitive enzyme—DDAH.

5. Chronic pharmacological inhibition of eNOS or genetic silencing of eNOS gene in mice leads to increased arterial pressure and vascular remodeling. NO induces the relaxation of vascular smooth muscle cells and regulates natriuresis in kidney.

6. An impairment of endothelium-dependent relaxations is present in atherosclerotic vessels even before vascular structural changes occur and represent the reduced eNOS-derived NO bioavailability. eNOS-deficient mice kept on high-cholesterol diet are prone to severe atherosclerosis.

7. The dual role of eNOS as a source of both, NO and super oxide, may account for its protective properties in certain experimental conditions of the ischemia-reperfusion model, or be detrimental in others.

8. NO demonstrates antiproliferative effect on smooth muscle cells (prevention of restenosis after balloon injury) and an antiapoptotic action on endothelial cells (promotion of re-endothelization after injury).

## REFERENCES

1. Cosentino F, Luscher TF. Maintenance of vascular integrity: role of nitric oxide and other bradykinin mediators. Eur Heart J 1995;16:K4–K12.
2. Govers R, Rabelink TJ. Cellular regulation of endothelial nitric oxide synthase. Am J Physiol Renal Physiol 2001;280:F193–F206.

3. Kibbe M, Billiar T, Tzeng E. Inducible nitric oxide synthase and vascular injury. Cardiovasc Res 1999;43:650–657.

4. Forstermann U, Boissel JP, Kleinert H. Expressional control of the constitutive isoforms of nitric oxide synthase (NOS I and NOS III). FASEB J 1998;10:773–790.

5. Palmer RM, Ashton DS, Moncada S. Vascular endothelial cells synthesize nitric oxide from L-arginine. Nature 1988;333:664–666.

6. Abu-Soud HM, Stuehr DJ. Nitric oxide synthases reveal a role for calmodulin in controlling electron transfer. Proc Natl Acad Sci USA 1993;90:10,769–10,772.

7. Raman CS, Li H, Martasek P, Kral V, Masters BS, Poulos TL. Crystal structure of constitutive endothelial nitric oxide synthase: a paradigm for pterin function involving a novel metal center. Cell 1998;95:939–950.

8. Sessa WC, Garcia-Cardena G, Liu J, et al. The Golgi association of endothelial nitric oxide synthase is necessary for the efficient synthesis of nitric oxide. J Biol Chem 1995;270:17,641–17,644.

9. Liu J, Garcia-Cardena G, Sessa WC. Biosynthesis and palmitoylation of endothelial nitric oxide synthase: mutagenesis of palmitoylation sites, cysteines-15 and/or -26, argues against depalmitoylation-induced translocation of the enzyme. Biochemistry 1995;34:12,333–12,340.

10. Boo YC, Jo H. Flow-dependent regulation of endothelial nitric oxide synthase: role of protein kinases. Am J Physiol Cell Physiol 2003;285:C499–C508.

11. Fleming I, Fisslthaler B, Dimmeler S, Kemp BE, Busse R. Phosphorylation of Thr(495) regulates Ca(2+)/calmodulin-dependent endothelial nitric oxide synthase activity. Circ Res 2001;88:E68–E75.

12. Hirata K, Kuroda R, Sakoda T, et al. Inhibition of endothelial nitric oxide synthase activity by protein kinase C. Hypertension 1995;25:180–185.

13. Simons K, Toomre D. Lipid rafts and signal transduction. Nat Rev Mol Cell Biol 2000;1:31–39.

14. Li H, Brodsky S, Basco M, Romanov V, De Angelis DA, Goligorsky MS. Nitric oxide attenuates signal transduction: possible role in dissociating caveolin-1 scaffold. Circ Res 2001;88:229–236.

15. Fleming I, Bauersachs J, Schafer A, Scholz D, Aldershvile J, Busse R. Isometric contraction induces the Ca2+-independent activation of the endothelial nitric oxide synthase. Proc Natl Acad Sci USA 1999;96:1123–1128.

16. Ohno M, Gibbons GH, Dzau VJ, Cooke JP. Shear stress elevates endothelial cGMP. Role of a potassium channel and G protein coupling. Circulation 1993;88:193–197.

17. Massion PB, Balligand JL. Modulation of cardiac contraction, relaxation and rate by the endothelial nitric oxide synthase (eNOS): lessons from genetically modified mice. J Physiol 2003;546:63–75.

18. Richter K, Buchner J. Hsp90: chaperoning signal transduction. J Cell Physiol 2001;188:281–290.

19. Garcia-Cardena G, Fan R, Shah V, et al. Dynamic activation of endothelial nitric oxide synthase by Hsp90. Nature 1998;392:821–824.

20. Noris M, Morigi M, Donadelli R, et al. Nitric oxide synthesis by cultured endothelial cells is modulated by flow conditions. Circ Res 1995;76:536–543.

21. Marsden PA, Heng HH, Scherer SW, et al. Structure and chromosomal localization of the human constitutive endothelial nitric oxide synthase gene. J Biol Chem 1993;268:17,478–17,488.

22. Robinson LJ, Weremowicz S, Morton CC, Michel T. Isolation and chromosomal localization of the human endothelial nitric oxide synthase (NOS3) gene. Genomics 1994;19:350–357.

23. Vaziri ND, Wang XQ. cGMP-mediated negative-feedback regulation of endothelial nitric oxide synthase expression by nitric oxide. Hypertension 1999;34:1237–1241.

24. Lüscher TF, Noll G. The pathogenesis of cardiovascular disease: role of the endothelium as a target and mediator. Atherosclerosis 1995;118:S81–S90.

25. Vanhoutte PM. How to assess endothelial function in human blood vessels. J Hypertens 1999;17:1047–1058.

26. Pronai L, Ichimori K, Nozaki H, Nakazawa H, Okino H, Carmichael AJ, Arroyo CM. Investigation of the existence and biological role of L-arginine/nitric oxide pathway in human platelets by spin-trapping/EPR studies. Eur J Biochem 1991;202:923–930.

27. Paschenko SV, Khramtsov VV, Skatchkov MP, Plyusnin VF, Bassenge E. EPR and laser flash photolysis studies of the reaction of nitric oxide with water soluble NO trap Fe(II)-proline-dithiocarbamate complex. Biochem Biophys Res Commun 1996;225:577–584.

28. Malinski T, Taha Z. Nitric oxide release from a single cell measured in situ by a porphyrinic-based microsensor. Nature 1992;358:676–678.

29. Alonso D, Radomski MW. Nitric oxide, platelet function, myocardial infarction and reperfusion therapies. Heart Fail Rev 2003;8:47–54.

30. Beckman JS, Beckman TW, Chen J, Marshall PA, Freeman BA. Apparent hydroxyl radical production by peroxynitrite: implications for endothelial injury from nitric oxide and superoxide. Proc Natl Acad Sci USA 1990;87:1620–1624.

31. Brown AS, Moro MA, Masse JM, Cramer EM, Radomski M, Darley-Usmar V. Nitric oxide-dependent and independent effects on human platelets treated with peroxynitrite. Cardiovasc Res 1998;40:380–388.

32. Pou S, Pou WS, Bredt DS, Snyder SH, Rosen GM. Generation of superoxide by purified brain nitric oxide synthase. J Biol Chem 1992;267:24,173–24,176.

33. Kawashima S, Yokoyama M. Dysfunction of endothelial nitric oxide synthase and atherosclerosis. Arterioscler Thromb Vasc Biol 2004;24:998–1005.

34. Cosentino F, Barker JE, Brand MP, et al. Reactive oxygen species mediate endothelium-dependent relaxations in tetrahydrobiopterin-deficient mice. Arterioscler Thromb Vasc Biol 2001;21:496–502.

35. Cooke JP. NO and angiogenesis. Atheroscler Suppl 2003;4:53–60.

36. Vallance P, Leone A, Calver A, Collier J, Moncada S. Endogenous dimethylarginine as an inhibitor of nitric oxide synthesis. J Cardiovasc Pharmacol 1992;20 Suppl 12:S60–S62.

37. MacAllister RJ, Fickling SA, Whitley GS, Vallance P. Metabolism of methylarginines by human vasculature; implications for the regulation of nitric oxide synthesis. Br J Pharmacol 1994;112:43–48.

38. Dayoub H, Achan V, Adimoolam S, et al. Dimethylarginine dimethylaminohydrolase regulates nitric oxide synthesis: genetic and physiological evidence. Circulation 2003;108:3042–3047.

39. Droge W. Free radicals in the physiological control of cell function. Physiol Rev 2002;82:47–95.

40. Gerzer R, Bohme E, Hofmann F, Schultz G. Soluble guanylate cyclase purified from bovine lung contains heme and copper. FEBS Lett 1981;132:71–74.

41. Ignarro LJ, Wood KS, Wolin MS. Regulation of purified soluble guanylate cyclase by porphyrins and metalloporphyrins: a unifying concept. Adv Cyclic Nucleotide Protein Phosphorylation Res 1984;17:267–274.

42. Tschudi MR, Barton M, Bersinger NA, et al. Effect of age on kinetics of nitric oxide release in rat aorta and pulmonary artery. J Clin Invest 1996;98:899–905.

43. Moreau P, Takase H, Kung CF, van Rooijen MM, Schaffner T, Lüscher TF. Structure and function of the rat basilar artery during chronic nitric oxide synthase inhibition. Stroke 1995;26:1922–1928.

44. Kung CF, Moreau P, Takase H, Luscher TF. L-NAME hypertension alters endothelial and smooth muscle function in rat aorta. Prevention by trandolapril and verapamil. Hypertension 1995;26:744–751.

45. Deng A, Baylis C. Locally produced EDRF controls preglomerular resistance and ultrafiltration coefficient. Am J Physiol 1993;264:F212–F215.

46. Ito S, Arima S, Ren YL, Juncos LA, Carretero OA. Endothelium-derived relaxing factor/nitric oxide modulates angiotensin II action in the isolated microperfused rabbit afferent but not efferent arteriole. J Clin Invest 1993;91:2012–2019.

47. Mattson DL, Roman RJ, Cowley AW Jr. Role of nitric oxide in renal papillary blood flow and sodium excretion. Hypertension 1992;19:766–769.

48. Lüscher TF, Raij L, Vanhoutte PM. Endothelium-dependent vascular responses in normotensive and hypertensive Dahl rats. Hypertension 1987;9:157–163.

49. Cosentino F, Katusic ZS. Tetrahydrobiopterin and dysfunction of endothelial nitric oxide synthase in coronary arteries. Circulation 1995;91:139–144.

50. Cosentino F, Patton S, d'Uscio LV, et al. Tetrahydrobiopterin alters superoxide and nitric oxide release in prehypertensive rats. J Clin Invest 1998;101:1530–1537.

51. Feron O, Kelly RA. The caveolar paradox: suppressing, inducing, and terminating eNOS signaling. Circ Res 2001;88:129–131.

52. Blair A, Shaul PW, Yuhanna IS, Conrad PA, Smart EJ. Oxidized low density lipoprotein displaces endothelial nitric-oxide synthase (eNOS) from plasmalemmal caveolae and impairs eNOS activation. J Biol Chem 1999;274:32,512–32,519.

53. Hirata K, Miki N, Kuroda Y, Sakoda T, Kawashima S, Yokoyama M. Low concentration of oxidized low-density lipoprotein and lysophosphatidylcholine upregulate constitutive nitric oxide synthase mRNA expression in bovine aortic endothelial cells. Circ Res 1995;76:958–962.

54. Laufs U, La Fata V, Plutzky J, Liao JK. Upregulation of endothelial nitric oxide synthase by HMG CoA reductase inhibitors. Circulation 1998;97:1129–1135.

55. Oemar BS, Tschudi MR, Godoy N, Brovkovich V, Malinski T, Luscher TF. Reduced endothelial nitric oxide synthase expression and production in human atherosclerosis. Circulation 1998;97:2494–2498.

56. Aji W, Ravalli S, Szabolcs M, et al. L-arginine prevents xanthoma development and inhibits atherosclerosis in LDL receptor knockout mice. Circulation 1997;95:430–437.

57. Kauser K, da Cunha V, Fitch R, Mallari C, Rubanyi GM. Role of endogenous nitric oxide in progression of atherosclerosis in apolipoprotein E-deficient mice. Am J Physiol Heart Circ Physiol 2000;278:H1679–H1685.
58. Suda O, Tsutsui M, Morishita T, et al. Long-term treatment with N(omega)-nitro-L-arginine methyl ester causes arteriosclerotic coronary lesions in endothelial nitric oxide synthase-deficient mice. Circulation 2002;106:1729–1735.
59. Knowles JW, Reddick RL, Jennette JC, Shesely EG, Smithies O, Maeda N. Enhanced atherosclerosis and kidney dysfunction in eNOS(–/–)Apoe(–/–) mice are ameliorated by enalapril treatment. J Clin Invest 2000;105:451–458.
60. Kuhlencordt PJ, Gyurko R, Han F, et al. Accelerated atherosclerosis, aortic aneurysm formation, and ischemic heart disease in apolipoprotein E/endothelial nitric oxide synthase double-knockout mice. Circulation 2001;104:448–454.
61. Shi W, Wang X, Shih DM, Laubach VE, Navab M, Lusis AJ. Paradoxical reduction of fatty streak formation in mice lacking endothelial nitric oxide synthase. Circulation 2002;105:2078–2082.
62. Ozaki M, Kawashima S, Yamashita T, et al. Overexpression of endothelial nitric oxide synthase accelerates atherosclerotic lesion formation in apoE-deficient mice. J Clin Invest 2002;110:331–340.
63. Ohashi Y, Kawashima S, Hirata K, et al. Hypotension and reduced nitric oxide-elicited vasorelaxation in transgenic mice overexpressing endothelial nitric oxide synthase. J Clin Invest 1998;102:2061–2071.
64. Kawashima S, Yamashita T, Ozaki M, et al. Endothelial NO synthase overexpression inhibits lesion formation in mouse model of vascular remodeling. Arterioscler Thromb Vasc Biol 2001;21:201–207.
65. van Haperen R, de Waard M, van Deel E, et al. Reduction of blood pressure, plasma cholesterol, and atherosclerosis by elevated endothelial nitric oxide. J Biol Chem 2002;277:48,803–48,807.
66. Kurose I, Kubes P, Wolf R, et al. Inhibition of nitric oxide production. Mechanisms of vascular albumin leakage. Circ Res 1993;73:164–171.
67. Fischer S, Clauss M, Wiesnet M, Renz D, Schaper W, Karliczek GF. Hypoxia induces permeability in brain microvessel endothelial cells via VEGF and NO. Am J Physiol 1999;276:C812–C820.
68. Spiecker M, Darius H, Kaboth K, Hubner F, Liao JK. Differential regulation of endothelial cell adhesion molecule expression by nitric oxide donors and antioxidants. J Leukoc Biol 1998;63:732–739.
69. Cosentino F, Luscher TF. Endothelial dysfunction in diabetes mellitus. J Cardiovasc Pharmacol 1998;32:S54–S61.
70. Stratton IM, Adler AI, Neil HA, et al. Association of glycaemia with macrovascular and microvascular complications of type 2 diabetes (UKPDS 35): prospective observational study. BMJ 2000;321:405–412.
71. Meraji S, Jayakody L, Senaratne MP, Thomson AB, Kappagoda T. Endothelium-dependent relaxation in aorta of BB rat. Diabetes 1987;36:978–981.
72. Mayhan WG, Simmons LK, Sharpe GM. Mechanism of impaired responses of cerebral arterioles during diabetes mellitus. Am J Physiol 1991;260:H319–H326.
73. Abiru T, Watanabe Y, Kamata K, Miyata N, Kasuya Y. Decrease in endothelium-dependent relaxation and levels of cyclic nucleotides in aorta from rabbits with alloxan-induced diabetes. Res Commun Chem Pathol Pharmacol 1990;68:13–25.
74. Giugliano D, Ceriello A, Paolisso G. Oxidative stress and diabetic vascular complications. Diabetes Care 1996;19:257–267.
75. Nishikawa T, Edelstein D, Du XL, et al. Normalizing mitochondrial superoxide production blocks three pathways of hyperglycaemic damage. Nature 2000;404:787–790.
76. Wiernsperger NF. Oxidative stress as a therapeutic target in diabetes: revisiting the controversy. Diabetes Metab 2003;29:579–585.
77. Wolff SP, Bascal ZA, Hunt JV. Autoxidative glycosylation: free radicals and glycation theory. Prog Clin Biol Res 1989;304:259–275.
78. Yim MB, Yim HS, Lee C, Kang SO, Chock PB. Protein glycation: creation of catalytic sites for free radical generation. Ann N Y Acad Sci 2001;928:48–53.
79. Creager MA, Luscher TF, Cosentino F, Beckman JA. Diabetes and vascular disease: pathophysiology, clinical consequences, and medical therapy: Part I. Circulation 2003;108:1527–1532.
80. Cosentino F, Hishikawa K, Katusic ZS, Luscher TF. High glucose increases nitric oxide synthase expression and superoxide anion generation in human aortic endothelial cells. Circulation 1997;96:25–28.

81. Cosentino F, Eto M, De Paolis P, et al.. High glucose causes upregulation of cyclooxygenase-2 and alters prostanoid profile in human endothelial cells: role of protein kinase C and reactive oxygen species. Circulation 2003;107:1017–1023.

82. Radomski MW, Palmer RM, Moncada S. An L-arginine/nitric oxide pathway present in human platelets regulates aggregation. Proc Natl Acad Sci USA 1990;87:5193–5197.

83. Radomski MW, Palmer RM, Moncada S. Characterization of the L-arginine:nitric oxide pathway in human platelets. Br J Pharmacol 1990;101:325–328.

84. Malinski T, Radomski MW, Taha Z, Moncada S. Direct electrochemical measurement of nitric oxide released from human platelets. Biochem Biophys Res Commun 1993;194:960–965.

85. Luscher TF, Diederich D, Siebenmann R, et al. Difference between endothelium-dependent relaxation in arterial and in venous coronary bypass grafts. N Engl J Med 1988;319:462–467.

86. Yang ZH, Diederich D, Schneider K, et al. Endothelium-derived relaxing factor and protection against contractions induced by histamine and serotonin in the human internal mammary artery and in the saphenous vein. Circulation 1989;80:1041–1048.

87. Jugdutt BI. Nitric oxide and cardioprotection during ischemia-reperfusion. Heart Fail Rev 2002;7: 391–405.

88. Tsao PS, Aoki N, Lefer DJ, Johnson G 3rd, Lefer AM. Time course of endothelial dysfunction and myocardial injury during myocardial ischemia and reperfusion in the cat. Circulation 1990;82:1402–1412.

89. Jones SP, Girod WG, Palazzo AJ, et al. Myocardial ischemia-reperfusion injury is exacerbated in absence of endothelial cell nitric oxide synthase. Am J Physiol 1999;276:H1567–H1573.

90. Bell RM, Yellon DM. The contribution of endothelial nitric oxide synthase to early ischaemic preconditioning: the lowering of the preconditioning threshold. An investigation in eNOS knockout mice. Cardiovasc Res 2001;52:274–280.

91. Sumeray MS, Rees DD, Yellon DM. Infarct size and nitric oxide synthase in murine myocardium. J Mol Cell Cardiol 2000;32:35–42.

92. Yang XP, Liu YH, Shesely EG, Bulagannawar M, Liu F, Carretero OA. Endothelial nitric oxide gene knockout mice: cardiac phenotypes and the effect of angiotensin-converting enzyme inhibitor on myocardial ischemia/reperfusion injury. Hypertension 1999;34:24–30.

93. Flogel U, Decking UK, Godecke A, Schrader J. Contribution of NO to ischemia-reperfusion injury in the saline-perfused heart: a study in endothelial NO synthase knockout mice. J Mol Cell Cardiol 1999;31:827–836.

94. Kanno S, Lee PC, Zhang Y, et al. Attenuation of myocardial ischemia/reperfusion injury by superinduction of inducible nitric oxide synthase. Circulation 2000;101:2742–2748.

95. Xuan YT, Tang XL, Qiu Y, et al. Biphasic response of cardiac NO synthase isoforms to ischemic preconditioning in conscious rabbits. Am J Physiol Heart Circ Physiol 2000;279:H2360–H2371.

96. Wang Y, Guo Y, Zhang SX, et al. Ischemic preconditioning upregulates inducible nitric oxide synthase in cardiac myocyte. J Mol Cell Cardiol 2002;34:5–15.

97. Guo Y, Jones WK, Xuan YT, et al. The late phase of ischemic preconditioning is abrogated by targeted disruption of the inducible NO synthase gene. Proc Natl Acad Sci USA 1999;96:11,507–11,512.

98. Sonveaux P, Martinive P, DeWever J, et al. Caveolin-1 expression is critical for vascular endothelial growth factor-induced ischemic hindlimb collateralization and nitric oxide-mediated angiogenesis. Circ Res 2004;95:154–161.

99. Janssens S, Flaherty D, Nong ZX, et al. Human endothelial cell nitric oxide synthase gene transfer inhibits vascular smooth muscle cell proliferation and neointima formation after balloon injury in rats. Circulation 1998;97:1274–1281.

100. Zhang H, Hannon GJ, Beach D. p21-containing cyclin kinases exist in both active and inactive states. Genes Dev 1994;8:1750–1758.

101. Tanner FC, Yang Z, Duckers E, Gordon D, Nabel GJ, Nabel EG. Expression of cyclin-dependent kinase inhibitors in vascular disease. Circ Res 1998;82:396–403.

102. Tanner FC, Meier P, Greutert H, Champion C, Nabel EG, Luscher TF. Nitric oxide modulates expression of cell cycle regulatory proteins: a cytostatic strategy for inhibition of human vascular smooth muscle cell proliferation. Circulation 2000;101:1982–1989.

103. Dimmeler S, Haendeler J, Nehls M, Zeiher AM. Suppression of apoptosis by nitric oxide via inhibition of interleukin-1beta-converting enzyme (ICE)-like and cysteine protease protein (CPP)-32-like proteases. J Exp Med 1997;185:601–607.

# III  DIAGNOSIS OF RESTENOSIS

# 15 The Use of Pressure Gradient in the Diagnosis of Restenosis

*Volker Klauss, MD*
*and Nico H. J. Pijls, MD, PhD*

## CONTENTS

## INTRODUCTION

The limitation of coronary angiography to assess the functional significance of coronary stenosis as well as coronary restenosis has been recognized for years *(1,2)*. It is well known that the angiographic assessment of an epicardial lesion correlates poorly with its physiological relevance *(3,4)*. Coronary angiography with its inherent limitations may not reliably predict whether a stenosis produces ischemia *(5)*. In addition, the determination of the severity of stenoses varies significantly among observers. In one study, experienced operators disagreed 30% of the time when deciding on the number of coronary arteries with a 70% stenosis *(6)*. Despite these limitations the decision for performing an intervention is often based on the angiographic appearance of a coronary lesion. It is known from many angiographic studies that revascularization rate increases after scheduled control angiography meaning that repeat intervention is more often based on morphological criteria, i.e., quantitative coronary angiography or solely "eye balling" than on physiological considerations *(7)*. Furthermore, as restenosis, which means in most of the cases in-stent restenosis may occur as a diffuse, proliferative process, the assessment of the hemodynamic significance is even more complex by angiography alone.

From: *Contemporary Cardiology: Essentials of Restenosis: For the Interventional Cardiologist*
Edited by: H. J. Duckers, E. G. Nabel, and P. W. Serruys © Humana Press Inc., Totowa, NJ

Given this limited accuracy of morphological methods to assess true stenosis severity, diagnosis of restenosis by angiography is even more disputable. In the view of the risk of a second restenosis, the higher costs of a reintervention (i.e., brachy therapy or drug eluting stents), potential procedural complications, and the lower long-term benefit, it is imperative that the decision of performing an intervention in a restenotic lesion is combined with objective evidences of myocardial ischemia.

In the present chapters, the potential of intracoronary pressure measurements for the diagnosis of restenosis will be discussed. As the vast majority of clinical studies dealing with intracoronary pressure measurements have been performed in *de novo* lesions the results and observations to restenotic lesions are extended where it seems possible. For conceptual reasons as illustrated later the focus will be on more details of the principle of fractional flow reserve than on the determination of coronary pressure gradient alone.

## DEFINITION OF FRACTIONAL FLOW RESERVE

The concept of fractional flow reserve has been developed as an invasively determined index of the functional severity of coronary stenosis *(8)*. Fractional flow reserve is defined as the ratio of maximum blood flow to the myocardium in the presence of a stenosis in the supplying coronary artery to the theoretical maximum flow in the absence of the stenosis *(9)*. This ratio represents the fraction of maximum flow that can be maintained in spite of the presence of this stenosis. In the clinical context the index of fractional flow reserve indicates to what extent maximum blood flow in a stenosed coronary vessel can be improved by a coronary intervention.

The determination of fractional flow reserve by pressure measurements requires the induction of maximal hyperemia. Only at maximum vasodilation, corresponding to maximum coronary and myocardial hyperemia, myocardial resistance is minimal and constant and blood flow is proportional to driving pressure. In the presence of a coronary stenosis, perfusion pressure over the myocardium and thus maximum attainable blood flow to the myocardium will be affected to the same proportion under hyperemic conditions. Thus, fractional flow reserve can be calculated by comparing the mean coronary pressure distal to a stenosis, as measured with pressure wire, with the proximal coronary pressure, as measured with the guide wire *(10)*.

Fractional flow reserve has several and unique features compared with other physiological indices. First, this index is independent of changes in systemic blood pressure, heart rate, or myocardial contractility *(11)*. Second, the normal value of fractional flow reserve is one in all patients and in all coronary arteries *(12)*. Third, it considers the contribution of collateral circulation *(13)*. Fourth, it can be applied in single and multivessel disease. Furthermore, a fractional flow reserve of less than 0.75 accurately identifies lesions associated with inducible myocardial ischemia *(14)*. Fianally, fractional flow reserve accounts for the extension of the perfusion territory of the stenotic artery: two identical stenoses with a different perfusion territory yield different values of fractional flow reserve, thus correctly matching the supplying artery to the area to be perfused. In a practical setting, fractional flow reserve can be derived easily from the ratio of mean distal coronary artery pressure to mean aortic pressure under maximal vasodilation by means of a 0.014-in. pressure guide wire (Fig. 1).

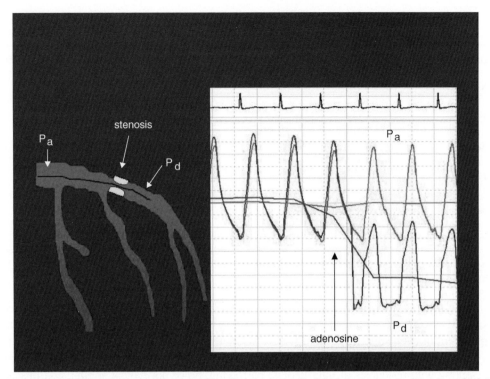

**Fig. 1.** Fractional flow reserve can be derived easily by means of a 0.014-in. pressure guide wire, which is placed distally to a stenosis of questionable hemodynamic relevance. By inducing maximal vasodilation with intravenous adenosine in this example, fractional flow reserve can be calculated by the ratio of mean distal coronary artery pressure (Pd) to mean aortic pressure (Pa). (Please *see* insert for color version.)

## CLINICAL VALIDATION OF FRACTIONAL FLOW RESERVE

Although not all theoretical concerns regarding the limitation of direct physiological measurements can be completely satisfied, the clinical validation strongly supports the value of intracoronary pressure measurement. In patients, the validation of physiological criteria has been established by population correlations with clinically accepted norms of several types of ischemic stress provocation *(15–18)*. In a landmark study, Pijls and colleagues *(14)* compared fractional flow reserve in 45 patients with intermediate lesions with bicycle exercise testing, nuclear perfusion imaging, and stress echocardiography. In all 21 patients in whom the fractional flow reserve was less than 0.75, at least one non-invasive test demonstrated inducible ischemia and reversed to normal after treatment. In 21 of the 24 patients in whom the fractional flow reserve was 0.75 or higher, there was no inducible ischemia on any of the noninvasive tests. The sensitivity, specificity, and concordance of fractional flow reserve were 88%, 100%, and 93%, respectively.

Although the first validation studies were performed in selected patients more recent studies confirmed consistently good correlations between fractional flow reserve cut-off values and noninvasive stress tests also in patients with multivessel disease and previous myocardial infarction (Table 1). Thus, sensitivity and specificity of fractional flow reserve vary between 69 and 100%, respectively. The cut-off value of fractional flow reserve for identifying reversible ischemia in these studies was consistently between 0.72 and 0.75, underlining the diagnostic accuracy of this index.

Table 1
Validation Studies Comparing FFR With Noninvasive Stress-Testing

| Study | Patients | Noninvasive tests | FFR | Sensitivity (%) | Specificity (%) |
|-------|----------|-------------------|-----|-----------------|-----------------|
| De Bruyne B et al. (9) | 60, SVD, no MI | Exercise ECG | 0.72 | 100 | 69 |
| Pijls NH et al. (25) | 45, SVD, no MI | Exercise ECG, DSE, SPECT | 0.75 | 88 | 100 |
| Chamuleau et al. (17) | 127, 2VD, no MI | SPECT | 0.74 | 69 | 79 |
| De Bruyne et al. (18) | 57, SVD, MI | SPECT | 0.75 | 82 | 87 |
| Usui et al. (26) | 167, MVD, MI | SPECT | 0.75 | 79 | 79 |

MI, myocardial infarction; SVD, single vessel disease; 2VD, Two-vessel-disease; MVD, multivessel disease; DSE, dobutamine stress echocardiography; SPECT, single photon computed tomography; ECG, electrocardiography.

To summarize there is enough evidence based on multiple validation studies that fractional flow reserve is a reliable index for indicating or excluding reversible ischemia at least equivalent or even superior to noninvasive stress test, such as exercise-electrocardiogram, myocardial scintigraphy, and dobutamine stress-echocardiography. Thus, in patients presenting with restenosis of intermediate narrowing, no or not typical angina, and missing or not conclusive stress tests, the decision whether to perform a revascularization can be based on the result of intracoronary pressure measurement immediately. Especially, in patients with debortable in-stent restenosis—many stents show some intimal hyperplasia without meaning that this is associated with any ischemia—demonstration of reversible ischemia is paramount before embarking in questionable brachytherapy or placing a drug eluting stent within the other stent.

## PRACTICAL SET-UP OF PRESSURE MEASUREMENTS IN THE CATHETERIZATION LABORATORY

No major adaptations are necessary in a catheterization laboratory to perform intracoronary pressure measurements on a routine basis. Currently, two microsensor-tipmanometer wires with a diameter of a standard guide wire are available. Each is connected through a cable to its specific interface, which indicates the pressure values (distal coronary and aortic) and—depending on the system—the corresponding pressure curves. Both interfaces are normally connected to the registration system of the cath lab. The quality of these pressure guide wires is nowadays similar to standard guide wires with respect to torquability and access to the lesion. Thus, for an experienced angiographer a pressure guide wire can be used as a first line wire and all manipulations and exchange procedures can be performed in a regular way.

Although the use of a regular guiding catheter is recommended because the inner coating allows for better torque control there is growing experience with the use of regular 4°F and 6°F diagnostic catheters (19). A crucial point as alluded to before is the induction a maximum hyperemia. Once the wire with sensor is distal to the lesion or segment of interest, a maximum hyperemic stimulus should be administered for a complete physiological evaluation. Multiple studies reported on the effect of different stimuli given either intracoronarily or intravenously (20–22). Generally, long acting drugs, such as papaverine, should be used if the intracoronary line is preferred; for intravenous application, adenosine or ATP are recommended. The most convincing mode to demonstrate the location of a lesion is a so-called pullback curve, also named as "physiological road map" of a coronary artery (Fig. 2). During maximum hyperemia the sensor is slowly pulled back from the distal position in the vessel to the ostium. The pullback curve also allows the detection of multiple lesions within one vessel or the presence of diffuse disease. It is therefore strongly recommended to perform pressure measurements in a standardized way by means of pressure pullback curves. Having the interface permanently installed in the cath lab, a diagnostic procedure can simply be extended by a physiological evaluation within a few minutes and thus applied on a routine basis by every operator.

## APPLICATION OF PRESSURE MEASUREMENTS IN THE DIAGNOSIS OF RESTENOSIS

In the present chapter, several cases will be shown in whom the application of pressure measurements was used for assessing the hemodynamic relevance of in-stent restenosis.

In the first case, a 50-yr-old man was scheduled for 6-mo control angiogram. Initially, a proximal left anterior descending coronary artery (LAD) lesion was treated with stent. The follow-up angiography revealed a moderate in-stent restenosis (Fig. 3), the patient was asymptomatic at that time. Many operators would probably have treated this restenosis with another percutaneous coronary intervention (PCI) including expensive procedures, such as brachytherapy or drug eluting stents. In this case, a pressure wire was used in combination with intravenous adenosine and showed a only mildly impaired fractional flow reserve clearly indicating no need for any revascularization procedure. The next case was a 64-yr-old male with former bypass surgery. Eight months ago the ostium of the venous graft to a small obtuse marginal branch was treated with stent implantation (bare metal stent). He presented with diffuse symptoms interpreted as angina by the referring physician. A myocardial scintigraphy was not conclusive so finally a diagnostic angiography was performed revealing a in-stent restenosis of the ostial stent of the graft (Fig. 4). By pressure measurements fractional flow reserve was 0.91 indicating no need for another PCI procedure in this graft.

A 58-yr-old male was scheduled for PCI of the LAD. Nine months ago the right coronary artery has been treated with a stent, 3 mo ago an in-stent restenosis was dilated with angioplasty alone. Before targeting the LAD a control angiogram of the RCA showed a mild-to-moderate restenosis again. Pressure measurement indicated a reduced but not clearly pathological fractional flow reserve (FFR) (Fig. 5). Pressure measurements of the lesions of the left coronary artery showed functionally diffused disease with clearly pathological FFR values in the LAD and first diagonal branch. The treatment of this patient was finally switched to bypass surgery, based on the results of the pressure measurement. As demonstrated in these cases, coronary pressure measurement is a helpful tool to evaluate the hemodynamic relevance of an instent restenosis, which is most often impossible to assess alone by angiographic means. Pressure measurements help to confirm the appropriateness of an intervention or to avoid on the other side additional interventions.

## COST-EFFECTIVENESS OF FRACTIONAL FLOW RESERVE

In a recent study, the cost-effectiveness of measuring fractional flow reserve in patients with intermediate lesions was assessed by use of decision analysis model *(23)*. Although the model assumptions were made for patients with single coronary vessel

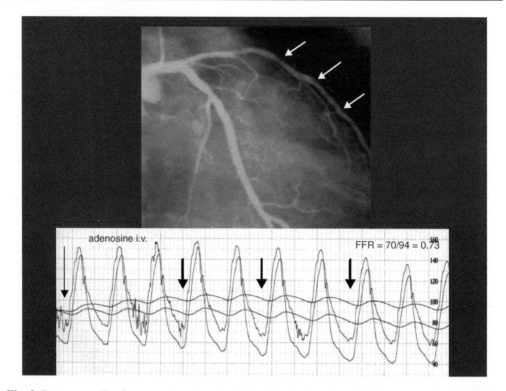

**Fig. 2.** Pressure-pullback curve, also named as "physiological road map" of a coronary artery. During maximum hyperemia the sensor is slowly pulled back from the distal position in the vessel to the ostium. The pullback curve allows the detection of multiple lesions within one vessel or the presence of diffuse disease as in the present example. This patient had typical angina and a positive single photon computed tomography on the anterior wall. The LAD is occluded and the pressure measurements of the diagonal branch showed a pathological FFR, which is owing to diffuse disease but not circumscript lesions. That means that an intervention at the angiographic lesion sites marked by the arrows will not really lead to a better functional result.

disease and *de novo* lesions, the differences in costs of each of the strategies compared with fractional flow reserve measurements illustrates the potential impact of the use of pressure measurements in restenotic lesions. On-line pressure measurements in case of intermediate lesions and no previous functional study was compared with a nuclear stress testing strategy and a strategy of stenting of all lesions. As the result of this study, immediate pressure measurements saved $1795 per patient compared with delayed noninvasive stress testing and $3830 compared with the stent strategy. Quality-adjusted life expectancy was similar among the 3 strategies, but the cost per quality adjusted life year for the nuclear stress testing strategy was substantial (>$800,000/quality adjusted life year). Keeping in mind that this model was applied in a patient subset not including patients with restenosis, the differences between the strategies are so pronounced that essential changes in a model with restenotic lesions might not be expected. This analysis war performed from a societal perspective. From a hospital perspective, each strategy might be attractive, depending on the reimbursement system.

## LIMITATIONS

Fractional flow reserve is limited by its reliance on achieving maximal hyperemia. If maximal hyperemia does not occur, the pressure gradient across a stenosis will be

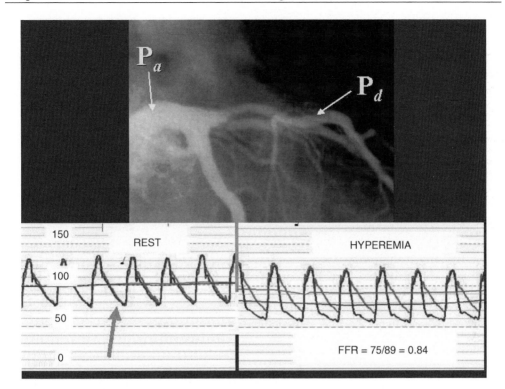

**Fig. 3.** A 50-yr-old man was scheduled for control angiography. Six months before, a proximal LAD lesion was treated with stent. The present angiogram revealed an in-stent restenosis, the angiographic severity was similar to that of the index procedure. Many operators would probably have treated this restenosis with another PCI, including expensive procedures, such as brachytherapy or drug eluting stents. In this case, a pressure wire was used in combination with intravenous adenosine and showed a only mildly impaired fractional flow reserve clearly indicating no need for any revascularization procedure. (Please *see* insert for color version.)

underestimated and the fractional flow reserve overestimated. For these reasons, careful and adequate administration of the vasodilating agent, particularly when using the intracoronary route, is critical. Intravenous adenosine is considered the reference standard for inducing hyeremia, but the added expense for the medication might be prohibitive. However, in hospitals with own pharmacies adenosine for the intravenous application can be provided at very low costs. Fractional flow reserve is furthermore affected by significant microvascular disease. Because achieving maximal hyperemia when measuring the pressure distal to stenosis is critical to accurately assess fractional flow reserve, a dysfunctional microcirculation secondary to, for example, diabetes can impair the microvascular vasodilator capacity. This can result in what one initially might consider an overestimation of the fractional flow reserve. However, the fractional flow reserve measurement continues to provide useful information about the epicardial lesion in this setting: a fractional flow reserve higher than 0.75 implies the absence of myocardial ischemia and the lack of need for revascularization.

Although the decision on the interventional treatment of a restenosis can be based on the result of pressure measurements currently there is a lack of the data on the safety of deferring an intervention. But whether the interventional treatment of a restenosis is decided by use of fractional flow reserve or by means of a noninvasive test by none of these tests the natural course of an individual restenosis can be determined.

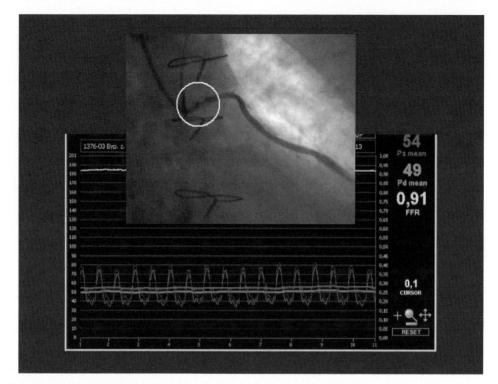

**Fig. 4.** Angiogram of a venous graft to a small obtuse marginal branch, which was treated with stent implantation (bare metal stent) 8 mo ago. The patient presented with diffuse symptoms inter-pretated as angina by the referring physician. A myocardial scintigraphy was not conclusive so finally a diagnostic angiography was performed revealing a in-stent restenosis of the ostial stent of the graft. By pressure measurements fractional flow reserve was 0.91 indicating no need for another PCI procedure in this graft. (Please *see* insert for color version.)

Thus, the decision to perform a PCI should primarily be based on the result of either stress test and not on the nature of the lesion itself. Having convincing data on the prognostic impact of postinterventional fractional flow reserve measurements after coronary stenting such data are missing for treating a restenotic lesion *(24)*. Although the importance of the functional result of any intervention might be assessed, cur-rently the contribution to the long-term outcomes in restenotic lesions is not known. Furthermore, the widespread use of fractional flow reserve measurements in most European countries is limited by the price of the pressure guide wire combined with the lack of reimbursement as a specific procedure. Additional studies are necessary to con-vince health insurances and hospital administrations that the use of fractional flow reserve is cost-effective and might even lower the costs when the method is adequately integrated in the diagnostic algorithm.

## CONCLUSIONS

Recognizing the above limitations fractional flow reserve can be performed easily, rapidly, and safely in patients with coronary artery disease. By its diagnostic accuracy this index can be used for on-line clinical decision making in patients with de-novo and restenotic lesions to decide on repeat intervention on one hand and to avoid unnecessary

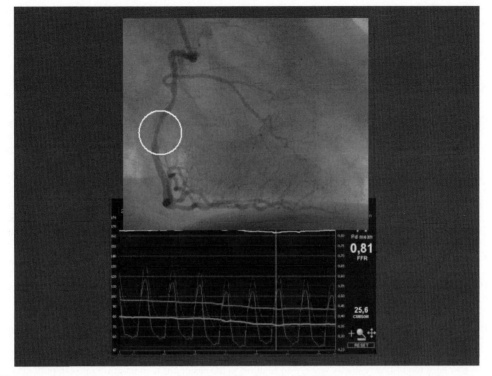

**Fig. 5.** A 58-yr-old male was scheduled for PCI of the LAD. Nine months ago the right coronary artery has been treated with a stent, 3 mo ago an in-stent restenosis was dilated with angioplasty alone. Before targeting the LAD a control angiogram of the RCA showed a mild-to-moderate restenosis again. Pressure measurement indicated a borderline pathological FFR. Pressure measurements of the lesions of the LCA showed functionally diffuse disease with clearly pathological FFR values in the LAD and first diagonal branch. The treatment of this patient was finally switched to bypass surgery, based on the results of the pressure measurement. (Please *see* insert for color version.)

revascularization on the other side. This applies especially when the hemodynamic significance of the lesion is questionable and no noninvasive functional evaluation has been performed or a test has been performed with a nonconclusive result.

## REFERENCES

1. Topol E, Nissen S. Our preoccupation with coronary luminology. The dissociation between clinical and angiographic findings in ischemic heart disease. Circulation 1995;92:2333–2342.
2. Kern M, De Bruyne B, Pijls-Nico HJ. From research to clinical practice: current role of intracoronary physiologically based decision making in the cardiac catheterization laboratory. J Am Coll Cardiol 1997;30:613–620.
3. White CW, Wright CB, Doty DB. Does visual interpretation of the coronary arteriogram predict the physiologic importance of a coronary stenosis? N Engl J Med 1984;310:819–824.
4. Bartunek J, Sys SU, Heyndrickx GR, Pijls NHJ, DeBruyne B. Quantitative coronary angiography in predicting functional significance of stenoses in an unselected patient cohort. J Am Coll Cardiol 1995;26:328–334.
5. Marcus ML, Skorton DJ, Johnson MR, Collins SM, Harrison DG, Kerber RE. Visual Estimates of percent diameter coronary stenosis: A battered gold standard. J Am Coll Cardiol 1988;11:882–885.
6. DeRouen TA, Murray JA, Owen W. Variability in the analysis of coronary arteriograms. Circulation 1977;55:324–328.
7. Ruygrok PN, Melkert R, Morel M-A, et al. Does six month follow-up angiography influence clinical management and outcome? J Am Coll Cardiol 2004;34:1507–1511.

8. Pijls-Nico HJ, Van Gelder B, Van der Voort P, et al. Fractional flow reserve. A useful index to evaluate the influence of an epicardial coronary stenosis on myocardial blood flow. Circulation 1995;92: 3183–3193.

9. DeBruyne B, Bartunek J, Sys SU, Heyndrickx GR. Relation between myocardial fractional flow reserve calculated from coronary pressure measurements and exercise-induced myocardial ischemia. Circulation 1995;92:3183–3193.

10. Pijls-Nico HJ, Kern MJ, Yock PG, De Bruyne B. Practice and potential pitfalls of coronary pressure measurement. Catheter Cardiovasc Interv 2000;49:1–16.

11. De Bruyne B, Bartunek J, Sys SU, Pijls NH, Heyndrickx GR, Wijns W. Simultaneous coronary pressure and flow velocity measurements in humans. Feasibility, reproducibility, and hemodynamic dependence of coronary flow velocity reserve, hyperemic flow versus pressure slope index, and fractional flow reserve. Circulation 1996;94:1842–1849.

12. De Bruyne B, Hersbach F, Pijls NH, et al. Abnormal epicardial coronary resistance in patients with diffuse atherosclerosis but "Normal" coronary angiography. Circulation 2001;104:2401–2406.

13. Pijls NH, van Son JA, Kirkeeide RL, De Bruyne B, Gould KL. Experimental basis of determining maximum coronary, myocardial, and collateral blood flow by pressure measurements for assessing functional stenosis severity before and after percutaneous transluminal coronary angioplasty. Circulation 1993;87:1354–1367.

14. Pijls NH, De Bruyne B, Peels K, et al. Measurement of fractional flow reserve to assess the functional severity of coronary-artery stenoses. N Engl J Med 1996;334:1703–1708.

15. Bartunek J, Marwick TH, Rodrigues AC. Dobutamine-induced wall motion abnormalities: correlations with myocardial fractional flow reserve and quantitative coronary angiography. J Am Coll Cardiol 1996;27:1429–1436.

16. Fearon WF, Takagi A, Jeremias A, et al. Use of fractional myocardial flow reserve to assess the functional significance of intermediate coronary stenoses. Am J Cardiol 2000;86:1013–1014, A10.

17. Chamuleau SA, Meuwissen M, Eck-Smit BL, et al. Fractional flow reserve, absolute and relative coronary blood flow velocity reserve in relation to the results of technetium-99m sestamibi single-photon emission computed tomography in patients with two-vessel coronary artery disease. J Am Coll Cardiol 2001;37:1316–1322.

18. De Bruyne B, Pijls-Nico HJ, Bartunek J. Fractional flow reserve in patients with prior myocardial infarction. Circulation 2001;104:157–162.

19. Legalery P, Seronde MF, Meneveau N, Schiele F, Bassand JP. Measuring pressure-derived fractional flow reserve through four French diagnostic catheters. Am J Cardiol 2004;91:1075–1078.

20. DeBruyne B, Pijls NHJ, Barbato E, et al. Intracoronary and intravenous adenosine 5′-triphosphate, adenosine, papaverine, and contrast medium to assess fractional flow reserve in humans. Circulation 2004;107:1877–1883.

21. Lopez-Palop R, Saura D, Pinar E, et al. Adequate intracoronary adenosine doses to achieve maximum hyperaemia in coronary functional studies by pressure derived fractional flow reserve: a dose response study. Heart 2004;90:95–96.

22. Casella G, Leibig M, Schiele TM, et al. Are high doses of intracoronary adenosine an alternative to standard intravenous adenosine for the assessment of fractional flow reserve? Am Heart J 2004;148:590–595.

23. Fearon WF, Yeung A, Lee DP, Yock P, Heidenreich PA. Cost-effectiveness of measuring fractional flow reserve to guide coronary interventions. Am Heart J 2003;145:882–887.

24. Pijls NH, Klauss V, Siebert U, et al. Coronary pressure measurement after stenting predicts adverse events at follow-up: a multicenter registry. Circulation 2002;105:2950–2954.

25. Pijls-Nico HJ, De Bruyne B, Peels K. Measurement of fractional flow reserve to assess the functional severity of coronary-artery stenoses. N Engl J Med 1996;334:1703–1708.

26. Usui Y, Chikamori T, Yanagisawa M, et al. Reliability of pressure-derived myocardial fractional flow reserve in assessing coronary artery stenosis in patients with previous myocardial infarction. Am J Cardiol 2003;92:699–702.

# 16 The Use of Radio Isotopes in the Diagnosis of Vascular Proliferative Disease

*Giedrius Davidavicius, MD,*
*Ganesh Manoharan, MBBCh, MD, MRCPI,*
*and William Wijns, MD, PhD*

## CONTENTS

## INTRODUCTION

Every patient undergoing percutaneous revascularization is at risk for developing coronary restenosis. Six months after the initial procedure, recurrence of the luminal narrowing at the site of intervention occurs in up to 35% of cases after conventional balloon angioplasty (percutaneous transluminal coronary angioplasty [PTCA]) and 19% after stenting using bare-metal stents *(1)*.

Restenosis is considered to be a complex set of responses to arterial injury. As assessed by intravascular ultrasound studies, the prevailing mechanism of restenosis after stand-alone PTCA is arterial remodeling, with late vessel contraction being responsible for 60% of late lumen loss *(2)*, whereas in-stent restenosis predominantly results from accelerated neointimal tissue proliferation *(3)*.

Although the use of drug-eluting stents *(4)* has significantly reduced in-stent restenosis rates, specific lesion, and patient subsets remain prone to restenosis, which may cause ischemia and negatively affect prognosis. This is particularly the case in patients with diabetes in whom the combination of microalbuminuria and silent ischemia identifies a subgroup of asymptomatic subjects who are at high-risk for future cardiac events *(5,6)*.

From: *Contemporary Cardiology: Essentials of Restenosis: For the Interventional Cardiologist*
Edited by: H. J. Duckers, E. G. Nabel, and P. W. Serruys © Humana Press Inc., Totowa, NJ

Hence, in daily clinical practice, it is important to differentiate ischemia whether caused by restenosis after an initially successful revascularization procedure or further progression of atherosclerosis. Stress myocardial perfusion imaging (MPI) is a clinically important tool, which can identify ischemic regions of myocardium, yield information about patient prognosis, and evaluate the presence of residual ischemia after revascularization. This information can be important for the selection of patients who require further angiographic evaluation and subsequent repeat revascularization. According to recent guidelines (7,8), MPI is useful both in symptomatic and in asymptomatic patients, in whom MPI can be performed routinely at 6 mo after percutaneous coronary intervention (PCI).

In this chapter, the current status, indications, timing and predictive accuracy of MPI using radioisotopes in assessing restenosis are reviewed in patients after PCI. A number of innovative approaches to molecular imaging of the atherosclerotic process will also be mentioned briefly.

## MPI WITH RADIONUCLIDES

Currently, the most commonly used noninvasive imaging technique for the detection of myocardial ischemia caused by severe coronary atherosclerosis is MPI using single-photon emission computed tomography (SPECT). Several radioactive flow tracers labeled with photon emitting atoms, such as thallium-201 ($^{201}$Tl) or one of the technetium-99m ($^{99m}$Tc)-labeled agents (sestamibi, tetrofosmin) are widely used in clinical practice.

### Flow Tracers

$^{201}$Tl is a cationic element with biological properties similar to those of potassium. It is cyclotron produced and emits mercury X-rays (88%) and γ-rays at 135, 165, and 167 keV (12%). $^{201}$Tl has a relatively long half-life (physical half-life is 74 h and biological half-life is 58 h). Following intravenous administration, its initial distribution is proportional to regional myocardial blood flow and depends on extraction fraction into the myocyte, which is high (~85%) at normal flow rates. $^{201}$Tl images obtained early after injection reflect the flow-dependent initial distribution and thus regional myocardial blood flow. In addition, myocardial viability can be assessed by images taken 2–24 h after injection that show tracer distribution in the potassium pool. In case of severe coronary artery stenosis, the initial uptake of $^{201}$Tl during exercise and the washout from the ischemic tissue is reduced in contrast to normal myocardium. Subsequently, ischemic perfusion defect fills-in over time because of the prolonged accumulation of $^{201}$Tl. Infarcted myocardium is characterized by significantly lower initial uptake in comparison with normal myocardium, without redistribution.

$^{99m}$Tc-labeled perfusion agents (tetrofosmin or sestamibi) are lipophilic, cationic complexes, which emit γ-rays at 140 keV with a physical half-life of 6 h. $^{99m}$Tc tetrofosmin exhibits slow myocardial clearance without evidence of delayed redistribution. It accumulates in mitochondria. The initial distribution of $^{99m}$Tc tracers following intravenous injection is proportional to regional blood flow. Both agents enter the myocyte by passive diffusion and bind stably to intracellular membranes. $^{99m}$Tc-labeled tracers show improved image contrast and resolution over $^{201}$Tl.

## Stress MPI by SPECT

The appropriate methodology to perform exercise, adenosine or dipyridamole SPECT MPI has been described extensively elsewhere *(7,8)*. [201]Tl SPECT imaging is done within 10 min after stress, and repeated 3–4 h later for redistribution imaging.

For patients who cannot exercise, pharmacological stress provides more reliable test results than ineffective exercise. To identify areas of reversible ischemia with the [99m]Tc tracers, separate injections at rest and with stress have to be undertaken; usually this is accomplished by using either 2-d protocol, in which the stress and resting studies are performed on separate days, or a same-day study, in which the [99m]Tc-labeled imaging agent is given at rest and again several hours later, at peak stress. Evaluation of ventricular wall systolic function and measurement of the left ventricular ejection fraction can be done with electrocardiography-gated images *(9)*.

## Image Acquisition and Analysis

Both [99m]Tc tracers and [201]Tl SPECT studies are imaged with a tomographic $\gamma$-camera centered on the heart. Images can be evaluated using a qualitative approach (visual interpretation of stress and rest tomograms), which is less reproducible and less specific than a semiquantitative analysis *(10)*.

Quantitative analysis of SPECT studies has been particularly helpful in objectively demonstrating improvement in regional perfusion after PTCA. Specificity of MPI increases when using a quantitative approach in which a polar map representing maximal pixel values is obtained from the myocardial wall. The polar maps are divided into segments and the values are averaged within each segment. The segment with the highest average value is set to 100%, and all other segments are normalized to that segment. The values for each segment represent the percent maximal uptake of the tracer. Pixels in which tracer uptake varied more than 2.5 standard deviation in comparison with normal mean values were considered abnormal. Vascular territories represented areas of myocardium subtended by specific vessels: antero-septal, anterior, antero-lateral, and apical areas for the left anterior descending coronary artery, inferior area for the right coronary artery, postero-lateral area for the left circumflex coronary artery.

Widely accepted scoring systems are as follows:

- *Normal*: homogeneous uptake of the radiopharmaceutical throughout the myocardium.
- *Defect*: a myocardial area with reduced uptake, intensity can vary from slightly reduced to almost absent activity.
- *Reversible defect*: a defect that is present on the initial stress images and is no longer present or to a lesser degree on resting or delayed images. Improvement over time on [201]Tl imaging is referred to as "redistribution."
- *Fixed defect*: a defect that is unchanged on both stress and rest images. This finding indicates infarcted area and scar tissue.
- *Reverse redistribution*: the initial stress images are either normal or show a defect, whereas the delayed or rest images show a new defect or a more severe defect. Initial excess accumulation of tracer is followed by rapid clearance from the scar tissue. The significance of this pattern remains controversial.

In the specific situation of post-PCI MPI, the tracer distribution in the vascular territory of dilated arteries can be also classified as:

1. Normal;
2. Stress-induced perfusion defect with complete normalization at rest (reversible defect);

3. Stress-induced perfusion defect with incomplete normalization at rest (partially reversible defect); and

4. Perfusion defect at stress without significant improvement at rest (persistent defect). In general, a reversible defect (b or c) is indicative of restenosis in patients treated with PCI *(10,11)*.

## IMAGING THE VASCULAR PROLIFERATIVE DISEASE PROCESS

The clinical diagnostic and prognostic evaluation of coronary artery disease has benefited considerably from the application of radionuclide imaging techniques. The main areas of research involve quantification of nutrient myocardial perfusion and molecular imaging. Clearly, the ability to image the vascular wall and to identify atherosclerotic lesions noninvasively would yield useful information that could potentially affect patient management strategy, for instance, through the early detection of preclinical atherosclerosis, the identification of vulnerable or metabolically active plaque before their clinical manifestation as an acute coronary syndrome.

### Quantitative Positron Emission Tomography

With positron emission tomography (PET), quantitative assessment of perfusion and coronary flow reserve has become possible. Several potential applications of PET could be of interest for both research and practice, such as the assessment of myocardial perfusion in the early stages of coronary artery disease, the identification of endothelial dysfunction, and monitoring of disease progression or regression.

The myocardial perfusion features attributable to mild "nonsignificant" coronary atherosclerosis can be defined by quantitative PET *(12)*. MPI using stress PET demonstrated the graded, longitudinal, base-to-apex perfusion abnormality in the presence of diffuse coronary atherosclerosis without the presence of angiographically significant lesions (Fig. 1).

It was proposed to use this finding as a noninvasive marker of diffuse coronary atherosclerosis. In addition, quantification of coronary flow reserve can demonstrate endothelial dysfunction and its reversal. Restoration of normal myocardial perfusion and perfusion reserve after treatment with statins, a phenomenon that relates to improved endothelial function, can be detected and monitored by PET *(13)*.

Other investigators who used quantitative PET showed that abnormal microcirculatory function is present in smokers in the absence of obstructive disease of the epicardial coronary arteries. The endothelial function is altered because of increased oxidative stress and impaired microcirculation responsiveness and vasomotion, which can be restored with antioxidant therapy *(14)*.

### Molecular Imaging

Atherosclerosis is a chronic systemic disease of elastic and muscular arteries with continuously ongoing immuno-inflammatory interaction between the vessel wall and blood components. Disease progression is characterized by development of endothelial dysfunction, infiltration of intimal layer by lipids, and inflammatory cells with consequent process of fibrosis *(15)*. At the cellular level endothelial dysfunction precipitates conversion of smooth muscle cells from contractile to the synthetic phenotype with subsequent proliferation and migration to the vascular intima, followed by platelet aggregation and release of growth factors.

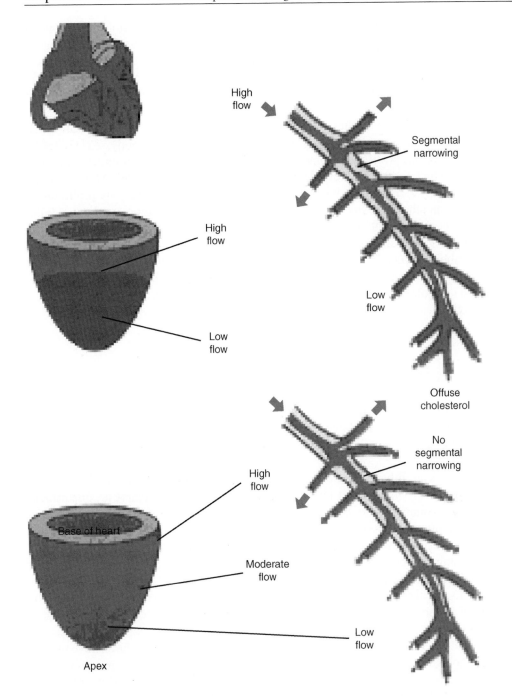

**Fig. 1.** Longitudinal, base-to-apex myocardial perfusion abnormality caused by diffuse coronary artery narrowing compared with segmental perfusion defects caused by localized stenoses *(12)*.

The relatively low resolution of nuclear imaging does not permit morphological imaging of the atherosclerotic plaque itself. However, functional imaging of the atherosclerotic wall has been proposed and tested using different strategies. Functional imaging uses various radioisotopes targeting specific cells or pathophysiological stages, such as proliferating smooth muscle cells, macrophages, lipids, or cholesterol content within the atherosclerotic lesion, or overlying thrombotic components. Several antigens known to uniquely target subintimal macrophages or the proliferating smooth muscle cells can be localized by radiolabeled monoclonal antibodies. Restenosis after PCI and allograft-related vascular disease are associated with accelerated proliferation of smooth muscle cells (16).

One of the feasibility studies performed by Narula et al. (17) demonstrated that $99^mTc$-based immuno imaging using a Fab' fragment of an antibody, Z2D3 (IgM), specifically identifies proliferating smooth muscle cells in the intima of human atheroma and rapidly detects atherosclerotic lesions in an experimental model. Mouse/human chimeric antibody Z2D3 (IgM) binds an antigen expressed exclusively by proliferating SMCs of human atheroma. In another experimental report, the authors used the radiolabeled purine analog, $99^mTc$-diadenosine tetraphosphate and its analog $99^mTc$-AppCHCIppA for noninvasive visualization of experimentally induced atherosclerotic lesions in rabbit aorta (18). The tracer accumulated within 15–30 min in atherosclerotic lesions whereas very low levels of accumulation were observed in normal tissues in the control group. Molecular imaging using $^{111}$Indium-Z2D3 was able to detect the proliferating smooth muscle cells 1 wk after stent placement in the swine model (19).

## MPI IN PATIENTS AFTER PCI

Radionuclide MPI should be seen as one of many available techniques that shape the management strategy of patients undergoing revascularization. Imaging of flow disturbances in patients with recurrent chest discomfort after PCI can serve as a gatekeeper for further invasive study. Radionuclide MPI can indeed provide objective evidence of myocardial ischemia, characterize, and localize its extent and indicate the likely presence of restenosis.

Unlike the case with experimental molecular approaches, restenosis can only be detected using MPI when vessel obstruction is severe enough to cause an impairment of maximal coronary blood flow with subsequent reduction of the coronary flow reserve. In addition, restenosis can manifest itself by recurrence of clinical symptoms and abnormal response to exercise stress electrocardiography. However, the presence or absence of angina pectoris has a low sensitivity for the detection of restenosis and myocardial ischemia following PCI (20–25).

Indeed, the recurrent manifestation of chest pain after PCI correlates poorly with the presence of restenosis (20–26). The positive predictive value of recurrent symptoms to identify restenosis ranges from 48 to 92%, whereas the range of negative predictive values varies between 70 and 98%. Even exercise-induced chest pain is an insensitive marker of angiographic restenosis (21). The specificity of chest pain is low because numerous noncardiac causes can cause chest discomfort. Incomplete revascularization or progression of atherosclerosis in the remote vascular territories also contributes to recurrent symptoms in the absence of restenosis at the dilated sites. Thus, the symptomatic status is not a powerful predictor of restenosis.

Likewise, the ECG response to exercise stress seems to be of limited sensitivity after PCI. Many patients have uninterpretable ST segment abnormalities at baseline or seem to be unable to reach maximal heart rates. The exercise electrocardiogram was predictive of neither recurrent angina nor restenosis (22–28). Lastly, silent clinical presentation of restenosis is quite common in the post-PCI patient population. The fact that approx

50% of patients with angiographic restenosis have no angina supports the performance of MPI in combination with clinical evaluation *(20)*. Stress MPI has higher sensitivity, specificity, and accuracy for the identification of restenosis than clinical symptoms alone or symptoms combined with stress ECG changes. Hence, the decision to repeat coronary angiography should be predominantly based on the clinical findings when supported by abnormal stress MPI *(29)*.

Although angiography remains the gold standard for measuring luminal narrowing and establishing the diagnosis of restenosis, routine repeat angiography is no longer performed after uneventful PCI. Routine angiography increases the number of revascularization procedures whereas rates of death and myocardial infarction (MI) are similar to those observed in patients randomized to undergo clinically-driven angiography *(30)*.

In clinical practice the decision to perform repeat angiography is taken when the patient has acute chest pain suggestive of abrupt vessel closure and when angina recurs within 4–9 mo after PCI. The emergence of noninvasive coronary angiography using either magnetic resonance imaging or multislice-computed tomography may offer new opportunities for the noninvasive assessment of coronary anatomy *(31)*. The improved image quality and the shorter acquisition time that can be achieved with the last generation multislice-computed tomography equipment (up to 64 slices) may affect the current follow-up strategy in patients after coronary revascularization *(32)*.

To which extent these techniques will affect the use or completely replace radionuclide MPI in the future remains to be determined. At present, the large body of evidence that demonstrates the value of MPI in patients after PCI was focused on evaluating clinically important issues such as:

1. Assessment of effectiveness of dilatation using balloon angioplasty or stenting in the myocardial territory supplied by the dilated vessel. Immediate changes in perfusion can be detected in the treated vessel territory using pre- and post-PCI imaging.
2. Assessment of the diagnostic performance of MPI in identifying restenosis, disease progression, and prediction of restenosis propensity.
3. Evaluation of prognosis.

### *Assessment of Effectiveness of PCI by MPI*

An accurate determination of the immediate functional result of revascularization can be achieved by performing MPI before and shortly after successful PCI, as demonstrated by the expected improvement in perfusion in the territory of the dilated artery. A change in myocardial perfusion toward normal in the territory of the dilated artery was observed in the majority of patients within the first week after successful PCI.

Hirzel et al. *(33)* showed that before PCI, myocardial perfusion abnormalities related to stenotic artery were present in 90% of patients. $^{201}$Tl tracer concentration in the territories of culprit arteries averaged 73 ± 2% of maximal tracer uptake. PCI resulted in augmentation of the relative $^{201}$Tl tracer concentration to 87 ± 2% of maximal activity ($p < 0.001$). Similar data were reported by Kanemoto *(34)* with an increase in $^{201}$Tl uptake from 72.9 ± 8.4 to 79.9 ± 11.7% ($p < 0.001$). DePuey et al. *(35)* showed that an improvement in myocardial perfusion can be achieved in 76% of patients within 1–2 d after successful PCI. The highest improvement in segmental $^{201}$Tl radionuclide uptake was achieved in the territories subtended by the most severely stenotic vessels, when the most noticeable enlargement in minimal luminal diameter was achieved. However, residual abnormalities on MPI (Fig. 2) can still be present early after successful PCI despite an angiographically optimal appearance of the epicardial vessel *(36–39)*.

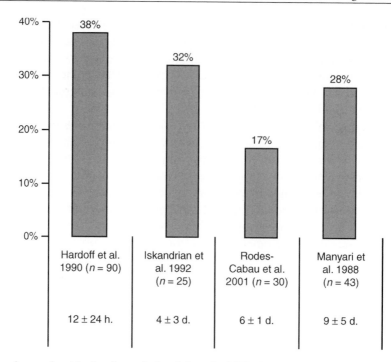

**Fig. 2.** Prevalence of residual early perfusion defects by MPI after stand-alone balloon PCI or stented angioplasty. Delay between PCI and MPI as indicated.

It appears that the early performance of MPI (within 1 wk after PCI) is limited by the high numbers of the segments with persistent decrease in tracer uptake. The causes for disagreement between results of MPI showing a reversible perfusion defect and optimal result by angiography were largely investigated. Particularly with stand-alone balloon PCI, pseudosuccesses are possible because of insufficient dilatation, dissection, elastic recoil of the vessel or distal embolization. Besides, endothelial and microvascular dysfunction with impaired coronary flow reserve can be present in patients with diffuse coronary atherosclerosis *(38,40,41)*.

Earlier studies were performed after stand-alone plain balloon angioplasty. Meanwhile stented angioplasty is performed in more than 80% of cases. Stent implantation results in larger luminal diameters and lower residual stenosis with elimination of elastic recoil. Only few reports have examined the impact of stent implantation on early postprocedural MPI. Rodes-Cabau *(38)* demonstrated the presence of abnormal perfusion scans in 17% of treated vascular territories 6 ± 1 d after successful stent implantation. The number of myocardial segments with reduced tracer uptake is lower but still present after stenting in comparison with reported data after plain balloon PCI (Fig. 2).

The incidence of reversible perfusion defects in the treated vascular territory can be as high as 54% following successful PCI or atherectomy and in 43% of patients within 48 h after stenting *(41)*. Using intracoronary ultrasound, investigators found that ischemic defects were associated with higher residual stenosis and higher plaque burden. However, there was significant overlap in residual stenosis values between patients with and without perfusion defects. The authors concluded that there are "additional mechanisms capable of impairing myocardial blood flow, such as endothelial dysfunction as a possible cause of perfusion defects following PCI."

Progressive reversal of microvascular dysfunction was felt to be responsible for the normalization of flow reserve over the weeks following coronary angioplasty, as indicated by quantitative PET measurements *(40)*. Why does flow reserve increase less than expected immediately after PCI given a good angiographic result? Various possibilities can be considered: resting flow is increased, the arteriolar bed does not dilate maximally or maximal flowthrough the epicardial vessel is impaired. The trauma induced by PCI to the vessel wall may induce the release of vasoconstrictor substances or embolization of debris limiting vasodilatation of the distal vasculature. Finally, the resting blood flow may increase because of a transient inability of the distal arteriolar bed to autoregulate in response to a sudden restoration of a normal perfusion pressure. Hence, a high incidence of false-positive myocardial perfusion abnormalities immediate after angioplasty could be related to delayed recovery of coronary flow reserve. This phenomenon might lead to an abnormal perfusion scan, even in the absence of recurrent stenosis of the epicardial conductance vessels.

Invasive intracoronary hemodynamic studies help to understand these discordant findings between MPI and angiography. Wilson et al. *(42)* showed that

1. Despite angiographically successful dilatation, coronary flow reserve remained abnormal in 55% of patients;
2. Flow reserve correlated poorly with lumen patency by angiography; and
3. It normalized in all patients who had no angiographic evidence of restenosis at 7.5 mo.

The author's group showed that altered vessel conductance by diffuse atherosclerosis could contribute to stress-induced myocardial ischemia and flow maldistribution on perfusion scintigrams *(43)*. This can be demonstrated by the presence of a continuous decline in pressure within coronary artery along the nonstenotic vessel length during hyperemia. Thus, even after effective dilatation of a focally stenotic segment of the epicardial coronary arteries, regional perfusion can remain impaired because of diffuse atherosclerosis of the conductance vessels and/or abnormal microvascular and resistive distal vessel function.

## Assessment of the Diagnostic Performance of MPI in Identifying Restenosis, Disease Progression, and Prediction of Propensity for Restenosis

Numerous MPI studies performed at various time-points after PCI have attempted to predict the occurrence of restenosis at late follow-up.

### PREDICTION OF DEVELOPMENT OF LATE RESTENOSIS WHEN MPI IS PERFORMED DURING THE FIRST WEEK AFTER PCI

The relationship between early reversible perfusion defects detected by MPI with subsequent development of early and late restenosis by angiography was extensively evaluated. A number of reports showed that the finding of a residual reversible perfusion defect early post-PCI was predictive for subsequent restenosis *(27–29,36,37,39,44–46)*.

For example, Hardoff et al. *(36)* found a reversible [201]Tl perfusion defect in 38% (39 out of 104) of myocardial regions supplied by the successfully dilated coronary vessel (90 consecutive patients) and identified a subset of patients at high risk of late (6–12 mo) angiographic restenosis (sensitivity 77%, specificity 67%). In contrast, late coronary restenosis developed in only 11% (7 of 65) of vessels and in 14% (5 of 37) of patients with a nonischemic [201]Tl scintigram on the first day after PCI. Therefore, it was stated that a reversible perfusion defect early after PCI and postangioplasty residual coronary narrowing are significant independent predictors of late restenosis *(36)*.

Few more recent studies have evaluated the effectiveness of early MPI in predicting late development of restenosis in patients after a coronary stent implantation. In a small series, stress $^{99m}$Tc-tetrofosmin MPI, using SPECT and performed at 6 ± 1 d after stented angioplasty, had a specificity of 94%, a sensitivity of 50%, and positive and negative predictive values of 75% and 84%, respectively, for the prediction of restenosis *(29)*. Investigators concluded that although these residual ischemic defects were associated with a high angiographic restenosis rate, the presence of normal MPI did not exclude late recurrence, as half of angiographic in-stent restenoses occurred in patients without residual ischemic defects at the time of early imaging.

## PREDICTION OF DEVELOPMENT OF LATE RESTENOSIS WHEN MPI IS PERFORMED 4 WK AFTER PCI

Prediction of future restenosis and consequent adverse events by thallium imaging performed within the first month after balloon angioplasty has been investigated by several authors *(27,46,52)*. For instance, Wijns et al. *(27,28)* showed that the presence of a reversible, exercise-induced defect within 4 wk after clinically successful PCI was predictive of the recurrence of angina in 66% of patients in whom it occurred with a negative predictive value of 83%. Stuckey et al. *(47,48)* performed quantitative exercise MPI at 2 wk after PCI in 68 asymptomatic patients of whom 23 (34%) patients developed recurrent angina at 10 mo follow-up. Abnormal MPI was a significant predictor of recurrent angina. MPI was abnormal in only 9% of patients who remained asymptomatic throughout the follow-up period. However, only nine of 23 patients with recurrent angina (39%) had abnormal MPI at 2 wk.

Again, Manyari et al. *(41)* pointed out that abnormal MPI soon after PCI does not necessarily reflect residual coronary stenosis or restenosis because perfusion in the territory of the dilated coronary artery progressively improves and completely normalizes by 3.3 mo. In 43 patients without evidence for previous MI before PCI and no signs of restenosis at 6–9 mo follow-up angiography, exercise thallium MPI was performed before PCI and repeated at 9 ± 5 d, 3.3 ± 0.6 mo, and 6.8 ± 1.2 mo. The sequential follow-up showed that initial perfusion defects normalized completely at 3.3 mo with no additional scintigraphic improvement demonstrable in the 6–9 mo studies.

As both hemodynamic and scintigraphic studies have demonstrated that perfusion abnormalities can persist for several days and weeks after PCI and resolve spontaneously, early MPI should not be used for restenosis prediction.

## IDENTIFICATION OF RESTENOSIS (LATE AFTER PCI)

Optimal timing for noninvasive detection of restenosis should be based on the time-course of neointimal proliferation, as known from sequential angiographic studies (Fig. 3).

Several reports *(29,49–54)* have indicated the ability of SPECT 201Tl imaging to accurately diagnose restenosis (Table 1). Hecht et al. *(49)* studied 116 patients who underwent SPECT imaging 6.4 ± 3.1 mo after PCI and 1-wk before repeat coronary angiography. Sensitivity, specificity, and accuracy values for the detection of restenosis were 93, 77, and 86%, respectively. The authors concluded that MPI imaging can be used to identify the treated vessel as causing recurrent ischemia against progression of atherosclerosis in other vessels.

More recently, Galassi et al. *(29)* applied exercise $^{99m}$Tc SPECT for detection of restenosis in 594 myocardial regions corresponding to 107 vascular territories in 97 patients following stented angioplasty. By MPI 94 reversible defects were present.

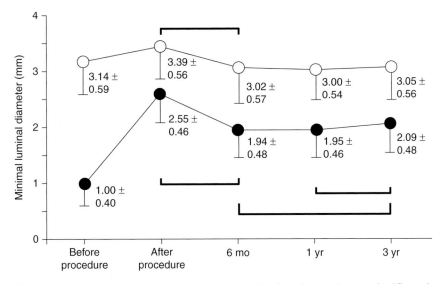

**Fig. 3.** The reduction is luminal diameter occurs during the first 6 mo whereas significant improvement can take place from 1 to 3 yr. For restenosis identification purposes, MPI is the best performed after 6 mo as the probability for further restenosis development is limited *(48)*.

Thirty-three of 107 (31%) vascular territories showed "in-stent" restenosis. Using stress SPECT, the identification of restenosis was obtained with a sensitivity of 82%, a specificity of 84%, and a predictive accuracy of 83%. The accuracy of the test was not affected by the achievement of maximal heart rate during exercise. Therefore, it was concluded that stress tetrofosmin SPECT imaging can identify in-stent restenosis more accurately than clinical symptoms and electrocardiographic changes. Abnormal MPI studies in the absence of in-stent restenosis are sometimes to be related to side branch stenosis or occlusion.

Interestingly, SPECT imaging seems to be more accurate for the diagnosis of restenosis after stented than after balloon angioplasty. One explanation could be that stents were used preferentially in larger vessels that supply larger areas of myocardium and yet, more easily detectable by noninvasive imaging when ischemic.

In conclusion, accurate identification of restenosis by MPI is achievable by stress-rest MPI using reversibility of stress defects as the diagnostic criterion.

### SPECIFIC ISSUES: INFARCT REGIONS AND MULTIVESSEL DISEASE

In the study by Kosa et al. *(52)*, the assessment of restenosis in previously infarcted regions (*n* = 48) yielded a lower sensitivity and specificity of 64% and 72%, respectively. Here, quantitative analysis might preferable to visual analysis by allowing the detection of more subtle perfusion changes in the infarcted territory. Sensitivity is lower in vessels subtending previously infarcted myocardium (Table 2).

In patients with multivessel disease, the rate of restenosis after multivessel intervention is considered to be higher *(54)*. Patient outcome and prognosis will be worse if restenosis develops in two or three vessels causing a large segment of the myocardium to become at risk of ischemia. The main limitation of MPI SPECT in multivessel patients is that only the most severely ischemic segments can be detected, as a result of the relative nature of MPI. Diagnostic performance will thus be affected by completeness of revascularization (Table 3). Nevertheless, in patients with multivessel disease and complete revascularization, the sensitivity of MPI was significantly higher than

Table 1
Results of MPI for the Detection of Restenosis After PCI

| Author | Year | No. of patients | Method used | Time after PTCA | Sensitivity | Specificity | Accuracy | Definition of restenosis (diameter reduction) |
|--------|------|-----------------|-------------|-----------------|-------------|-------------|----------|-----------------------------------------------|
| Hecht et al. | 1990 | 116 | 201Tl SPECT | | 93 | 77 | 86 | >50 |
| DePuey et al. | 1989 | 40 | 99mTc SPECT | | 86 | 84 | | >50 |
| Milan et al. | 1996 | 37 | 99mTc SPECT | | 88 | 78 | 83 | >50 |
| Kosa et al. | 1998 | 82 | 201Tl and 99mTc SPECT | 210 ± 130 d | 79 | 78 | 79 | >50 (100% of stents) |
| Galassi et al. | 2000 | 97 | 99mTc SPECT | 128 ± 41 d | 82 | 84 | 83 | >50 (100% of stents) |
| Milavetz et al. | 1998 | 218 | 201Tl or 99mTc SPECT | | 95 | 73 | 88 | >70 |
| Beygui et al. | 2000 | 179 | 201Tl SPECT | 6 ± 2 mo | 63 | 77 | 71 | >50 (16% of stents) |

SPECT, single-photon emission computed tomography.

Table 2
Restenosis Detection by MPI in Coronary Arteries Adjacent to Infarcted Myocardium

| Author | Modality | Sensitivity (%) | | Specificity (%) | | Accuracy (%) | |
|---|---|---|---|---|---|---|---|
| | | Infarct-related vessels | Noninfarct-related vessels | Infarct-related vessels | Noninfarct-related vessels | Infarct-related vessels | Noninfarct-related vessels |
| Beygui F. et al. | SPECT | 71 | 56 | 63 | 81 | 67 | 74 |
| Galassi et al. | $^{99m}$Tc SPECT | 88 | 76 | 71 | 95 | 76 | 89 |
| Kosa et al. | $^{201}$Tl/$^{99m}$Tc | 64 | 100 | 72 | 82 | 70 | 85 |

Table 3
The Detection of Restenosis by MPI in Patients With Multiple Vessel Disease After Complete vs Incomplete Revascularization

| Author | Modality | Sensitivity (%) | | Specificity (%) | | Accuracy (%) | |
|---|---|---|---|---|---|---|---|
| | | Partial | Complete | Partial | Complete | Partial | Complete |
| Hecht et al. | $^{201}$Tl SPECT | 93 | 93 | 77 | 76 | 85 | 87 |
| Galassi et al. | $^{99m}$Tc SPECT | 63 | 100 | 81 | 86 | 75 | 91 |
| Beygui et al. | $^{201}$Tl SPECT | 67 | 62 | 57 | 84 | 60 | 76 |

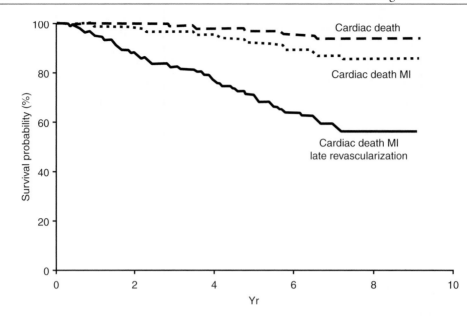

**Fig. 4.** Long-term event rate in patients with normal left ventricular function after PCI: The Kaplan-Meier survival curves for survival free of cardiac death, cardiac death/MI, cardiac death/MI/late revascularization.

that of the presence of angina or exercise testing *(54)*. Other investigators noted that incomplete coronary revascularization increased the sensitivity of MPI whereas the specificity decreased *(28,49)*. The resolution of the imaging modality may not be high enough to distinguish ischemia. Because of disease elsewhere in the body it results in restenosis from ischemia.

### *Evaluation of Long-Term Prognosis After PCI: The Prognostic Value of MPI*

Stress MPI was shown to convey very strong prognostic information in patients with coronary artery disease. Several studies have specifically been designed to evaluate the prognostic value of MPI in patients after successful PCI *(26,55–57)*. The results demonstrate that stress-rest SPECT MPI performed beyond the time of restenosis window does bear longer term prognostic value, which is superior to exercise stress testing and symptoms.

Clinical and angiographic outcomes up to 10 yr after PCI and stenting are favorable, with low rate of repeat revascularization at the treated site *(55)*. Therefore, patients without residual ischemia and good left ventricular function after successful PCI represent a low-risk population subgroup (Fig. 4).

Conversely, the patients with detectable ischemia at stress-rest SPECT MPI had an increased rate of cardiac death, MI, and need for repeat revascularization at long-term follow-up in comparison with patients without ischemia *(55–59)*. There was a high incidence (31%) of silent ischemia in patients with ischemic stress MPI scans *(26,55,58)*. Multivariate analysis allows to identify predictors of poor outcome *(55,57,59)*. Summed stress score at MPI is a robust measure of total ischemia and is significantly associated ($p = 0.047$) with the hard end points of cardiac death or MI (Table 4).

Table 4
Univariate Associations Between Variables Derived From Exercise and MPI Imaging With Cardiac Death or MI and With Late PCI/CABG (>2–3 mo After MPI)

| Author | Variable | $\chi^2$ | p-value | Hazard ratio | 95% CI |
|---|---|---|---|---|---|
| Ho et al. | Summed stress score | 3.1 | 0.078 | 0.98 | 0.96–1 |
| | Summed reversibility score | 1 | <0.312 | 1.03 | 0.98–1.08 |
| | Duke score | 9.2 | <0.002 | 0.94 | 0.91–0.98 |
| Acampa et al. | Summed stress score | 3.9 | <0.05 | 1 | 1–1.1 |
| | Summed difference score | 30.9 | <0.001 | 1.4 | 1.2–1.6 |
| | Duke score | 1 | NS | 1 | 0.9–1.1 |

In a series of 152 patients studied 5 mo after stented angioplasty, a strong relationship between ischemic defects and major cardiac events has been demonstrated, irrespective of the symptomatic status *(60)*. Acampa et al. *(57)* showed that extent and severity of reversible perfusion defects at SPECT (summed difference score) strongly predicts event-free survival late after PCI. The cumulative probability of event-free survival after 55 mo was 89% in patients without ischemia and 27% in those with ischemia ($p < 0.001$). The incidence of cardiac events was higher in patients with ischemic perfusion scans irrespective of the presence or absence of angina pectoris. The question how long the patient remains at low risk was answered by Hachamovitch et al. *(59)*. In a study of 7376 consecutive patients with a normal exercise or adenosine myocardial perfusion scintography study, the investigators showed that a normal MPI study confers good prognosis for up to 1.8 yr. Another issue relates to the significance of silent ischemia after PCI *(60)*. As already mentioned, the presence of ischemia on stress MPI—rather than the symptomatic status—is a strong predictor for future adverse cardiac events *(55)*.

## SUMMARY STATEMENTS

- Patients with recurrent typical angina pectoris less than 6 mo after PTCA should undergo coronary angiography.
- Decisions to perform revascularization in patients with restenosis should be based not only on the presence of restenosis at angiography, but rather on the results of functional testing using MPI or surrogate invasive techniques.
- High-risk asymptomatic patients with decreased left ventricular function, multivessel disease, proximal left anterior descending disease, previous sudden cardiac death, diabetes mellitus, hazardous occupations, and suboptimal PCI results should undergo MPI during follow-up, irrespective of symptomatic status.
- Stress MPI should be performed in asymptomatic patients after uncomplicated, angiographically successful PCI if the exercise ECG is abnormal.
- Atypical symptoms after revascularization can be evaluated by stress MPI.
- If angina recurs more than 6 mo after PTCA, stress MPI can be used to assess the extent and location of ischemia, as progression of native coronary disease rather than in-stent restenosis is likely.
- The ability of MPI to diagnose restenosis and to differentiate it from the progression of coronary disease can assist in the management of these patients.
- Given the high incidence of silent ischemia in patients with restenosis, stress-rest MPI enables to stratify patients in high- and low-risk subgroups.
- Coronary angiography is superfluous in patients with normal MPI scans, which is predictive of a good long-term prognosis.
- The presence of a reversible defect at MPI is related to increased probability of subsequent cardiac events, prompting a more aggressive therapeutic approach to these patients.

## CONCLUSIONS

Currently, MPI has been shown to be the most reliable technique to follow patients who have undergone revascularization. Stress-rest MPI after revascularization is particularly helpful in clinical decision making for identifying causes of recurrent chest pain as well as in high-risk asymptomatic patients. At present, guidelines do not recommend to perform systematic stress MPI test in patients after PTCA *(7,8)*. However, if there is an indication for stress testing, stress MPI is superior to exercise stress testing on the basis of its ability to predict hard cardiac events and patient outcome.

# 17 Magnetic Resonance Imaging for Restenosis

*Robert Jan M. van Geuns, MD, PhD
and Timo Baks, MD*

## INTRODUCTION

Magnetic resonance imaging (MRI) of the coronary arteries is a difficult subject. Owing to the motion of the heart during contraction and respiration artefact free imaging needs extremely fast techniques that MRI does not fully qualify yet. However, constant progress is made *(1)* and with electrocardiography triggering and respiratory motion correction techniques, submilliter resolution can be achieved with reasonable acquisition times *(2)*. Only one study focussed on the use of magnetic resonance (MR) coronary angiography techniques for the detection of restenosis after coronary angioplasty *(3)*. In this study, in which 118 patients after percutaneous transluminal coronary angioplasty were investigated, sensitivity for restenosis detection was 73% (11/15) and specificity was 49%. Overall accuracy was 53% for MRI, which was significantly ($p = 0.014$) lower compared with electron beam computed tomography. Unfortunately, MR coronary angiography of restenosis is currently hindered by the obligatory use of coronary artery stents to decrease the incidence of restenosis. Still MRI for the detection of restenosis is being performed using different alternative techniques and this subject will be reviewed in this chapter.

## SAFETY OF STENTS

Coronary artery stents have demonstrated their efficacy as additional treatment in angioplasty, initially for treatment of abrupt vessel closure or dissection, but later also for reducing restenosis as demonstrated in the STRESS and BENESTENT studies *(4,5)*.

From: *Contemporary Cardiology: Essentials of Restenosis: For the Interventional Cardiologist*
Edited by: H. J. Duckers, E. G. Nabel, and P. W. Serruys © Humana Press Inc., Totowa, NJ

Since then stents have been used in more than 80% of percutaneous coronary intervention (PCI) procedures in 2000 and presently this approaches 100%. As most stents are produced of 316 low-carbon Stainless steel, safety in MRI scanners has always been an issue. First, the magnetic field deploys a force on the stent depending on the static magnetic field strength (usually 1 or 1.5 T, in the future 3 T) and the applied gradients during the examination (6), the materials used (degree of ferromagnetism), the mass of the implant used, and the location and orientation relative to the magnetic field. These induced forces may in theory lead to displacement of the stent. Nevertheless these forces are much smaller then those used during implantation or those that the stents experience during motion of the heart at the time of contraction (7). The second issue is heating because stents are closed loops of conductive low-ferromagnetism materials and rapid changing magnetic forces can induce electrical currents that can cause local heating. Thermal injuries during MR examination associated with electrical monitoring devices have been described (8). Radiofrequency (RF) pulses used are a second source of heating. Several studies have evaluated the heating effects in MR scanners, in one study on a nitinol-based guidewire, temperature rose by a maximum of 48°C in a phantom (9,10). Heating of MR tracking catheters has also been reported (11), although to a lesser degree. Studies on coronary artery stents on the other hand showed a maximum rise of 0.3°C in one study (12) and no significant heating effects in another (7,13,14). This is explained by the length of the conducting material used and by flow phantoms that allow some cooling by continuous refreshment of the blood within the stent.

MRI after stent implantation is considered to be safe once endothelialization has occurred (15), because endothelialization presumably opposes possible dislodgement (16,17). Actual patient information on the Internet by the American Heart Association advises to postpone MR imaging till 4 wk after the procedure. On the contrary, the American Heart Association Diagnostic and Interventional Catheterization Committee does not preclude MRI in the presence of coronary stents when it is clinically indicated (18). Additionally, Gerber et al. (19) have demonstrated in a retrospective clinical trial the safety of MRI within 8 wk (median of 18 d) after stent implantation in 111 patients; no stent thrombosis or cardiac death occurred within 30 d. Recent studies in celltransplantation mostly treated with PCI including stent implantation, using repetitive MRI measurements (TOPCARE-AMI and BOOST, mean 4.7 and 3.5 d postPCI, respectively) showed no adverse events (20,21). Supported by these last studies no restrictions on MRI after coronary stent implantation are applied in the institution.

## STENT RELATED ARTEFACTS

Currently, the majority of coronary stents are nonferromagnetic and considered MRI safe as explained earlier, but stents remain the source of image artefacts owing to local magnetic field inhomogeneities and provoked eddy currents in the conductive material of the stent, hampering image interpretation. The size of the artefacts is dependent on the materials and imaging sequences used. Here in principle Spin-echo techniques and its derivatives show significant smaller artefacts than gradient echo-sequences (7). Comparing 14 different stents lumen was visible in all except one colbalt stent, and in 10 of the 14 stents artificial lumen narrowing was less than 33%, using a contrast enhanced magnetic resonance angiography sequences that can be considered standard for noncoronary angiography (22). Best results were obtained with Nitinol (a nickel–titanium alloy) and Tantalum stents, although within the Nitinol stents a variable appearance was observed depending on the stent geometry. Artefacts are reduced by

Table 1
Sensitivity and Specificity of MR Coronary Flow Measurements
for the Detection of Restenosis After PCI

| Restenosis | Year | Treatment | Patients | Sign | Sensitivity | Specificity |
|---|---|---|---|---|---|---|
| Hundley | 2000 | Ballon | 17 | ≤50% | 82 | 100 |
| Saito | 2001 | Stent | 10 | – | – | – |
| Nagel | 2003 | Stent | 38 | ≥75% | 83 | 94 |

using short echo-times wherein the shorter echo-times in gradient-echo sequences can compensate for the increased sensitivity of GE imaging to field inhomogeneities. Besides the materials and techniques used it was shown that the angle β to B0 was the main factor that influenced the artefact size, with a larger angle increasing the artefact in a nonlinear relationship (23–25). As artefacts hamper lumen visualization on most MRA and all MR coronary angiography techniques after current stent treatment, alternative analysis techniques and stent material and design are being investigated.

## MR FLOW MEASUREMENTS

A very attractive tool in MRI is the ability to noninvasive measure flow with dedicated MR flow sensitive techniques. This has been used to quantify valve regurgitation and stenosis (26) and is frequently used in congenital heart disease (27). The same technique has been used to quantify flow in the coronary arteries and detection of flow-limiting stenosis in native coronary arteries (28–30) and bypass grafts (31–33) using vasodilatators. In these settings a reasonable sensitivity and specificity for graft function has been obtained. Hundley et al. (34) used these flow techniques to measure flow reserve in patients with recurrent angina after balloon angioplasty. For a flow reserve of less than 2, 100% and 82% sensitive and 89% and 100% specific, detecting a luminal diameter narrowing of less than or equal to 70% and 50%, respectively was achieved (Table 1). The same approach was used by Saito et al. (35) for the detection of instent restenosis, with the modification that flow was measured just distal from the stent to avoid the imaging artefact related to stainless steel stents. They demonstrated that flow could accurately be measured just distal to the stent (Fig. 1). Nagel et al. (36) studied 38 patients after successful PCI with stent deployment with this approach and coronary flow velocity reserve with MRI similar to Doppler results ($r = 0.87$), with a mean relative difference of 7.5%. Using a threshold of 1.2 for coronary flow velocity reserve, a sensitivity of 83% with a specificity of 94% was achieved for more than or equal to 75% stenoses. In both these studies imaging was limited to the proximal vessels and left anterior descending coronary arteries were nearly exclusively included, additionally, patients with suspected microvasculare disease were excluded.

## MR COMPATIBLE (TRANSPARENT) STENTS

Metallic stents signal attenuation within the stent is caused by RF (RF shielding) of the metallic stent material. Induced eddy currents in the stent may also lead to a lower nominal RF excitation angle inside the stent (37,38). Only with large-diameter nitinol stents in the iliac arteries have sufficiently small artefacts been reported to allow diagnostic follow-up, either by standard MRA (39) or by increasing the excitation angle of the MRA sequence (23). As the material of stent is of great influence on stent artefact,

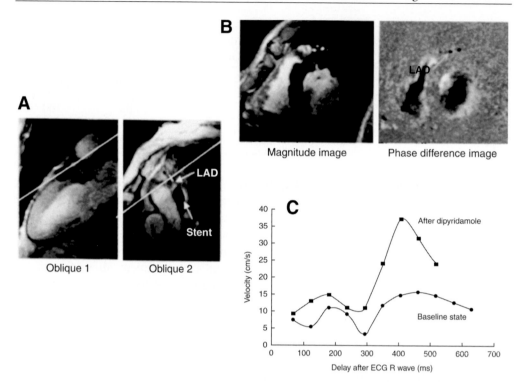

**Fig. 1. (A)** Definition of slice location for MRI blood flow measurements in the LAD artery on double oblique scout magnetic resonance imaging (MRI) images. **(B)** Magnitude and phase-difference images acquired with fast velocity-encoded cine MRI acquisition. **(C)** MRI blood flow velocity curves in the LAD artery before and after intravenous injection of dipyridamole. Reproduced from ref. *35.*

a quest for metal alloys with minimal artefacts was started to develop a truly MR transparent stent. One alloy consisting of copper (75%), silver (8%), platinum (2%), gold (14%), and palladium (1%) was proposed to minimize susceptibility artefacts *(40)*. The examined prototypes of fully MR-compatible MRI stents allowed artefact-free visualization of the stent lumen with phase-contrast and contrast-enhanced T1-weighted angiography, as well as phase-contrast flow measurements in the stented area *(41)*.

As copper can induce an inflammatory reaction causing in-stent restenosis, the large amount in this alloy is worrying, but biocompatible coatings of the MR stent may solve this problem. Another alloy proposed by van Dijk et al. *(42)* consists mainly of palladium and silver and is iron- and nickel-free. The mechanical properties of ABI alloy resemble Stainless steel. Using 2D and 3D gradient echo sequences artefacts of this ABI alloy stent was significantly smaller than Nitinol or Tantalum stent. So far only a simple helix has been built out of this material.

The BIOTRONIK absorbable metal stent (BIOTRONIK, Bulach, Switzerland) is a magnesium alloy stent that undergoes degradation over 2- to 3-mo period after deployment. This stent is reported compatible with MR angiography. As the stent is absorbable their use does not require prolonged antiplatelet therapy and neointimal proliferation, restenosis, and chronic inflammation may be reduced. Recently, results from a first-in-man BEST BTK trial, in which absorbable metal stents were implanted below the knee were reported (EuroPCR2004). Between December 2003 and January 2004, 63 patients with critical limb ischemia were enrolled just before limb amputation

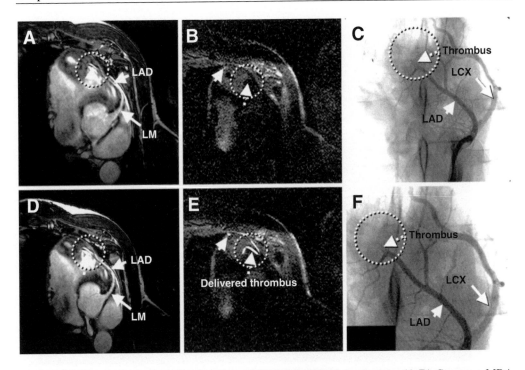

**Fig. 2.** In vivo magnetic resonance imaging of Gd-labeled fibrinogen clots. **(A,D)** Coronary MRA before (A) and after (D) thrombus delivery. On both scans, no apparent thrombus is visible (circle). **(B,E)** Black-blood inversion recovery TFE scans before (B) and after (E) clot delivery (same view as A and D). After thrombus delivery (E), 3 bright areas are readily visible (arrows and circle), consistent with location of thrombus. No apparent thrombus was visible on prethrombus (B) images (arrow and circle). **(C)** X-ray angiogram confirming MR finding of thrombus in mid-LAD (circle). **(F)** Magnified view of C. LM indicates left main. Reproduced from ref. *43.*

(Rutherford 4 and 5). At 3 mo, 89% of the stented vessels remained patent and a randomized trial is planned by the company. One limitation is that the magnesium alloy is not visible on fluoroscopy, which is partly resolved by two markers on the balloon that guide the procedure. With this kind of stent, instent thrombus has been identified for the first time noninvasively *(43)* (Fig. 2).

Another interesting approach to visualize the stent lumen is to use the stent as a receiver coil itself *(44)*. To achieve this stents need to be designed to act as active resonant structures at the Larmor frequency of the MR system. The stents thus acted as local RF signal amplifiers. The first generation used a coaxial cable to transport the signal to the scanner system. However, such a cable-based approach for high-resolution in-stent imaging is invasive and thus is limited to the time of the intervention. Follow-up studies would be difficult to achieve, because the approach requires electrical contact between the stent and the MR scanner, and hence repeated invasive access. In a more sophisticated way, Quick et al. *(45)* employed the principle of inductive coupling wherein the B(1) fields of the stents were coupled to that of an outside surface coil. Thus, the signal from the stent antenna could be wireless and received by a surface coil connected to the MR system (Fig. 3). This concept has been tested in vitro and in vivo and a near 30 times improvement in signal intensity in the stent lumen has been demonstrated. Unfortunately, several limitations are to be noted. First, low flip angle sequences were necessary as transmit flip angles were also amplified and artefacts were introduced owing to inhomogeneity of the B1 field of the stent.

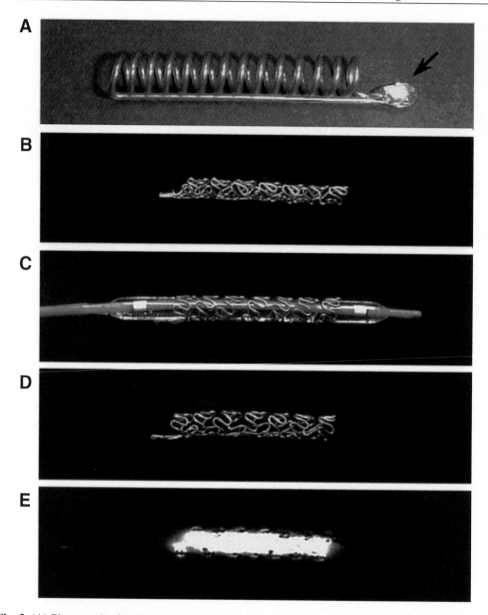

**Fig. 3. (A)** Photograph of a solenoidal stent prototype (length 35 mm, inner diameter 4 mm). The 14-turn solenoidal stent mesh was tuned with a chip capacitor (arrow) to the resonant frequency of the scanner. **(B)** Photograph of a balloon-expandable self-resonant stent prototype (length 28 mm, inner diameter before/after expansion 1.8/4 mm); stent in the folded state, **(C)** stent mounted on a 5F balloon catheter (balloon $40 \times 4$ mm$^2$) after full inflation of balloon, **(D)** fully deployed stent, and **(E)** MR image acquired with the stent immersed in an NaCl phantom acquired with the following sequence: FLASH 2D sequence, TR/TE = 200/11 ms, flip = 2°, FOV = $60 \times 60$ mm$^2$, matrix = $512 \times 512$, slice = 2 mm$^2$, time = 1:44 min, in-plane resolution $117 \times 117$ m$^2$. Reproduced from ref. *45.*

Additionally, the use of RF-intensive sequences potentially by this amplification can lead to local concentration of RF energy (hot spots) in the vicinity of the stent, which could result in heating of surrounding tissues. Decoupling, i.e., detuning of the resonant structure during RF transmission, would decrease the potential risk of RF heating, and can be achieved passively by incorporation of additional electronic elements (e.g., crossed diodes) in the design. Second, optimal stent design for balloon-expandable delivery is more difficult and the redesigned solenoidal design with a zigzag pattern of the stent wire resulted in local signal cancellations (Fig. 3). Third, the stents should be coated with a polymer to guarantee electric isolation from the surrounding tissue and blood, otherwise electricity and therefore signal may be lost. One author performed a study on heating of coronary artery stents with the intention to induce cell necrosis and thereby restenosis *(46)*. Afterwards with maximum energy power output they were able to raise the temperature of the stent to 80°C with necrosis on microscopy.

## SUMMARY

In the past coronary artery stents where regarded as possible contraindications for MRI. Additional safety studies have resolved this issue and MRI is now frequently performed even within the first days of implantation. Artefacts related to the stent hinder image interpretation but flow measurement just distal of a stent have proven to be able to detect significant instent restenosis. More recent development includes MR transparent stents and in the future, stent might serve as local imaging coils to increase signal to noise ratio.

## REFERENCES

1. van Geuns RJ, Wielopolski PA, de Bruin HG, et al. Magnetic resonance imaging of the coronary arteries: techniques and results. Prog Cardiovasc Dis 1999;42:157–166.
2. Stuber M, Botnar RM, Danias PG, et al. Double-oblique free-breathing high resolution three-dimensional coronary magnetic resonance angiography. J Am Coll Cardiol 1999;34:524–531.
3. Ropers D, Regenfus M, Stilianakis N, et al. A direct comparison of noninvasive coronary angiography by electron beam tomography and navigator-echo-based magnetic resonance imaging for the detection of restenosis following coronary angioplasty. Invest Radiol 2002;37:386–392.
4. Schatz RA, Baim DS, Leon M, et al. Clinical experience with the Palmaz-Schatz coronary stent. Initial results of a multicenter study. Circulation 1991;83:148–161.
5. Serruys PW, de Jaegere P, Kiemeneij F, et al. A comparison of balloon-expandable-stent implantation with balloon angioplasty in patients with coronary artery disease. Benestent Study Group. N Engl J Med 1994;331:489–495.
6. Shellock FG. Biological effects and safety aspects of magnetic resonance imaging. Magn Reson Q 1989;5:243–261.
7. Hug J, Nagel E, Bornstedt A, Schnackenburg B, Oswald H, Fleck E. Coronary arterial stents: safety and artifacts during MR imaging. Radiology 2000;216:781–787.
8. Dempsey MF, Condon B. Thermal injuries associated with MRI. Clin Radiol 2001;56:457–465.
9. Konings MK, Bartels LW, Smits HF, Bakker CJ. Heating around intravascular guidewires by resonating RF waves. J Magn Reson Imaging 2000;12:79–85.
10. Liu CY, Farahani K, Lu DS, Duckwiler G, Oppelt A. Safety of MRI-guided endovascular guidewire applications. J Magn Reson Imaging 2000;12:75–78.
11. Wildermuth S, Dumoulin CL, Pfammatter T, Maier SE, Hofmann E, Debatin JF. MR-guided percutaneous angioplasty: assessment of tracking safety, catheter handling and functionality. Cardiovasc Intervent Radiol 1998;21:404–410.
12. Shellock FG, Shellock VJ. Metallic stents: evaluation of MR imaging safety. AJR Am J Roentgenol 1999;173:543–547.
13. Friedrich MG, Strohm O, Kivelitz D, et al. Behaviour of implantable coronary stents during magnetic resonance imaging. Int J Cardiovasc Intervent 1999;2:217–222.
14. Strohm O, Kivelitz D, Gross W, et al. Safety of implantable coronary stents during 1H-magnetic resonance imaging at 1.0 and 1.5 T. J Cardiovasc Magn Reson 1999;1:239–245.
15. Roubin GS, Robinson KA, King SB 3rd, et al. Early and late results of intracoronary arterial stenting after coronary angioplasty in dogs. Circulation 1987;76:891–897.
16. Shellock F. Pocket Guide to MR Procedures and Metallic Objects: Update 2001. Lippincott Williams & Wilkins, Philadelphia, PA, 2001.
17. Jost C, Kumar VV. Are Current Cardiovascular Stents MRI Safe? J Invasive Cardiol 1998; 10:477–479.

18. Levine GN, Kern MJ, Berger PB, et al. Management of patients undergoing percutaneous coronary revascularization. Ann Intern Med 2003;139:123–136.

19. Gerber TC, Fasseas P, Lennon RJ, et al. Clinical safety of magnetic resonance imaging early after coronary artery stent placement. J Am Coll Cardiol 2003;42:1295–1298.

20. Britten MB, Abolmaali ND, Assmus B, et al. Infarct remodeling after intracoronary progenitor cell treatment in patients with acute myocardial infarction (TOPCARE-AMI): mechanistic insights from serial contrast-enhanced magnetic resonance imaging. Circulation 2003;108:2212–2218.

21. Wollert KC, Meyer GP, Lotz J, et al. Intracoronary autologous bone-marrow cell transfer after myocardial infarction: the BOOST randomised controlled clinical trial. Lancet 2004;364:141–148.

22. Lenhart M, Volk M, Manke C, et al. Stent appearance at contrast-enhanced MR angiography: in vitro examination with 14 stents. Radiology 2000;217:173–178.

23. Meyer JM, Buecker A, Schuermann K, Ruebben A, Guenther RW. MR evaluation of stent patency: in vitro test of 22 metallic stents and the possibility of determining their patency by MR angiography. Invest Radiol 2000;35:739–746.

24. Bartels LW, Smits HF, Bakker CJ, Viergever MA. MR imaging of vascular stents: effects of susceptibility, flow, and radiofrequency eddy currents. J Vasc Interv Radiol 2001;12:365–371.

25. Meyer JM, Buecker A, Spuentrup E, et al. Improved in-stent magnetic resonance angiography with high flip angle excitation. Invest Radiol 2001;36:677–681.

26. Caruthers SD, Lin SJ, Brown P, et al. Practical value of cardiac magnetic resonance imaging for clinical quantification of aortic valve stenosis: comparison with echocardiography. Circulation 2003;108:2236–2243.

27. Simpson IA, Chung KJ, Glass RF, Sahn DJ, Sherman FS, Hesselink J. Cine magnetic resonance imaging for evaluation of anatomy and flow relations in infants and children with coarctation of the aorta. Circulation 1988;78:142–148.

28. Clarke GD, Eckels R, Chaney C, et al. Measurement of absolute epicardial coronary artery flow and flow reserve with breath-hold cine phase-contrast magnetic resonance imaging. Circulation 1995;91: 2627–2634.

29. Hundley WG, Lange RA, Clarke GD, et al. Assessment of coronary arterial flow and flow reserve in humans with magnetic resonance imaging. Circulation 1996;93:1502–1508.

30. Davis CP, Liu PF, Hauser M, et al. Coronary flow and coronary flow reserve measurements in humans with breath-held magnetic resonance phase contrast velocity mapping. Magn Reson Med 1997; 37:537–544.

31. Hoogendoorn LI, Pattynama PM, Buis B, et al. Noninvasive evaluation of aortocoronary bypass grafts with magnetic resonance flow mapping. Am J Cardiol 1995;75:845–848.

32. Galjee MA, van Rossum AC, Doesburg T, Hofman MB, Falke TH, Visser CA. Quantification of coronary artery bypass graft flow by magnetic resonance phase velocity mapping. Magn Reson Imaging 1996;14:485–493.

33. Langerak SE, Kunz P, de Roos A, Vliegen HW, van Der Wall EE. Evaluation of coronary artery bypass grafts by magnetic resonance imaging. J Magn Reson Imaging 1999;10:434–441.

34. Hundley WG, Hillis LD, Hamilton CA, et al. Assessment of coronary arterial restenosis with phase-contrast magnetic resonance imaging measurements of coronary flow reserve. Circulation 2000; 101:2375–2381.

35. Saito Y, Sakuma H, Shibata M, et al. Assessment of coronary flow velocity reserve using fast velocity-encoded cine MRI for noninvasive detection of restenosis after coronary stent implantation. J Cardiovasc Magn Reson 2001;3:209–214.

36. Nagel E, Thouet T, Klein C, et al. Noninvasive determination of coronary blood flow velocity with cardiovascular magnetic resonance in patients after stent deployment. Circulation 2003;107: 1738–1743.

37. Maintz D, Kugel H, Schellhammer F, Landwehr P. In vitro evaluation of intravascular stent artifacts in three-dimensional MR angiography. Invest Radiol 2001;36:218–224.

38. Bartels LW, Bakker CJ, Viergever MA. Improved lumen visualization in metallic vascular implants by reducing RF artifacts. Magn Reson Med 2002;47:171–180.

39. Juergens KU, Tombach B, Reimer P, Vestring T, Heindel W. Three-dimensional contrast-enhanced MR angiography of endovascular covered stents in patients with peripheral arterial occlusive disease. AJR Am J Roentgenol 2001;176:1299–1303.

40. Buecker A, Spuentrup E, Ruebben A, Gunther RW. Artifact-free in-stent lumen visualization by standard magnetic resonance angiography using a new metallic magnetic resonance imaging stent. Circulation 2002;105:1772–1775.

41. Buecker A, Spuentrup E, Ruebben A, et al. New metallic MR stents for artifact-free coronary MR angiography: feasibility study in a swine model. Invest Radiol 2004;39:250–253.
42. van Dijk LC, van Holten J, van Dijk BP, Matheijssen NA, Pattynama PM. A precious metal alloy for construction of MR imaging-compatible balloon-expandable vascular stents. Radiology 2001;219:284–287.
43. Botnar RM, Perez AS, Witte S, et al. In vivo molecular imaging of acute and subacute thrombosis using a fibrin-binding magnetic resonance imaging contrast agent. Circulation 2004;109:2023–2029.
44. Quick HH, Ladd ME, Nanz D, Mikolajczyk KP, Debatin JF. Vascular stents as RF antennas for intravascular MR guidance and imaging. Magn Reson Med 1999;42:738–745.
45. Quick HH, Kuehl H, Kaiser G, Bosk S, Debatin JF, Ladd ME. Inductively coupled stent antennas in MRI. Magn Reson Med 2002;48:781–790.
46. Floren MG, Gunther RW, Schmitz-Rode T. Noninvasive inductive stent heating: alternative approach to prevent instent restenosis? Invest Radiol 2004;39:264–270.

# 18 Coronary Imaging With Multislice Spiral Computed Tomography

*Koen Nieman, MD, PhD*

## INTRODUCTION

In the past decade, the introduction of noninvasive coronary imaging using different imaging modalities such as magnetic resonance imaging (MRI), electron beam computed tomography (EBCT), and multislice spiral computed tomography (MSCT) has been witnessed. Nonmechanical EBCT was developed in the 1970s and is characterized by the absence of a rotating gantry. Instead, an electron beam is projected along a 216° tungsten target ring, positioned in the lower part of the gantry, from which X-ray is created on electron impact. The emitted X-rays pass through the patient and are collected by the detector ring on the opposite side of the gantry. Cross-sectional images can be acquired with a temporal resolution of 100 ms. For cardiac imaging, the acquisition is triggered prospectively by the patient's ECG. Per cardiac cycle one or more 1.5 or 3 mm slices are acquired, whereas the rest remain at the same longitudinal position. EBCT has been applied mostly for the quantification of coronary calcium. In the 1990s, with the use of intravenous contrast media, this modality was used for coronary and bypass angiography, myocardial perfusion imaging, and ventricular function evaluation. Scanners with double detector rings and an image acquisition time of 50 ms are currently under evaluation.

In 1993, promising results in comparison with conventional angiography were published using two-dimensional (2D) MRI to image the coronary arteries *(1)*. Various scanning techniques, free-breathing and breath-hold, 2D and three-dimensional (3D), have been evaluated for the assessment of the coronary arteries. Other applications of

From: *Contemporary Cardiology: Essentials of Restenosis: For the Interventional Cardiologist*
Edited by: H. J. Duckers, E. G. Nabel, and P. W. Serruys © Humana Press Inc., Totowa, NJ

cardiac MRI include assessment of ventricular performance and myocardial perfusion, with and without physical or pharmacologically induced stress, imaging of infarctions, and coronary plaques (2). In 1998, four-slice spiral CT with a sufficient rotation speed for cardiac imaging was introduced, which showed promising results for coronary imaging. Currently, 16- and even 4-slice MSCT scanners with a rotation time less than 400 ms offer noninvasive coronary angiography with a very good accuracy for the detection of coronary obstruction in comparison with conventional angiography.

## CARDIAC CT

### *Data Acquisition*

Cardiac imaging with MSCT is performed using retrospective ECG-gating (Fig. 1). The heart is scanned continuously during a number of heart cycles, after which axial slices during the same cardiac phase are reconstructed using the recorded ECG. With a gantry rotation time of 420 ms the temporal resolution, using a half-rotation reconstruction algorithm, is 210 ms (3). When scanning data of the same position derived from consecutive cycles combined to reconstruct an image, the effective temporal resolution can be further improved. Compared with other invasive and noninvasive cardiac imaging techniques the temporal resolution is still modest and in patients with a high heart rate the use of β-blockers is recommended to improve the image quality. In the absence of contraindications, an oral dose of a short-acting β-blocker, for instance 100 mg metoprolol, is sufficient to lower the heart rate to an acceptable level (Fig. 2).

Today's scanners are equipped with up to 16 parallel detector rings with an individual detector width of 0.5–0.75 mm depending on the scanner type. This results in a near-isotropic resolution, which means an equal resolution in all three spatial dimensions, of approx $0.5 \times 0.5 \times 0.5$ mm$^3$. Although 4-slice scanners required a long breath-hold of up to 40s to acquire all data, 16-slice scanners cover the heart in 15–20 s only. The short breath-hold time makes the acquisition more comfortable, limits the occurrence of involuntary respiration, and minimizes the heart rate acceleration induced by breath holding. Contrast bolus of an iodine containing contrast medium is injected intravenously. To deliver a high and compact contrast dose, a saline bolus chaser can be injected immediately after the contrast medium. The scan is automatically initiated as soon as the head of the contrast medium is detected in the aortic root.

### *Image Reconstruction*

As mentioned previously, images are reconstructed retrospectively, synchronized to the patient's ECG. Because data is acquired continuously with an overlapping scan protocol, sets of axial slices can be reconstructed during any cardiac phase. Generally, a number of image sets are reconstructed at slightly varying time positions within the diastole. The most optimal dataset is then further processed to evaluate the coronary arteries. Although the minimal axial slice width is 0.5–0.75 mm, the effective reconstructed slice thickness can be increased to 1 mm to improve the contrast-to-noise. An overview of the characteristics of MSCT coronary angiography can be found in Table 1.

### *Postprocessing and Analysis*

If the reconstruction interval is set at 0.6 mm one angiogram will consist of more than 200 images, which is cumbersome to evaluate slice-by-slice. To facilitate the evaluation of CT angiography various postprocessing tools have been developed. The use

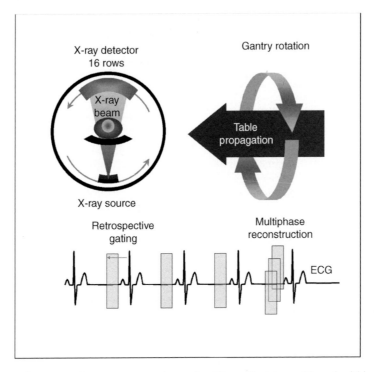

**Fig. 1.** Computed tomography coronary angiography. The patient is positioned within the scanner gantry and the X-ray tube and detectors rotate on opposite sides. While the tube and detectors rotate, the table with the patient is transported at a constant speed through the gantry. Retrospectively, images are reconstructed using isocardiophasic computed tomography data acquired during a sequence of cardiac cycles. Within this R-to-R interval, the reconstruction window can be placed at any position, allowing multiphasic reconstruction.

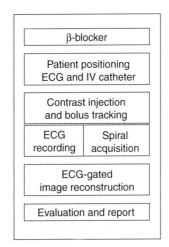

**Fig. 2.** Computed tomography coronary angiography scan protocol.

of thin-slab maximum intensity projections, which are a selective 2D display of the structures with a high CT value, including contrast medium or calcified tissues within a selected slab. It allows for quick assessment of the data set, but is less effective when other highly attenuating material, such as calcium or metal stents are in the proximity

Table 1

Diagnostic Performance of 4- and 16-Slice MSCT to Detect Coronary Stenosis,
With Conventional Coronary Angiography as Reference Standard

| | N | Evaluation | Excl | Sens | Spec | PPV | NPV | Sens[a] |
|---|---|---|---|---|---|---|---|---|
| 4-slice MSCT | | | | | | | | |
| Nieman et al. | 31 | Segment-based | 27% | 81% | 97% | 81% | 97% | 68% |
| Achenbach et al. | 64 | Branch-based | 32% | 85% | 76% | 56% | 93% | 55% |
| | | | 32% | 91% | 84% | 59% | 98% | 58% |
| Knez et al. | 43 | Segment-based | 6% | 78% | 98% | 84% | 96% | 51% |
| Vogl et al. | 64 | Segment-based | 28% | 75% | 99% | 92% | 98% | NR |
| Kopp et al.[b] | 102 | Segment-based | 15% | 86% | 96% | 76% | 98% | 86% |
| | | | | 93% | 97% | 81% | 99% | 93% |
| Giesler et al.[c] | 100 | Branch-based | 29% | 91% | 89% | 66% | 98% | 49% |
| Nieman et al.[c] | 78 | Segment-based | 32% | 84% | 95% | 67% | 98% | 63% |
| 16-slice MSCT | | | | | | | | |
| Nieman et al. | 58 | Branch-based | 0 | 95% | 86% | 80% | 97% | 95% |
| Ropers et al. | 77 | Branch-based | 12 | 92% | 93% | 79% | 97% | 85% |

Excl, percent excluded segments/branches; Sens, sensitivity; Spec, specificity; PPV and NPV, positive and negative predictive value with respect to the assessable segments/branches.
[a]Sensitivity including missed lesions in nonassessable segments/branches.
[b]Results by two observers, without consensus reading.
[c]Studies include patients from earlier publications.

of the vessel. In these situations multiplanar reconstructions, which are 2D cross-sections at a freely selectable position or angle, provide a more accurate view on the lumenal integrity of the vessel (Fig. 3).

3D reconstructions of the coronary arteries, from an external or internal (virtual endoscopy) perspective allow an overview of the coronary morphology, and its relation to the cardiac anatomy (Fig. 4). Findings can be presented to referring physicians and the myocardial region affected by an obstruction is easily visualized. 3D reconstructions are less suited for initial assessment of the coronary lumen, particularly in the presence of stents and calcified plaque tissue. Image artefacts can occasionally go unnoticed when using advanced postprocessing techniques. Confirmation of a detected lesion on the original source images is therefore recommended.

## CTA Characteristics

Cardiac and coronary imaging with tomographic modalities differ substantially from conventional X-ray projection angiography with selective contrast enhancement of the coronary arteries. Intravenous contrast enhancement results in opacification of all cardiac cavities including the cardiac veins, great vessels, and lung circulation. More than in conventional angiography, highly attenuating material other than contrast medium, appears as the brightest structures in the images. Metal objects such as stents, pacemaker leads and sternal wires, and vascular clips after surgery appear as the most attenuating material on the CT angiogram. Also calcified tissues, which apart from the chest wall can be found in the aorta, cardiac valves, coronary arteries, and the pericardium, have an attenuation that exceeds that of contrast enhanced blood in the coronary arteries.

Whereas conventional angiography produces a large series of images of the entire coronary artery during a number of heart cycles, an MSCT image consist of combined

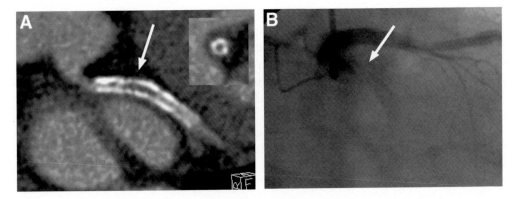

**Fig. 3.** Stent occlusion. Computed tomography **(A)** and conventional angiography **(B)** of an occluded stent (arrow) in the left circumflex branch. The dark material within the bright stent structure appears to be thrombotic material.

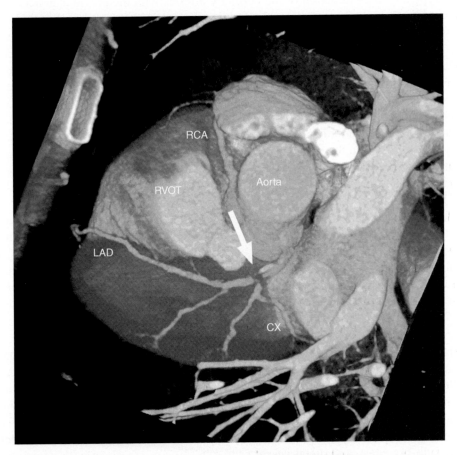

**Fig. 4.** Multislice spiral computed tomography coronary angiogram. Multislice spiral computed tomography coronary angiogram of a patient with a significant stenosis (arrow) at the bifurcation of the left main branch. LAD, left anterior descending; CX, circumflex; RCA, right coronary artery; RVOT, right ventricular outflow tract.

data that was collected during a number of cardiac cycles. This results in an apparent interruption of the vessel in case of arrhthmia. Because only a single phase of the cardiac cycle is imaged, no investigation about the coronary flow is possible and the differentiation between a short occlusion or severe stenosis cannot always be made. Intracoronary calcium can obscure the coronary lumen and lead to overestimation of the vessel obstruction. The improved spatial resolution of 16-slice MSCT has to a certain extent reduced the interpretability of severely calcified coronary arteries. Advantages of MSCT is the fact that a true cross-sectional vessel area can be measured. Besides the coronary lumen, other tissues surrounding the vessel lumen are visualized by CT. Apart from the already mentioned calcium, also noncalcified atherosclerotic material can be visualized by CT.

## DETECTION OF CORONARY STENOSIS

### 4-Slice MSCT

According to a number of studies, the most recent generation of MSCT scanner are able to reliably image the coronary arteries and allow detection of stenotic disease *(4,5)*. Typically, the evaluation of the coronary arteries with the previous generation of 4-slice MSCT scanners, as well as other noninvasive modalities has been limited to the proximal and middle segments of the major coronary branches. Distal segments and side branches were excluded because the small size and limited contrast enhancement resulted in insufficient image quality and precluded evaluation. Of the proximal and middle segments only 70% to 80% of all available segments could be interpreted by 4-slice MSCT, which significantly limited the clinical value of the techniques *(6–10)*. The reason for nonaccessibility is often multifactorial and includes calcifications, cardiac or respiratory motion, and adjacent contrast filled structures blending with the coronary artery segments. When the image quality was sufficient, the sensitivity to detect stenotic disease ranged between 75% and 90%, the specificity between 85% and 90% (Table 2).

Initial studies showed a diagnostic accuracy of 4-slice MSCT that was similar to EBCT. EBCT appears more robust at higher heart rates, whereas MSCT could better assess smaller segments because of its high image resolution and low image noise. In a patient with a higher heart rate motion artefacts, particularly in the right coronary artery, should not be avoided in all cases. Two studies evaluated the diagnostic accuracy of MSCT in relation to the heart rate and found that the image interpretability and diagnostic accuracy to detect significant lesions in patients with a low heart rate was significantly better *(11,12)*. Therefore, the use of medication to reduce the heart rate is advocated in these patients.

### 16-Slice MSCT

The current 16-slice spiral CT scanners are equipped with more and thinner detectors and the means for faster rotation. This has substantially improved in the image quality and robustness of CT coronary angiography, and made the procedure easier to perform. Contrary to most 4-slice CT protocols, all studies with 16-slice technology included routine use of β-blockers to further reduce motion artefacts. In two published studies, the image interpretability has increased to approx 90%, including all branches, larger side-branches, and distal vessel segments. In a comparison with conventional angiography by Nieman et al. *(5)* a sensitivity to identify significantly stenosed branches (down to a vessel diameter size of 2 mm) was reported as 95%, with a specificity of 86%, without exclusion of any segments owing to suboptimal image quality *(4)*.

Table 2
Scanner Parameters of ECG-Synchronized of 16-Slice MSCT Coronary Angiography

| Parameter | 16-slice spiral CT (Sensation 16, Siemens, Germany) |
| --- | --- |
| Detector collimation | $16 \times 0.75$ mm$^2$ |
| Rotation time | ≤420 ms |
| Contrast volume | 100 mL iodine containing contrast medium + 50 mL saline (bolus chaser) |
| Respiratory synchronization | Inspiratory breath-hold |
| Cardiac synchronization | Retrospective ECG-gating |
| Temporal resolution | 105–210 ms |
| Scan time | 15–20 s |

Ropers et al. performed a similar study (minimal vessel diameter size 1.5 mm), but excluded 12% of the nonevaluable segments from evaluation. They reported a sensitivity of 92% and a specificity of 93% (Table 2).

## PLAQUE IMAGING

Initially, the major application of cardiac CT was detection and quantification of coronary calcium, for the prediction of stenosis, and future cardiac events. Besides these calcified particles, current MSCT technology allows visualization of noncalcified plaque tissue as well (Fig. 5). Early studies in ex vivo material as well as in in vivo, have shown a correlation between the histological plaque composition and the measured CT attenuation. Highly attenuating calcified plaques are easily recognized on CT. One study has shown that plaques that were qualified as lipid-rich appear to have a significantly different CT attenuation, compared with plaques that are qualified as predominantly fibrous according to intracoronary angiography (13). With the current spatial resolution, more detailed information, for instance the thickness of the fibrous cap, is not possible. Detection and evaluation of preclinical and clinical atherosclerotic plaque burden in different stages of development may become an important application of CT coronary angiography. Further studies are needed to establish the reliability and reproducibility of this application.

## IMAGING OF CORONARY ARTERIES WITH STENTS

Whereas the feasibility and diagnostic accuracy of MSCT imaging has been described extensively regarding the assessment of regular coronary arteries, the usefulness of MSCT in patients who underwent coronary intervention is hardly documented. Patients who undergo PCI will often need repeated coronary angiography either owing to restenosis of the stented segment, or progression of disease in other coronary segments. Today, only a fraction of patients undergo PCI without the use of stents. Particularly, these patients would benefit from a noninvasive technique to visualize the coronary artery system. Achenbach et al. showed that EBCT, in comparison with conventional coronary angiography, had a high sensitivity for the detection of stenosis after PCI, in cases without stent placement (14).

### Stent Characteristics

Most stents used today are made of stainless steel. The assessment of stented coronary arteries is complicated by the high X-ray attenuating of the stent material.

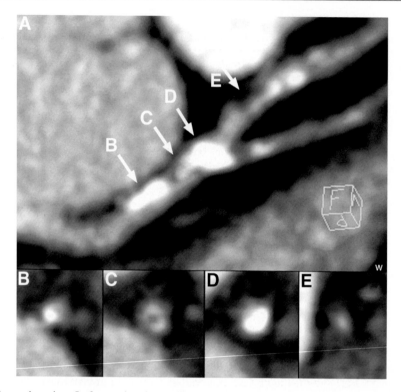

**Fig. 5.** Plaque imaging. Left anterior descending coronary artery and diagonal branch with diffuse atherosclerotic disease. Consecutive cross-sections (**B–E**) show the variation in plaque size and substance. Mixed calcified and noncalcified plaque can be observed in plane **C**.

Although they can be barely visible on conventional X-ray film, their appearance on CT is explicit. The CT attenuation values, or Hounsfield units, of the stent material exceeds that of any natural material in or around the heart, which gives them a bright appearance on the CT images. On CT, the thickness of the stent struts is increased compared with their actual size, which is called the blooming effect (Fig. 6). This phenomenon has been confirmed by in vitro studies of immobile stents and therefore cannot be explained by motion blurring alone *(15)*. A number of factors are responsible for the increased size. Because the diameter of the stent struts measures only a fraction of the in-plane spatial resolution of most MSCT scanners, partial voluming will occur. Furthermore, the slightly widened slice-sensitivity profile in spiral scanning, as well as the beam hardening, which is the change of the X-ray spectrum as it passes through the body, might be responsible for the blooming effect of highly attenuating objects such as stents.

The blooming effect of the stents extends in all in-plane directions. As a result the vessel lumen adjacent to the stent is not well assessable. The blooming effect is related to the spatial resolution and remains limited to the direct vicinity of the stent, which is why stents in larger noncoronary vessels are better assessable than coronary stents (Fig. 7). Particularly in smaller coronary branches little artifact-free lumen remains. The severity of the artifact varies with the type and the spatial resolution of the CT scanner, the patient's heart rate, and the material and amount of material used in the stent.

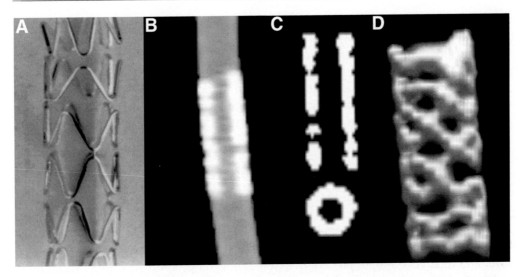

**Fig. 6.** In vitro stent imaging. Photograph **(A)** and in vitro computed tomography scan of a 4-mm coronary stent. Positioned within a contrast-enhanced silicon tube, the blooming effect causes the stent struts to appear larger, and the lumen within the stent narrowed **(B)**. Long- and short-axis cross-section of the stent **(C)**. Three-dimensional reconstruction of the stent **(D)**.

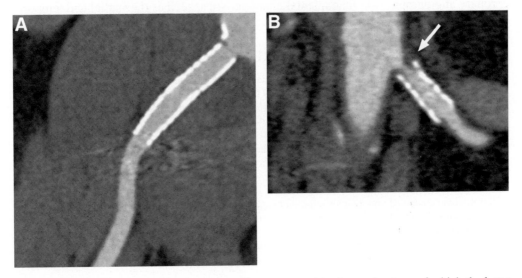

**Fig. 7.** Nonardiac stents. Large stents in the iliac artery and in the renal artery, of which the latter shows a stenosis at the proximal side (arrow).

## Role of MSCT After Stenting

Using a 16-slice MSCT scanner and sufficient slow heart rate coronary arteries with stents are reasonably well assessable. Although no large comparative studies have been published, there seems to be consensus about the ability of MSCT to recognize complete stent occlusion. Contrary to the assessment of coronary arteries without stents, the detection of moderate stenosis appears less accurate, owing to the previously mentioned image artifacts. The blooming artifact also limits qualification of the plaque material within the stent. Other subtle irregularities in the proximity of the stent, such as mild neo-intimal hyperplasia, stent malapposition, tissue prolaps, are obscured by the metal artefacts. In patients who previously underwent PCI, the role of CT seems at this point limited to detection of progression of obstruction in the coronary segments without stents, detection of stenosis near the edges of the stent, and detection of in-stent occlusion and perhaps high-grade stenosis. In the future, better stent visualization may be possible with further improvement of the spatial resolution by implementation of even thinner detector rings, dedicated image processing, and the use of less radiopaque stent materials.

## CONCLUSION

In the recent years considerable progress has been made in the development of non-invasive imaging of the coronary arteries. Multislice spiral CT is currently the most accurate noninvasive angiographical modality for the detection of coronary stenosis. Despite the use of radiation and contrast media, MSCT coronary angiography is a fast, safe, and relatively simple procedure. Although advancements in scanner technology will expectedly improve the assessment of coronary arteries with stents, the role of MSCT after percutaneous coronary intervention is for the time limited to exclusion of complete stent obstruction and evaluation of coronary artery disease in the remaining nonstented segments. To further improve the quality and quantitative potential of MSCT coronary angiography, the fundamental characteristics, such as the spatial and temporal resolution need to be further optimized.

## REFERENCES

1. Manning WJ, Li W, Edelman RR. A preliminary report comparing magnetic resonance coronary angiography with conventional angiography. N Engl J Med 1993;328–832.
2. Fayad ZA, Fuster V, Nikolaou K, Becker CR. Computed tomography and magnetic resonance imaging for noninvasive coronary angiography and plaque imaging. Current and potential future concepts. Circulation 2002;106:2026–2034.
3. Nieman K, Cademartiri F, Lemos PA, Raaymakers R, Pattynama PMT, de Feyter PJ. Reliable noninvasive coronary angiography with fast submillimeter multislice spiral computed tomography. Circulation 2002;106:2051–2054.
4. Ropers D, Baum U, Pohle K, et al. Detection of coronary artery stenoses with thin-slice multi-detector row spiral computed tomography and multiplanar reconstruction. Circulation 2003;107:664–666.
5. Nieman K, Oudkerk M, Rensing BJ, et al. Coronary angiography with multi-slice computed tomography. Lancet 2001;357:599–603.
6. Achenbach S, Giesler T, Ropers D, et al. Detection of coronary artery stenoses by contrast-enhanced, retrospectively electrocardiographically-gated, multislice spiral computed tomography. Circulation 2001;103:2535–2538.
7. Knez A, Becker CR, Leber A, et al. Usefulness of multislice spiral computed tomography angiography for determination of coronary artery stenoses. Am J Cardiol 2001;88:1191–1194.
8. Vogl TJ, Abolmaali ND, Diebold T, et al. Techniques for the detection of coronary atherosclerosis: multi-detector row CT coronary angiography. Radiology 2002;223:212–220.
9. Kopp AF, Schröder S, Kuettner A, et al. Non-invasive coronary angiography with high resolution multidetector-row computed tomography: results in 102 patients. Eur Heart J 2002;23:1714–1725.
10. Giesler T, Baum U, Ropers D, et al. Noninvasive visualization of coronary arteries using contrast-enhanced multidetector CT: influence of heart rate on image quality and stenosis detection. Am J Roentgenol 2002;179:911–916.
11. Nieman K, Rensing BJ, van Geuns RJM, et al. Non-invasive coronary angiography with multislice spiral computed tomography: impact of heart rate. Heart 2002;88:470–474.
12. Schroeder S, Kopp AF, Baumbach A, et al. Noninvasive detection and evaluation of atherosclerotic coronary plaques with multislice computed tomography. J Am Coll Cardiol 2001;37:1430–1435.

13. Achenbach S, Moshage W, Bachmann K. Detection of high-grade restenosis after PTCA using contrast-enhanced electron beam CT. Circulation 1997;96:2785–2788.

14. Nieman K, Cademartiri F, Raaijmakers R, Pattynama P, de Feyter P. Noninvasive angiographic evaluation of coronary stents with multi-slice spiral computed tomography. Herz 2003;28:136–142.

15. Flohr T, Stierstorfer K, Bruder H. New technical developments in multislice CT, Part 2: Sub-millimeter 16-slice scanning and increased gantry rotation speed for cardiac imaging. RöFo, Fortschr Röntgenstr 2002;174:1022–1027.

# IV    THERAPY OF RESTENOSIS

# 19 Pharmacotherapy of Restenosis

*Pim J. de Feyter* MD, PhD
*and Georgios Sianos* MD, PhD

## CONTENTS

## INTRODUCTION

Restenosis has been recognized as the main limitation of coronary balloon angioplasty since its introduction in 1978. The main causes were the constrictive vessel remodeling (acute and chronic) and the neointimal hyperplasia. The coronary stents were introduced in 1986 and reduced restenosis from 30–40% to 15–20% in certain type of lesions by eliminating the vessel remodeling. The advent of drug-eluting stents in 2000 reduced restenosis even further to single digit numbers (5–8%), by eliminating the formation of neointimal hyperplasia. Despite these significant improvements restenosis has not been eradicated, whereas the long-term outcome after drug-eluting stent implantation with potential delayed restenosis, remains unknown. Furthermore, the reported randomized drug-eluting stent trials investigated mainly patients with selected simple lesions and the outcome in more complex patients with bifurcations, long lesions, in small vessels or in diabetics still remains largely unknown. In this chapter, the use of systemic drug therapy to prevent restenosis after coronary balloon angioplasty, or after coronary stent implantation will be reviewed.

## PHARMACOTHERAPY FOR RESTENOSIS AFTER BALLOON ANGIOPLASTY: THE EARLIER STUDIES

In the eighties and earlier nineties many pharmacological agents have been investigated in over 25,000 patients in more than 60 trials (Table 1) (*1*). The drugs tested, targeted

From: *Contemporary Cardiology: Essentials of Restenosis: For the Interventional Cardiologist*
Edited by: H. J. Duckers, E. G. Nabel, and P. W. Serruys © Humana Press Inc., Totowa, NJ

Table 1
Pharmacological Agents Against Postballoon Angioplasty Restenosis

Aspirin
Ticlopidin
Thromboxane $A_2$ inhibitors
Prostacyclin
Anticoagulants (warfarin, heparin, enoxaparin, reviparin, hirudin, certoparin, fraxiparin)
Steriods
Calcium antagonists (nifedipine, verapamil, diltiazem, amlodipine)
ACE-inhibitors (cilazapril, fosinopril)
Trapidil
Fish oil
Statins (lovastatin, fluvastatin, pravastatin)
Serotonin antagonists
Angiopeptin
Nitric oxide donors
Antioxidants (probucol, tocopheral)
Antiproliferative (colchicine, tranilast, cilostazol)
β-blocker (carvedilol)
Vitamins (multivitamins, β-carotene, vitamins C and E)

various pathophysiological mechanisms including platelet activation and aggregation, thrombus formation, smooth muscle cell proliferation, inflammation, and matrix metabolism but did not address the important component of late constrictive vessel remodeling. The tested agents failed to reduce restenosis, despite the promising results in animal models and in some cases in initial pilot human trials. The reasons for failure are various, such as inadequate dosage, inappropriate timing of treatment, ineffective agents, or use of agents aimed to the wrong restenosis mechanisms. Probably, the most important reason was the inability to achieve adequate drug levels at the angioplasty site.

## PHARMACOTHERAPY FOR RESTENOSIS AFTER BALLOON ANGIOPLASTY: THE LATER STUDIES

The systemic pharmacological approach for the prevention of restenosis following balloon angioplasty continued and several pharmacological agents were tested even after the introduction of stent implantation.

Data from studies in animals had demonstrated that antioxidants had a beneficial effect on both cell proliferation and arterial remodeling after balloon angioplasty, an action attributed to interfere with the oxidation of the low-density lipoprotein (2). Small studies in humans with the antioxidant probucol were promising and were confirmed in a large randomized study (3). Three hundred seventeen patients were treated with probucol starting 1 mo before angioplasty and continued for 6 mo postprocedure. An extra dose of 1000 mg probucol was also administered 12 h before angioplasty. Significant reduction in restenosis rate was observed (20.7% vs 38.9%, $p = 0.003$) as well as in the need for repeated angioplasty (11.2% vs 26.6%, $p = 0.009$) in the probucol group. Unfortunately, unwanted side effects, such as 40% reduction of high-density lipoprotein levels, and the prolongation of the QTc interval, led to the abandon of this pharmacological approach and probucol was not marketed.

AGI-1067 is a metabolically stable compound of probucol with proposed safer profile compared with probucol. A randomized study, the CART (Canadian antioxidant restenosis trial)-1, investigated the efficacy of AGI-1067 in 305 patients postangioplasty (stents were used in 85% of the patients) *(4)*. Indeed, AGI-1067 reduced the restenosis rate, although it did not prolong the QTc interval, it caused significant reduction in HDL levels varying from 4.4 to 18.7% with increasing dosages. A new trial, the CART-2 should provide a more definite answer regarding the safety and efficacy of this new compound.

The efficacy of lowering of plasma homocysteine levels to reduce the restenosis after balloon angioplasty was tested in a randomized trial of 100 control patients vs 105 patients treated with a combination of folic acid (1 mg), vitamin B12 (400 µg), and pyridoxine (10 mg) for 6 mo after successful coronary angioplasty *(5)*. The minimum lumen diameter was significantly larger in the folate treatment group $1.72 \pm 0.76$ vs $1.45 \pm 0.88$ ($p = 0.02$). Restenosis was also significantly reduced (19.6% vs 37.6%, $p = 0.01$) as well as the need for target lesion revascularization (10.8% vs 22.3%, $p = 0.047$). However, in this trial approx 60% of the cases a coronary stent was implanted and a subanalysis showed that in these patients there was only a trend in reduction of restenosis whereas in balloon-treated patients this effect was statistically significant.

Oral rapamycin treatment for recalcitrant restenosis, i.e., in patients with failed radiation therapy for in-stent restenosis, demonstrated no benefit following balloon angioplasty, and adverse drug effects were frequent *(6)*.

## PHARMACOLOGICAL TREATMENT TO PREVENT IN-STENT RESTENOSIS

A wide variety of pharmacological treatments have been investigated for the prevention of in-stent restenosis (Table 2) *(7–20)*. The majority of these trials were negative. A few small studies with Enoxaparin (local drug delivery), Prednison for 45 d in patients with signs of ongoing inflammation (high C-reactive protein levels) or Cilastozol were positive. However, the small number of patients enrolled in these studies, precluded definitive conclusions regarding the efficacy of these drugs. Furthermore, local drug delivery is rather cumbersome and precludes widespread use.

## PHARMACOLOGICAL TREATMENT FOR PREVENTION OF MAJOR ADVERSE EVENTS AFTER STENT-IMPLANTATION

Thrombotic processes are thought to be responsible for the development of ischemic events following percutaneous coronary intervention. The activation and aggregation of platelets can be inhibited by platelet glycoprotein IIb/IIIa antagonists *(21)*. The evaluation of oral Xemilofiban in controlling thrombotic events-trial (EXCITE) tested the hypothesis that 6-mo oral administration of Xemilofiban, an oral glycoprotein IIb/IIIa receptor antagonist would decrease death, myocardial infarction, and the need for urgent revascularization after percutaneous coronary intervention *(22)*. A total of 7232 patients were randomized to either placebo ($n = 2414$), 10 mg Xemilofiban ($n = 2400$), or 20 mg Xemolofiban ($n = 2418$). Stent implantation was performed in approx 75% of the patients. The rate of death, myocardial infarction or urgent revascularization at 6 mo was not statistically different between the three groups, 13.5, 13.9, and 12.7%, respectively as well as death and myocardial infarction.

Tranilast is an anti-inflammatory agent and interferes with the proliferation and migration of vascular smooth muscle cells. Tranilast was shown to be effective for the

Table 2
Pharmacological Treatment to Prevent In-Stent Restenosis or Major Adverse Cardiac Events

| Trial | Compound | Active Rx | | | Control | | | |
|---|---|---|---|---|---|---|---|---|
| | | $n$ | RR (%) (6 m) | MACE (%) | $n$ | RR (%) (6 m) | MACE (%) | |
| Trappist | Trapidil 500 mg | 154 | 31 | 22 | 158 | 24 | 20 | ns |
| Eraser | Abciximab bolus + infusion | 154 | 19 | 21 | 71 | 12 | 25 | ns |
| ISAR-3 | Roxithromycine 500 mg 28 d | 506 | 31 | 26 | 504 | 29 | 23 | ns |
| Polonia | Enoxaparin (local delivery) | 50 | 10 | 8 | 50 | 24 | 22 | $p = 0.05$ |
| HIPS | Heparin (local delivery) | 88 | 20 | 25 | 91 | 14 | 23 | ns |
| Italics | Antisense c-myc (local delivery) | 42 | 34 | 29 | 43 | 39 | 28 | ns |
| Impress | Prednison 45 d (high levels CRP) | 41 | 7 | 7 | 42 | 33 | 33 | $p = 0.001$ |
| Lee | Prednisolone iv | 70 | 18 | 7 | 70 | 19 | 7 | ns |
| Kamishirado | Cilastazol | 65 | 13 | 7 | 65 | 31 | 12 | $p = 0.05$ |
| Park | Cilastozol 6 mo | 201 | 27 | 20 | 208 | 23 | 13 | ns |
| Suzuki | L-arginine (local delivery) | 25 | 9 | na | 25 | 21 | na | ns |
| Presto | Tranilast | 1598 | 33 | 16 | 420 | 33 | 16 | ns |
| Meurice | Quinapril (DD genotype) | 46 | 37 | 24 | 45 | 24 | 16 | ns |
| Neuman | Abciximab (AMI) | 200 | 31 | 20 | 200 | 31 | 24 | ns |

RR, restenosis rate; MACE, major adverse coronary events; AMI, acute myocardial infarction; C-RP, C-reactive protein; m, months.

reduction of restenosis in a small angiographic trial *(23)*. The prevention of restenosis with Tranilast (PRESTO) trial investigated the efficacy of Tranilast 600 or 900 mg daily for 1 or 3 mo for the prevention of death, myocardial infarction, or ischemia-driven target vessel revascularization (combined end point) at 9 mo after percutaneous intervention *(17)*. In approx 85% of the patients a stent was implanted. A total of 11,484 patients were enrolled in the study. Placebo (*n* = 2298), Tranilast 600 mg (*n* = 2306), and 900 mg (*n* = 2280) for 1 mo and tranilast 600 mg (*n* = 2300) and 900 mg (*n* = 2300) for 3 mo. The primary end point occurred in 15.8% of the patients in the placebo group, and in 15.5% and 16% of the patients in the 1 mo and 3 mo Tranilast groups, respectively. There was no difference in outcome between the groups that received the 600 or 900 mg.

Statins are not associated with reduction of restenosis after balloon angioplasty *(24–28)* but may, in accordance with their beneficial effects on major cardiac adverse events in primary and secondary prevention trials, have a beneficial effect on the clinical outcome in patients who underwent a successful first percutaneous coronary intervention. The LIPS-trial (lescol intervention prevention study) tested this hypothesis *(29)*. Sixteen hundred seventy seven patients were enrolled; 844 received 80 mg Fluvastatin and 833 were on placebo. The MACE rate (death, myocardial infarction, and reintervention) was significantly reduced in the fluvastation group (26.7% vs 21.4%) during a mean follow-up period of 3.9 yr (RR 0.78 [0.64–0.95]). This outcome was even more striking when patients with early reintervention were excluded; 16% for the Fluvastatin group vs 22.5% for the placebo group (RR 0.67 [0.54–0.84]).

Chronically increased blood sugar levels are associated with accelerated progression of coronary artery disease and higher likelihood for restenosis. Careful blood sugar control might reduce the incidence of restenosis in these patients. This hypothesis was tested in a nonrandomized study of 179 diabetic patients and a control group of 60 nondiabetic patients. A hemoglobin A1c level of 7% or lower was used as marker of optimal glycemic control. Diabetic patients with optimal glycemic control had reduced incidence of repeat revascularization at 12 mo after balloon angioplasty or stenting compared with diabetic patients with poor glycemic control (15% vs 34%, respectively *p* = 0.02) and almost similar to nondiabetic patients (18%) *(30)*.

## REFERENCES

1. Chan AW, Moliterno DJ. Restenosis: the clinical issues. In: Topol, ed. Textbook of Interventional Cardiology. WB Saunders, Philadelphia, PA, 2003, pp. 415–454.
2. Carew TE, Schwenke DC, Steinberg D. Antiatherogenic effect of probucol unrelated to its hypocholesterolemic effect: evidence that antioxidants in vivo can selectively inhibit low density lipoprotein degradation in macrophage-rich fatty streaks and slow the progression of atherosclerosis in the Watanabe heritable hyperlipidemic rabbit. Proc Natl Acad Sci USA 1987;84:7725–7729.
3. Tardif JC, Cote G, Lesperance J, et al. Probucol and multivitamins in the prevention of restenosis after coronary angioplasty. Multivitamins and Probucol Study Group. N Engl J Med 1997;337:365–372.
4. Tardif JC, Gregoire J, Schwartz L, et al. Effects of AGI-1067 and probucol after percutaneous coronary interventions. Circulation 2003;107:552–558.
5. Schnyder G, Roffi M, Pin R, et al. Decreased rate of coronary restenosis after lowering of plasma homocysteine levels. N Engl J Med 2001;345:1593–1600.
6. Brara PS, Moussavian M, Grise MA, et al. Pilot trial of oral rapamycin for recalcitrant restenosis. Circulation 2003;107:1722–1724.
7. Serruys PW, Foley DP, Pieper M, Kleijne JA, de Feyter PJ. The TRAPIST Study. A multicentre randomized placebo controlled clinical trial of trapidil for prevention of restenosis after coronary stenting, measured by 3-D intravascular ultrasound. Eur Heart J 2001;22:1938–1947.
8. The ERASER Investigators. Acute platelet inhibition with abciximab does not reduce in-stent restenosis (ERASER study). Circulation 1999;100:799–806.

 9. Neumann F, Kastrati A, Miethke T, et al. Treatment of Chlamydia pneumoniae infection with roxithromycin and effect on neointima proliferation after coronary stent placement (ISAR-3): a randomised, double-blind, placebo-controlled trial. Lancet 2001;357:2085–2089.

10. Kiesz RS, Buszman P, Martin JL, et al. Local delivery of enoxaparin to decrease restenosis after stenting: results of initial multicenter trial: Polish-American Local Lovenox NIR Assessment study (The POLONIA study). Circulation 2001;103:26–31.

11. Wilensky RL, Tanguay JF, Ito S, et al. Heparin infusion prior to stenting (HIPS) trial: final results of a prospective, randomized, controlled trial evaluating the effects of local vascular delivery on intimal hyperplasia. Am Heart J 2000;139:1061–1070.

12. Kutryk MJ, Foley DP, van den Brand M, et al. Local intracoronary administration of antisense oligonucleotide against c-myc for the prevention of in-stent restenosis: results of the randomized investigation by the Thoraxcenter of antisense DNA using local delivery and IVUS after coronary stenting (ITALICS) trial. J Am Coll Cardiol 2002;39:281–287.

13. Versaci F, Gaspardone A, Tomai F, et al. Immunosuppressive Therapy for the Prevention of Restenosis after Coronary Artery Stent Implantation (IMPRESS Study). J Am Coll Cardiol 2002; 40:1935–1942.

14. Cheol Whan Lee MD, Jei-Kun Chae MD, Hee-Young Lim, et al. Prospective randomized trial of corticosteroids for the prevention of restenosis after intracoronary stent implantation. Am Heart J 1999;138:60–63.

15. Kamishirado H, Inoue T, Mizoguchi K, et al. Randomized comparison of cilostazol versus ticlopidine hydrochloride for antiplatelet therapy after coronary stent implantation for prevention of late restenosis. Am Heart J 2002;144:303–308.

16. Suzuki T, Hayase M, Hibi K, et al. Effect of local delivery of L-arginine on in-stent restenosis in humans. Am J Cardiol 2002;89:363–367.

17. Holmes DR, Jr, Savage M, LaBlanche JM, et al. Results of Prevention of Restenosis with Tranilast and its Outcomes (PRESTO) trial. Circulation 2002;106:1243–1250.

18. Meurice T, Bauters C, Hermant X, et al. Effect of ACE inhibitors on angiographic restenosis after coronary stenting (PARIS): a randomised, double-blind, placebo-controlled trial. Lancet 2001;357(9265): 1321–1324.

19. Neumann FJ, Kastrati A, Schmitt C, et al. Effect of glycoprotein IIb/IIIa receptor blockade with abciximab on clinical and angiographic restenosis rate after the placement of coronary stents following acute myocardial infarction. J Am Coll Cardiol 2000;35:915–921.

20. Park SW, Lee CW, Kim HS, et al. Effects of cilostazol on angiographic restenosis after coronary stent placement. Am J Cardiol 2000;86:499–503.

21. Lefkovits J, Plow EF, Topol EJ. Platelet glycoprotein IIb/IIIa receptors in cardiovascular medicine. N Engl J Med 1995;332:1553–1559.

22. O'Neill WW, Serruys P, Knudtson M, et al. Long-term treatment with a platelet glycoprotein-receptor antagonist after percutaneous coronary revascularization. EXCITE Trial Investigators. Evaluation of Oral Xemilofiban in Controlling Thrombotic Events. N Engl J Med 2000;342:1316–1324.

23. Tamai H, Katoh O, Suzuki S, et al. Impact of tranilast on restenosis after coronary angioplasty: tranilast restenosis following angioplasty trial (TREAT). Am Heart J 1999;138:968–975.

24. O'Keefe JH, Jr, Stone GW, McCallister BD, Jr, et al. Lovastatin plus probucol for prevention of restenosis after percutaneous transluminal coronary angioplasty. Am J Cardiol 1996;77:649–652.

25. Weintraub WS, Boccuzzi SJ, Klein JL, et al. Lack of effect of lovastatin on restenosis after coronary angioplasty. Lovastatin Restenosis Trial Study Group. N Engl J Med 1994;331:1331–1337.

26. Sahni R, Maniet AR, Voci G, Banka VS. Prevention of restenosis by lovastatin after successful coronary angioplasty. Am Heart J 1991;121:1600–1608.

27. Bertrand ME, McFadden EP, Fruchart JC, et al. Effect of pravastatin on angiographic restenosis after coronary balloon angioplasty. The PREDICT Trial Investigators. Prevention of Restenosis by Elisor after Transluminal Coronary Angioplasty. J Am Coll Cardiol 1997;30:863–869.

28. Serruys PW, Foley DP, Jackson G, et al. A randomized placebo-controlled trial of fluvastatin for prevention of restenosis after successful coronary balloon angioplasty; final results of the fluvastatin angiographic restenosis (FLARE) trial. Eur Heart J 1999;20:58–69.

29. Serruys PW, de Feyter P, Macaya C, et al. Fluvastatin for prevention of cardiac events following successful first percutaneous coronary intervention: a randomized controlled trial. JAMA 2002;287:3215–3222.

30. Corpus RA, George PB, House JA, et al. Optimal glycemic control is associated with a lower rate of target vessel revascularization in treated type II diabetic patients undergoing elective percutaneous coronary intervention. J Am Coll Cardiol 2004;43(1):8–14.

# 20 Brachytherapy

*Ron Waksman, MD*

## CONTENTS

## INTRODUCTION

Postangioplasty restenosis has been the major limitation confronting interventional cardiology. The three major components of restenosis following balloon angioplasty are identified as an exuberant cellular proliferation and matrix synthesis (intimal hyperplasia) triggered by injury to the vessel wall *(1–4)*, acute elastic recoil immediately following balloon deflation, and late vascular contraction (remodeling) resulting in a decrease in total vessel diameter *(5–8)*. Coronary stenting eliminates elastic recoil and vessel contraction by acting as a mechanical scaffold within the vessel, thus reducing the restenosis rate *(9,10)*. Stents, however, are associated with a higher degree of proliferative response and increase in lumen late loss *(11)*.

With the use of stents in nearly 90% of coronary intervention, in-stent restenosis (ISR), once it occurs, is the major challenge in prevention and treatment. Conventional treatments, such as repeat balloon angioplasty, ablative treatment with atherectomy devices, laser angioplasty or cutting balloon have been disappointing, with recurrence rates averaging 25–50% for focal restenosis and up to 65% for diffuse restenosis.

Ionizing radiation occurs in many forms ranging from lightly ionizing X-rays, electrons, and β- or γ-rays, to more densely ionizing neutrons, α-particles, and other heavy particles. Vascular brachytherapy has emerged as a promising means for reducing the restenosis recurrence rate. For years, the growth-inhibiting properties of ionizing radiation have been used successfully to control benign proliferative disorders, such as keloid formation, ophthalmic pterygium, macular malformations, A-V malformations,

From: *Contemporary Cardiology: Essentials of Restenosis: For the Interventional Cardiologist*
Edited by: H. J. Duckers, E. G. Nabel, and P. W. Serruys © Humana Press Inc., Totowa, NJ

and heterotopic ossification *(12,13)*. Based on this experience, vascular brachytherapy, the intravascular delivery of radiation, was viewed as a viable solution to inhibit neointimal hyperplasia. In 1965, before the angioplasty and restenosis era, Friedman et al. *(14)* reported the use of Iridium-192 (Ir-192), 14 Gray (Gy) delivered intraluminally to the injured aorta of cholesterol fed rabbits, and demonstrated inhibition of smooth muscle cell proliferation and intimal hyperplasia in the irradiated atherosclerotic arteries.

Vascular brachytherapy following angioplasty for the prevention of restenosis was introduced in 1992 by several investigators who performed a series of preclinical studies and demonstrated consistently profound reduction of neointima formation following balloon injury *(15–36)*. In these experiments, the radiation was delivered into the vessel wall either by high-dose rate using catheter-based systems, or by low-dose rate radioactive implants, such as radioactive stents. The results of these preclinical trials were encouraging and facilitated the initiation of the feasibility clinical trials first in the peripheral arteries, later in coronary arteries through pivotal trials, and then onto commercialization of the technology for clinical use in Europe in 1999. In November 2000, the Food and Drug Administration (FDA) approved vascular brachytherapy for ISR. Today vascular brachytherapy offers clinicians an opportunity to provide effective treatment for patients with ISR. Other indications are still pending based on the results of ongoing trials.

## THE CLINICAL TRIALS

The clinical investigation for the role of vascular brachytherapy as a standard therapy for the prevention of restenosis has been launched with clinical trials both in the peripheral and coronary systems.

### *The Peripheral System (Frankfurt and Vienna)*

Liermann and Schopohl from Frankfurt, Germany were pioneers in determining the effect of endovascular radiation on restenosis in the peripheral arteries in a 1990 study utilizing endovascular radiation in patients with ISR at the saphenous femoral artery (SFA). In this study, 29 patients who developed restenosis at the SFA following stent implantation underwent directional atherectomy or balloon dilatation, which was followed by endovascular radiation. The source was Ir-192 and the dose was 12 Gy prescribed to the vessel wall delivered into a noncentering 5 Fr delivery closed-end lumen catheter through a high-dose rate MicroSelectron-HDR afterloader (Nucletron-Odelft, Veenendaal, The Netherlands). The patients tolerated the radiation treatment well and the investigators reported a patency rate of 75% in the treated lesions at 5-yr follow-up without any documentation of adverse event related to this therapy *(37,38)*. Another important trial using the same radiation system and similar radiation protocol following percutaneous transluminal coronary angioplasty (PTCA) to the SFA and the popliteal arteries was conducted in 113 patients in Vienna. This group reported 50% reduction in the clinical restenosis rate of the irradiated group vs control *(39)*. Minar et al. continued with a series of registries and randomized studies. Among them were Vienna I-V, which used intravascular γ-radiation as adjunct therapy to angioplasty of lesions in superficial femoral arteries to optimize the dosing and to investigate the utility of the technology for stented arteries. A list of SFA trials is shown in Table 1.

### *Peripheral Artery Radiation Investigational Study*

The Peripheral Artery Radiation Investigational Study (PARIS) was a prospective, randomized, double-blind, multicenter study designed to compare the long-term (1-yr)

Table 1
Superficial Femoral Artery Radiation Trials

| Study | Number of patients | Randomized | Center catheter | Dose Gy | At mm | Patency (%) |
|---|---|---|---|---|---|---|
| Frankfurt | 40 | – | – | 12 | 3 | 82 |
| Vienna 1 | 10 | – | No | 12 | 3 | 60 |
| Vienna 2 | 113 | Yes | No | 12 | r + 0 | 72 |
| Vienna 3 | 134 | Yes | Yes | 18 | r + 2 | 77 |
| Vienna 4 | 33 | No | Yes | 14 | r + 2 | 76[a] |
| Vienna 5 | 98 | Yes | Yes | 14 | r + 2 | 88 |
| Swiss 4 arm | 346 | Yes | Yes | 12 | r + 2 | 83 |
| Paris pilot | 40 | No | Yes | 14 | r + 2 | 88 |
| PARIS | 200 | Yes | Yes | 14 | r + 2 | 76 |

[a]Excluding thrombosis cases.

effects of balloon angioplasty with high-dose brachytherapy (14 Gy) to the effects of balloon angioplasty alone in patients with intermittent claudication owing to stenosis of the femoral-popliteal arteries. Two hundred patients were available for analysis (104 in the brachytherapy group, 96 in the placebo group). Patients were followed up for 12 mo with clinical visits at 1, 6, and 12 mo. There was no significant difference in minimal lumen diameter (MLD), percent diameter stenosis, late loss, or the number of total occlusions. Brachytherapy did not improve the restenosis rate or the functional symptoms in patients with intermittent claudication compared with balloon angioplasty treatment *(40)*.

## The Coronary System

β- and γ-radiation were studied for the treatment of ISR, whereas only β sources examined the potential of this therapy in the treatment of *de novo* lesions. Following is a summary of the clinical trials conducted thus far with β- and γ-emitters.

## TRIALS OF γ-RADIATION

### The Venezuelan Experience

The first study of intracoronary radiation (IRT) performed in human coronary arteries was an open label, feasibility and safety study conducted in Caracas, Venezuela by Condado et al. Between July 1994 and January 1995, 21 patients (22 lesions) were treated with IRT with an Ir-192 source after routine PTCA for unstable angina. Serial quantitative coronary angioplasty (QCA) detected a binary restenosis rate of 28.6% ($n = 6$) at 6 mo and remained the same at 5 yr (Fig. 1). The late loss (0.29 mm) and loss index (0.25) did not change and remained low at 2, 3, and 5 yr. Angiographic complications included four aneurysms (two procedure related and two occurring within 3 mo). At 2 yr, only one aneurysm increased in size (46 vs 27 mm$^2$); and at 3 and 5 yr, all aneurysms remained unchanged. No other angiographic complications were observed. There were no adverse events, such as death or myocardial infarction (MI). None of the patients developed complications or illnesses that could be related to the effects of the radiation *(41)*.

### γ-Radiation for ISR

The Checkmate™ System, from Cordis Corporation, is the first γ-intravascular brachytherapy radiation system for treating ISR in patients with coronary artery disease.

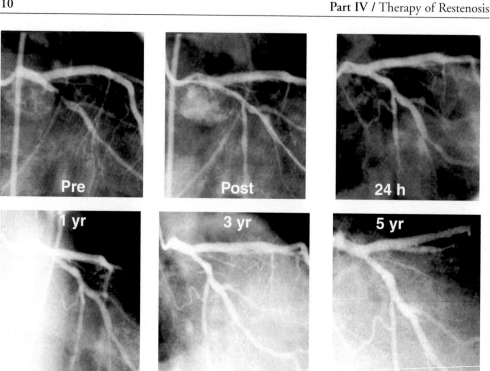

**Fig. 1.** Intracoronary radiation 5-yr follow-up.

The only γ-emitter used for the prevention of restenosis in clinical trials is Iridium-192 (Ir-192). The efficacy of Ir-192 in reducing clinical and angiographic restenosis in patients with ISR has been confirmed by a number of studies, including two single-center trials, Scripps Coronary Radiation to Inhibit Proliferation Poststenting (SCRIPPS) and Washington Radiation for In-Stent restenosis Trial (WRIST); and multicenter trials, γ-I and γ-II; and AngioRad™ Radiation Technology for In-Stent restenosis Trial In native Coronaries (ARTISTIC). All of these trials were performed using a manual delivery system with a noncentering catheter with either intravascular ultrasound (IVUS)-based or fixed depth dosimetry (Table 2).

### Scripps Coronary Radiation to Inhibit Proliferation Poststenting I–IV

SCRIPPS was the first randomized trial that evaluated the safety and efficacy of intra-coronary γ-radiation given as adjunctive therapy to stents. In this study, 26 of 55 patients were randomized to receive Ir-192 utilizing a ribbon (19–35 mm) delivered in a noncen-tered, closed-end lumen catheter at the treatment site, whereas 29 of the 55 patients were randomized to placebo. The prescribed dose was 8–30 Gy with a dwell time of 20–45 min. The initial angiographic follow-up obtained at 6.8 mo showed significantly lower angio-graphic restenosis rates (≥50% stenosis of the luminal diameter) in the Ir-192 group (17% vs 54%, $p = 0.01$). Three-year angiographic follow-up obtained in 37 patients revealed restenosis in 33.3% of the radiation patients compared with 63.6% in the placebo group, ($p < 0.05$). A subgroup analysis of the 35 patients who were enrolled in the trial owing to ISR, has shown a 70% reduction in the recurrence rate in the irradiated group vs the placebo group *(42,43)*. There were no evident clinical complications resulting from the radiation

Table 2
Clinical Trials for ISR Using Catheter-Based Systems with γ-Radiation

| Study name | Design | Dose (Gy) | Results |
|---|---|---|---|
| SCRIPPS | Single center, double-blind, randomized of 55 patients with restenosis | 8–30 to media by IVUS | Clinical benefits maintained at 5 yr |
| SCRIPPS IV | Double-blind, randomized study of 358 patients | 14 vs 17 at 2 mm from the source | Modest but significant 36% decrease in restenosis at 8 mos, 41% decrease in MACE in 17 Gy group |
| WRIST | Single center, double-blind, randomized of 130 patients with ISR (100 natives, 30 vein grafts) | 15 at 2 mm for vessels 3–4 mm. 18 for vessels more than 4 mm | MACE significantly reduced. Reduction in need for repeat TLR and TVR at 5 yr |
| SVG WRIST | Multicenter, double-blind, randomized of 120 patients with ISR | 14 or 15 at 2 mm for vessels 4 mm. 15 at 2.4 mm for vessels more than 4 mm | At 3 yr, irradiated points have lower TLR and TLR-MACE rates |
| Long WRIST | Two center, double-blind, randomized of 120 patients with ISR lesions (36–80 mm) | 15 at 2 mm for vessels 3–4 mm | 42% MACE in irradiated patients compared with 63% in placebo group |
| Long WRIST HD | Single center, registry of 120 patients with ISR. Lesions (36–80 mm) | 18 at 2 mm for vessels 3–4 mm | MACE rate further reduced to 22%. Late thrombosis—9% |
| WRIST 12 | 120 patients with diffuse ISR in natives and coronaries—12 mo of clopidogrel | 14 at 2 mm | Late thrombosis rate of 3.3%. Lower TLR and MACE rates than those treated with 6 mo of therapy |
| Integrilin WRIST | 300 patients – 150 assigned to eptifibatide (Integrilin) and 150 to heparin only | 15 at 2 mm | Clinical composite end points at 30 d similar between the two groups—4.7% (Integrilin) vs 4% (heparin only) |
| γ-I | Multicenter, randomized double blind study of 252 patients with ISR | 8–30 to media by IVUS | Irradiated patients show significant reduction of restenosis—21.6 vs 50.5% |

*(Continued)*

**Table 2** *(Continued)*

| Study name | Design | Dose (Gy) | Results |
|---|---|---|---|
| γ-II | Multicenter, registry of 125 patients with ISR | 14 at 2 mm | Similar to γ-I MACE and TLR were reduced by 36% and 48%, respectively, as compared with placebo |
| γ-V | Multicenter registry of 600 patients. With 12 mo clopidogrel for new stent and 6 mo for nonstent | 14 at 2 mm | N/A |
| ARTISTIC I | Multicenter, double-blind, randomized of 115 patients with in-stent restenosis | 12-15-18 at 2 mm | At 3 yr, MACE is 22.8% in the irradiated group compared with 24.1% in the placebo group |
| ARTISTIC II | Multicenter study of 340 patients | 18 at 2 mm | At 9 mo, irradiated patients have an acute procedural success rate of 86.9% compared with placebo—92.3% |
| CURE | A registry of 120 patients with in-stent restenosis considered unsatisfactory candidates for CABG or medical therapy | 14 at 2 mm | Enrollment extended. Clinical follow-up available for initial 120 patients. 31% TVR and 33% MACE at 6 mo |

treatment, and clinical benefits were maintained at 5 yr, with a significant reduction in the need for target lesion revascularization (TLR) ($p = 0.03$). Limitations of this trial included the small sample size and an uneven distribution of baseline clinical characteristics. SCRIPPS II for ISR in diffuse lesions (30–80 mm) and SCRIPPS III with prolonged antiplatelet therapy (ATP) (6–12 mo of Plavix®) followed the original SCRIPPS study and have shown that radiation is effective for diffuse lesions, prolonged platelet therapy reduces late thrombosis, and additional stenting is to be avoided.

In SCRIPPS IV, the objective was to compare the safety and efficacy of a 21.4% increase, from 14 to 17 Gy, of γ-radiation in patients with ISR. This was a double-blind, randomized trial utilizing 14 Gy vs 17 Gy at 2 mm from the source. Three hundred fifty-eight patients were included from two sites. Inclusion criteria included in-stent restenotic native and SVG lesions up to 75 mm in length. End points were late loss, restenosis, TLR, target vessel revascularization (TVR), and major adverse cardiac event (MACE) rates. A 21.4% increase in γ-radiation dose (from 14 to 17 Gy) resulted in 18% reduction in restenosis (in-lesion),

26% reduction in late loss (in-lesion), 44% reduction in TLR, 36% reduction in TVR, 41% reduction in MACE, and 75% reduction in total occlusions.

## WRIST SERIES

### *Original WRIST*

The Original Washington Radiation for In-Stent Restenosis (WRIST) is the first in a series of studies designed to evaluate the effectiveness of radiation therapy in patients with ISR. In these studies, γ-radiation was delivered through a ribbon with different trains of radioactive (Ir-192) seeds, which was inserted manually into a closed-end lumen catheter. In the initial WRIST study, 130 patients (100 patients with native coronaries and 30 patients with saphenous vein grafts [SVG]), with in-stent restenotic lesions (up to 47 mm in length) were blindly randomized to receive either Ir-192 or placebo. Angiographic restenosis (27% vs 56%, $p = 0.002$) and TVR (26% vs 68%, $p < 0.001$) were reduced at 6 mo in IRT patients. Between 6 and 60 mo, IRT compared with placebo patients had more TLR (IRT = 21.6% vs placebo = 4.7%, $p = 0.04$) and TVR (IRT = 21.5% vs placebo = 6.1%, $p = 0.03$). At 5 yr, the MACE rate was significantly reduced with IRT (46.2% vs 69.2%, $p = 0.008$). In WRIST, patients with ISR treated with IRT using Ir-192 had a reduction in the need for repeat TLR and TVR at 6 mo and at 5 yr *(44)*.

### *Saphenous Vein Grafts WRIST*

Saphenous vein graft (SVG)-WRIST is an FDA-approved, double-blind, randomized trial that evaluated 120 patients postcoronary bypass surgery with diffuse lesions of ISR in SVG. In this study, after treating the lesion, a noncentered, closed-end lumen catheter was positioned at the treated site, and patients randomly received a ribbon with either Ir-192 or with nonradioactive seeds delivered by hand. Different ribbons consisting of 6, 10, and 14 seeds were used to cover lesions <47 mm in length. The prescribed radiation doses were 14 or 15 Gy at a 2 mm radial distance from the center of the source in vessels with a diameter of 4 mm. For vessels >4 mm in diameter, 15 Gy at 2.4 mm was prescribed. Angiographic restenosis (21% vs 44%, $p = 0.005$) and TVR (18% vs 55%, $p < 0.001$) were dramatically reduced at 6 mo in IRT patients. At 12 mo, IRT compared with placebo patients had less TLR (17% vs 57%, $p < 0.001$) and TVR (28% vs 62%, $p < 0.001$). At 36 mo clinical follow-up, patients receiving IRT continued to have markedly lower TLR and TLR-MACE rates when compared with controls *(45)*.

### *Long WRIST/Long WRIST High Dose*

One hundred and twenty patients with diffuse ISR in native coronary arteries (lesion length 36–80 mm) were randomized for either radiation with Ir-192 with 15 Gy at 2 mm from the source axis or placebo. After enrollment, 120 additional patients with the same inclusion criteria were treated with Ir-192 with 18 Gy and included in the Long WRIST High Dose registry. ATP was initially prescribed for 1 mo and was extended to 6 mo in the last 60 patients of the Long WRIST High Dose registry. At 6 mo, the binary angiographic restenosis rates were 73%, 45%, and 38% in the placebo, 15 Gy and 18 Gy radiated groups, respectively ($p < 0.05$) (Fig. 2). At 1 yr, the primary clinical end point of MACE was 63% in the placebo group and 42% in the radiated group with 15 Gy ($p < 0.05$). The MACE rate was further reduced with 18 Gy (22%, $p < 0.05$ vs 15 Gy).

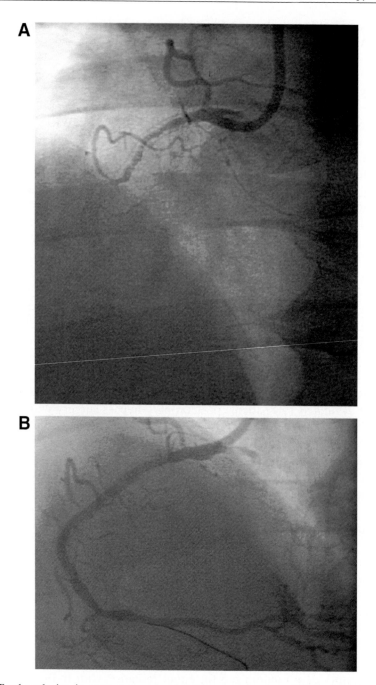

**Fig. 2. (A)** Total occlusion in-stent restenosis of right coronary artery. **(B)** Final angiographic result postradiation. **(C)** Six-mo follow-up angiography.

Late thrombosis was 12%, 15%, and 9% in the placebo group, 15 Gy group with 1 mo APT and 18 Gy group with 6 mo of APT, respectively. It was concluded that vascular brachytherapy with Ir-192 is safe and reduces the rate of recurrent restenosis in diffuse ISR. Efficacy of brachytherapy on angiographic and clinical outcomes are enhanced with a radiation dose of 18 Gy and prolonged APT *(46)*.

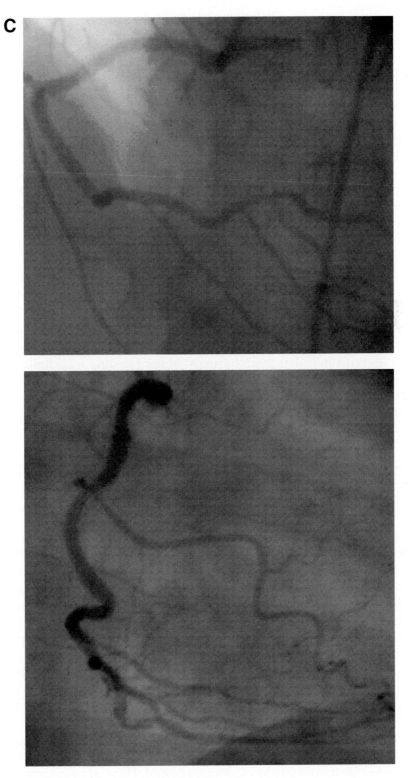

**Fig. 2.** *(Continued)*

## WRIST 12/WRIST Plus

In WRIST 12, about 120 consecutive patients with diffuse ISR in native coronaries and vein grafts with lesions <80 mm in length underwent PTCA, laser ablation, or rotational atherectomy. Additional stents were placed in 39 patients (33%). After the intervention, a ribbon with different trains of radioactive Ir-192 seeds was positioned to cover the treated site, and a dose of 14 Gy to 2 mm was prescribed. Patients were discharged with clopidogrel and aspirin for 12 mo and followed up clinically. The cardiac clinical event rates at 15 mo were compared with the γ-treated ($n = 120$) patients of the WRIST Plus study (only 6 mo of ATP). Whereas the late thrombosis rates were similar (3.3% for the group given 12 mo of ATP vs 4.2% for the group given 6 mo, $p = 0.72$), the group treated with 12 mo of ATP had a rate of 21% for MACE and 20% for TLR compared with 36% ($p = 0.01$) and 35% ($p = 0.009$), respectively, in patients who were treated with only 6 mo of clopidogrel (47).

## Integrilin WRIST

Integrilin WRIST aimed to study the impact of GPIIb/IIIa inhibitor (eptifibatide) as adjunct therapy to IRT for patients with ISR. In the study using Ir-192, 150 patients were assigned to eptifibatide (Integrilin) and 150 patients to heparin only. Clinical composite end points at 30 d were similar between the patients treated with and without eptifibatide (4.7% vs 4%, $p = 0.78$). There was a similarity in the non-Q-wave MI rates between the eptifibatide and control groups. Major bleeding was similar in patients treated with and without eptifibatide. Overall, the use of eptifibatide as adjunct therapy for patients with ISR who are treated with IRT did not impact the clinical outcome at 30 d (48).

## γ-TRIALS

This is a series of trials utilizing the Checkmate system (Cordis, Miami, FL) for the treatment of ISR.

## γ-I

γ-I is a multicenter, randomized, double-blind trial of 252 patients with ISR, which assessed the feasibility, safety, and efficacy of intracoronary γ-radiation (Ir-192) ribbon hand-delivered using IVUS to guide dosimetry (dose range between 8 and 30 Gy). Six-month angiographic results obtained in 111 patients (84.7%) in the Ir-192 group and in 103 patients (85.1%) in the placebo group, revealed significant reductions in the in-stent (21.6% vs 50.5%, $p < 0.005$) and in-lesion (32.4% vs 55.3%, $p = 0.01$) restenosis rates of the radiation arm vs control. Patients who derived the highest benefit were those with long lesions and/or diabetes. There was a 43% reduction in restenosis for lesions longer than 30 mm, and a 62% reduction in restenosis for diabetic patients (75.9% vs 36.1%). After 9 mo, the composite primary end point of death, MI, emergency bypass surgery and revascularization procedures of the target lesion was significantly lower in the irradiated arm (28.2% vs 43.8% in the placebo group, $p = 0.02$).

Clinical events demonstrated a reduction in the TLR rate from 42.1% to 24.4%. The rate of death (3.12 vs 0.8, $p = 0.17$) and the rate of acute MI (9.9% vs 4.1%, $p = 0.09$), however, were higher in the irradiated group vs control. These complications were related in part to the late thrombosis phenomenon, which was more frequent in patients treated with radiation therapy than with placebo (5.3% vs 0.8%, $p = 0.07$). All patients in the Ir-192 group who presented with late thrombosis had new stents placed within the in-stent target lesion at the time of the procedure, but none of the patients who had late thrombosis died during the study period *(49)*. This trial demonstrated the efficacy of intracoronary γ-radiation for the prevention of the recurrence of ISR, and increased awareness regarding the correlation between late thrombosis and an increased risk of MI.

## γ-II

γ-II is a registry of 125 patients who were treated for the same inclusion/exclusion criteria as γ-I, but with a fixed dosimetry of 14 Gy at 2 mm from the center of the source. The treated lesions in γ-II were more heavily calcified, whereby 45% of patients required rotational atherectomy in contrast to 26% of patients in the original γ-I. Despite the differences in lesions, the results between γ-I and II were remarkably similar. γ-II patients had lower MLD after the procedure, perhaps owing to increased lesion complexity and the fact that fewer stents were placed in γ-II patients, as compared with γ-I. There was a 52% in-stent and a 40% in-lesion reduction in restenosis frequency. TLR rates were reduced by 48% and MACE were reduced by 36%. The late thrombosis rate was 4% at 270 d with only 8 wk of ATP *(50)*.

### AngioRad Radiation Technology for In-Stent Restenosis Trial in Native Coronaries I/II

The ARTISTIC I study examined the benefits of using a flexible, 30 mm Ir-192 wire source (AngioRad System, Vascular Therapies, United States Surgical Corporation, Norwalk, CT) in 115 patients. Fifty-eight patients were randomized to a nonradioactive placebo wire and 57 to a radioactive source wire. The source was not delivered in one patient. At 3 yr, clinical follow-up data were available in 53.4% (31/58) of the control patients and in 66.7% (38/57) of irradiated patients. Placebo patients had a cumulative MACE rate of 24.1%, whereas in the AngioRad group, it was 22.8% *(51)*.

The purpose of ARTISTIC II was to determine the safety and efficacy of the AngioRad System in inhibiting ISR as measured by a composite clinical end point at 9 mo posttreatment. Three hundred forty patients were included: 236 patients with 236 lesions were enrolled and treated with the AngioRad System at 11 clinical sites. The control group included 104 patients with 104 lesions enrolled and treated (without radiation) previously at seven clinical sites in the ARTISTIC I and WRIST studies. The Kaplan-Meier estimate of freedom from target vessel failure (TVF) for the placebo group was 52%, whereas in the irradiated group it was 85.5%. The acute results showed that patients treated with the AngioRad device had an acute procedural success rate of 86.9% and patients in the control group had an acute procedural success rate of 92.3% *(52)*.

## CLINICAL TRIALS OF β-RADIATION

There are three systems of β-emitters currently in use: the β-Cath™ System (Novoste Corporation, Norcross, GA) (Fig. 3), the Guidant GALILEO™ (Fig. 4), Intravascular Radiotherapy System (Guidant Corporation, Houston, TX), and the radiation delivery system™ (RDX) (Radiance Medical, San Diego, CA) (Fig. 5). Large-scale clinical studies testing the effectiveness of β-radiation for restenotic (Table 3) and *de novo*

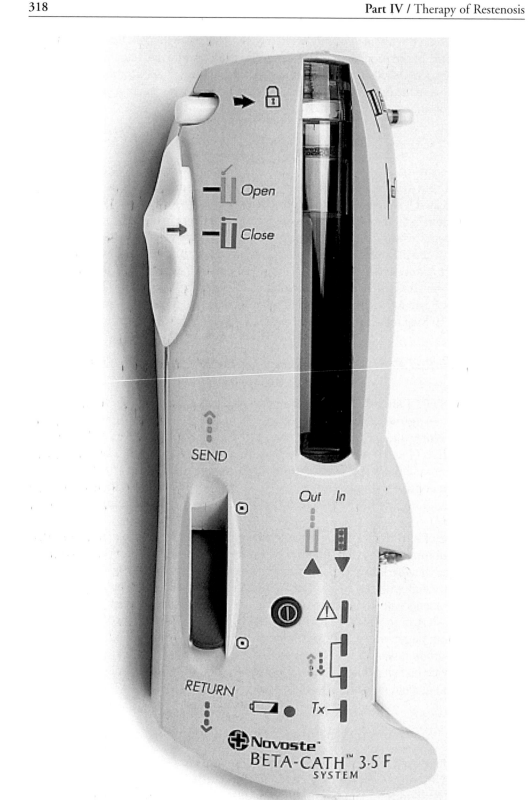

**Fig. 3.** β-Cath™ system (Novoste Corporation, Norcross, GA).

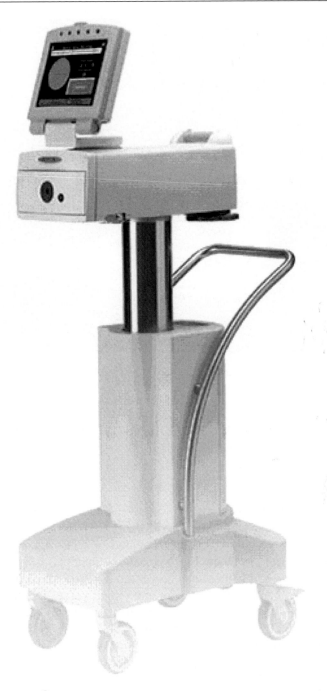

**Fig. 4.** Guidant GALILEO® III intravascular radiotherapy system (Guidant Corporation, Houston, TX).

lesions (Table 4) have paralleled the encouraging results of γ-radiation. Important early studies included the Geneva trial *(53)* and the dose-finding study β Energy Restenosis Trial (BERT), which used Y-90 *(54)*. In these studies, radiation was delivered safely with low rates of angiographic binary restenosis. The β Radiation in Europe registry used Sr/Y-90 (Novoste system). In the initial 149 patients, 6-mo and 1-yr rates of TVR

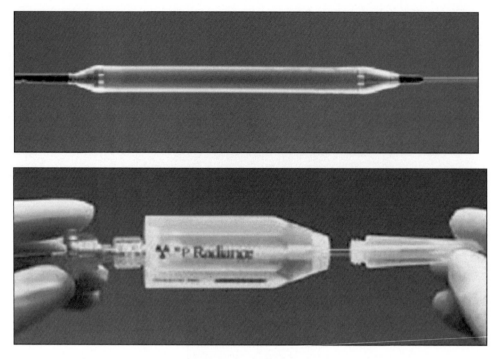

**Fig. 5.** RDX™ radiation delivery system (Radiance Medical, San Diego, CA).

with PTCA were 22% and 31%, respectively *(55)*. Using P-32, proliferation reduction with vascular energy trial (PREVENT) *(56)* demonstrated a reduced late loss index and binary restenosis with active treatment.

## β-*CATH*

The β-Cath system trial was the first prospective, randomized, multicenter trial investigating the use of vascular brachytherapy for the prevention of restenosis in *de novo* lesions using a 30 mm Sr/Y-90 source train in conjunction with stand alone balloon angioplasty, or provisional stent placement in which balloon angioplasty was suboptimal *(57)*.

The primary end point of the study was 8-mo TVF (death, MI, and TVR). The inclusion criteria included a single lesion and single vessel intervention with a *de novo* or restenotic lesion >50% (by visual assessment) in vessels between 2.7 and 4 mm reference vessel diameter (RVD). The radiation dose prescription point was calculated at 2 mm from center of source axis: 16.1 Gy in RVD ≥2.7 to ≤3.3 mm and 20.7 Gy in RVD > 3.3 to ≤ 4 mm. Baseline demographic and angiographic characteristics were similar between groups.

Comparison of placebo and radiation treatment from pooled PTCA and stent groups (ATP ≥ 60 d) showed equivalent 8-mo TLR (15.4% vs 13.7%, $p = 0.37$) and TVF/MACE (20.6% vs 18.7%, $p = 0.40$). This β-Cath study was the first to identify the higher-than-expected rate of late stent thrombosis when radiation was used with new stent implantation. The primary clinical end point, TVF, was not shown to be significantly lower in the combined radiation arms compared with combined placebo arms. Secondary analyses of β-radiation in the PTCA branch showed a 34.6% reduction for Sr/Y-90 in TVF/MACE ($p = 0.06$), and a 37.6% reduction for Sr/Y-90 in lesion segment restenosis rate ($p = 0.003$).

Table 3
Clinical Trials for ISR Using Catheter-Based Systems With β-Radiation

| Study name | Design | Isotope and dose (Gy) | Results |
|---|---|---|---|
| β WRIST | 50 patients with ISR in native coronaries | 20.6 Gy at 1 mm from the balloon surface | Clinical benefit maintained at 2 yr Reduction in TLR, TVR, and MACE compared with placebo |
| INHIBIT | Multicenter, randomized of 332 patients | P-32, 20 Gy at 1 mm into vessel wall | Binary restenosis reduced by 50% (analysis segment) and 55% in MACE |
| START | Multicenter, randomized study of 476 patients | Sr/Y-90, 18-23 Gy at 2 mm | Reduction in TLR, TVR, and MACE (35%) in the irradiated group. No late thrombosis seen |
| START 40/20 | 207 patient registry that mirrored START | Sr/Y-90, 18-23 Gy at 2 mm | 44% reduction in restenosis compared with 36% in irradiated arm of START |
| BRITE | Feasibility study of 32 patients with in-stent restenotic lesions less than 25 mm | P-32, 20 Gy at 1 mm from the balloon | Binary restenosis 0% in stented segment and 7.5% in analysis segment |
| BRITE II | Randomized study of 429 patients with ISR | P-32, 20 Gy at 1 mm | ISR 10.9% and geographic miss 8.5% at 9 mo |
| SVG BRITE | 49 patients—24 de novo and 25 SVG ISR lesions | P-32, 20 Gy at 1 mm | 1-yr TVR of 8% and 13% angiographic restenosis |
| 4R | 50 South Korean patients with ISR | Re-188, 15 Gy at 1 mm into the vessel wall | 6-mo angiographic restenosis rate was 10.4% |
| GALILEO INHIBIT | International multicenter registry of 120 patients | P-32, 20 Gy at 1 mm into vessel wall | Binary restenosis reduced by 74% in stented segment and by 27% in analysis segment |

The results in angiographic restenosis were disparate in the combined stent branches, a 28.9% reduction for Sr/Y-90 in lesion segment restenosis rate ($p = 0.004$) and a 30% increase for Sr/Y-90 in the analysis segment ($p = 0.004$).

The paradox of positive treatment effect for Sr/Y-90 seen in lesion segment analysis and the negative treatment effect of Sr/Y-90 seen in the analysis segment likely explains

Table 4
Clinical Trials Using Catheter-Based Systems With β-Emitters in Coronaries
for *De Novo* Lesions

| Study name | Design | Isotope and dose (Gy) | Results |
|---|---|---|---|
| GENEVA | Open label in 15 patients after PTCA | Y-90, 18 Gy to surface of balloon | Demonstrated feasibility and safety for *de novo* lesions. Restenosis rate 40% |
| BERT | Open label, feasibility study of 23 patients in two centers | Sr/Y-90 12, 14, or 16 Gy to 2 mm | Restenosis rate of 15% with late loss of 10% |
| β-Radiation in Europe | European registry of 150 patients | Sr/Y-90 14, 18 Gy to 2 mm from source | 6-mo and 1-yr TVR with PTCA were 22% and 31%, respectively |
| BETA-CATH | Multicenter, randomized study of 1455 patients post-PTCA and provisional stenting | Sr/Y-90 14 or 18 Gy to 2 mm | 240-d TVF rate of 14.2% Restenosis rate 31% |
| Dose Finding | European, multicenter study in 183 patients after PTCA | Y-90 9, 12, 18, or 32 Gy to 1 mm | Marked reduction in restenosis in nonstented arteries after 18 Gy administration |
| PREVENT | Multicenter, randomized, sham-controlled study of 105 patients with *de novo* or restenotic lesions | P-32 16-20-24 Gy to 1 mm | 22.4% restenosis at 6 mo. MACE 16% at 1 yr |
| BRIDGE | Multicenter, randomized trial of 112 patients | P-32, 20 Gy at 1 mm | At 1 yr, TVR and MACE rates were 20.4% and 25.9% vs 12.1% and 17.2% in the irradiated and control groups, respectively |
| ECRIS | Randomized, controlled trial of 225 patients | Re-188, 22.5 Gy at 0.5 mm tissue depth | At 6 mo, binary restenosis, TVR, and late loss were significantly lower in the irradiated group |

the negative treatment effect of Sr/Y-90 on clinical restenosis in stents, and merits further investigation. Geographic miss (inadequate radiation coverage of the interventional injury) may have contributed to the negative results of Sr/Y-90. The overall positive results in the lesion segment analysis and the strong trends in the clinical outcomes in the PTCA branch suggest a potential role for Sr/Y-90 radiation in the treatment of *de novo* coronary lesions if the increase of restenosis in the "analysis segment" can be solved.

## β-*Energy Restenosis Trial*

BERT is a feasibility study approved by the FDA limited to 23 patients in two centers (Emory and Brown Universities). The study was designed to test the $^{90}$Sr/Y source delivered by hydraulic system (Novoste Corp. Norcross, GA) *(54)*. The prescribed doses in this study were 12, 14, or 16 Gy and the treatment time did not exceed 3.5 min. The radiation was successfully delivered to 21 of 23 patients following conventional PTCA without any complications or adverse events at 30 d. At follow-up, two patients at 6 mo and one patient at 9 mo underwent repeat revascularization to the target lesion. One patient underwent stent implantation to a segment proximal to the irradiated site. Angiographic follow-up at 6 mo assessed by QCA detected late loss of 10% with a late loss index of 5%. The Canadian arm of this study included 30 patients from the Montreal Heart Institute utilizing the same system under the same protocol *(57)*. At 6 mo follow-up, the angiographic restenosis rate was 10% with negative late loss and late loss index. IVUS analysis of this cohort demonstrated larger lumen at 6 mo follow-up with reduction of the wall area. The European arm of the BERT (BERT 1.5) was conducted at the Thoraxcenter in Rotterdam, The Netherlands in an additional 30 patients who were treated successfully with balloon angioplasty. Angiographic restenosis in this cohort was higher than reported in the United States and Canada trials *(58)*.

## *Proliferation Reduction With Vascular Energy Trial*

PREVENT was a prospective, randomized, sham-controlled, multicenter study of 105 patients with *de novo* (70%) or restenotic (30%) lesions who were randomized to either placebo or 3 different doses of β-radiation (16, 20, and 24 Gy to a depth of 1 mm in the artery wall) ($^{32}$P) to prevent restenosis after PTCA or stenting. The binary restenosis rate at 6-mo angiographic follow-up was 8.2% at the target site for the radiation treated group vs 39.1% for the control group ($p = 0.001$). Restenosis at the target site plus adjacent segments was 22.4% for patients who received treatment vs 50% for the control group ($p = 0.02$) *(56)*. Long-term (12-mo) MACE (death, MI, and TLR) occurred in 13 patients in the brachytherapy group (16%) and in six control patients (24%, $p = NS$). If TVR is included, MACE occurred in 26% vs 32% ($p = NS$), respectively. The occurrence of MI owing to thrombotic events after discharge happened in seven patients who received radiotherapy and in none in the control group. Stenosis adjacent to the target site contributed significantly to the diminution of the clinical benefit. Prolonged ATP and a reduced use of new stents at the time of radiation may minimize these complications. Therefore, β-radiation with a P-32 source wire and a centering catheter is safe and effective in reducing neointimal formation within the target site in patients undergoing PTCA.

## *Dose-Finding Study Group*

The Dose-Finding Study Group was a prospective, randomized, multicenter, dose-finding trial. The primary objective was to determine the effect of 9, 12, 15, and 18 Gy of β-radiation (Yttrium-90) at a tissue depth of 1 mm on restenosis rates after PTCA in *de novo* lesions. Secondary objectives included safety and technical performance of the device. Of the 183 patients randomized, 181 received the prescribed doses of β-radiation: 45 received 9 Gy, 45 received 12 Gy, 46 received 15 Gy, and 45 received 18 Gy. Stenting after radiation was required in 47% of the patients because of residual stenosis or major dissection. At 6-mo angiographic follow-up, a significant dose-dependent benefit was evident. There was abrupt thrombosis or late occlusion of the target vessel in 4 out of 120 (3.3%) patients who were treated with only balloon angioplasty and in 7 of the 49 (14.3%) patients who received new stents. There was only one death in the 18 Gy group. In conclusion, this study demonstrated a marked reduction in restenosis in nonstented arteries after administration of 18 Gy of β-radiation, especially in patients who underwent plain balloon angioplasty, suggesting that β-radiation therapy should be evaluated as an adjunctive to PTCA (59).

## β-WRIST

β-WRIST examined the efficacy of β-radiation for prevention of ISR, with similar design to the original WRIST study. This registry included 50 patients who were treated for ISR in native coronaries, 2.5–4 mm in diameter with lesions <50 mm in length. β-radiation using a $^{90}$Y source was administered using a centering catheter and an afterloader system. Clinical outcomes were compared between these patients and those of the original WRIST cohort (randomized to either placebo or $^{192}$Ir). Angiographic restenosis at 6 mo in β-WRIST was 22% with a late total occlusion rate of 12%. Compared with the historical control group of WRIST, β-WRIST patients demonstrated a 58% reduction in the rate of TLR and 53% reduction in TVR at 6 mo ($p < 0.001$). No differences were detected in comparison with the γ-radiated patients of WRIST. The clinical benefit was maintained at 2-yr follow-up with β-radiation reducing TLR (42% vs 66%, $p = 0.016$), TVR (46% vs 72%, $p = 0.009$) and MACE (46% vs 72%, $p = 0.008$) compared with placebo. The efficacy of β- and γ-emitters for the treatment of ISR appeared similar at longer term follow-up (60).

## START/START 40/20

A pivotal multicenter, randomized trial, START (STents And Radiation Therapy), involved 476 patients in over 55 centers throughout the United States and Europe, and was designed to determine the efficacy and safety of the β-Cath system for the treatment of ISR. Patients were randomized to either placebo or an active radiation train 30 mm in length. The inclusion criteria were single ISR lesions >50% (by visual assessment) in native coronary target vessels between 2.7 and 4 mm in diameter. The target lesion (≤20 mm) required treatment with a 20 mm balloon and a 30 mm source train.

In radiated patients, the mean lesion length was 16.3 mm in arteries 2.8 mm in diameter. After successful angioplasty, these patients were treated with the β-Cath system containing $^{90}$Sr/Y seeds, delivering β-radiation through a closed-end lumen catheter. The dose prescribed at a point 2 mm from center of source axis was based on visual assessment of RVD; 18.4 Gy in RVD ≥2.7 to ≤3.3 mm and 23 Gy in RVD >3.3 to ≤4 mm. The duration of ATP was initially based on operator preference and was modified in early 1999 to at least 90 d of clopidogrel (75 mg/QD) following recommendations from the β-Cath Trial Data Safety Monitoring Board, where late thrombosis as a complication of brachytherapy was first recognized.

At 8 mo, angiographic restenosis rates in the irradiated segments were 24% vs 46% in the placebo group ($p < 0.001$). In the irradiated group, TLR was 13% as compared with 22% in control ($p = 0.008$), with similar reductions of TVR (16% vs 24%,

42. Teirstein PS, Massullo V, Jani S, et al. Catheter-based radiotherapy to inhibit restenosis after coronary stenting. N Engl J Med 1997;336:1697–1703.

43. Teirstein PS, Massullo V, Jani S, et al. Two-year follow-up after catheter-based radiotherapy to inhibit coronary restenosis. Circulation 1999;99:243–247.

44. Waksman R, Ajani AE, White RL, et al. Five-year follow-up after intracoronary gamma radiation therapy for in-stent restenosis. Circulation 2004;109:340–344.

45. Rha SW, Kuchulakanti PK, Pakala R, et al. Three year follow-up after intracoronary gamma radiation for in-stent restenosis in saphenous vein grafts. Cath Cardio Interv 2005;65:257–262.

46. Waksman R, Cheneau E, Ajani AE, et al. Washington Radiation for In-Stent Restenosis Trial for Long Lesions Studies. Intracoronary radiation therapy improves the clinical and angiographic outcomes of diffuse in-stent restenotic lesions: results of the Washington Radiation for In-Stent Restenosis Trial for Long Lesions (Long WRIST) Studies. Circulation 2003;107:1744–1749.

47. Waksman R, Ajani AE, Pinnow E, et al. Twelve versus six months of clopidogrel to reduce major cardiac events in patients undergoing gamma-radiation therapy for in-stent restenosis: Washington Radiation for In-Stent restenosis Trial (WRIST) 12 versus WRIST PLUS. Circulation 2002;106:776–778.

48. Waksman R, Ajani AE, Gruberg L, et al. The use of IIB/IIIA inhibitors in patients with in-stent restenosis treated with intracoronary gamma radiation: integrilin WRIST. Cath Cardio Interv 2004;62:162–166.

49. Leon MB, Teirstein PS, Moses JW, et al. Localized intracoronary gamma-radiation therapy to inhibit the recurrence of restenosis after stenting. N Engl J Med 2001;344:250–256.

50. Ajani AE, Kim HS, Waksman R. Clinical trials of vascular brachytherapy for in-stent restenosis: update. Cardiovasc Radiat Med 2001;2:107–113.

51. Waksman R, Bhargava B, Chan RC, et al. Intracoronary radiation with gamma wire inhibits recurrent in-stent restenosis. Cardiovasc Radiat Med 2001;2:63–68.

52. Kereikas DJ, Waksman R, Mehra A, et al. Multi-center experience with a novel Ir-192 vascular brachytherapy device for in-stent restenosis: final results of the AngioRad™ T radiation therapy for in-stent restenosis intracoronaries II (ARTISTIC II) trial. J Am Coll Cardiol 2003;41:49A.

53. Verin V, Urban P, Popowski Y, et al. Feasibility of intracoronary beta-irradiation to reduce restenosis after balloon angioplasty. A clinical pilot study. Circulation 1997;95:1138–1144.

54. King SB 3rd, Williams DO, Chougule P, et al. Endovascular beta-radiation to reduce restenosis after coronary balloon angioplasty. Results of the beta energy restenosis trial (BERT). Circulation 1998;97:2025–2030.

55. Sianos G, Kay IP, Costa MA, Regar E, et al. Geographical miss during catheter-based intracoronary beta-radiation: incidence and implications in the BRIE study. J Am Coll Cardiol 2001;38:415–420.

56. Raizner AE, Oesterle SN, Waksman R, et al. Inhibition of restenosis with β-emitting radiotherapy report of the proliferation reduction with vascular energy trial (PREVENT) Circulation 2000;102:951–958.

57. Waksman R, Raizner A, Popma JJ. Beta emitter systems and results from clinical trials. state of the art. Cardiovasc Radiat Med 2003;4:54–63.

58. Bonan R, Arsenault A, Tardif JC, et al. Beta energy restenosis trial, Canadian Arm. Circulation 1997;96:I-219.

59. Verin V, Popowski Y, deBruyne B, et al. Endoluminal beta-radiation therapy for the prevention of coronary restenosis after balloon angioplasty. N Engl J Med 2001;344:243–249.

60. Waksman R, Bhargava B, White L, et al. Intracoronary beta radiation therapy inhibits recurrence of in-stent restenosis. Circulation 2000;101:1895–1898.

61. Popma J. Late clinical and angiographic outcomes after use of $^{90}$Sr/$^{90}$Y beta radiation for the treatment of in-stent restenosis: results from the $^{90}$Sr treatment of angiographic restenosis (START) trial. J Am Coll Cardiol 2000;36:311–312.

62. Waksman R, Raizner AE, Yeung AC, Lansky AJ, Vandertie L. Localized intracoronary beta radiation therapy to inhibit recurrence of in-stent restenosis. Lancet 2002;359:551–557.

63. Waksman R, Buchbinder M, Reisman M, et al. Balloon-based radiation therapy for treatment of in-stent restenosis in human coronary arteries: results from the BRITE I study. Catheter Cardiovasc Interv 2002;57:286–294.

64. Stone GW, Mehran R, Midei M, et al. Usefulness of beta radiation for de novo and In-Stent restenotic lesions in saphenous vein grafts. AJC 2003;92:312–314.

65. Park S-W, Kong M-K, Moon DH, et al. Treatment of diffuse in-stent restenosis with rotational atherectomy followed by radiation therapy with a rhenium-188-mercaptoacetyltriglycine-filled balloon. J Am Coll Cardiol 2001;38:3:631–637.

66. Serruys PW, Wijns W, Sianos G, et al. Direct stenting versus direct stenting followed by centered beta-radiation with IVUS-guided dosimetry and long-term antiplatelet treatment; results of a randomized trial (the BRIDGE trial). J Am Coll Cardiol 2004;44:528.

67. Höher M, Wöhrle J, Wohlfrom M, et al. Intracoronary beta-irradiation using a rhenium-188 filled balloon catheter—a randomized trial in patients with *de novo* and restenotic lesions. Circulation 2003;7:3022.

68. Sabaté M, Pimentel G, Prieto C, et al. Intracoronary brachytherpay after stenting in diabetic patients: results of a randomized study. J Am Coll Cardiol 2004;44:520–527.

69. Moses J. IRIS trials low-activity 32-P stent. Advances in Cardiovascular Radiation Therapy III, Washington, DC, 1999:387–388.

70. Serruys PW, Kay IP. I like the candy, I hate the wrapper: the (32)P radioactive stent [editorial]. Circulation 2000;101:3–7.

71. Wexberg P, Siostrzonek P, Kirisits C, et al. High activity radioactive BX -stents for reduction of restenosis after coronary interventions: the Vienna P-32 dose response study. Circulation 1999;100: I-156.

72. Wardeh A, Wijns W, Albiero R, et al. Angiographic follow-up after 32-P beta emitting radioactive "cold ends" Isostent implantation. Results from Aalst, Milan and Rotterdam. Circulation 2000;102: II-442.

73. Waksman R, Bhargava B, Mintz GS, et al. Late total occlusion after intracoronary brachytherapy for patients with in-stent restenosis. J Am Coll Cardiol 2000;36:65–68.

74. Costa MA, Sabat M, van der Giessen WJ, et al. Late coronary occlusion after intracoronary brachytherapy. Circulation 1999;100:789–792.

75. Sabate M, Serruys PW, van der Giessen WJ, et al. Geometric vascular remodeling after balloon angioplasty and beta-radiation therapy: A three-dimensional intravascular ultrasound study. Circulation 1999;100:1182–1188.

76. Kim HS, Waksman R, Cottin Y, et al. Edge stenosis and geographical miss following intracoronary gamma radiation therapy for in-stent restenosis. J Am Coll Cardiol 2001 15;37:1026–1030.

# 21

# Preclinical Data of Eluting Stents

*Antonio Colombo, MD*
*and Alaide Chieffo, MD*

## INTRODUCTION

The concept of using stents coated with agents that could potentially inhibit neointimal hyperplasia has emerged and drug-eluting stents (DES) represent one of the fastest growing fields in interventional cardiology today. Different animal models have been used in order to test the safety and efficacy of DES. The drug-eluting coatings contain antimitotic (e.g., sirolimus [SRL], SRL analogs, paclitaxel, and actinomycin), anti-inflammatory (e.g., dexamethasone [DEX]), prohealing (e.g., 17β-estradiol and endothelial progenitor cells [EPC]), immunosuppressive (SRL, tacrolimus, everolimus, mycophenolic acid [MPA]) agents. These compounds are often blended with synthetic polymers that act as drug reservoirs and elute the active agent over a period of several weeks or months. Local drug delivery has been demonstrated in preclinical studies to achieve higher tissue concentrations of the drug that is applied to the vessel at the precise site and at the time of vessel injury.

Recently, the concept of gene-eluting stents has been introduced using naked plasmid DNA encoding for human vascular endothelial growth factor (VEGF)-2 resulting in significant reduction in neointima formation with acceleration, rather than inhibition of re-endothelialization.

From: *Contemporary Cardiology: Essentials of Restenosis: For the Interventional Cardiologist*
Edited by: H. J. Duckers, E. G. Nabel, and P. W. Serruys © Humana Press Inc., Totowa, NJ

DES represents the third revolution in the field of interventional cardiology following balloon angioplasty (percutaneous coronary angioplasty [PTCA]) and the implantation of bare-metal stents (BMS). Although stents significantly reduce restenosis when compared with balloon angioplasty, they have not eliminated restenosis and in-stent restenosis (ISR) as intimal hyperplasia (1) became a new clinical challenge. Experimental evidence exists for four major phases, that leads to neointimal formation in the treated vessel segment:

1. Thrombus formation at the injury site;
2. Inflammation;
3. Proliferation and migration of smooth muscle cells (SMC); and
4. Extracellular matrix formation.

Oral administration of drugs to prevent the restenotic process leads to insufficient drug concentration to the target site (2). In recent years, the knowledge of biomolecular aspects of cell cycle regulation has made possible the development of a tailored approach to cell proliferation and to different phases of the restenotic process (3).

The concept of local drug delivery through DES couples the biological and mechanical solutions necessary to maximize the angiographic result and facilitate the vessel repair from the injury caused by stent implantation itself. At the same time, local drug-delivery, using drug-eluting stents, offers the advantage of allowing high local concentrations of drug at the treatment site, whereas minimizing systemic toxic effects.

Currently, there are three different approaches of binding pharmacologically active compounds on coronary stents. The first approach consists in binding the drug by a polymer on the stent surface. Other approaches are to either bind the drug by an inorganic stent coating (permanent or bioabsorbable) or to directly load the drug on the stent surface without a coating (on stent approach).

## RESTENOSIS AFTER ANGIOPLASTY AND AFTER STENTING: TWO DIFFERENT MECHANISMS

Based on the experiences derived from experimental animal models, cell culture, human pathological evidence, as well as angiographic, angioscopic, and intravascular ultrasound observations, the sequence of events that take place in the artery and that characterize the restenotic process, can be divided into three phases:

1. A first phase of elastic recoil, usually occurring within 24 h of the procedure.
2. A second phase of mural thrombus formation and organization associated with inflammatory infiltrate at the site of vascular injury in the subsequent 2 wk. In this phase, immediately after stent implantation, activation, adhesion, aggregation, and deposition of platelets and neutrophils occurs. The platelet thrombus formed can even become large enough to occlude the vessel. Within hours, the thrombus at the injured site becomes fibrin-rich and also fibrin/red cell thrombus adheres to the platelet mass. From day 3 the thrombus is covered by a layer of endothelial-like cells and intense cellular infiltration begins at the injury site with monocytes (which become macrophages after migration into the mural thrombus) and lymphocytes. In the process, these cells progressively migrate deeper into the mural thrombus and vessel wall.
3. A third phase of cell activation, proliferation, and extracellular matrix formation, which usually lasts from 2 to 3 mo. In this phase, SMC from different vessel wall layers proliferate and migrate and thereafter reabsorb the residual thrombus until all of it is gone and replaced by neointimal cells. For several weeks, proliferating activity can be detected in the endothelial layer, the intimal layer, the medial layer, and in the adventitia.

4. Thereafter a more or less quiescent fourth state will ensue, characterized by further build-up of extracellular matrix.

Several factors may influence the production of neointimal volume, including the amount of platelet-fibrin thrombus at the injury site, the total number of SMC within the neointima, and the amount of extracellular matrix elaborated by neointimal cells. Limiting one of those steps, either individually or in combination, might reduce the neointimal response following mechanical injury.

The development of stents seemed the most logical solution to the problem of restenosis following angioplasty. If it is assumed that restenosis following angioplasty is initially caused by vessel constriction (remodeling), the insertion of a stent appeared its most simple solution. The truth of the matter is that vessel constriction is one among different elements leading to restenosis following angioplasty, but not to restenosis following stent implantation.

Vascular remodeling has assumed to have a great importance as a cause of coronary restenosis in the last few years in non-stented patients *(4)*. Following coronary angioplasty, three different remodeling responses have been described:

1. Compensatory enlargement *(5)*;
2. Absence of compensation; or
3. Vascular constriction.

Although mechanisms of chronic remodeling are poorly understood, several explanations have been postulated to explain the late lumen narrowing after PTCA: fibrosis of the vessel wall underlying the lesion, rearrangement of extracellular matrix composition and structure, and response to increased shear stress *(6)*. It has been also reported that $\alpha_v\beta_3$ integrin may regulate contraction of the vessel wall *(7)*. The integrins may therefore play a role in active contraction, as well as migration of SMC.

Animal studies indicate that after PTCA, stretching of the adventitia may result in the proliferation and synthesis of extracellular matrix by myofibroblasts within the adventitia itself, with consequently scar-like contraction and compression of the underlying vascular wall, *(8,9)*. This mechanism, however, does not seem relevant for late lumen narrowing in human coronary arteries subjected to stent implantation.

The potential impact of neointimal hyperplasia and geometric remodeling on restenosis requires further studies. Methods to prevent constrictive remodeling or to promote compensatory enlargement should be investigated.

## PATHOPHYSIOLOGY OF IN-STENT RESTENOSIS

ISR is mainly caused by neointimal hyperplasia *(1,10,11)*. Vessel injury by an angioplasty balloon or stent struts leads to the activation of platelets and mural thrombus formation *(12–14)*. The presence of vascular injury, mural thrombus, and a metallic foreign body activates circulating neutrophils and tissue macrophages *(14–16)*. These cellular elements release cytokines and growth factors that activate SMC *(17,18)*. Upregulation and expression of genes that regulate cell division, lead to cell proliferation *(19)*. Production of matrix metalloproteinases (MMP) is also upregulated, leading to remodeling of the extracellular matrix *(20)* and initiating SMC migration *(21,22)*. The end result of this cascade of events is the uncontrolled proliferation and migration of SMC around the vessel intima and the deposition of extracellular matrix material and migration, which often lead to significant luminal narrowing 3–6 mo after percutaneous coronery intervention (PCI) *(23,24)*.

In the *first wave* (1–4 d after vessel injury), medial SMC from the site of injury and possibly from adjacent areas are activated and stimulated by the triggering factors mentioned earlier. In addition to mitogenic factors released by endothelial cells, stretching of the arterial wall is a potent stimulus for SMC activation and growth. Once activated, SMC undergo characteristic phenotypic transformation from a "contractile" to a "synthetic" form, which is responsible for the production of extracellular matrix, rich in chondroitin sulfate and dermatan sulfate, seen in the first 6 mo after injury. The *second wave* (3–14 d after vessel injury) and the *third wave* (14 d to months after vessel injury) are respectively characterized by the migration of SMC through breaks in the internal elastic lamina into the intima, the local thrombus, and SMC proliferation, followed by extracellular matrix formation. Those events are characterized by complex interactions between growth factors, second messengers, and gene-regulatory proteins, resulting in a phenotypic change from a quiescent state to a proliferative one. The peak of proliferation is observed 4–5 d after balloon injury, but the duration of migration is not known, nor it is known whether a phase of cellular replication is required before SMC migration. Few studies have been done to identify the matrix molecules involved in the migration into the intima. Proteoglycans may also be important for the formation of neointima. SMC migration presumably requires degradation of the basement membrane surrounding the cells. Several MMPs, including tissue type plasminogen activator, plasmin, MMP-2, and MMP-9, may be responsible for this process *(25,26)* and the administration of a protease inhibitors reduces SMC migration into the intima. Cell migration is probably initiated by recognition of extracellular matrix proteins by a family of cell surface adhesion receptors known as integrins *(27)* whose selective blockage has been demonstrated to inhibit SMC migration and reduce neointimal formation.

As SMC decrease their proliferation rate, they begin to synthesize large quantities of proteoglycan matrix. The extracellular matrix production continues for up to 20–25 wk and over time it is gradually replaced by collagen and elastin, whereas the SMC turn into quiescent cells. The resulting neointima is made up of a fibrotic extracellular matrix with few cellular constituents. The endothelial cells proliferate and cover the denuded area and begin to produce large quantities of heparan sulfate and nitric oxide (NO), both of which inhibit SMC proliferation.

Also, the restored level of blood flow seems to be a crucial factor in the development of neointimal hyperplasia *(28–30)*. It has been postulated that wall shear stress (WSS) could be important causative factor. Recently, the causal relationship between WSS and neointimal hyperplasia formation in stents has been studied by locally increasing WSS with a flow divider placed in the center of the stent *(31)*. Using this model, the local increase in WSS was accompanied by a local reduction of neointimal hyperplasia and a local reduction in inflammation and injury, providing a direct evidence for a modulating role of shear stress in in-stent neointimal hyperplasia.

It is not clear why in some cases these reparative processes may lead to an excess in tissue growth, causing reduction of the lumen of the vessel, whereas in other instances the amount of hyperplasia remains limited. At present, there is increasing evidence that these genetic factors and local factors, such as injury to the external elastic lamina, may play a role in increasing these reparative processes *(32,33)*.

## ANIMAL MODELS

Animal models are considered the cornerstone to test strategies in order to develop treatments for pathological conditions and to understand pathophysiological mechanisms of diseases. The ideal animal model for therapy testing should be readily available, inexpensive to purchase and to maintain, and easy to handle *(34)*. Moreover, it should mimic the human pathophysiology of neointimal proliferation and remodeling. Several animal models have been developed during the last decade in attempt to reproduce restenotic lesions and find a therapeutic strategy to reduce neointima formation. Unfortunately, despite several models of restenosis have been evaluated in the last 15 y, there appeared to be no perfect animal model for human restenosis. Common models include the rat carotid air desiccation or balloon endothelial denudation model *(35,36)*, the rabbit femoral or iliac artery balloon injury model with or without cholesterol supplementation *(37)* and the porcine injured carotid *(38,39)* and coronary artery model.

The most common used animal model of ISR is the porcine coronary artery injury model. The histopathological features of neointima obtained in porcine models closely resemble the human neointima, and the amount of neointimal thickening is proportional to injury severity *(34,39)*. This has allowed the creation of an injury–neointima relationship that can be used to evaluate the response to different therapies. Maximal neointimal hyperplasia is induced in pigs by 4 wk after injury by an angioplasty balloon or coronary stent *(40)*. The amount of neointimal hyperplasia in this animal model is correlated to the degree of injury in the vessel wall. However, the repair process in the pig coronary arterial injury model using normal coronary arteries is certainly more rapid and may be different from the response to balloon angioplasty that characterize human coronary atherosclerotic plaques.

Another animal model of ISR is the rabbit iliac artery model *(41,42)*. In this model, rabbits are fed with a hypercholesterolemic diet for several weeks before performing the injury by an angioplasty balloon, reproducing similar pathological changes to those observed in human coronary arteries after stent implantation *(37,42)*. The hypercholesterolemic rabbit model has been criticized for the high level of hyperlipidemia required for the development of lesions. The latter results in a large macrophage foam cell component, which resemble fatty streaks rather than human restenotic lesions.

One of the oldest and most investigated models is the rat carotid artery model. The rat has several logistical advantages over other species. The rat carotid artery is commonly used for injury by balloon denudation: SMC proliferation peaks usually at 3 wk resulting in the formation of neointima. However, the morphology of normal rat corotid arteries differs considerably from humans: the artery wall has no vasa vasorum and contains a much thinner subintimal layer and a smaller percentage of elastin in the media *(34)*. The rat model, based on these elastic arteries, does not develop severe stenotic neointimal lesions, and is therefore these very permissive in term of efficacy of pharmacological interventions.

Animal models are certainly important in understanding the arterial reaction to coronary interventions and are essential for testing new treatment modalities for restenosis. The capacity of animal models of stenting to predict human responses depends on its similarity of the stages of healing in animals and humans. The main difference between animal and human response to arterial repair appears to lie in the temporal response to healing that is prolonged in humans compared with the animals *(43)*.

## COMPARISON OF VASCULAR HEALING IN ANIMALS AND HUMANS

In a morphometric analysis of 40 human stents collected at necropsy, it has been demonstrated that peak neointimal thickness occurs between 6 mo and 1 y *(43)*. In contrast, neointimal formation in stented pig coronary artery has been shown to be maximal at 1 mo. Consequently, the response to healing after placement of a bare-metal stent in a human coronary artery is five to six times longer than in pigs or rabbits. One explanation for the delayed arterial healing in humans is the underlying atherosclerotic process, as the arterial intervention in animals are usually performed in young adults and the stent is located in healthy vessels. It has also been postulated that the differential rate of healing between animals and humans could be proportional to the longevity of the species.

At 1 mo, after the implantation of DES (either SRL-eluting stent [SES] or paclitaxel-eluting stent [PES]) in pig and rabbit arteries, delayed healing with persistent fibrin deposition, variable inflammation, and incomplete endothelization was detected. The histological findings of DES at 1 mo in pig coronary arteries compared with BMS showed a 2 or 3 wk delay in healing. Late studies at 90 or 180 d with either paclitaxel (pig and rabbit) or sirolimus (pig), eluting stents showed complete neointimal healing, absence of fibrin and inflammation, and fully endothelialized luminal surface *(43)*.

## DRUG-ELUTING STENTS

Oral administration of drugs to prevent the restenotic process has not had a significant impact on restenosis rates *(2)* due to the lack of effect of systemically administered agents may have been inadequate drug concentrations at the site of stent implantation. The limited success of these agents in decreasing rates of ISR, coupled with side effects, prompted the development of DES.

Currently, there are three different approaches of binding pharmacologically active compounds to coronary stents. The first approach consists of binding the drug by a polymer on the stent surface. Other approaches are to either bind the drug by an inorganic stent coating (permanent or bioabsorbable) or to directly load the drug on the stent surface without a coating (on stent approach).

Biocompatible materials currently under investigation are thought to be less thrombogenic and inflammatory, and are thereby potentially able to reduce neointimal hyperplasia *(23,24)*. These materials include inert coatings, such as carbon, gold, and silicon carbide. Because of its biocompatibility phosphorylcholine (PC), a neutrally charged phospholipid polymer found on animal plasma membranes has also generated some interest. Despite these theoretical and experimental advantages, no clinical study performed in humans has so far demonstrated a reduced thrombogenicity or a better biocompatibility as evidenced by a reduction in local reaction (tissue growth). The DES may contain antimitotic (e.g., SRL, SRL analogs, paclitaxel, and actinomycin), anti-inflammatory (e.g., DEX), prohealing (e.g., 17 β-estradiol and EPC), and immunosuppressive (SRL, tacrolimus, everolimus, MPA) agents (Table 1).

These agents are often blended with synthetic polymers that act as drug reservoirs and elute the active agent over a period of several weeks or months. Unfortunately, many of these synthetic polymers appear to induce an exaggerated inflammatory response and neointimal hyperplasia in animal models *(44,45)*. An exception to this early experience is represented by poly-L-lactate acid (PLA) bioabsorbable coating polymer *(46)*. The potential benefits of this absorbable polymer are its restriction to

Table 1
DES Agents

| Agent | Class | Action at the dosage proposed | Current clinical stent platform |
|---|---|---|---|
| Estradiol | Prohealing | Inhibition of SMC proliferation and acceleration of re-endothelialization | BiodivYsio PC |
| Endothelial progenitor cell | Prohealing | Acceleration of re-endothelialization | BiodivYsio PC Genous R-Stent |
| Corticosteroids | Anti-inflammatory | Decrease migration and functional capability of the cells of inflammation | BiodivYsio PC |
| Paclitaxel | Antimitotic | Altering the equilibrium between microtubules and α-and β- tubulin by favoring the formation of abnormally stable microtubules | Taxus Nir Flex Taxus Express Taxus Libertè |
| Sirolimus | Antimitotic | *Antiproliferative* Inhibition of SMC migration and proliferation *Immunosuppressive* Blockage of T- and B-lymphocomplex by both calcium-dependent and calcium-independent pathways. Inhibition of proliferation of peripheral blood mononuclear cells and mast cells in response to various stimuli | Cypher Bx Velocity Cypher select |
| Everolimus | Sirolimus analog | *Immunosuppressive* Blocks growth-driven transduction signals in the T-cell response to alloantigen | Challenge S-Stent Champion Stent Bio-absorbable PLA polymer |
| Biolimus | Sirolimus analog | Inhibition of SMC migration and proliferation | S-Stent Bio-absorbable PLA polymer |
| ABT-578 | Sirolimus analog | Inhibition of SMC migration and proliferation | Endeavor PC ZoMaxx PC |
| MPA-eluting stent | Immuno-suppressive | Immunosuppressive inhibition of *de novo* purine synthesis | Duraflex Stent |
| VEGF-2 | Growth factor | Reductions in neointima formation with acceleration of re-endothelialization | BiodivYsio PC Plasmid DNA encoding for VEGF-2 |

the outer surface of each strut (so that drug and polymer are not exposed to flowing blood in the arterial lumen) and the eventual degradation of the polymer to carbon dioxide and water, which are free of any toxic byproducts *(46)*. Thus, the stent design "guarantees" that there will be complete elimination of the drug from the stent over a finite period of time without drug retention, which could pose a threat for late adverse events months to years after implantation.

Recently, the concept of gene-eluting stents has been introduced using naked plasmid DNA encoding for human VEGF-2 (Table 1) *(47)*.

## DES BIOCOMPATIBLE MATERIALS

In vitro and in vivo studies reported that PC, a neutral phospholipid found on animal cell membranes is extremely biocompatible (23,24). Metal stents coated with PC are well tolerated in porcine coronary arteries, but do not seem to inhibit neointimal hyperplasia (48). Anyway, this biopolymer is also capable of acting as a drug reservoir for programmed elution of a second agent.

## DES WITH PROHEALING AGENTS

### Estradiol

17β-estradiol (17β-E) was administrated 72 h before balloon injury, using a model of carotid balloon injury in ovariectomized rats (49). In this model, it was demonstrated that adventitial activation contributes to the vascular injury response and that estrogens reduce this contribution. Similarly, in a pig model of coronary PTCA, the efficacy of locally delivered 17β-E was assessed in inhibiting neointimal hyperplasia after PTCA (50). On morphometric study, the arterial segments treated with 17β-E demonstrated significantly less neointimal proliferation (neointimal area, percent neointima, neointima/media area) compared with arteries treated with vehicle alone or PTCA only. Immunohistochemistry showed decreased SMC proliferative activity in 17β-E-treated arteries. Using the same animal model, the effect of locally delivered 17β-E during angioplasty on endothelial function was also studied (51). After 4 wk, the improvement in endothelial function was assessed by angiography following intracoronary acetylcholine infusion and by immunohistochemistry. Locally delivered 17β-E significantly enhanced re-endothelialization and endothelial function after PTCA, possibly by improving the expression of eNOS.

Recently, the effect of a 17β-E-eluting stent was reported on neointimal formation in a porcine model (52). Each artery of six pigs was randomized to a control, low-dose, or high-dose 17β-E-eluting stent. All animals were sacrificed at 30 d for histopathological analysis. There was a 40% reduction in intimal area in the high-dose stents compared with control stents (for high dose vs control, $p < 0.05$). There was complete endothelial regeneration at 30 d and a similar inflammatory response to stenting on histopathology in all the stent groups. This is the first study to show that 17β-E-eluting stents are associated with reduced neointimal formation without affecting endothelial regeneration in the pig model of ISR.

### Endothelial Progenitors Cells

EPC originate from bone marrow and circulate through the blood stream. In a novel bioengineered stent design, these circulating EPCs are captured and immobilized to the stent by an antibody coating directed toward CD34, a marker of these cells. In vitro and in vivo studies have suggested that on-stent cell delivery of EPCs could be a novel therapeutic device for re-endothelialization or endothelium lining or paving at an atherosclerotic arterial wall, resulting in the prevention of in-stent thrombus formation and ISR as well as the rapid formation of normal tissue architecture (53,54). EPC capture coating has been reported to reduce significantly neointima area and percent (%) stenosis if compared with bare-metal stent at 28 d and to be safe and feasible for treatment of coronary artery disease (55).

# DES WITH CORTICOSTEROIDS

Several research groups examined whether stents coated with corticosteroids inhibit neointimal hyperplasia in animals. Although DEX-coated stents reduced the inflammatory reaction induced by a synthetic polymer, the effect on neointimal hyperplasia was minimal in two studies in pigs *(56,57)*.

In contrast, De Scheerder and colleagues *(58)* reported that methylprednisolone-coated stents had an inhibitory effect on polymer-induced inflammation and restenosis at 6 wk compared with controls. Overall, the results of animal studies investigating corticosteroid-coated stents and their effect on neointimal hyperplasia have been unimpressive.

# DES WITH ANTIMITOTIC AGENTS

The equivocal results with corticosteroid-coated stents in inhibiting neointimal proliferation led several investigators to evaluate the efficacy of stent-based delivery of other antimitotic agents.

## *Sirolimus (Rapamycin)*

SRL, a natural macrolide antibiotic with potent antiproliferative effects on vascular SMC was first approved by the US Food and Drug Administration in 1999 for use as an antirejection agent following organ transplantation *(59)*. The key mechanism of SRL action is entry into target cells and binding to the cytosolic immunophilin FK-binding protein (FKBP)-12 to form a SRL FKBP-12 complex that interrupts signal transduction, thereby interfering with protein synthesis. The binding to the cytosolic receptor FKBP-12 blocks an enzyme denominated mammalian target of rapamycin-kinase. This substance upregulates p27 levels and inhibits the phosphorylation of retinoblastoma protein, resulting in a cell cycle arrest at the G1–S transition *(60)*. Therefore, this drug exhibits not only a potent immunosuppressive (FKBP blockade) but also antiproliferative properties.

### IMMUNOSUPPRESSIVE PROPERTIES

In numerous in vitro studies, SRL has shown to block T- and B-lymphocomplex formation by both calcium-dependent and -independent pathways *(61–63)*; and was reported to be as potent as tacrolimus, but about 70 times more potent than cyclosporine, in inhibiting calcium-dependent B-cell proliferation.

Furthermore, SRL was reported to inhibit calcium-independent B-cell production unresponsively to both tacrolimus and cyclosporine *(64–68)* and to inhibit proliferation of peripheral blood mononuclear cells and mast cells in response to various stimuli *(69,70)*.

Although specific data regarding the immunosuppressive properties of the SES are needed from human studies, in vivo animal studies indicate some anti-inflammatory properties for the SES. Inflammation score and SMC proliferation was significantly lower at 30 d after implantation of SES than a bare-metal control stent in porcine coronary arteries (0.12 vs 0.97, $p < 0.0001$) *(71)*. The inflammation for the SES (containing 185 µg SRL) was also about one-third of that for a DEX-eluting stent, but this difference was not statistically significant. Moreover, in this model, vascular injury led to increased production of monocyte chemoattractant protein-1 and interleukin-6, whereas stents eluting SRL or DEX reduced expression of these cytokines. This anticytokine effect of the SES may have resulted from antiproliferative activity and reduced cytokine production by SMC.

## ANTIPROLIFERATIVE PROPERTIES

Sirolimus inhibits in vitro SMC proliferation, induced by basic fibroblast growth factor or platelet-derived growth factor (PDGF) and inhibits migration of stimulated pig, rat, mouse, and human VSMC, as outlined in several reviews *(60,72)* whereas tacrolimus showed no significant influence on PDGF-stimulated migration of cultured rat and human SMC *(73)*. Furthermore, SRL inhibited PDGF-stimulated proliferation of human VSMC with potency approx 80 times more than that of tacrolimus, yet SRL inhibited cultured endothelial cell growth about 20,000 times more potently than tacrolimus. Although, these preliminary findings raise the possibility that a SES could be associated with a higher risk of delayed endothelial regrowth and subsequent late thrombosis than a stent containing tacrolimus, this is unlikely to be clinically signifi-cant because in vivo *(71)* and clinical trials *(74)* suggest a low risk of late thrombosis with the SES.

Several studies in experimental animal models have assessed in vivo the antiprolif-erative effects of the SES. In animal models, SES-containing 6–1200 μg of sirolimus markedly reduced neointimal area by 23–52% and mean percent stenosis by 27–46%, compared with bare-metal or polymer-coated control stents, 28–30 d after stent implantation *(42,71,75,76)*. Using a porcine models a significant decrease in mean neointimal area was reported 30 d after insertion of a slow-release SES (180 μg) *(76)*. This antirestenotic effect was, however, not maintained 90 and 180 d after stent implantation. Mean neointimal area at these time-points was not markedly different for slow- and rapid-release SES (180 μg) and BMS, suggesting delayed cellular proliferation with the SRL preparations. Long-term effects of SES warrants further investigation, as it may have a major clinical bearing on the efficacy of stenting, re-endothelialization and late thrombosis.

SES (64–196 μg) decreases neointimal formation in a dose-dependent manner: low-dose SRL was associated with a 23% reduction in neointimal area and 45% reduction with high-dose sirolimus, respectively, not statistical significant ($p = $ NS) and statistical signif-icant ($p < 0.05$) vs controls *(75)*. Using a porcine model, the efficacy of stent-based delivery of SRL (185 μg) alone or in combination with dexamethasone (DEX) (350 μg) were evaluated to reduce in-stent neointimal hyperplasia *(71)*. In the same study, bio-compatibility studies were conducted using either porcine or canine models *(71)*. The tissue level of sirolimus (SRL) was $97 \pm 13$ ng/artery, with a stent content of $71 \pm 10$ μg at 3 d. At 7 d, proliferating cell nuclear antigen and retinoblastoma protein expression were reduced 60 and 50%, respectively, by the SES. After 28 d, the mean neointimal area was $2.47 \pm 1.04$ mm$^2$ for the SRL alone and $2.42 \pm 1.04$ mm$^2$ for the combina-tion of SRL and DEX compared with the bare-metal stents ($5.06 \pm 1.88$ mm$^2$, $p < 0.0001$) or DEX-coated stents ($4.31 \pm 3.21$ mm$^2$, $p < 0.001$), resulting in a 50% reduc-tion of percent in-stent stenosis. These findings contrast with the more pronounced effect, which was found with human implantation. In addition, the late catch-up phe-nomena reported at 6 mo in the pig model was not found in subsequent human trials with long-term follow-up *(77,78)*. Similarly, actinomycin did not achieve the same encouraging results, as in animal models, when used in humans and the "ACTinomycin-d eluting stent Improves Outcomes by reducing Neointimal hyperplasia" (the ACTION) trial had to be stopped after the enrolment of the first 90 patients as a result of an unac-ceptably high target lesion revascularization rate *(79)*.

In vivo animal studies reported adequate endothelial regrowth 14–28 d after SES implantation *(66,75)* suggesting a low risk of late thrombosis. In a mouse model, it has been recently investigated whether rapamycin could reduce neointima formation in vein graft disease *(80)*. In the treatment group, 100 μg or 200 μg of rapamycin were applied locally in pluronic gel. The control group did not receive local treatment. Grafts were harvested at 1, 2, 4, and 6 wk and underwent morphometric analysis as well as immunohistochemical analysis. Treatment with 100 or 200 μg rapamycin showed a dose-dependent reduction of intimal thickness. The difference of intimal thickness of 200 μg. In the treated animals compared with controls was statistically significant at 1 and 2 wk. Immunohistochemically, the reduction of intimal thickness was associated with a decreased amount of infiltration of $CD^{8+}$ cells and a decreased amount of metallothionein positive cells in the rapamycin-treated grafts.

## *SRL Analogs*

### EVEROLIMUS

Everolimus is an immunosuppressive macrolide bearing a stable 2-hydroxyethyl chain substitution at position 40 on the SRL (rapamycin) structure. Everolimus was developed in an attempt to improve the pharmacokinetic characteristics of SRL, particularly to increase its oral bioavailability. Everolimus blocks growth-driven transduction signals in the T-cell response to alloantigen and thus acts at a later stage than the calcineurin inhibitors, cyclosporine and tacrolimus *(81–83)*.

It has been evaluated whether orally administered everolimus inhibits in-stent neointimal growth in rabbit iliac arteries *(84)*. The rabbits were randomized to receive orally everolimus (group 1: 1.5 mg/kg/d starting 3 d before stenting and reduced to 1 mg/kg/d from days 14 to 28, group 2: everolimus 1.5 mg/kg given 1 day before stenting followed by 0.75 mg/kg/d for 28 d) or matching placebo for each group. Stents were deployed in both iliac arteries, and arteries were harvested at 28 d after stenting. Both everolimus treatment groups significantly reduced in-stent neointimal growth (46% reduction and 42% reduction in intimal thickness in groups 1 and 2, respectively). In group 2 everolimus-treated animals, the neointima was healed or healing, characterized by stent struts covered by a thin neointima, overlying endothelial cells, and only small foci of fibrin. Scanning electron microscopy showed more than 80% stent surface endothelialization in group 2 everolimus-treated rabbits.

Everolimus-eluting stent has been tested in a porcine model of restenosis *(85)*. Five bare stents and five everolimus-eluting stent were implanted in 10 coronary arteries of five pigs. The pigs were killed at 90 d. Histopathology showed persisting voids around the struts of everolimus-eluting stents consistent with the presence of surface polymer. Despite this, the vessels showed evidence of complete healing with no difference in intimal inflammation, fibrin deposition, or matrix formation between the two groups. There was near complete endothelialization in all sections *(85)*.

### BIOLIMUS

Biolimus A9 is a rapamycin analog highly lipophilic, which has been shown to inhibit SMC proliferation in vitro *(86)*. The Biolimus A9 drug-eluting stent system has a bioabsorbable polymer, which has been demonstrated in vitro to elute faster into release medium than SRL *(86)*. In a porcine coronary model, a significant decrease in area stenosis, intimal thickness, and intima media ratio have been demonstrated at 28 d, in biolimus-eluting stents vs control base, metal stents (Fig. 1). Nonsignificant inflammation was reported in biolimus-eluting stents and the drug/polymer matrix was completely reabsorbed *(86)*.

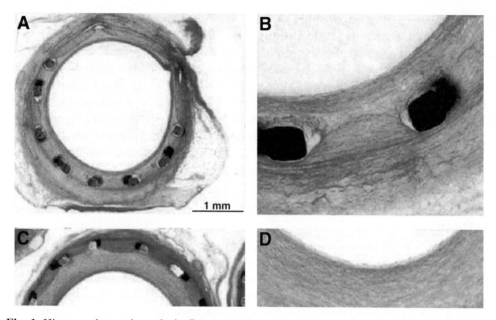

**Fig. 1.** Histomorphometric analysis. Representative cross-sectional histology of Biolimus A9 stent (**A,B**) and control stent (**C,D**) at 28-d follow-up.

## ABT-578

ABT-578 is a new synthetic analog of rapamycin, designed to inhibit SMC proliferation—a key contributor to restenosis—by blocking the function of the mammalian target of rapamycin cell-cycle regulatory protein. Given these pharmacodynamics, ABT-578 was considered beneficial for intracoronary delivery to arrest the process responsible for neointimal hyperplasia after angioplasty and stenting *(87)*. Among the next generation of DES will be a stent that uses the nonbioabsorbable polymer PC to release ABT-578 *(46)*. ABT-578-PC-coated stent implantation in a porcine model showed a 43% decrease in neointimal area, 46% reduction of neointimal thickness, and 24% increase in lumen size compared with control stents *(88)*.

### *Paclitaxel*

The anticancer properties of paclitaxel (Taxol, Bristol-Myers Squibb, New York, NY) were demonstrated in a program launched by the National Cancer Institute in 1963 *(89)*. In 1971, paclitaxel was identified as the active compound extracted from the bark of the Pacific yew *Taxus brevifolia (89)*. Paclitaxel was initially used in the treatment of resistant breast and ovarian cancer. The binding of paclitaxel to tubulin results in blockade of cell division in the $G_0/G_1$ and $G_2/M$ phases of the cell cycle *(90,91)*. When the compound is attached to tubulin this protein loses its flexibility and can no longer disassemble. This effect is obtained by altering the equilibrium between microtubules and α- and β-tubulin by favoring the formation of abnormally stable microtubules *(92,93)*. This mechanism of action, the prevention of microtubule deconstruction, is distinct from previously identified antimitotic agents (colchicine, methotrexate, vinca alkaloids) which act by inducing microtubule disassembly *(94,95)*.

In addition to this major action, paclitaxel acts at a multifunctional level as an anti-inflammatory, antiproliferative, antimigratory, antisecretory compound that also antagonizes extracellular matrix production. It is important to differentiate the effects of paclitaxel at low vs high doses *(96)*. At low doses, the drug blocks progression through the $G_0$–$G_1$ interphase and the $G_1$–S phase. The cell maintains cytostasis at $G_1$. This action occurs through induction of *p53-p21* tumor suppressor genes. At high doses, paclitaxel blocks cell cycle progression at the $G_2$/M (mitotic arrest) and at M/$G_1$ phase (postmitotic arrest). These two conditions may lead to cell death or apoptosis. The cytostatic effect of paclitaxel can be demonstrated in vitro with the Comet assay (DNA electrophoresis), which demonstrates the integrity of the nucleus *(97–99)*.

Paclitaxel was tested as an antirestenotic agent for the first time using a rat model of balloon angioplasty *(100)*. In this model, systemic administration of paclitaxel resulted in a 70% reduction in neointimal proliferation. Moreover, these effects were achieved at measured blood levels 100 times lower than those obtained with doses effective against cancer *(100)*. Important findings came from the evaluation of the dose-dependent effects of paclitaxel on neointima formation utilizing a cell culture model for human arterial smooth muscle and endothelial cells *(101)*. A sustained antiproliferative effect during a 14 d period was demonstrated following administration of a wide range of doses. Furthermore, except at very high drug concentrations ($\geq$50 µmol/L), cell exposure to paclitaxel did not result in signs of acute toxicity or apoptotic cell death (nucleus fragmentation, DNA breaks, or both). Importantly, at low doses of paclitaxel (<0.1 µmol/L) growth of endothelial cells was less inhibited than that of SMC, whereas at higher doses (0.1–10 µmol/L), comparable inhibitory effects were found on both cell lines.

Local application of paclitaxel in the rabbit carotid artery following balloon injury demonstrated inhibition of neointima formation 4 wk after intervention, without toxic or allergic side effects or adverse influence on re-endothelialization. In a rabbit model, utilizing a double balloon for local drug delivery, administration of paclitaxel (10 mL of a concentration of 10 µmol/L) reduced neointimal proliferation by 47% compared with control vehicle delivery, which was accompanied by an increase in total vessel area of 33% after 8 wk compared with only balloon dilatation *(102)*. The extent of stenosis in paclitaxel-treated animals was significantly reduced compared with balloon-dilated control animals ($p = 0.0012$, 1, 4, and 8 wk after intervention: 14.6, 24.6, and 20.5%, vs 24.9, 33.8, and 43.1%, respectively). Marked vessel enlargement compared with balloon-dilated control animals could be observed ($p = 0.0001$, total vessel area after 1, 4, and 8 wk: paclitaxel group: 1.983, 1.700, and 1.602 mm$^2$, control: 1.071, 1.338, and 1.206 mm$^2$, respectively). In this model, the rate and extent of re-endothelialization was also not significantly different between paclitaxel-treated and control animals. Before the in vivo study, delivery efficiency was determined with radiolabeled paclitaxel in porcine hearts. Tubulin staining and electron microscopy revealed changes in microtubule assembly, which were limited to the intimal area.

Following these encouraging early results the next step has been to coat a metallic stent with this compound. A metallic stent was wrapped with a polylactide copolymer to serve as a vehicle for local drug delivery (about 200 µg/stent) *(103)*. In a rabbit model, the neointimal area following implantation of the paclitaxel-coated stent at 4 wk was reduced by 50% ($p = 0.004$), and at 8 wk by 60% ($p = 0.003$) compared with the control. Compared with the 8 wk results, at 6 mo there was only a 12% increase in the neointimal area in the arteries of the animals in which the paclitaxel-coated stents were implanted. However, endothelial coverage of the paclitaxel-coated stent was still incomplete at 180 d. Endothelial cells covered 2.7 quadrants in the control group as compared to one in the paclitaxel-coated stents. Notably, when only the vessel without previous cell denudation was examined, there was no difference between control and paclitaxel-coated stents.

These results may be contrasted with experiments in which local stent-based paclitaxel delivery was accomplished without a polymer vehicle. The effect of different doses of paclitaxel placed on a stent utilizing an immersion technique without a polymer was investigated in minipigs *(104)*. The treatment effects were evaluated at 4 wk after stenting with no paclitaxel, 0.2 μg/stent, 15 μg/stent, and 187 μg/stent. A dose-dependent decrease in neointima formation was found, with a 39.5% reduction in neointimal area in the high-dose animals vs the controls, and a 90.4% increase in luminal area because of concurrent media thinning and vessel expansion. Vessel wall dilatation accounted for 42% of the luminal increase at high dose and for 36% at intermediate dose. Reduction in media thickness partially accounted for the increase in lumen area. Excessive fibrin deposition filled the gaps between the stent struts and the media in the high-dose group, and endothelialization was scant.

The effect of a biodegradable polymer containing 1.5, 8.6, 20.2, and 42 μg of paclitaxel per stent on intimal hyperplasia was also assessed in a rabbit model *(105)*. In accordance to previous studies, the authors found a dose-dependent reduction in neointimal thickness (present only at the 20.2 and 42 μg doses) at 4 wk. Histological evaluation revealed incomplete healing and the presence of areas of inflammation and necrosis, particularly in animals treated with the higher dosage stents. Here also a catch-up at 90 d was described of late restenosis formation in the paclitaxel groups to that of the control. Whether the lack of sustained effect is because of the animal model used or a persistent inflammatory trigger created by the polymer, the suboptimal release kinetics, or a true lack of sustained effect is unclear.

The combination of a NO donor and a paclitaxel-NO donor conjugate coated on a vascular stent was recently tested in a rabbit iliac artery model of stenosis as a potential therapy for restenosis *(106)*. Paclitaxel was conjugated with a NO donor at the 7-position to give compound 7. An adamantane-based NO donor 14 was synthesized and combined with 7 to provide a burst of NO in the first few critical hours following injury to the vessel wall. Both 7 and 14 demonstrated antiproliferative activity and antiplatelet activity. Stents were coated with a layer of a polymer containing test compounds. The total amount of NO eluted from the stents after a 6 h implantation in the rabbit iliac artery was 35, 95, and 69% of the original content for the stents coated with 7, 14, and the combination of 7 and 14, respectively. The antistenotic activity of 7 and 14 was determined in a 28-d rabbit model with two control groups (uncoated stents and polymer-coated stents) and two study groups (paclitaxel-coated stents and stents coated with the combination of 7 and 14). Polymer-coated stents caused inflammation and increased stenosis by 39% when compared with the uncoated stents. The stents coated with the combination of 7 and 14 behaved similarly to the uncoated stents: 41% better than the polymer-coated stents and 34% better than the paclitaxel-coated stents. These data indicate a beneficial effect of adding NO to an antiproliferative agent (paclitaxel) and suggest a potential therapeutic combination for the treatment of stenotic vessel disease.

In contrast, contrast media have been used to delineate the contour of coronary arteries, but also have been proposed as a matrix for an antiproliferative drug in order to prevent restenosis. In cell culture experiments (bovine VSMC), 60-min incubation with contrast agent–taxane formulations (iopromide–paclitaxel, iopromide–protaxel) has been reported to inhibit VSMC proliferation over 12 d in a concentration-dependent fashion *(107)*.

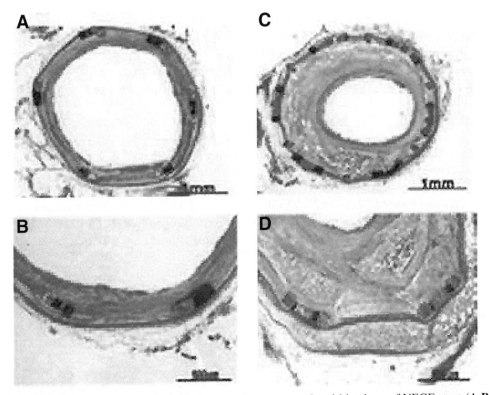

**Fig. 2.** Histomorphometric analysis. Representative cross-sectional histology of VEGF stent **(A,B)** and control stent **(C,D)** at 3-mo follow-up.

Shorter incubation times of 10 and 3 min showed similar efficacy. For in vivo investigation, 16 stents were implanted into the coronary arteries of eight pigs using a 1.3–1 overstretch ratio. A control group received iopromide 370 alone, whereas the treatment group was injected with an iopromide–protaxel formulation at a dose of 74 μmol/L, which is far below protaxel levels inducing systemic toxicity. After 28 d, the treatment group showed a 34% reduction of the neointimal area. It was provided that using a contrast agent as solvent for a taxane constitutes a new drug delivery mechanism able to inhibit ISR in the porcine restenosis model.

In order to further test, the efficacy of paclitaxel added to the contrast agent iopromide in the prevention of restenosis, 34 stents were implanted into the left anterior descending and circumflex coronary arteries of 17 pigs, using a 1.2:1 overstretch ratio *(108)*. The unsupplemented contrast agent iopromide-370 was used as a control; the treatment groups were treated with 80 mL intracoronary iopromide plus either 100 or 200 μmol/L paclitaxel, or 80 mL intravenous iopromide plus 200 μmol/L paclitaxel. A short time incubation (3 min) almost completely inhibited VSMC proliferation, for up to 12 d. Whereas intravenous paclitaxel had no effect, intracoronary application of paclitaxel reduced late lumen loss. Histomorphometry revealed a corresponding dose-dependent reduction of the neointimal area and restenosis by intracoronary iopromide paclitaxel. This study provided evidence that intracoronary application of a taxane dissolved in a contrast medium profoundly inhibits ISR. This novel, widely feasible approach may be suited for the prevention of restenosis in a broad spectrum of interventional treatment regimens.

## MPA-Eluting Stent

MPA is a cytostatic immunosoppressive agent, which inhibits *de novo* purine synthesis *(109)*. It is indicated for the prophylaxis of organ rejection in patients receiving allogenic renal, cardiac, or hepatic transplants. MPA-eluting stent reduced significantly the intimal area and percent stenosis as compared to bare-metal stents in a porcine model at 28 d *(55)*.

## Gene-Eluting Stents

Recently, local delivery through a gene-eluting stent of naked plasmid DNA encoding for human VEGF-2 was assessed whether this approach could achieve similar reductions in neointima formation with acceleration rather than inhibition of re-endothelialization *(47,110–112)*. VEGF-2 plasmid (100 or 200 μg/stent)-coated stents vs uncoated stents were implanted in a randomized, blinded fashion in iliac arteries of 40 normocholesterolemic, and 16 hypercholesterolemic rabbits *(47)*. After 10 d, re-endothelialization was nearly complete and significantly higher in VEGF-stent group as compared to control stents. At 3 mo, intravascular ultrasound analysis revealed that lumen cross-sectional area was significantly more (4.2 vs 2.27 mm$^2$, $p < 0.001$) in VEGF stents compared with control stents in hypercholesterolemic rabbits. Morphometric analysis showed, in hypercholesterolemic animals, more neointimal lesion cross-sectional area and percent area stenosis in control stents whereas lumen cross-sectional area was significantly improved in the VEGF-stented vessels at 3 mo (Fig. 2). Moreover, transgenic expression was detectable in the vessel wall along with improved functional recovery with a 2.4-fold increase in NO production. This strategy addressed the liability common to all current strategies of restenosis prevention and may be considered as stand-alone or combination therapy. Additional preclinical or clinical investigations of VEGF plasmid coated stents for local gene delivery are warranted.

## REFERENCES

1. Hoffmann R, Mintz GS, Dussaillant GR, et al. Patterns and mechanisms of in-stent restenosis. A serial intravascular ultrasound study. Circulation 1996;94:1247–1254.
2. Holmes DR, Jr, Savage M, LaBlanche JM, et al. Results of Prevention of REStenosis with Tranilast and its Outcomes (PRESTO) trial. Circulation 2002;106:1243–1250.
3. Braun-Dullaeus RC, Mann MJ, Dzau VJ. Cell cycle progression: new therapeutic target for vascular proliferative disease. Circulation 1998;98:82–89.
4. Schwartz RS, Topol EJ, Serruys PW, Sangiorgi G, Holmes DR, Jr. Artery size, neointima, and remodeling: time for some standards. J Am Coll Cardiol 1998;32:2087–2094.
5. Kakuta T, Currier JW, Haudenschild CC, Ryan TJ, Faxon DP. Differences in compensatory vessel enlargement, not intimal formation, account for restenosis after angioplasty in the hypercholesterolemic rabbit model. Circulation 1994;89:2809–2815.
6. Isner JM. Vascular remodeling. Honey, I think I shrunk the artery. Circulation 1994;89:2937–2941.
7. Mogford JE, Davis GE, Platts SH, Meininger GA. Vascular smooth muscle alpha v beta 3 integrin mediates arteriolar vasodilation in response to RGD peptides. Circ Res 1996;79:821–826.
8. Lafont A, Guzman LA, Whitlow PL, Goormastic M, Cornhill JF, Chisolm GM. Restenosis after experimental angioplasty. Intimal, medial, and adventitial changes associated with constrictive remodeling. Circ Res 1995;76:996–1002.
9. Shi Y, Pieniek M, Fard A, O'Brien J, Mannion JD, Zalewski A. Adventitial remodeling after coronary arterial injury. Circulation 1996;93:340–348.
10. Farb A, Sangiorgi G, Carter AJ, et al. Pathology of acute and chronic coronary stenting in humans. Circulation 1999;99:44–52.
11. Farb A, Weber DK, Kolodgie FD, Burke AP, Virmani R. Morphological predictors of restenosis after coronary stenting in humans. Circulation 2002;105:2974–2980.

# 22 Clinical Data of Eluting Stents

*Marco A. Costa, MD, PhD,*
*Alexandre Abizaid, MD, PhD,*
*Amanda G. M. R. Sousa, MD, PhD,*
*and J. Eduardo Sousa, MD, PhD*

## CONTENTS

## INTRODUCTION

Stents were introduced into clinical practice in the late 1980s. Subsequently, the Belgian Netherlands STENT and the Stent Restenosis Study trials established the "stent era" in coronary revascularization *(1,2)*, despite an subacute thrombosis (SAT) rate of 3.7%, and more vascular bleeding complications with stents vs balloon angioplasty. Major advances in stent technologies have occurred in the past decades. Stent design has been altered to afford more flexibility, higher radial strength, lower profile, and minimal metallic coverage. Efforts are now directed at coating a stent with single or

From: *Contemporary Cardiology: Essentials of Restenosis: For the Interventional Cardiologist*
Edited by: H. J. Duckers, E. G. Nabel, and P. W. Serruys © Humana Press Inc., Totowa, NJ

multiple bioactive antirestenosis agents, which is delivered uniformly to the underlying tissue, namely drug-eluting stents (DES). Recent clinical data (Table 1), which will be discussed in this chapter, have demonstrated the potential of these new stent technologies to become the predominant revascularization strategy in the near future. The list of promising DES technologies is long. Many of these devices were supported by sound basic science data, but only a few have proven clinical feasibility (Table 1). Based on the mechanism of action of the biological compound and its target in the restenotic process, DES were grouped as immunosuppressive, antiproliferative, anti-inflammatory, antithrombotic, and prohealing. Some agents, such as sirolimus, may affect multiple targets in the restenotic process but will be discussed under a single category.

## STENTS ELUTING ANTI-INFLAMMATORY AGENTS

Clinical data utilizing anti-inflammatory-eluting stents are limited. The study of antirestenosis with BiodivYsio dexamethasone-eluting stent (STRIDE) study was a phase II, multicenter registry conducted in Europe. Stents were immersed on-site in a solution of dexamethasone. Sixty patients with *de novo* lesions were treated with these dexamethasone-eluting stents. At 6-mo follow-up, angiographic binary restenosis (>50% diameter stenosis at follow-up) was 13.3% and late loss (the difference between the minimal luminal diameter postprocedure and the minimal luminal diameter at follow-up) was 0.45 mm$^3$. Another registry, the dexamethasone loaded stents in small coronary vessels to prevent restenosis (DELIVER) study enrolled 30 patients to test the feasibility of dexamethasone-eluting stents (average dose of 0.27 µg/mm$^2$ of stent) for the treatment of small coronary arteries. This stent has been approved for clinical use in Europe.

## STENTS ELUTING IMMUNOSUPPRESSIVE AGENTS

Xenobiotic molecules (rapamycin, FK506, cyclosporine, and analogs) and antimetabolites (mycophenolate mofetil) have been tested.

## SIROLIMUS-ELUTING STENTS

### De Novo *Lesion*

#### FIRST-IN-MAN

The first clinical experience with sirolimus-eluting stent (SES) was initiated in 1999 and involved 45 patients with native coronary artery disease and angina *(4,5)*. Two different formulations of SES were used (slow release [SR], $n = 30$ and fast release [FR], $n = 15$). Virtual absence of neointimal proliferation was documented by serial intravascular ultrasound (IVUS) and angiography at all time-points (4, 6, 12, and 24 mo) *(6)*. There were three nontarget vessel revascularizations after 2 yr. Among patients treated with SR-formulation stents, there were only two target lesion revascularizations (TLR). One of these patients received an uncoated stent distal to the SES 18 mo after the index procedure. Five months later, the patient returned with restenosis of the uncoated stent, which also involved the SES. The second patient had a 51% DES lesion proximal to the stent. Both patients were successfully treated with the implantation of new SES. Another patient with a vulnerable plaque depicted by IVUS at 1-yr follow-up had an abrupt vessel occlusion at 14 mo. One cannot rule out the possibility of stent thrombosis, but this event appears to be caused by the rupture of the vulnerable plaque, which

Table 1
DES Tested Clinically

| Drug | Stent | Manufacturer | Clinical trials | In-stent[a] late loss, (mm) | In-stent[a] restenosis (%) |
|------|-------|--------------|-----------------|------------------------------|-----------------------------|
| Sirolimus (Rapamycin) | BX Velocity™ | Cordis, Jonhson and Johnson | FIM | 0.16 (SR), −(0.02 (FR) | 0 |
| | | | RAVEL | −0.01 | 0 |
| | | | SIRIUS | 0.14 | 2 |
| | | | ISR Registry | 0.36 | 4 (Brazil cohort) |
| | | | SECURE, ARTS-2, | | |
| | | | FREEDOM, | | |
| | | | EC-SIRIUS, | | |
| | | | RESEARCH | | |
| | | | e-CYPHER | | |
| | | | REALITY | | |
| | | | E CYPHER | | |
| | | | S.T.L.L.R | | |
| Taxane | QuaDS™ | QUANAN | SCORE Registry | | 0 |
| | | QUANAN | SCORE Randomized | 0.35 | 6.4 |
| | | QUANAN/ Boston scientific | ISR Registry | 0.47 | 13 |
| Paclitaxel (Taxol) | NIR™ | Boston scientific | TAXUS I | 0.36 | 0 |
| | NIRx™ Comformer | | TAXUS II | 0.31 (SR), 0.30 (MR) | 2.3 (SR), 4.7% (MR) |
| | | | TAXUS III | 0.44 | 16 |
| | Express™, Express 2™ | | TAXUS IV | 0.39 | 5.5 |
| | Supra G™ | Cook | ASPECT | 0.29 (HD) | 4 (HD) |
| | | | | 0.57 (LD) | 12 (LD) |
| | V-Flex plus/Logic™ | | ELUTES | 0.1 (HD) | 3.1% (HD) |
| | | | | 0.47–0.5 (ID) | 11.8–13.5 (ID) |
| | | | | 0.7 (LD) | 20 (LD) |
| | Logic PTX™ | Guidant/cook | PATENCY | | 38 |
| | Multi-Link Panta™ | | DELIVER | 0.81 | 14.9 |

(Continued)

355

Table 1 (*Continued*)

| Drug | Stent | Manufacturer | Clinical trials | In-stent[a] late loss, (mm) | In-stent[a] restenosis (%) |
|---|---|---|---|---|---|
| Actinomycin D | Multi-Link Tetra™ | Guidant | ACTION | 1.02 (LD) 0.93 (HD) | 25 (LD) 15 (HD) |
| Everolimus | S Stent™ | Biosensor/guidant | FUTURE, FUTURE II | 0.10 0.12 | 0 0 |
| Dexamethasone | | Abbott | STRIDE | 0.45 | 13.3 |
| Estrogen | BiodivYsio™ | | EASTER | 0.57 | 10 |
| Batimastat | | | | | |
| Angiopeptin | | | BRILLIANT | 0.88 | 21 |
| ABT-578 | S7™, S660™, Driver™ | Medtronic | ENDEAVOR | 0.33 | 2.1 |
| Mycophenoloic Acid | Duraflex™ | Avantec Vascular Devices | IMPACT | 1.04 (FR) 0.94 (SR) | 12% (both formulations) |
| CD-34 Antibody | R Stent™ | Orbus Neich MT | HEALING | | |

SR, slow release; FR, fast release; LD, low dose; HD, high dose.
[a]Follow-up period varies considerably between trials (≥4 mo-follow-up).

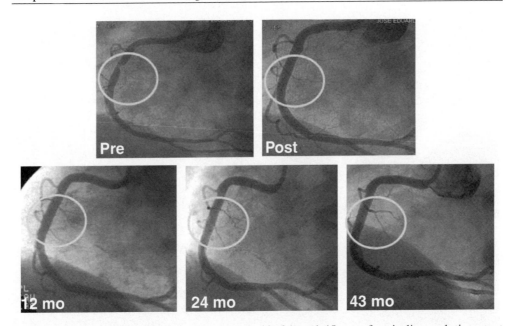

**Fig. 1.** Sequential angiography follow-up at 4, 12, 24, and 45 mo of a sirolimus-eluting stent implanted in the midright coronary artery.

was documented by IVUS 2 mo earlier. The first-in-man (FIM) operators were not allowed to implant more than 1 SES per patient, which limited the ability to completely cover the entire lesion in some patients. In addition, 65% of the lesions were predilated with a balloon longer than the stent length, which invariably produced injury in segments not "protected" by the medication, similar to "geographical miss" during brachytherapy. These findings may indicate the need for complete stent coverage of the entire atherosclerotic plaque and traumatized segments that may be prone to intimal hyperplasia or plaque progression. One should not expect restenosis to occur if a diligent implantation technique with appropriate selection of stent size for various plaque morphologies and lengths is applied. Finally, it must be realized that progression of atherosclerosis will still occur in untreated coronary segments. The 4-yr angiographic follow-up of the FIM study was completed recently and preliminary data showed sustained results with minimal intimal hyperplasia after SES (Figs. 1 and 2). This pioneer investigation provides unique long-term data on SESs, and allays any concern about a potential late "catch-up" of restenosis or late side effects.

## RANDOMIZED COMPARISON OF A SIROLIMUS-ELUTING STENT WITH A STANDARD STENT FOR CORONARY REVASCULARIZATION (RAVEL)

RAVEL was the first randomized trial to compare SR SESs (Cypher™) with bare BX Velocity stents for revascularization of single, *de novo* lesions in native coronary arteries *(7)*. The trial included 238 patients at 19 medical centers in Europe and Latin America. Patients received aspirin indefinitely and clopidogrel or ticlopidine for 2 mo. In-stent late loss was significantly lower in the sirolimus-stent group (−0.01 mm) than in the standard-stent group (0.80 mm, $p < 0.001$). None of the patients in the sirolimus-stent group had binary restenosis, and the incidence of MACE was 5.8% in the sirolimus-stent group after 1 yr. Importantly, no episodes of stent thrombosis occurred. A subgroup

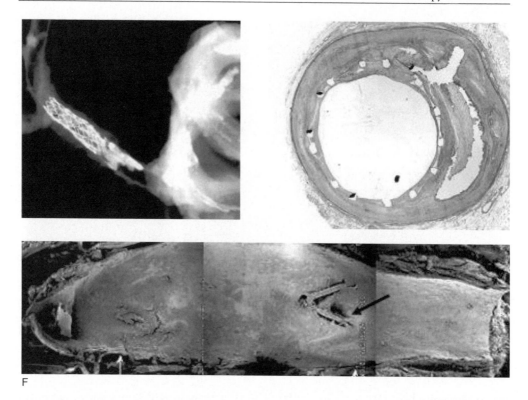

F

**Fig. 2.** Widely patent sirolimus-eluting stent in the right coronary artery (left upper panel). Light microscopic section demonstrated a thin healed intimal hyperplasia (right, upper panel). Scanning electron microscopy (SEM, bottom panel) showed more than 95% endothelized stent surface, with uncovered stent strut at a branch point (arrow). (Please *see* insert for color version.)

analysis of diabetic patients enrolled in the RAVEL trial showed a similar late loss in nondiabetics (−0.03 mm) and diabetic (0.07 mm) treated with SES. There was no restenosis in the SES groups (diabetic and nondiabetic) compared with a 42% rate in the diabetic population assigned to bare metal stents *(8)*.

### UNITED STATES MULTICENTER, RANDOMIZED, DOUBLE-BLIND STUDY OF THE SES IN DE NOVO NATIVE CORONARY LESIONS (SIRIUS)

Patients (*n* = 1100) with *de novo* coronary disease were randomized to receive SR sirolimus-eluting (Cypher) stent or bare BX Velocity stents at 53 United States sites *(9)*. Multiple stents were implanted in 27.4% of the patients (mean of 1.4 stents/patient). In-stent late loss was 0.17 mm and in-lesion late loss was 0.25 mm. After 9 mo, 10.5% of the patients receiving the Cypher stent reached the primary end point of target vessel failure as compared with 19.5% in the control group. In the sirolimus group, in-stent restenosis was 2%, and in-lesion restenosis was 9.1%. As a result, the FDA approved the Cypher for clinical use in April 2003. The 2-yr follow-up results of the SIRIUS trial demonstrated the long-term safety and efficacy of SES (Kereiakes DJ, MD personal communication, 2003).

The European and Canadian SIRIUS trial (E, C-SIRIUS) randomized 350 patients with similar baseline characteristics of the United States SIRIUS study *(10)*. In the E-SIRIUS, multiple stents were implanted in 170 (48%) patients. At 8 mo, there were lower incidence of binary restenosis (5.9 vs 42.3%, $p = 0.0001$) and need for target-lesion revascularizations (4 vs 20.9%, $p < 0.0001$) in the SESs compared with control stents.

## *In-Stent Restenosis Studies*

The in-stent restenosis registry involved 41 patients treated in Brazil ($n = 25$) and in the Netherlands ($n = 16$). This was an open-label safety study involving only patients with single vessel in-stent restenotic lesions. In the Brazilian cohort, all vessels were patent at the time of 12-mo follow-up angiography *(11)*. Late loss averaged 0.36 mm in-stent. One of the 25 patients developed in-stent restenosis at 1-yr follow-up. There were no deaths, stent thromboses, or repeat revascularizations. The Rotterdam cohort included a more complex group of patients. In this group, 19% of the patients had previous brachytherapy failure, and one transplant heart patient was treated. There were two deaths, one late thrombosis, one vessel occlusion, and two in-lesion restenosis. The same investigators later reported similar outcomes for patients with *de novo* and in-stent restenosis lesions treated with SESs *(12,13)*. In the United States, the preapproval compassionate-use of SESs (SECURE) protocol involved patients ($n = 252$) with in-stent restenosis who have failed other approved therapies, such as radiation therapy and coronary artery bypass surgery. Preliminary data show the majority (79.3%) of this extremely high-risk population free of events at 6-mo follow-up.

## SIROLIMUS ANALOGS ELUTING STENTS

The FUTURE I study randomized 42 nondiabetic patients to be treated with everolimus-eluting stent (Challenge™, $n = 27$) vs bare metal stent ($n = 15$). There was no in-stent restenosis and 0.11-mm late loss was observed at 6 mo follow-up in the treated group. The FUTURE II study enrolled 64 patients, including diabetics. There was no restenosis and in-stent late loss was 0.12 mm in the treated group ($n = 21$) at 6-mo follow-up (Grube E, personal communication 2003). Taken together, these pilot investigations demonstrated the potential of everolimus-eluting stent to prevent restenosis.

The Driver™ cobalt alloy stent (Medtronic, Santa Rosa, CA) coated with phosphorylcholine and 10 µg ABT-578 per mm stent length has been tested in patients ($n = 100$) with *de novo*, short coronary stenoses (ENDEAVOR trial). One patient (1%) had subacute thrombosis, and another one underwent repeat target vessel revascularization at 4-mo follow-up. Late loss averaged 0.33 mm at 4-mo follow-up, which suggests the potential of this novel DES to prevent restenosis.

## TACROLIMUS-ELUTING STENTS

The endovascular investigation determining the safety of new tacrolimus eluting stent grafts registry, which included 15 patients with saphenous vein graft disease and the preliminary safety evaluation of nanoporous tacrolimus-eluting stent study, which included 30 patients with *de novo* lesions treated with tacrolimus-eluting stents have failed to demonstrate a clinical benefit of these technologies to prevent restenosis.

## MYCOPHENOLIC ACID-ELUTING STENT

Mycophenolic acid is the active metabolite of mycophenolate mofetil and has both antineoplastic and immunosuppressive properties. The IMPACT study included 150 patients with *de novo* coronary lesions and tested SR (45 d) and fast release (15 d) stents coated with 4.5 μm of mycophenolic acid/mm² vs bare Duraflex™ stents. Preliminary results suggest no differences in angiographic outcomes between groups.

## STENTS ELUTING ANTIPROLIFERATIVE AGENTS

A number of antineoplastic medications have been considered for the prevention of restenosis. Paclitaxel and its derivatives have been the most investigated compounds of this group.

## PACLITAXEL-ELUTING STENTS

Many different platforms using polymer coating or surface modifications to adhere paclitaxel onto the stents have been utilized during the last 2 yr.

### De Novo *Lesions*

The QuaDS™ DES (Quanam Medical Corp) was the first DES, implanted in human coronary artery. This slotted tube stent had 50% of its surface area covered by multiple nonbiodegradable polyacrylate sleeves that release 7-hexanoyltaxol (called QP2 or taxane). Approximately 800 μg of the drug was loaded per 2.4 mm of sleeve length, such that 13-mm-long stents have a total drug dose of 2400 μg and 17-mm-long stents contained 3200 μg of taxane *(14)*. This registry enrolled 26 patients randomly assigned to receive drug-loaded stents (*n* = 13, 14 stents) or bare stents (*n* = 13, 18 stents). At 18-mo follow-up, there was no binary restenosis in the drug-eluting group. Study to compare restenosis rate between QueST and QuaDS-QP2 (SCORE) trial was a randomized study conducted in 15 sites in Europe to test the effectiveness of the QuaDDs-QP2 stent *(15)*. The trial was interrupted prematurely after the enrollment of 266 patients because of a high incidence of stent thrombosis (9.4%) and myocardial infarction (14.5%) in the eluting-stent group. These clinical events were probably related to poor stent design and extremely high concentrations of taxane.

## POLYMER-BASED TAXOL-ELUTING STENTS

### TAXUS I

This study evaluated the safety of the SR polymer coated NIRx™ Conformer stent loaded with 85 μg of paclitaxel (1 μg/mm²). Sixty-one patients with short (<15 mm), *de novo* coronary lesions were randomized to either drug-eluting or bare stent. In-stent late loss was 0.36 mm in the DES group vs 0.71 mm in control group. At 1-yr, MACE was 3% in the eluting-stent vs 10% in the uncoated-stent group *(16)*. There were no reports of death, stent thrombosis TLR, or binary restenosis in the drug-eluting group.

### TAXUS II

This triple-blinded, randomized, multicenter trial tested the efficacy of 2 formulations of paclitaxel-eluting NIRx Conformer stent to treat patients with short, *de novo* coronary lesions *(17)*. The study included 536 patients divided into 4 groups: 267 were treated with either bare (*n* = 136) or SR (*n* = 131)-eluting stents, whereas 269 were treated with bare (*n* = 134) or moderate-release eluting stents (MR, *n* = 135). All eluting stents were coated with the Translute™ polymer loaded with 1 μg of paclitaxel/mm².

Clopidogrel (75 mg QID) was administered for 6 mo. Binary in-stent restenosis rates were 2.3% (SR) and 4.7% (MR) vs 17.9% and 20.2% in the control groups, respectively. Late loss was 0.31 mm (SR) and 0.30 mm (MR) in the eluting-stent groups. Percent neointimal hyperplasia volume was markedly reduced in the eluting groups (SR = 7.85% and MR = 7.84%) vs control (23.17% and 20.54%, respectively). There were no late stent thromboses or aneurysms up to 6 mo *(17)*.

## *TAXUS IV*

The TAXUS IV trial randomized 1314 patients (73 United States sites) with *de novo* coronary lesions to be treated with a single SR polymeric paclitaxel-eluting TAXUS™ stent (*n* = 662) or conventional bare metal stent (*n* = 652). Patients with reference vessel diameter between 2.5 and 3.75 mm, and lesion length between 10 and 28 mm were included. Clopidogrel was prescribed for 6 mo postprocedure. The incidence of SAT was 0.3% at 30 d and 0.6% at 6 mo in the TAXUS arm. Angiographic follow-up at 9 mo were performed in 559 patients overall. In-stent late loss was 0.39 mm, in-stent restenosis was 5.5% and in-lesion restenosis was 7.9% in the TAXUS arm. After 12 mo, 6.8% of the patients receiving the TAXUS stent underwent repeat TVR as compared with 16.7% in the control group. The FDA is reviewing the TAXUS IV data and approval for clinical use is expected early in 2004.

### *In-Stent Restenosis*

## TAXUS III

This feasibility study utilized SR taxol-eluting NIRx Conformer platform for the treatment of patients with in-stent restenosis and was conducted at 2 sites in Europe, enrolling 30 patients. The protocol allowed the implantation of up to 2 (15 mm) eluting stents. In-stent late loss averaged 0.54 mm after 6 mo and MACE rate was 29% at 12 mo *(18)*.

## NONPOLYMER-BASED TAXOL-ELUTING STENTS

### *European Evaluation of Paclitaxel Eluting Stent (ELUTES)*

This study compared the V-Flex™ stent loaded with 4 different doses of paclitaxel (0.2, 0.7, 1.4, and 2.7 µg /mm²) vs bare metal stents for the treatment of *de novo* coronary lesions. Stents were directly impregnated with paclitaxel without a polymer. Patients (*n* = 190) were randomized evenly among the 5 groups. A dose-dependent effect on in-stent late loss was observed: 0.1 mm in the high-dose group, 0.47 and 0.5 mm in intermediate-dose groups, and 0.7 mm in both low-dose and control groups. One-year MACE were similar between groups *(19)*.

### *Asian Paclitaxel-Eluting Clinical Trial (ASPECT)*

This randomized study compared Supra-G™ stents directly impregnated with two different doses of paclitaxel (1.3 and 3.1 µg/mm²) vs bare metal stents. Patients (*n* = 177) with *de novo* coronary lesions were treated with single stents. Antiplatelet therapy was administered for 6 mo. In 37 patients, cilostazol was used in place of clopidogrel or ticlopidine. In-stent late loss was 0.29 mm in the high-dose group, compared with 0.57 in low-dose group and 1.04 mm in the bare stent group and restenosis rates were 4%, 12%, and 27% for the high-dose, low-dose, and control groups, respectively. Overall, 1-yr MACE-and TLR-rates were similar among all groups. However, 4 of the

12 patients receiving the high-dose eluting stents who were also receiving cilostazol, had stent thrombosis *(20)*.

The PATENCY study compared Logic PTX™, paclitaxel-eluting stents (2 µg/mm$^2$), with bare stents in *de novo* coronary lesions. A total of 50 patients were enrolled in 2 United States sites. Clopidogrel was administered for 3 mo. There were no stent thrombosis up to 9 mo, but restenosis rates were similar in the two groups (38% in the eluting-stent group and 35% in the control arm) (Heldman A, MD, unpublished data, 2002). The DELIVER trial (*n* = 1043) compared nonpolymeric paclitaxel-eluting stents (3 µ/mm$^2$) vs bare metal stents. Angiographic data at 9-mo follow-up failed to demonstrate any antirestenosis effect of nonpolymeric paclitaxel-eluting stents. Late loss was 0.81 mm and 15% of patients had restenosis in the treated arm (O'Neill W, MD personal communication, 2003).

## ACTINOMYCIN-ELUTING STENTS

The ACTION study was designed to test the safety, feasibility, and effectiveness of two different doses of actinomycin-eluting Tetra™ stents (Guidant Corporation, Santa Clara, CA) for the treatment of *de novo*, short coronary lesions. Six-month angiographic late loss was 1.02 mm in the low dose (2.5 µ/mm$^2$), 0.93 mm in the high dose (3 µ/mm$^2$) actinomycin-eluting stents compared with 0.75 mm in the control group (Serruys PW, personal communication, 2003).

## ANGIOPEPTIN-ELUTING STENTS

Somatostatin, an angiopeptin analog has been shown to reduce tissue response to several growth factors including platelet-derived growth factor, basic fibroblast, and insulin-like growth factors. The first human experience with angiopeptin-eluting stent, an open-label registry, tested the feasibility of angiopeptin-eluting BiodivYsio™ stents in 13 patients with coronary *de novo* lesions (SWAN). Thirteen stents were loaded with 22 µg of angiopeptin and 1 stent was loaded with 126 µg of the drug. There was no in-hospital or 30-d MACE (Kwok O.H., MD, unpublished data, 2002). Long-term follow-up data are pending.

## STENT-ELUTING EXTRACELLULAR MATRIX MODULATORS

Extracellular matrix constitutes a major component of the restenotic lesion and therefore represents a potential target for antirestenosis therapy. Matrix metalloproteinases (MMP), particularly MMP-2 (72-kD type IV collagenase) and MMP-9 (92-kD type IV collagenase), have the ability to digest collagen and facilitate smooth muscle cell migration. Batimastat, a nonspecific MMP inhibitor has been tested to prevent restenosis. The Batimastat antirestenosis trial utilizing the biodivYsio local delivery phosphoryl-choline-stent (BRILLIANT-I) was a multicenter registry designed to test the feasibility of batimastat-eluting stents to treat *de novo* coronary lesions in 173 patients. Safety was demonstrated, but late loss was 0.88 mm and 21% of the patients developed binary restenosis (De Scheerder, MD, unpublished data, 2002).

## PROHEALING ELUTING STENTS

The promotion of healing in the vascular endothelium may be a more natural and, consequently, safer approach to the prevention of restenosis.

## NITRIC OXIDE-ELUTING STENTS

The NOBLESSE trial ($n = 45$) tested the Genic Stent System (Blue Medical Devices, Helmont, The Netherlands) coated with Oxygen Free Radical scavenger conjugated with Poly-Ester-Amide (PEA) coating. There were no clinical events and late loss was 0.69 mm at 4 mo after the procedure (Constantini C, personal communication 2003).

## ESTRADIOL-ELUTING STENTS

Estradiol may improve vascular healing, reduce smooth muscle cell migration and proliferation and promote local angiogenesis. Estrogen and Stent to Eliminate Restenosis (EASTER) was a single center feasibility study testing 17-β estradiol-eluting BiodivYsio stents in 30 patients with *de novo* coronary lesions. Stents were loaded on-site by immersion in a solution of estradiol. The average concentration was 2.54 $\mu g/mm^2$ of stent. Late loss was 0.32 mm in-lesion and 0.57 mm in-stent. IVUS detected neointimal hyperplasia was 23.5%. At 6 mo, there were no deaths or stent thrombosis, and only 1 patient underwent repeat revascularization. These studies demonstrated the feasibility and safety of "prohealing" DES, but a potent antirestenotic effect of such agents remains to be demonstrated. Taking advantage of recent discoveries on the presence of circulating progenitor endothelial cells *(21)*, the ongoing HEALING study is testing the R stents™ (Orbus Neich Medical Technologies, Fort Lauderdale, FL) coated with antibodies to CD34 receptors on progenitor cells. This technology would enhance the development of a functioning endothelium monolayer and ultimately prevent thrombosis and restenosis.

The DES devices compiled earlier represent only a cross-section of upcoming technologies. Soon, stents eluting statins, trapidil, cytochalasin D, methotrexate, or the combination of multiple agents (i.e., hirudin plus iloprost and heparin plus sirolimus) will be exposed to clinical testing. Novel stents designed for local drug-delivery have also been developed. The Conor MedSystems MedStent *(22)* has individual polymer inlays that can be loaded with different agents and provide controlled spatial-and temporal-drug release. Pilot clinical investigations testing the Conor stent loaded with different formulations of paclitaxel have been initiated in Europe.

## REAL WORLD CLINICAL DATA

Whether the excellent results observed in pivotal clinical trials, which involved selected populations treated in experienced academic clinical sites, can be achieved in daily practice without the attendant risk of stent thrombosis and other undesirable side effects has been questioned. CYPHER received CE Mark approval in April 2002. More recently, polymer-based Paclitaxel-eluting Express™ (PES) stents (TAXUS, Boston Scientifc Corporation) became available in Europe. In the United States, the FDA approved the CYPHER stent in April 2003, and the TAXUS stent in early 2004. A number of postmarket studies are evaluating the utilization of these DES in more challenging lesions and patient subsets. The Rapamycin-Eluting Stent Evaluated At Rotterdam Cardiology Hospital (RESEARCH) started immediately after the stent became available in Europe. The investigators adopted a unique policy of using the SES as the default strategy for all PCI procedures performed at the Thoraxcenter. Approximately 68% of patients included in this registry would have been excluded from earlier clinical trials because of previous coronary surgery, in-stent restenosis, acute myocardial infarction or need for multivessel stenting, among other risk factors. Outcomes of the first 508 patients with *de novo* lesions treated exclusively with SES were compared with 450 patients treated with bare metal stents in the 6-mo period immediately before the availability of DES *(23)*. Patients with chronic total occlusion, in-stent restenosis, bifurcation lesions, or those treated with more than 3 stents or more than 36 mm total stent length received clopidogrel for at least 6 mo. At 1 yr, the risk of major cardiac events was reduced by 38% compared with bare metal stents (9.7% vs 14.8%; $p < 0.01$) mainly owing to a 65% reduction in the risk of clinically driven repeat intervention after SES (3.7% vs 10.9%; $p < 0.01$ vs bare metal stent). Likewise most percutaneous coronary intervention (PCI) studies, the incidence of death or myocardial infarction was similar between both groups *(23)*.

The RESEARCH registry confirmed the effectiveness of SESs in a broad range of patient and lesion subsets. This study also provided evidence regarding the safety of this device in routine clinical practice. Among the patients treated with SES, only 2 (0.4%) presented with SAT in the first month after the procedure, vs 1.6% SAT rate in the bare stent group *(23)*. Usually, thrombosis rates (per patient) with bare metal stents range from 0.4% to 2.8%, with the higher incidences observed with multi-vessel stenting. The second phase of the RESEARCH registry, testing the paclitaxel-eluting stents as a default strategy for PCI, has been initiated, but long-term results on the first 543 patients are pending. The e-CYPHER is an ongoing multinational postmarketing surveillance registry involving 45 countries and 417 sites worldwide. Both on- and off-label use are recorded. A total of 8763 have been enrolled to date. The majority of patients were treated with clopidogrel for more than 3 mo, whereas 1/3 of patients received clopidogrel for less than 2 mo. There were 1.4 stents implanted per patient. Stents were deployed at 14.2 atm; postdilation was performed in 22% and direct stenting in 31% of patients (Guagliumi G, personal communication 2003). The incidence of SAT was only 0.95% in the first 2056 patients with complete 6-mo follow-up data. The overall MACE rate was 5.86% (death = 2.1%, MI = 1.45%, TLR = 2.38%) at 6-mo follow-up. The outcomes observed in this worldwide registry substantiate the findings of the RESEARCH study and allay any concerns regarding the safety of SES in "real world" clinical practice. The WISDOM registry is another web-based multinational registry. To date, approx 1000 patients treated with polymer-based PES have been enrolled in 26 sites (9 countries). The majority (91%) of the patients received a single PES and the mean total of stent length was 22 mm. Clopidogrel was prescribed for 6 mo. At 30 d, only 0.4% of patients had stent thrombosis.

## STENT DEPLOYMENT TECHNIQUE

Currently, the RESEARCH protocol, which mandated unconditional use of SES, represents a unique opportunity to understand the subtle, yet important, changes in deployment techniques in the "DES era" (Table 2). The number of stents (2.1 stents per patient), the total-stent length (38.7 mm), and the utilization of longer stents were higher in the SES group than in the bare stent group *(23)*, which reflects an attempt of the operators to cover completely the diseased and injured segments with the DES (i.e., "from normal to normal vessel")—the "Longer is Better" philosophy. The use of longer stent lengths and a high incidence of direct stenting (≥30%) were also noted in large multinational registries. Importantly, DES implantations were performed at high-inflation pressures (≥12 atm).

Table 2
Recommendations for DES Technique

| Potential problems | How to avoid |
| --- | --- |
| Coating disruption | Careful device handling |
| | Predilation in tight, calcified stenosis |
| Target lesion revascularization TLR | Balloon always shorter than the stent length |
| | Complete lesion coverage |
| | Avoid mechanical trauma outside the stented segment, namely longitudinal geographical miss. |
| | Avoid gap between stents[a] |
| | Proper stent sizing |
| Non-TLR target lesion revascularization | Appropriate patient selection |
| | Avoid trauma outside the target segment |
| | Cover the entire lesion |
| | If a second stent is require, use another DES drug-eluting stent[a] |
| Stent thrombosis | Proper stent sizing |
| | Proper stent expansion/apposition (>13 atm balloon inflation) |
| | Stent-high grade (≥C) residual dissections |
| | Prolonged dual antiplatelet therapy (minimal 3 mo) |

[a]Overlapping may not be safe for all DES.

In an attempt to address this very important issue of DES deployment technique (Table 2), the e-CYPHER S.T.L.L.R trial will enroll 1500 patients treated with SES in 50 United States clinical sites. All operators will follow specific criteria for stent deployment, particularly stent sizing and the procedure will be recorded entirely. Angiographic data will be transmitted "on-line" to an independent core laboratory, which will *prospectively* determine whether there was geographical miss *(24)* during stent deployment. Patients will be followed for 12 mo in order to define whether SES deployment technique affects acute and late outcomes.

## FUTURE DES INDICATIONS

The trend of frequent off label use of DES in daily practice was confirmed in e-CYPHER. It seems that operators worldwide have been encouraged to treat more complex anatomical and clinical situations. Despite the lack of controlled, randomized, scientific data, a large number of complex lesions, including left main (2%), chronic total occlusion (9.4%), bifurcation (8.6%), long lesions more than 30 mm (12.2%), restenosis (14.5%), and vein grafts (2.1%) have been treated in the e-CYPHER. Similar patient profile with high-risk characteristics was observed in the WISDOM registry.

The ARTS-2 and DIABETES studies will soon provide data on of the use of SES to treat multivessel disease and diabetic patients, respectively. Future randomized studies, testing the performance of these devices in acute myocardial infarction *(25)*, bifurcation lesions *(26)* , chronic total occlusions, in-stent restenosis, and bypass graft disease may further broaden clinical indications. Despite the economical and inventory constraints that certainly hindered a more prompt adoption of DES, this technology is likely to replace bare metal stents in the cathlab in the near future. However, operators should use caution when applying DES off label until results of randomized trials become available.

# REFERENCES

1. Fischman DL, Leon MB, Baim DS, et al. A randomized comparison of coronary-stent placement and balloon angioplasty in the treatment of coronary artery disease. Stent Restenosis Study Investigators. N Engl J Med 1994;331:496–501.
2. Serruys PW, de Jaegere P, Kiemeneij F, et al. A comparison of balloon-expandable-stent implantation with balloon angioplasty in patients with coronary artery disease. Benestent Study Group. N Engl J Med 1994;331:489–495.
3. Liu X, Huang Y, Hanet C, et al. Study of antirestenosis with the biodivYsio dexamethasone-eluting stent (STRIDE): a first-in-human multicenter pilot trial. Catheter Cardiovasc Interv 2003;60:172–178; discussion 179.
4. Sousa JE, Costa MA, Abizaid A, et al. Lack of neointimal proliferation after implantation of sirolimus-coated stents in human coronary arteries: A quantitative coronary angiography and three-dimensional Intravascular ultrasound study. Circulation 2001;103:192–195.
5. Sousa JE, Costa MA, Abizaid AC, et al. Sustained suppression of neointimal proliferation by sirolimus-eluting stents: one-year angiographic and intravascular ultrasound follow-up. Circulation 2001;104:2007–2011.
6. Sousa JE, Costa MA, Sousa AG, et al. Two-year angiographic and intravascular ultrasound follow-up after implantation of sirolimus- stents in human coronary arteries. Circulation 2003;107:381–383.
7. Morice MC, Serruys PW, Sousa JE, et al. A randomized comparison of a sirolimus-eluting stent with a standard stent for coronary revascularization. N Engl J Med 2002;346:1773–1780.
8. Abizaid A, Costa MA, Blanchard D, et al. Sirolimus-eluting stents inhibit neointimal hyperplasia in diabetic patients. Insights from the RAVEL trial. Eur Heart J 2004;25:107–112.
9. Moses JW, Leon MB, Popma JJ, et al. Sirolimus-eluting stents versus standard stents in patients with stenosis in a native coronary artery. N Engl J Med 2003;349:1315–1323.
10. Schofer J, Schluter M, Gershlick AH, et al. Sirolimus-eluting stents for treatment of patients with long atherosclerotic lesions in small coronary arteries: double-blind, randomised controlled trial (E-SIRIUS). Lancet 2003;362:1093–1099.
11. Sousa JE, Costa MA, Abizaid A, et al. Sirolimus-eluting stent for the treatment of in-stent restenosis: a quantitative coronary angiography and three-dimensional intravascular ultrasound study. Circulation 2003;107:24–27.
12. Degertekin M, Regar E, Tanabe K, et al. Sirolimus-eluting stent for treatment of complex in-stent restenosis: the first clinical experience. J Am Coll Cardiol 2003;41:184–189.
13. Degertekin M, Lemos PA, Lee CH, et al. Intravascular ultrasound evaluation after sirolimus eluting stent implantation for de novo and in-stent restenosis lesions. Eur Heart J 2004;25:32–38.
14. Honda Y, Grube E, de La Fuente LM, et al. Novel drug-delivery stent: intravascular ultrasound observations from the first human experience with the QP2-eluting polymer stent system. Circulation 2001;104:380–383.
15. Kataoka T, Grube E, Honda Y, et al. 7-hexanoyltaxol-eluting stent for prevention of neointimal growth: an intravascular ultrasound analysis from the study to compare restenosis rate between QueST and QuaDS-QP2 (SCORE). Circulation 2002;106:1788–1793.
16. Grube E, Silber S, Hauptmann KE, et al. TAXUS I: six- and twelve-month results from a randomized, double-blind trial on a slow-release paclitaxel-eluting stent for de novo coronary lesions. Circulation 2003;107:38–42.
17. Colombo A, Drzewiecki J, Banning A, et al. Randomized study to assess the effectiveness of slow- and moderate-release polymer-based paclitaxel-eluting stents for coronary artery lesions. Circulation 2003;108:788–794.
18. Tanabe K, Serruys PW, Grube E, et al. TAXUS III Trial: in-stent restenosis treated with stent-based delivery of paclitaxel incorporated in a slow-release polymer formulation. Circulation 2003;107:559–564.

19. Gershlick A, De Scheerder I, Chevalier B, et al. Inhibition of restenosis with a paclitaxel-eluting, polymer-free coronary stent: the European evaluation of paclitaxel eluting stent (ELUTES) trial. Circulation 2004;109:487–493.
20. Park SJ, Shim WH, Ho DS, et al. A paclitaxel-eluting stent for the prevention of coronary restenosis. N Engl J Med 2003;348:1537–1545.
21. Asahara T, Murohara T, Sullivan A, et al. Isolation of putative progenitor endothelial cells for angiogenesis. Science 1997;275:964–967.
22. Finkelstein A, McClean D, Kar S, et al. Local drug delivery via a coronary stent with programmable release pharmacokinetics. Circulation 2003;107:777–784.
23. Lemos PA, Serruys PW, van Domburg RT, et al. Unrestricted utilization of sirolimus-eluting stents compared with conventional bare stent implantation in the "real world." The rapamycin-eluting stent evaluated at Rotterdam cardiology hospital (RESEARCH) registry. Circulation 2004;109:190–195.
24. Sousa JE, Serruys PW, Costa MA. New frontiers in cardiology: drug-eluting stents: Part II. Circulation 2003;107:2383–2389.
25. Lemos PA, Saia F, Hofma SH, et al. Short- and long-term clinical benefit of sirolimus-eluting stents compared to conventional bare stents for patients with acute myocardial infarction. J Am Coll Cardiol 2004;43:704–708.
26. Colombo A, Moses JW, Morice MC, et al. Randomized Study to Evaluate Sirolimus-Eluting Stents Implanted at Coronary Bifurcation Lesions. Circulation 2004.

# 23    Biodegradable Stents

*Takafumi Tsuji, MD, Hideo Tamai, MD, and Keiji Igaki, PhD*

## CONTENTS

## THE ROLE OF STENTS IN PERCUTANEOUS CORONARY INTERVENTION

Percutaneous coronary intervention (PCI) is indispensable in the treatment of ischemic heart disease. In the early days of conventional balloon angioplasty, acute coronary occlusion as a result of coronary dissection or vessel recoil was observed immediately after PCI, and initial results were not satisfactory. Moreover, the long-term restenosis rate was 30–40%, and the recurrence of angina was a problem. In order to solve these problems, Sigwart et al. *(1)* developed a metallic stent, which was used clinically for the first time in 1986. As this pioneering work, the use of stents has become routine in the practice of PCI. Metallic stents are very effective in the prevention of acute coronary occlusion by coronary dissection or recoil of a vessel. Furthermore, the results of large clinical trials, such as STRESS and BENESTENT, suggested that metallic stents are also effective in the prevention of chronic restenosis *(2,3)*. Despite the success that has been achieved with metallic stents, there are also some important limitations. There is a risk of subacute thrombosis (SAT) until endothelial cells cover the surface of the metallic stent. Although the frequency of SAT has been lowered by the use of antiplatelet agents, such as ticlopidine, for at least 1 mo after stent implantation, SAT has not been completely eliminated. Moreover, in-stent restenosis in a complicated coronary lesion poses a significant clinical problem especially

From: *Contemporary Cardiology: Essentials of Restenosis: For the Interventional Cardiologist*
Edited by: H. J. Duckers, E. G. Nabel, and P. W. Serruys © Humana Press Inc., Totowa, NJ

with the expanding use of PCI to treat ischemic heart disease. Stents are thought to be required for about 12 mo to prevent lumen narrowing in response to chronic vessel remodeling. As metallic stents remain permanently implanted, there is concern about the deleterious effects of stents on the coronary vessels that may take several years to develop. Furthermore, metallic stents may serve as an obstacle for the treatment of in-stent restenosis.

## HISTORY OF THE BIODEGRADABLE STENT

Although stents made from biodegradable polymers, have been proposed for many years in order to overcome the limitations of metallic stents, progress in this area has been slow and biodegradable stents have not achieved widespread acceptance. Stack et al. *(4)* of Duke University developed the first biodegradable stent in the early 1980s. After these investigators tested several polymer materials, they produced a polymer stent made from poly-L-lactic acid (PLLA), and implanted the PLLA stents in the femoral artery of 11 dogs. Although in-stent occlusion was observed in one animal within 18 mo, stent thrombosis and neointimal hyperplasia were rarely observed in the other animals. Subsequently, many studies on the polymer stent were performed, and research that questioned the biocompatibility of PLLA was presented as the joint effort of three prominent institutions from 1992 to 1996 *(5)*. Although biocompatibility of PLLA material was already widely accepted in orthopedic procedures at that time *(6–9)*, biocompatibility of PLLA for the coronary arteries was regarded as problematic. Thereafter, polymer stents were developed using various materials with results that were not as good as metallic stents and thus, polymer stents were never used clinically.

## HISTORY OF THE IGAKI–TAMAI STENT

Initially, Tamai et al. selected polyglycolic acid (PGA) as a material for the polymer stent. PGA is a polymer that is hydrolyzed in the body and biodegraded within 3 mo, and the clinical utility of this material had already been demonstrated in applications, such as biodegradable sutures. The thread of PGA was woven in the shape of a mesh, and the PGA polymer stent was produced. A PGA stent was successfully implanted in dog coronary arteries for the first time in 1993, and in pig coronary arteries in 1994. In the study of dog coronary arteries, a PGA stent was implanted in the left anterior descending artery in 25 dogs, and coronary angiography (CAG) and pathological observation were performed up to 24 wk later. Thrombus occlusion of the stent was not observed in the coronary angiograms, and percent diameter stenosis (%DS) reached a maximum of 26% by the fourth week of follow-up. There was mild neointimal hyperplasia and a very slight foreign body reaction in the postmortem pathological examination.

Moreover, in the animals with 24 wk of follow-up, biodegradation of the stent strut was complete and inflammation was not observed. In contrast to these results, in the pig coronary arteries the PGA stent produced advanced stenosis and was insufficient as a stent. It is thought that pig coronary arteries have a restenosis response that is closer to human coronary arteries than dog coronary arteries. Therefore, it was decided to continue research using pig coronary arteries. As the peak of in-stent restenosis occurs within 6 mo in human coronary arteries, the stent material was changed to PLLA and additional stents were implanted in pig coronary arteries. PLLA is a polymer, which is hydrolyzed in the body and biodegraded within 24 mo. Although the mechanical

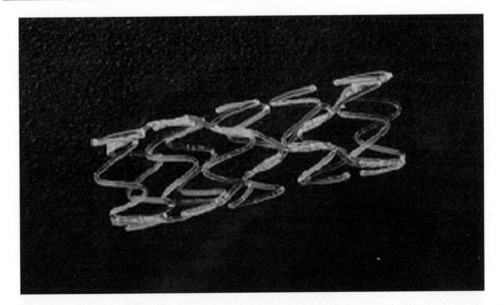

**Fig. 1.** The Igaki–Tamai stent is a self-expanding biodegradable polymer stent made from the thread of PLLA with the zigzag helical coil design.

strength of the biodegradable polymer stent is weakened as hydrolysis progresses, the mechanical strength of the PLLA stent is maintained for 12 mo after implantation. Initially, the PLLA polymer stent was woven from the thread of PLLA in the shape of a mesh and implanted in pig coronary arteries. The results were not satisfactory because neointimal hyperplasia was very high, peaking by the fourth week.

Histological examinations at the site of restenosis showed that neointimal hyperplasia was proportional to the degree of injury to the vessel wall, and it was thought that the cause of restenosis was vessel injury at the time of stent implantation. Subsequent to this work, a PLLA self-expanding coil stent (Igaki–Tamai stent, Fig. 1) was developed and research was resumed using pig coronary arteries *(10)*. Fourteen Igaki–Tamai stents and nine Palmaz-Schatz stents were implanted in pig coronary arteries and serial CAG was performed. In the sixth week, there was no significant difference in minimal lumen diameter (MLD) ($2.18 \pm 0.84$ mm vs $2.30 \pm 0.58$ mm, $p = 0.82$) and %DS ($24.2 \pm 19.8\%$ vs $15.9 \pm 15.6\%$, $p = 0.49$) between Igaki–Tamai stents and Palmaz–Schatz stents. The histological findings in pigs with the Igaki–Tamai stent showed that the lumen was large and there was mild neointimal hyperplasia in the second, sixth, and sixteenth week (Fig. 2).

## APPLICATION OF THE IGAKI–TAMAI STENT
## TO HUMAN CORONARY ARTERIES

The Igaki–Tamai stent is a self-expanding biodegradable polymer stent made from the thread of PLLA with a zigzag helical coil design. The thickness of the stent strut is 0.017 mm (0.007 in.), and the stent length is 12 mm. The stent is mounted on a balloon with a covered sheath and implanted at the lesion site by balloon expansion. Clinical application of the Igaki–Tamai stent was carried out for the first time following approval of the Ethics Committee of the hospital and written informed consent in September 1998. Ultimately, 84 PLLA stents were implanted in 63 lesions in 50 patients through

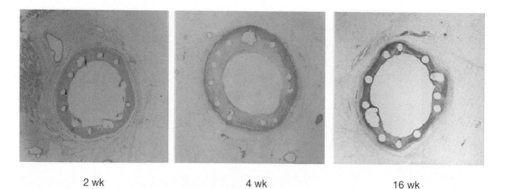

2 wk                         4 wk                         16 wk

**Fig. 2.** The histological findings after implantation of the Igaki–Tamai stent in pig coronary arteries. Findings are shown at 2, 4, and 16 wk after implantation.

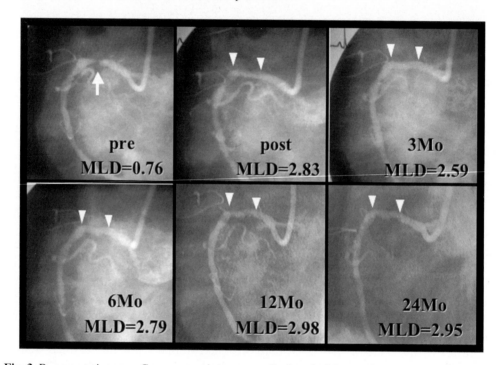

**Fig. 3.** Representative case. Coronary angiograms are displayed of the proximal right coronary artery in a 62-yr-old male. Angiograms are shown before the procedure, immediately after the procedure, and at 3, 6, 12, and 24 mo later.

April 2000 *(11)*. CAG (Fig. 3) and intravascular ultrasound (IVUS) (Figs. 4 and 5) were performed before and immediately after the procedure. Additional assessment by quantitative CAG and intracoronary ultrasound was performed 1 d, 3 mo, 6 mo, and 12 mo after the procedure. Aspirin (81 mg/d) and ticlopidine (200 mg/d) were administered as antiplatelet therapy for at least 1 mo after stent implantation.

Although stent implantation was successful in all cases, there was SAT in one case, and thus the in-hospital success rate was 98%. No other thrombotic occlusions were observed over 12 mo of follow-up. Major adverse cardiac events were evaluated and the major adverse cardiac events-free survival rate including target lesion revascularization was 84.2%. In the analysis by quantitative CAG, the reference diameter was 2.95 ± 0.46 mm

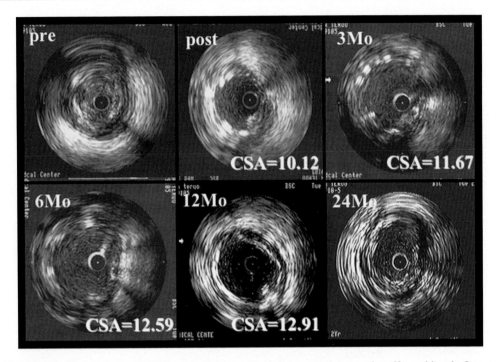

**Fig. 4.** Representative case. IVUS images of the proximal right contrary artery in a 62-yr-old male. Images are shown before the procedure, immediately after the procedure, and at 3, 6, 12, and 24 mo later.

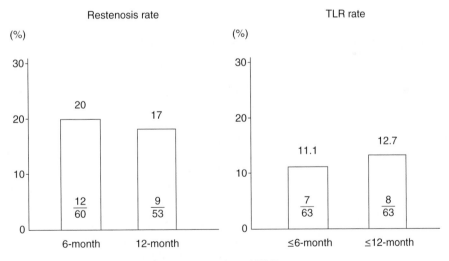
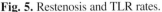

**Fig. 5.** Restenosis and TLR rates.

and the lesion length was $13.5 \pm 5.7$ mm. MLD before the procedure was $0.91 \pm 0.39$ mm, and the DS was $69 \pm 13\%$ MLD was $1.76 \pm 0.74$ mm and $2.16 \pm 0.52$ mm at 6 and 12 mo after the procedure, respectively. The DS was $38 \pm 22\%$ and $29 \pm 13\%$ at 6 and 12 mo, respectively. The restenosis rate was 20 and 17%, and the target lesion revascularization rate was 11 and 13% at 6 and 12 mo, respectively. These results are equivalent to those achieved with conventional metallic stents (Tables 1 and 2).

Table 1
In-hospital Results

| | |
|---|---|
| Initial success | |
|     Procedure success | : 84/84 (100%) |
|     Lesion success | : 63/63 (100%) |
|     Clinical success | : 49/50 (98%) |
| Complications | |
|     Death | : 0 |
|     QMI | : 1/50[a] (2%) |
|     Energent CABG | : 0 |
|     Re-PCI | : 1/50[a] (2%) |
|     Bleeding | : 0 |

[a]Same patient.

Table 2
One-Year Results

| | |
|---|---|
| Death | : 0 |
| QMI | : 1/50[a] (2%) |
| CABG | : 0 |
| Stent thrombosis | :1/50[a] (2%) |
| Re-PCI | |
|     6 mo | : 6/50 (12%) |
|     12 mo | : 7/50 (14%) |
| MACE-free rate (Kaplan-Meier) | : 84.2% |

[a]Same patient.

## TIME-COURSE OF IVUS FINDINGS AFTER IMPLANTATION OF THE IGAKI–TAMAI STENT

IVUS images of the Igaki–Tamai stents after implantation were similar to IVUS images of conventional metallic stents; there was high-echo contrast accompanied by multiple reflections where the stent struts made contact with the vessel wall. IVUS images 6 mo after implantation revealed neointimal hyperplasia inside the stent, but the stent struts still showed high-echo contrast. In the 19 patients that had serial IVUS through 24 mo of follow-up, the vessel area (VA) was 16.3 mm$^2$, the stent area (SA) was 6.8 mm$^2$, the lumen area (LA) was 4.7 mm$^2$, the plaque + media area (P + M) was 9.5 mm$^2$, and the neointimal area (NI) was 2.1 mm$^2$ at 6 mo. At 12 mo of follow-up, the VA was 15.6 mm$^2$, the SA was 6.8 mm$^2$, the LA was 5.3 mm$^2$, the P + M was 8.7 mm$^2$, and the NI was 1.5 mm$^2$. At 24 mo, the stent struts were difficult to distinguish with IVUS suggesting that the majority of the stent had biodegraded. A paired $t$-test showed that there were no significant changes in the VA and SA from 6 to 12 mo. However, the LA showed a tendency to expand ($p = 0.060$), and the P + M area and NI area were reduced significantly ($p = 0.011$ and $p = 0.021$, respectively) from 6 to 12 mo. These results indicate that the neointima was decreased by the time the stent biodegraded and suggest that biodegradation of the stent did not cause new neointimal hyperplasia. There was no reduction of the VA because of remodeling; the lumen was maintained, and the reduction of the intensity of the stent accompanying biodegradation did not have a negative influence on the lumen area.

# CONCLUSIONS

The Igaki–Tamai stent is a biodegradable polymer stent made from PLLA and has been shown to function adequately as a coronary stent. Recently, drug-eluting stents, which are coated with drugs, such as sirolimus *(12)* and paclitaxel *(13)*, have received a great deal of attention for their potential ability to prevent restenosis. The drug-eluting stent has a polymer coating attached to the metallic stent and the drug is contained in the polymer coating. As the Igaki–Tamai stent is made up entirely of polymer, this stent can hold more amount of drug than the polymer-coated metallic stent. Therefore, further prevention of restenosis can be expected with the development of a drug-eluting Igaki–Tamai stent. Additional research will be required to determine if biodegradable polymer stents can produce a dramatic improvement in the clinical results of PCI.

# REFERENCES

1. Sigwart U, et al. Intravascular stents to prevent occlusion and restenosis after transluminal angioplasty. N Engl J Med 1987;316:701–706.
2. Fischman DL, et al. A randomized comparison of coronary stent placement and balloon angioplasty in the treatment of coronary artery disease. N Engl J Med 1994;331:496–501.
3. Serruys PW, et al. A comparison of balloon-expandable stent implantation with balloon angioplasty in patients with coronary artery disease. N Engl J Med 1994;331:489–495.
4. Zidar J, et al. Biodegradable stents. In: Topol EJ, ed. Textbook of interventional cardiology, 2nd ed. WB Saunders, Philadelphia, PA, 1994, pp. 787–802.
5. Giessen WJ, et al. Marked inflammatory sequelae to implantation of biodegradable and non-biodegradable polymers in porcine coronary arteries. Circulation 1996;94:1690–1697.
6. Schkenraad JM, et al. Biodegradable hollow fibers for the controlled release of drugs. Biomaterials 1988;9:116–120.
7. Schakenraad JM, et al. Enzyme activity toward poly (L-lactic acid) implants. J Biomed Mater Res 1990;24:529–545.
8. Bos RRM, et al. Resorbable poly (L-lactide) plates and screws for the fixation of zygomatic fractures. J Oral Maxillofac Surg 1987;45:751–753.
9. Suganuma J, et al. Biological response of intramedullary bone to poly-L-lactic acid. J Appl Biomat 1993;4:13–27.
10. Tamai H, et al. A biodegradable poly-L-lactic acid coronary stent in the porcine coronary artery. J Interven Cardiol 1999;12:443–450.
11. Tamai H, et al. Initial and 6-month results of biodegradable poly-L-lactic acid coronary stents in humans. Circulation 2000;102:399–404.
12. Regar E, et al. Angiographic findings of the multicenter Randomized Study With the Sirolimus-Eluting Bx Velocity Balloon-Expandable Stent (RAVEL): sirolimus-eluting stents inhibit restenosis irrespective of the vessel size. Circulation 2002;106:1949–1956.
13. Liistro F, et al. First clinical experience with a paclitaxel derivate-eluting polymer stent system implantation for in-stent restenosis: immediate and long-term clinical and angiographic outcome. Circulation 2002;105:1883–1886.

# V  BIOTECHNOLOGY IN THE TREATMENT OF RESTENOSIS

# 24 Vascular Gene Therapy

*Gurpreet S. Sandhu, MD, PhD*
*and Robert D. Simari, MD*

## CONTENTS

## INTRODUCTION

The application of genetic treatments for vascular disease was conceived at a time when restenosis was the primary impediment to percutaneous intervention. Initial attempts to deliver vectors to the normal vasculature included plasmid and retroviral-based strategies *(1)*. These studies demonstrated the ability to transduce vascular cells albeit with low efficiency. The development of recombinant adenoviral vectors allowed for enhanced gene-transfer efficiency in normal and atherosclerotic arteries compared with nonviral and retroviral vectors *(2)*. The enhanced efficiency of adenoviral vectors allowed for the testing of therapeutic strategies to inhibit neointimal formation following arterial injury *(3,4)*. Although initial attempts to translate these early antiproliferative studies were stymied by concerns regarding the safety of adenoviral vectors and the lack of effective delivery catheters, clinical trials have recently begun in the US and Europe testing antiproliferative vascular gene-transfer strategies delivering pluripotent transgenes including those encoding for distinct isoforms of *nitric oxide synthase (5–7)*. Clinical targets in these initial studies include an array of vasculoproliferative disorders, including arterio-venous fistulae stenosis and restenosis following coronary stenting.

An alternative therapeutic strategy to directly modulate arterial remodeling following arterial injury tested the hypothesis that delivery of angiogenic peptides through gene transfer might enhance re-endothelialization and limit restenosis. Gene transfer of *vascular endothelial growth factor* (VEGF), a potent and specific secreted mitogen for endothelium was demonstrated to enhance re-endothelialization and reduce neointimal formation in animal models (Fig. 1) *(8)*. These pioneering studies by Jeffrey Isner took advantage of the potency and the secreted nature of the transgene product and used

From: *Contemporary Cardiology: Essentials of Restenosis: For the Interventional Cardiologist*
Edited by: H. J. Duckers, E. G. Nabel, and P. W. Serruys © Humana Press Inc., Totowa, NJ

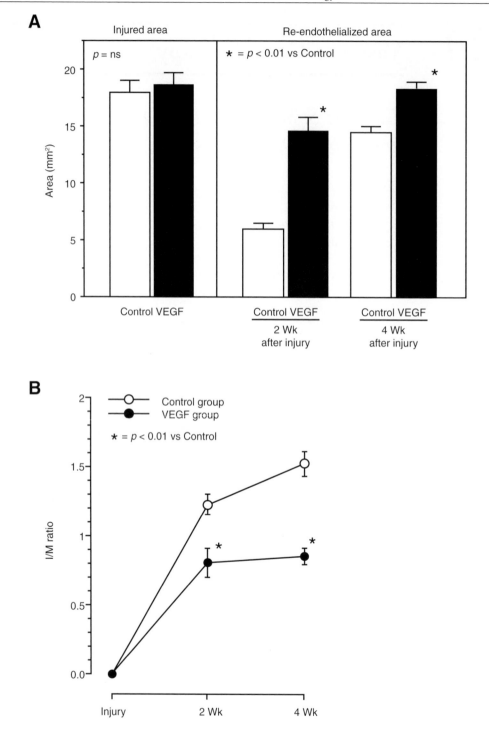

**Fig. 1.** Gene transfer of *VEGF* enhances re-endothelialization and reduces intimal formation. **(A)** Bar graph showing planimetric analysis of extent of re-endothelialization. Injured area was similar for animals in control group and in *VEGF*-treated group. Re-endothelialized area, indicated macroscopically by absence of blue dye stain, was more extensive in *VEGF*-treated animals than in control animals, at both 2 and 4 wk after injury. **(B)** Plot of ratio of intimal area to medial area (I/M ratio) at

"naked" DNA delivery without adjuvants. This approach was quickly advanced to clinical trials using plasmid delivery of a gene encoding for $VEGF_{165}$ into ischemic limbs (9).

Currently, with the use of drug-eluting stents, the application of genetic therapies for restenosis requires a broader view. The systemic prevention and stabilization of sites of vascular injury, the proximate cause of myocardial infarction, limb ischemia, and stroke are the most important targets for cardiovascular gene transfer. As such, restenosis following percutaneous coronary intervention remains a local and defined model for this broader view. This chapter will provide an overview of molecular technology used for vascular gene transfer and the requirements for translational success.

Central to any gene-transfer strategy is the choice of the therapeutic transgene to be expressed. (In following chapters, multiple therapeutic targets and associated transgenes will be discussed in detail.) Once a transgene is selected, the requirements for the extent and duration of expression necessitate selection of two additional central features, i.e., the vector to be used and the regulatory elements required. These critical features (vector and regulatory elements) are inherently linked in many important ways in terms of basic molecular and cellular biology. This interaction between regulatory elements and vectors will be discussed in terms of vascular gene transfer.

## VASCULAR GENE-TRANSFER VECTORS

The goal for any vascular gene-transfer strategy is the efficient transduction of vascular cells. The "holy grail" of vascular gene-transfer strategies would include systemic delivery of vectors that target specific vascular sites, such as sites of vascular injury or atherosclerosis. Short of that, local delivery, either through surgical dwell or with the use of delivery catheters, has been used to deliver genetic vectors to the vessel wall. Appropriate selection of delivery devices and methods of targeting and localization play an important role in the process of optimizing gene delivery. The choice of vector depends on the desired goal of the gene therapy as well as the structural and functional limitations imposed by the vector itself (10). Vectors vary in cell specificity, efficacy of tranduction, stability of integration and expression, toxicity, immunogenicity, and oncogenicity. To be effective vectors must not only survive systemic host-defense mechanisms, but must also cross several tissue and cellular barriers in an intact manner (Table 1).

Vectors may broadly be divided into viral and nonviral systems (Table 2). Plasmid DNA (11), with or without adjuvant molecules, has been the most commonly used nonviral system in the vasculature. The use of cosmids (12) and artificial chromosomes although possible have not been utilized in vessels. Adenoviruses, adeno-associated viruses (AAV), and retroviruses are the best-characterized viral vectors for the vasculature. Other vectors being studied as agents for gene therapy but not tested in the vasculature include herpes simplex virus, hepatitis A virus, pox virus, sindbis virus, Semliki forest virus, vaccinia virus, human papilloma virus, Epstein-Barr virus, and simian virus-40. The primary goal for all vectors is to achieve high degrees of transduction whereas avoiding immunogenicity and cellular toxicity.

---

**Fig. 1.** (Continued)   2 and 4 wk after injury. I/M ratio (1.23 ± 0.07) is significantly higher among 2-wk control animals than 2-wk animals treated with VEGF (0.81 ± 0.11, $p < 0.01$). Intimal thickening progressed in control group during subsequent 2 wk; in contrast, intimal thickening essentially ceased in VEGF-treated group. Consequently, I/M ratio at 4 wk was 1.60 ± 0.12 for control animals vs 0.86 ± 0.05 for VEGF-treated group ($p < 0.0001$).

Table 1
Barriers to Effective Vascular Gene Delivery

Systemic factors
  Vector neutralization by antibodies, plasma
  Nonefficient delivery systems
  Noneffective vector targeting
Vascular factors
  Low levels of vascular cell proliferation
  Extensive extracellular matrix including elastic laminae
  Adjacency to flowing blood
  Limited ability to occlude vessel
  Presence of side branches
Cellular factors (not limited to the vasculature)
  Lysosomal degradation of vectors
  Inefficient delivery of vector to the nucleus
Systemic factors
  Vector neutralization by antibodies, plasma
  Nonefficient-delivery systems
  Noneffective vector targeting
Vascular factors
  Low levels of vascular cell proliferation
  Extensive extracellular matrix including elastic laminae
  Adjacency to flowing blood
  Limited ability to occlude vessel
  Presence of side branches
Cellular factors (not limited to the vasculature)
  Lysosomal degradation of vectors
  Inefficient delivery of vector to the nucleus

# NONVIRAL VECTORS

## Plasmids

Plasmids are circular double-stranded DNA molecules without an external protein coat. These are occasionally referred to as "naked DNA." Plasmids were used in pioneering vascular gene-transfer studies *(1)*. Their advantages include their simplicity and low cost of their design and propagation *(13)*. Plasmids can accommodate large transgene inserts and have an episomal (nuclear but not chromosomal) location with minimal integration into the host genome. Immunogenicity and cellular toxicity both are generally low. However, the immunogenicity of plasmids depends on their nucleotide (CpG) content *(14)*. Drawbacks to the use of plasmids in vascular gene transfer include low-efficiency transduction and a short duration of transgene expression that is limited to a few days or weeks *(1)*. Attempts to improve transduction include combining plasmid DNA with adjuvants to enhance their stability and cellular uptake as well as the combined use of physical methods, such as electroporation or ultrasound.

## DNA–Liposome Complexes

Cationic and neutral lipids have the ability to self-aggregate into vesicles. This property is used to form liposomes that may be combined with inherently anionic DNA

Table 2
Characteristics of Vascular Gene-Transfer Vectors

| | Efficiency | Integration | Immunogenecity | Stability |
|---|---|---|---|---|
| "Naked" DNA | Low | Low | Variable | Days |
| DNA-liposomes | Low-mod | Low | Variable | Days |
| Retroviruses | Low | Likely | Low | Weeks |
| Adenoviruses | High | Low | High | Days–weeks |
| AAV | ??? | Low | Low | Months |

molecules *(15)*. These complexes provide the associated DNA some protection against nucleases and an enhanced ability to bind cellular membranes. Direct delivery of DNA–liposomes has been performed to deliver DNA to the vasculature *(1,16)*. Furthermore, the lipid coat can also be modified with ligands to facilitate receptor–ligand-mediated cell targeting and internalization *(17)*. Viral proteins, such as protein coat particles of hemagglutinating virus of Japan, when added to liposomes have been used to improve transfection efficiency *(18)*. Attempts to improve DNA delivery include the use of polylysine and polyethylenimine to form complexes with DNA *(19)*. In addition to external modifications, the genetic sequences of plasmids may be altered for effects beyond transgene expression. Fragments of the human papilloma virus or the Epstein-Barr virus have been engineered into plasmid-based vectors. These DNA sequences allow plasmids to be retained as episomes inside cells for longer periods of time. Each of these modifications has been used to address the inherent low efficiency and lack of stability and long-term expression of "naked" DNA.

### Physical Methods to Enhance Plasmid Delivery

In addition to local delivery of plasmids, physical methods have been used to enhance vascular plasmid uptake and gene transfer. These methods, including electroporation and sonoporation are designed to temporarily disrupt cellular membranes to enhance DNA delivery. Both methods have been used to deliver plasmids in vitro and in vivo. Electroporation requires direct access to the vessel to place electrodes *(20)*. Delivery of ultrasound to vessels could be potentially performed using percutaneous delivery (Fig. 2) *(21)*.

## VIRAL VECTORS

### Retroviruses

Because of their molecular simplicity and widescale in vitro use, murine retroviruses were originally used in early studies of vascular gene transfer *(1)*. These viruses have the ability to integrate in to the host genome, which may provide stable long-term expression *(22)*. These viruses are based on the Moloney murine leukemia virus from which the *gag*, *pol*, and *env* genes have been removed. The 3′ and 5′ long-terminal repeats (LTR) and additional regions that provide promoters and polyadenylation and packaging sequences allow for integration and reverse transcription.

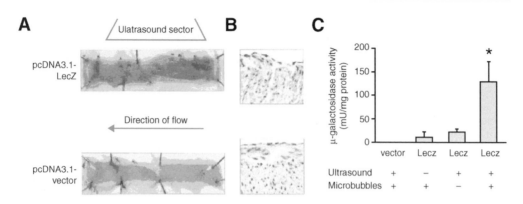

**Fig. 2.** Ultrasound-induced disruption of DNA3.1-*LacZ*-coated microbubbles improves gene delivery. PCAs were perfused with microbubbles loaded with pcDNA3.1-*LacZ* or control vector (2 µg/mL, perfusion: 2 mL/min) and exposed to ultrasound for 5 s. After 18 h, expression and activity of β-galactosidase were assessed as described in Methods. Representative photographs of vessels are shown in **A**; histochemical images are shown in **B**. **(C)** β-Galactosidase activity was quantified in homogenates of coronary arteries exposed to either pcDNA3.1-*LacZ* (2 µg/mL) or microbubbles loaded with pcDNA3.1-*LacZ* (2 µg/mL) or the control vector (pcDNA3.1, 2 µg/mL) in the presence or absence of ultrasound (5 s; flow rate, 2 mL/min). Data represent mean ± SEM, $n = 3$; *$p < 0.05$ vs all other treatments. (Please *see* insert for color version.)

Transduction with murine retroviruses is limited to replicating cells, thereby making them more suitable for ex vivo gene therapy or in vivo delivery to dividing cells. Transduction efficiency in the vasculature (with low levels of cellular replication) is usually low (<1%), but transgene expression may last months or longer. This feature has limited efforts for direct vascular gene transfer with murine retroviral vectors. Additionally, the potential for insertional mutagenesis has been a long-standing concern and this was highlighted by the occurrence of leukemia in two children treated with retrovirus-based gene therapy as part of the French adenosine deaminase-deficiency trial *(23)*.

To overcome the inability of infecting nondividing cells, lentiviral vectors derived from the human immunodeficiency virus-1 have been developed *(24)*. These vectors may provide long-term expression within quiescent cells, beneficial features for long-term vascular gene transfer. In vitro, these viruses may have advantages over adenoviruses or AAV. Lentiviral vectors have been delivered and tracked using magnetic resonance imaging in pig arteries (Fig. 3) *(25)*. Comparisons with other vectors have not been performed.

## *Adenoviruses*

The development of recombinant adenoviral vectors allowed for the preclinical testing of vascular gene-transfer strategies. Adenovirus serotypes 2 and 5 are among the best studied and the most commonly used of these DNA viruses *(26,27)*. Adenoviruses have a broad tropism for human cells that is determined in part by the nature of the capsid proteins. These capsid proteins may be altered by the addition of new ligands to improve targeting to specific tissues. Both proliferating as well as nonproliferating cells are infected with relatively high efficiency.

The 30–35 kb genome of these viruses is rendered replication incompetent by deleting the *E1* gene (necessary for viral replication), and can support a transgene up to 8 kb in size. The demonstration of vascular inflammation with first-generation vectors (*E1* deleted) led to the development of viruses with deletions in *E2* and *E4* (second generation) *(28,29)*. Additional deletions allow insert sizes up to 20–30 kb but necessitate the use of helper viruses in their production. These so-called "helper-dependent" or "gutted" vectors are incapable of replication in culture and require assistance from a helper virus that provides essential gene products to facilitate replication of the recombinant virus. These helper-dependent adenoviruses have a high efficiency of transfer, but can often be difficult to obtain in a pure form that is free of the helper virus.

Adenoviruses remain episomal with low levels of genomic integration. Drawbacks to their use include inflammation, as well as an induction of a humoral and cytotoxic T-lymphocyte-mediated immune response *(28,29)*. There have been concerns regarding increased neointima formation secondary to inflammation. An adenoviral vector was implicated in the first reported gene therapy-related death *(30)* in a University of Pennsylvania study. However, the titer used in that study was higher than those generally used in preclinical vascular studies or proposed vascular clinical trials. Transgene expression from first-generation vectors is usually limited to 2 or 3 wk and may be better suited for the therapy of restenosis or acute vascular injury rather than disorders requiring chronic long-term therapy. Delivery of helper-dependent vectors to the vasculature has not been reported.

### Adeno-Associated Viruses

AAV are members of the parvo virus family and are capable of transducing dividing as well as nondividing cells *(31)*. They are not known to cause any human disease, but up to 80% of adults demonstrate antibodies against AAV. The wild-type single-stranded DNA viruses preferentially integrate in chromosome 19 of the host genome. This specificity appears to be lost in recombinant AAV vectors and these are mostly retained intracellularly in an episomal form. AAV vectors may be less toxic than adenoviruses. However, these viruses have relatively small (5–6 kb) capacity for inserts and require helper viruses (or their equivalent) during production.

AAV delivery to the vasculature has been performed in vivo with variable results. This variability may be as a result of distinct delivery methods, models, or viral preparation. In spite of these differences, vascular delivery of AAV vectors has been shown to infect vascular cells with the potential of long-term transgene expression and less toxicity *(32,33)*.

## PROMOTERS FOR VASCULAR GENE TRANSFER

Successful transgene expression requires the presence of a promoter that is biologically functional in the desired target tissue. Promoters are genetic sequences that regulate the transcription of genes by binding and coordinating cellular factors (transcription factors) that are involved in the process. Early vectors were engineered to drive gene expression through strong viral promoters or the LTR of retroviruses. The requirement for regulation and tissue specificity has led to several innovative approaches toward promoter design. In general, promoters may be divided into constitutive, tissue specific, and regulatable. Multifunctional derivatives have also been constructed with increasing frequency. Promoter design is an important constituent in process of optimizing and

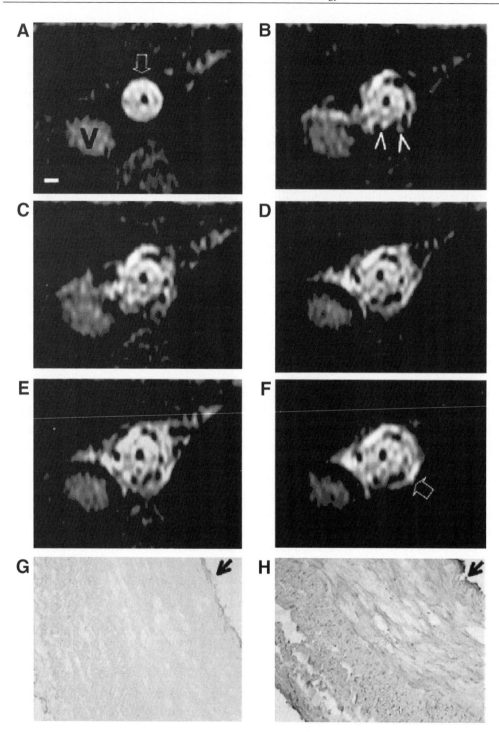

**Fig. 3.** High-resolution MR images of the gadolinium/GFP lentivirus delivery in the iliac artery of a pig. **(A)** Before gadolinium/GFP lentivirus infusion, the balloon is inflated with 3% Magnevist. The open arrow indicates the artery, and V, the vein. Scale = 1 mm. **(B–F)** During gadolinium/GFP lentivirus infusion from minute 3 to 15 (at 3–minute intervals), the arterial wall is enhanced by the gadolinium coming from the gene-infusion channels (arrowheads in B) of the gene delivery catheter. At minute 15, the arterial wall is enhanced as a ring (arrow in F). **(G,H)** Corresponding

controlling the location, magnitude, and duration of expression following successful gene transfer.

## Constitutive Promoters

These promoters by definition are always "on." Any gene driven by these promoters shall be expressed at a high rate determined by the strength of the promoter as well as the cellular milieu that it is placed within. Viral promoters, such as the cytomegalovirus (CMV) promoter, *(34)* have long been the prototype "gold standard" because they function across species in a wide variety of eukaryotic cells. These promoter DNA fragments are small in size and can readily be spliced adjacent a gene of interest placed in a variety of viral or nonviral transfer systems. Levels of expression of genes expressed by these viral promoters are also usually consistently high but may be downregulated by cellular factors. Retroviral long-terminal repeat sequences provide a similarly strong promoter function.

With further refinement in gene-transfer technology, it has become obvious that high levels of expression are not always necessary, and in some cases, also not desirable. This has lead to the use of weaker promoters derived from the human genes as well as other promoters that control constitutive genes in mature eukaryotic cells.

## Tissue-Specific Promoters

Tissue specificity may be engineered by utilizing tissue-specific promoters or their derivatives. They can be modified to provide intrinsic or extrinsic regulation through *cis-* or *trans*-acting molecules. Depending on the potency of the transgene, low levels of gene expression are often adequate to achieve the desired therapeutic goal. Vectors may be designed to provide tissue specificity either by means of being capable of targeting specific cell lines, or by means of carrying tissue-specific promoter systems *(35)*. The process of targeting vectors to specific cells or tissues is imprecise at best at the current time.

Most viral vectors have limited selectivity for vascular tissue. However, the simple placement of a promoter derived from a gene that is selectively expressed in either endothelial cells or smooth muscle will often result in transcriptional targeting. Endothelium has been successfully targeted by using promoters derived from the *vascular cell adhesion molecule-1, von Willebrand factor, endothelial nitric oxide synthetase, tyrosine kinase-2, fms like tyrosine kinase-1,* and *kinase-like domain receptor* genes. Promising tissue-specific promoters for targeting smooth muscle include those derived from the genes *sm22-α, calponin, caldesmon, desmin, sm-myosin heavy chain, sm-α actin,* and *telokin* (Fig. 4) *(36)*. Further characterization and molecular manipulation of these promoters shall likely yield smaller, functional fragments capable of being used for transcriptional targeting of gene therapy.

These tissue-specific promoters come with their unique challenges. Some may be thousands of base pairs in length, making them impractical for use in vectors with limited carrying capacity. Others may require the presence of additional enhancers and *cis*-acting sequences in order to provide the desired tissue specificity. In general, tissue specificity

**Fig. 3.** *(Continued)* immunohistochemistry in both control (G) and GFP-targeted (H) arteries. (H) GFP is detected as brown-colored precipitates through all layers of the intima (arrows) and media as well as the adventitia. Original magnification, × 200. (Please *see* insert for color version.)

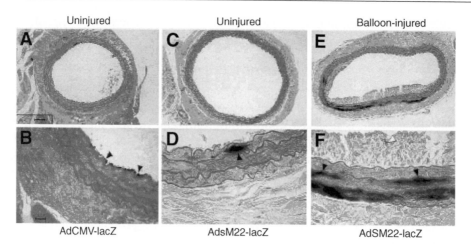

**Fig. 4.** *lacZ*-transgene expression in uninjured and balloon-injured rat carotid arteries infected with *AdSM22-lacZ* and *AdCMV-lacZ*. **(A–D)** Isolated segments of uninjured rat carotid arteries were infected with 109 plaque-forming unit (PFU) of either *AdSM22-lacZ* or the control *AdCMV-lacZ* virus. 7 d after infection, rats were killed, and the carotid arteries were removed and stained for β-galactosidase activity. **(A,B)** In uninjured arteries infected with *AdCMV-lacZ*, β-galactosidase activity (blue staining) was observed in endothelial cells (black arrowheads) and in rare cells located within the adventitia. **(C,D)** In uninjured arteries infected with the *AdSM22-lacZ* virus, β-galactosidase activity was observed in rare SMCs located within the superficial (abluminal) layer of the tunica media. No staining of endothelial cells was observed. **(E,F)** After anesthesia and intubation, the left and right carotid arteries of Sprague-Dawley rats were isolated and injured by dilatation with a Fogarty catheter. A 24-gauge intravenous catheter was introduced into the lumen of each isolated arterial segment and 109 PFU of *AdSM22-lacZ* was instilled for 5 min. β-Galactosidase activity was observed in the SMCs located within the superficial and deep layers of the tunica media (black arrowheads) and within rare cells located within the neointima (open arrowhead). Photomicroscopy was performed using a Zeiss Axiophot microscope (Carl Zeiss Thornwood, NY). Original magnification, A,C,E, × 10; B,D,F, × 40. (Please *see* insert for color version.)

may enhance the translation of preclinical gene-transfer studies by reducing transgene expression in nontarget tissues and its associated complications.

## *Regulatable Promoters*

The ability to precisely titrate the expression of a newly introduced gene remains a subject of intense investigation. Various approaches attempt to provide either extrinsic control through exogenously administered small molecules or through intrinsic autoregulation. Intrinsic autoregulation may be engineered by providing promoter and other DNA elements derived from genes that are normally induced during disease, or states of stress. As an example, *steroid response elements* have been used to enhance gene expression in response to stress. Various cytokine responsive systems have also been developed to respond to states of inflammation or disease.

Extrinsic regulation, mostly in the form of induction through small molecules like sirolimus or tetracycline, has shown promise in early studies *(37)*. The sirolimus analog (rapalog)-based system uses a novel approach to bring together engineered fragments of a DNA binding and a *trans*-activating domain in the presence of rapalog (Fig. 5). This results in the titratable creation of a functional transcription activator molecule. Similarly, RU 486, which can bind two split fragments of a progesterone receptor, has been used to create a functional transcription activator molecule in a manner similar to the rapalog system.

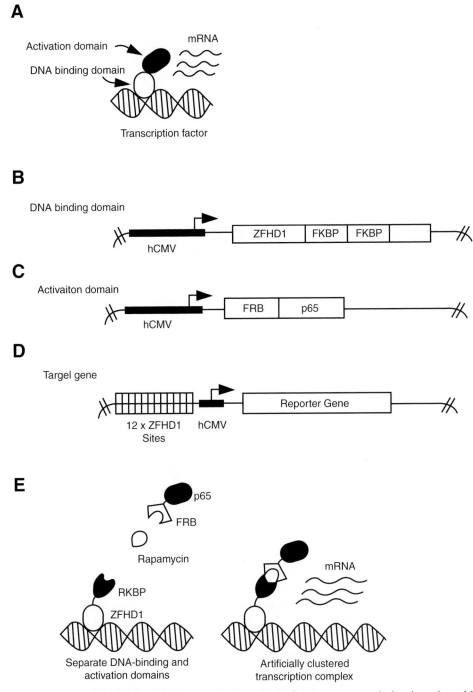

**A**

Activation domain

DNA binding domain

mRNA

Transcription factor

**B**

DNA binding domain

hCMV | ZFHD1 | FKBP | FKBP

**C**

Activaiton domain

hCMV | FRB | p65

**D**

Targel gene

12 x ZFHD1 Sites | hCMV | Reporter Gene

**E**

p65

FRB

Rapamycin

RKBP

ZFHD1

Separate DNA-binding and activation domains

mRNA

Artificially clustered transcription complex

**Fig. 5.** Rapamycin-regulated gene-expression system. For this system, transcription is activated by dimerization between proteins, one containing a DNA-binding protein and a second with a transcription activation domain (**A**). Plasmids encoding a *synthetic DNA-binding domain (ZFHD1)* fused to the FK506-binding protein (FKBP) (**B**) and the *NK-κB p65* transactivation domain fused to the FKBP-rapamycin-binding protein (FRB) (**C**) are cotransfected with a reporter gene (therapeutic gene) (**D**) containing binding sites for the DNA-binding fusion protein. In the presence of dimerizer, rapamycin, or FK1012, the two fusion proteins are able to interact and bring a *trans*-activation domain to the promoter through association with the DNA-binding domain, a process activating transcription (**E**). Human *CMV* (hCMV) promoter sequences are designated by filled boxes on the plasmid diagrams.

A goal of successful vector design is to provide a method of regulatable gene expression for human therapy. Significant progress has been made in all these aspects. However, each system contains elements that are foreign and may induce immunogenicity. Yet, ultimately, regulation of gene transfer in humans will provide important safety controls.

## THE INTERFACE OF VECTORS, PROMOTERS, AND THE FUTURE

The design of vectors and regulatory elements continues to evolve rapidly. Present day vectors, although successful in delivering transgenes, suffer from several limitations. The "holy grail" of vascular gene transfer would be nontoxic, targeted, regulatable vectors, which could be administered systemically and would be capable of chronic expression of transgenes. Currently, all vector systems fail to achieve these goals. However, hopeful opportunities are evident.

The derivation of recombinant viruses from pathogenic viruses often results in either direct toxic effects in the recipient, or triggers an immune reaction, which limits the utility of the vector as a gene-delivery system. This is particularly true of the adenovirus-derived vectors. These viruses, although providing a high-efficiency delivery platform, are unable to produce a therapeutic effect that lasts beyond a few days. Transgene size is also a concern, as many genes and regulatory sequences easily exceed the approx 8 kb insert size limit of these recombinant viruses. Helper-dependent adenovirus overcomes this size constraint, allowing for transcriptional targeting as well as capsid modification. Whether these vectors will allow for chronic expression of transgenes remains to be seen.

Retroviruses on the other hand provide a promise of stable genomic integration with low toxicity and immunogenicity. However, their predilection for insertion into active genes as well as the recent malignancies observed in children treated for severe combined immunodeficiency, have limited enthusiasm for this platform. Additional problems include a transgene size limited to less than 8 kb. There are also issues with the endogenous elements in the *LTR* sequences interfering with gene expression driven by internally added promoters. These vectors also have the disadvantage of infecting only the actively replicating cells. However, these vectors might provide stable transduction of vascular progenitors in vitro and subsequent delivery *(38)*. The lentiviral vectors based on human immunodeficiency virus-1 appear to overcome some of these limitations and are being evaluated for possible therapeutic use.

Plasmid DNA, which formed the basis of early trials, can carry much larger fragments of DNA but is hindered by poor stability, low-transfection efficiency, and transgene expression that is limited to a few days. The development of the various nonviral systems attempts to overcome these limitations by coating this naked DNA with lipids, polymers, or peptides. The incorporation of ligands to some of these synthetic polymer-based platforms and the use of physical delivery methods are promising developments that may improve the ability to target specific tissues using plasmids.

Systemic delivery of vectors is a long-term goal for vascular gene transfer. An exciting new development was recently published, demonstrating enhanced systemic targeting of AAV vectors displaying unique epitopes targeting endothelial cells *(39)*. Endothelial targeting peptides were discovered and displayed on AAV vectors to enhance systemic targeting

**A**

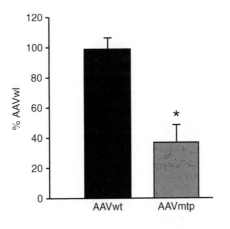

**B**

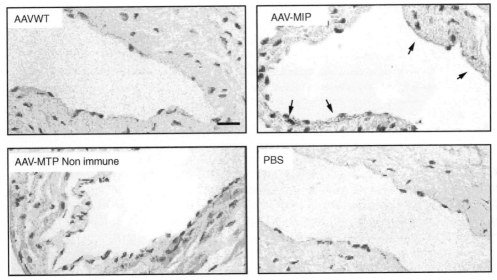

**Fig. 6.** AAV expressing targeting peptide (MTP) decreases liver uptake and increases systemic vascular targeting in vivo. **(A)** Transgene expression in liver homogenates 28 d after infusion of $3 \times 10^{11}$ GPs/mouse of AAVwt or AAVmtp. $*p < 0.05$ vs AAVwt. **(B)** Immunohistochemical detection of β-galactosidase expression in vena cava at 28 d after infusion. Representative sections from four animals/group. Arrows indicate examples of transgene-positive cells. Bar ≈ 20 μm (applicable to all panels). (Please *see* insert for color version.)

(Figs. 6 and 7). Studies like this, combined with the vast amount of genomic and proteomic data from vascular tissue will enhance opportunities for systemic delivery of vectors.

It is likely that in the near future current vectors will be optimized or it will be possible to design completely synthetic "vectors" that combine the desirable features of the various natural systems. The disease, which is targeted and the molecular biology

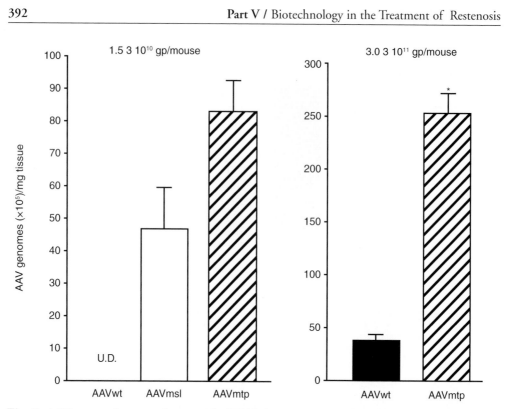

**Fig. 7.** AAV expressing targeting peptide (MTP) increases systemic vascular targeting in vivo. AAV organ distribution and vascular retargeting 28 d after infusion. AAV quantification in vena cava 28 d after infusion of $1.5 \times 10^{10}$ ($n$ = four mice/group; U.D., undetectable) or $3 \times 10^{11}$ GPs/mouse ($*p < 0.05$ vs AAVwt, $n$ = three mice/group).

of the vectors as well as methods for targeting will be understood better. The coming decade shall likely see the advent of these next generation systems, which shall provide high-efficiency platform for addressing the problem of restenosis. Yet, the ultimate goal of these therapies is a broader application to the prevention and stabilization of systemic vascular disease.

## REFERENCES

1. Nabel E, Plautz G, Boyce F, Stanley J, Nabel G. Recombinant gene expression *in vivo* within endothelial cells of the arterial wall. Science 1989;244:1342–1344.
2. Feldman L, Steg P, Zheng L, et al. Low-efficiency of percutaneous adenovirus-mediated arterial gene transfer in the atherosclerotic rabbit. J Clin Invest 1995;95:2662–2671.
3. Ohno T, Gordon D, San H, et al. Gene therapy for vascular smooth muscle cell proliferation after arterial injury. Science 1994;265:781–784.
4. Simari R, San H, Rekhter M, et al. Regulation of cellular proliferation and intimal formation following balloon injury in atherosclerotic rabbit arteries. J Clin Invest 1996;98:225–235.
5. von der Leyen HE, Dzau VJ. Therapeutic potential of nitric oxide synthase gene manipulation. Circulation 2001;103:2760–2765.
6. Kibbe MR, Billiar TR, Tzeng E. Gene therapy for restenosis. Circ Res 2000;86:829–833.
7. Kibbe MR, Tzeng E, Gleixner SL, et al. Adenovirus-mediated gene transfer of human inducible nitric oxide synthase in porcine vein grafts inhibits intimal hyperplasia. J Vasc Surg 2001;34: 156–165.
8. Asahara T, Chen D, Tsurumi Y, et al. Accelerated restitution of endothelial integrity and endothelium-dependent function after phVEGF165 gene transfer. Circulation 1996;94:3291–3302.

9.  Isner J, Pieczek A, Schainfeld R, et al. Clinical evidence of angiogenesis after arterial gene transfer of phVEGF165 in patients with ischaemic limb. Lancet 1996;348:370–374.
10. Verma IM, Somia N. Gene therapy—promises, problems and prospects. Nature 1997;389:239–242.
11. Wolff J, Malone R, Williams P, et al. Direct gene transfer into mouse muscle *in vivo*. Science 1990;247:1465–1468.
12. Hohn B, Koukolikova-Nicola Z, Lindenmaier W, Collins J. Cosmids. Biotechnology 1988;10:113–127.
13. Schatzlein AG. Non-viral vectors in cancer gene therapy: principles and progress. Anticancer Drugs 2001;12:275–304.
14. Reyes-Sandoval A, Ertl HC. CpG methylation of a plasmid vector results in extended transgene product expression by circumventing induction of immune responses. Mol Ther 2004;9:249–261.
15. Song YK, Liu F, Chu S, Liu D. Characterization of cationic liposome-mediated gene transfer in vivo by intravenous administration. Hum Gene Ther 1997;8:1585–1594.
16. Stephan DS, Yang ZY, San H, et al. A new cationic liposome DNA complex enhances the efficiency of arterial gene transfer *in vivo*. Human Gene Ther 1996;7:1803–1812.
17. Ogris M, Steinlein P, Carotta S, Brunner S, Wagner E. DNA/polyethylenimine transfection particles: influence of ligands, polymer size, and PEGylation on internalization and gene expression. AAPS Pharm Sci 2001;3:E21.
18. Dzau VJ, Mann MJ, Morishita R, Kaneda Y. Fusigenic viral liposome for gene therapy in cardiovascular diseases. Proc Natl Acad Sci USA 1996;93:11,421–11,425.
19. Wu GY, Wu CH. Receptor-mediated in vitro gene transformation by a soluble DNA carrier system. J Biol Chem 1987;262:4429–4432.
20. Matsumoto T, Komori K, Shoji T, et al. Successful and optimized in vivo gene transfer to rabbit carotid artery mediated by electronic pulse. Gene Ther 2001;8:1174–1179.
21. Teupe C, Richter S, Fisslthaler B, et al. Vascular gene transfer of phosphomimetic endothelial nitric oxide synthase (S1177D) using ultrasound-enhanced destruction of plasmid-loaded microbubbles improves vasoreactivity. Circulation 2002;105:1104–1109.
22. Buchschacher GL, Jr. Introduction to retroviruses and retroviral vectors. Somat Cell Mol Genet 2001;26:1–11.
23. Hacein-Bey-Abina S, von Kalle C, Schmidt M, et al. A serious adverse event after successful gene therapy for X-linked severe combined immunodeficiency. N Engl J Med 2003;348:255–256.
24. Brenner S, Malech HL. Current developments in the design of onco-retrovirus and lentivirus vector systems for hematopoietic cell gene therapy. Biochim Biophys Acta 2003;1640:1–24.
25. Yang X, Atalar E, Li D, et al. Magnetic resonance imaging permits in vivo monitoring of catheter-based vascular gene delivery. Circulation 2001;104:1588–1590.
26. Kovesdi I, Brough DE, Bruder JT, Wickham TJ. Adenoviral vectors for gene transfer. Curr Opin Biotechnol 1997;8:583–589.
27. Benihoud K, Yeh P, Perricaudet M. Adenovirus vectors for gene delivery. Curr Opin Biotechnol 1999;10:440–447.
28. Wen S, Schneider DB, Driscoll RM, Vassalli G, Sassani AB, Dichek DA. Second-generation adenoviral vectors do not prevent rapid loss of transgene expression and vector DNA from the arterial wall. Arterioscler Thromb Vasc Biol 2000;20:1452–1458.
29. Wen S, Driscoll RM, Schneider DB, Dichek DA. Inclusion of the E3 region in an adenoviral vector decreases inflammation and neointima formation after arterial gene transfer. Arterioscler Thromb Vasc Biol 2001;21:1777–1782.
30. Marshall E. Gene therapy death prompts review of adenovirus vector. Science 1999;286:2244–2245.
31. Grimm D. Production methods for gene transfer vectors based on adeno-associated virus serotypes. Methods 2002;28:146–157.
32. Lynch C, Hara P, Leonard J, Williams J, Dean R, Geary R. Adeno-associated virus vectors for vascular gene delivery. Circ Res 1997;80:497–505.
33. Rolling F, Nong Z, Pisvin S, Collen D. Adeno-associated virus-mediated gene transfer into rat carotid arteries. Gene Ther 1997;4:757–761.
34. Appleby CE, Kingston PA, David A, et al. A novel combination of promoter and enhancers increases transgene expression in vascular smooth muscle cells in vitro and coronary arteries in vivo after adenovirus-mediated gene transfer. Gene Ther 2003;10:1616–1622.
35. Nettelbeck DM, Jerome V, Muller R. Gene therapy: designer promoters for tumour targeting. Trends Genet 2000;16:174–181.

36. Kim S, Lin H, Barr E, Chu L, Leiden J, Parmacek M. Transcriptional targeting of replication-defective adenovirus transgene expression to smooth muscle cells *in vivo*. J Clin Invest 1997;100:1006–1014.
37. Robbins PD, Ghivizzani SC. Viral vectors for gene therapy. Pharmacol Ther 1998;80:35–47.
38. Griese DP, Ehsan A, Melo LG, et al. Isolation and transplantation of autologous circulating endothelial cells into denuded vessels and prosthetic grafts: implications for cell-based vascular therapy. Circulation 2003;108:2710–2715.
39. White SJ, Nicklin SA, Buning H, et al. Targeted gene delivery to vascular tissue in vivo by tropism-modified adeno-associated virus vectors. Circulation 2004;109:513–519. Epub 2004, Jan 2019.

# 25

# Antisense and ODN Transcription Factors in the Treatment of Vascular Proliferative Disease

*Nicholas Kipshidze,* MD, PhD,

*Mykola Tsapenko,* MD, PhD,

*George Dangas,* MD, PhD, *and Pat Iversen,* PhD

**CONTENTS**

## INTRODUCTION

Coronary artery disease is the most common cause of morbidity and mortality in industrialized countries. In recent decades, the number of coronary artery bypass graft surgery procedures has slowly declined owing to continued conversion to minimally invasive percutaneous transluminal coronary angioplasty (PTCA) and stent therapy *(1)*. However, negative vessel remodeling, vessel elastic recoil, and neointima proliferation as a result of a healing response to vessel injury leads to narrowing of the vessel lumen, thus leading to a high incidence (30–80%) of restenosis *(2)*. Introduction of the stent showed a significant decrease in vessel remodeling and elastic recoil at the site of intervention and clearly demonstrated the superiority of stent implantation to PTCA alone with respect to restenosis in *de novo* coronary lesions *(3,4)*. However, it was also evident that neointimal proliferation is not affected by stenting technique *(5)*.

From: *Contemporary Cardiology: Essentials of Restenosis: For the Interventional Cardiologist*
Edited by: H. J. Duckers, E. G. Nabel, and P. W. Serruys © Humana Press Inc., Totowa, NJ

Extensive use of coronary stents to prevent restenosis has produced a new disease: in-stent restenosis. Unfortunately, this complication continues to be difficult to prevent; regardless of the treatment strategy, the rate of in-stent restenosis (20–60% after bare metal stent implantation) is still unacceptably high, depending on vessel and patient bias *(2–4,6)*. This is particularly true in patients with diabetes and in some lesion subsets, such as bifurcated lesions, long diffuse lesions, and/or small vessels *(6)*. Despite significant advances in the treatment of cardiovascular disease, intimal hyperplasia remains the most common cause of early failure after revascularization. In addition to mechanical procedures, current treatment strategy on intimal hyperplasia includes two main approaches: inhibiting vascular smooth muscle cell (VSMC) proliferation and growth, as well as promoting re-endothelialization and augmenting endothelial functions, and stimulating the pathways that lead to VSMC apoptosis. The recent trend toward stent-based drug delivery explored the potential of antiproliferative drugs in the treatment and prevention of intimal hyperplasia. Several completed studies (RAVEL, SIRIUS [Sirolimus], TAXUS I–IV [Paclitaxel], ELUTE, ASPECT [Paclitaxel], and so on) showed the great potential of this approach in the treatment of in-stent restenosis. Further advances in vascular gene transfer have shown potential new treatment modalities for cardiovascular disease, particularly in the treatment of vascular restenosis.

## GENE THERAPY OF INTIMAL HYPERPLASIA

Gene therapy, which has been defined as the transfer of nucleic acids (either functional genes or oligonucleotides) to the somatic cells of an individual with a resulting therapeutic effect *(7)*, targets particular genes and thus appears to be more selective and suited to a site-specific treatment approach, as in the case of intimal hyperplasia, than conventional drug therapy. Moreover, vascular gene transfer can be used not only to overexpress or block therapeutically important proteins and correct genetic defects, but also to study various genes and experimentally test their role in the development of particular pathological conditions. Neointimal hyperplasia involves a complex interaction between multiple growth factors that promote VSMC migration and proliferation *(8–10)*. Platelet aggregation and simultaneous activation of smooth muscle cells (SMC) in the media immediately follow injury to the vessel wall. Within 24 h, DNA replication in the medial smooth muscle cells can be observed; in approx 4 d, migration of SMC from the media to the intima becomes apparent. In the intima, proliferation of SMC occurs for several days and stops in about 4 wk, even in the absence of endo-the-lial regeneration. Furthermore, synthesis and deposition of the extravascular matrix lead to intimal hyperplasia *(11,12)*.

Many molecular determinants of intimal hyperplasia have been identified. They involve the release of a host of cytokines and growth factors by platelets, leukocytes, and smooth muscle cells, which can induce the synthesis of gene products that stimulate VSMC migration and proliferation, thereby contributing to excessive intimal growth. Gene transfer studies (e.g., *eNOS, p53, kallikrein* gene, *herpes simplex virus-tk* with ganciclovir therapy, *cytosine deaminase* with 5-FC therapy, *tissue factor* pathway *inhibitor, adrenomedullin*, and *c-Myc* antisense) have shown the potential advantages of gene therapy in the prevention of intimal hyperplasia *(13–22)*. However, several hurdles must be overcome before gene-based stent therapy can be applied successfully in clinical trials. This includes increasing the efficiency of gene delivery through the atherosclerotic plaque; increasing intramural retention times; preventing the inflammatory reaction that stents coated with biodegradable polymers can elicit; overcoming the risk of systemic gene delivery; and accessing the adventitia through a percutaneous approach *(23)*.

## RATIONALE FOR USING ANTISENSE OLIGONUCLEOTIDES IN THE TREATMENT OF INTIMAL HYPERPLASIA

The first successful experience that used oligonucleotides to inhibit gene expression and virus replication was presented by Zamecnik and Stephenson in 1978 *(24)*. They synthesized a 13-mer oligodeoxynucleotide complementary to the 5′- and 3′- reiterated terminal sequences of the Rous Sarcoma virus 35S RNA and showed that exposure of infected fibroblasts to this oligomer led to a 99% decrease in reverse transcriptase activity in the medium, which also correlated with a decrease in cellular transformation. This study showed that such compounds might have a therapeutic advantage by specifically targeting genetic sequences that are critical to disease processes.

Three major classes of oligonucleotides exist: antisense sequences (commonly called antisense oligonucleotides, or oligodeoxy nucleotides [ODN]); antigen sequences; ribozymes and *cis*-element double-stranded decoy ODN. Antisense sequences are derivatives of nucleic acids (DNA or RNA sequences) that hybridize cytosolic messenger RNA (mRNA) strands through hydrogen bonding to complementary nucleic acid bases. Antigene sequences hybridize double-stranded DNA in the nucleus, forming triple helixes. Instead of inhibiting protein synthesis simply by binding to a single targeted mRNA, ribozymes combine enzymatic processes with the specificity of base pairing, creating a molecule that can incapacitate multiple targeted mRNAs *(25)*. Transfection of decoy ODN will result in attenuation of authentic *cis–trans* interaction, leading to the removal of *trans*-factors from the endogenous *cis*-elements, with subsequent modulation of gene expression *(26)*.

The antisense approach to inhibiting gene expression involves introducing oligonucleotides complementary to mRNA into cells to block any one of the following processes: uncoiling of DNA, transcription of DNA, export of RNA, DNA splicing, RNA stability, or RNA translation involved in the synthesis of proteins in cellular proliferation *(27)*. It includes the use of ODN, antisense mRNA, autocatalytic ribozymes, and the insertion of a section of DNA to form a triple helix. The inhibition of gene expression thus achieved is believed to be highly specific and is dependent on formation of the antiparallel duplex by complementary base pairing between the antisense DNA and the target mRNA, in which adenosine and thymidine or guanosine and cytidine interact through hydrogen bonding. This elegant specificity of the Watson-Crick base pairing between the ODN and the target mRNA may form the basis for a highly effective and specific therapeutic modality and might be used to eliminate the expression of any cellular protein *(28)*.

Oligonucleotides that are complementary or antisense to individual mRNA sequences bind to the particular sequence and prevent translation *(29)*. Once inside the cell, ODN binds to its target mRNA in the cytoplasm, nucleus, or both. This hybridization with the mRNA explains two main mechanisms of action of the oligonucleotides *(30,31)*. First, oligonucleotides have been suggested to exert steric interference *(32)* to ribosome binding and translation, or splice excision. Evidence for steric interference came from studies in which antisense to the 5′ cap of mRNA was found to be the most effective in inhibiting rabbit β-globin protein synthesis *(33)*; the 5′ cap is the site where a number of initiation factors bind for ribosome assembly, the unwinding of DNA, and ribosome translocation along the mRNA *(34)*.

Second, the effect of ODN is owing to induction of cleavage of mRNA by the nuclease *RNAse H* that specifically recognizes DNA-RNA duplexes *(35–37)*. ODN can also enter the nucleus where they may inhibit splicing *(38)*, preventing the process of pre-mRNA or mRNA, or block transport of the mRNA out of the nucleus. Introduction of oligonucleotides thus results in a reduction of specific mRNA and protein levels if mediated by *RNAse H*, or a reduction in specific protein levels if mediated by steric interference. It was also found that SMC proliferation could be inhibited by antisense oligomers through nonantisense mechanisms *(39)*. In this case, the presence of four contiguous guanosine residues (G-4 tract) within the oligonucleotide sequence caused a sequence-specific, but not antisense-dependent, antiproliferative effect.

## EFFICACY OF ANTISENSE OLIGONUCLEOTIDES IN THE INHIBITION OF SMC PROLIFERATION AND THE PREVENTION OF RESTENOSIS

Inhibition of several cellular proto-oncogenes including DNA binding protein c-Myb *(40,41)*, nonmuscle myosin heavy chain, proliferating-cell nuclear antigen (PCNA) *(42,43)*, platelet-derived growth factor *(44)*, basic fibroblast growth factor *(45)*, c-raf *(46)*, and c-Myc *(47,48)* have been shown to inhibit SMC proliferation in vitro; the efficacy of these oligomers has been confirmed in in vivo studies as well *(49–51)*. These in vitro and in vivo studies not only demonstrated efficacy of the ODN in the inhibition of SMC proliferation and intimal hyperplasia, but also revealed key points in the development of antisense therapy for arterial restenosis.

The combination of two different oligonucleotides has demonstrated an inhibitory effect on arterial intimal hyperplasia following balloon injury *(52)*. Even after single intraluminal delivery, the antisense oligomer combination directed against *PCNA* and *cell division cycle 2 kinase* (cdc2) was effective in suppressing neointima formation in the rat model of carotid artery balloon injury *(50)*. Another combination of ODNs, antisense *cdc2* and *cdk2* oligonucleotides, was successfully used by Abe et al. *(53)* to suppress neointimal SMC accumulation in vivo in the rat carotid artery. At the same time, Robinson et al. *(54)* demonstrated that single endoluminal delivery of *PCNA/cdc2* antisense oligonucleotides by porous balloon catheter does not affect neointima formation or vessel size in the pig coronary artery model of postangioplasty restenosis. The time frame of antisense ODN introduction to injured vessel may play an important role in the prevention of restenosis. Schmidt et al. *(55)* showed that rat carotid artery SMC proliferation begins 1–2 d after balloon catheter-induced injury, and entry of cells into the growth phase was completed within 3 d of injury. At the same time, minimally modified b-FGF-specific antisense ODN exerted its antiproliferative activity within this time frame. This strategy has also been successfully applied in the inhibition of various targets, such as c-cbl and c-src *(56)*, herpes simplex virus type-1 *(57)*, and c-Myc *(47)*.

Different structural types of antisense ODN demonstrate different efficacy and specificity in inhibiting targeted mRNA. Stein et al. *(58)* carried out cell-free translation studies to compare the efficacy and specificity of four antisense structural types: DNA, phosphorothioate DNA, 2′-O-methyl RNA, and morpholino oligonucleotides, a novel antisense oligonucleotide. It was shown that at low concentrations of antisense oligomer, all four types provide high specificity, but the morpholino oligos and 2′-O-methyl RNA afford better efficacy. At high oligomer concentrations, all four types provide high efficacy, but the morpholino oligos and 2′-0-methyl RNA provide substantially better specificity than the DNA and S-DNA. It was also shown that mRNA could discriminate between oligonucleotides that differ only by one or two bases *(30,58,59)*. Changes in a c-Myc antisense ODN sequence of only two bases resulted in almost complete loss of its activity *(59)*.

Frequent nonspecific effects may follow the use of antisense oligonucleotides. Some of these effects are sequence-specific, as described for 4-guanosine residue, which causes an aptamer effect leading to nonantisense dependent inhibition *(39)*. Although in vitro studies have clearly established that antisense oligomers can inhibit target genes without producing gross toxic effects on cultured cells, in vivo studies in *Xenopus* oocytes reveal that it is not possible to obtain specific cleavage of an intended target RNA without causing at least the partial destruction of many nontargeted RNA *(42)*. Despite the apparent success of antisense oligonucleotide therapy, several limitations of this technology have manifested. First, the ODN must effectively cross the cell membrane to reach the cytoplasm or nucleus (permeation). Once inside the cell, the ODN must be resistant to degradation (stability). Finally, the ODN must be able to bind specifically and with a high affinity to the RNA target to inhibit the desired gene (affinity and specificity) *(28,30)*.

Oligonucleotides are strongly negatively charged, which prevent them from passing the cell surface passively. Uptake of ODN appears to occur by receptor-mediated endocytosis and is determined by various factors including the length of the ODN, the total charge of the molecule, its lipid solubility, and the nucleotide concentration *(60,61)*. Naturally occurring nucleotide oligomers are easily and rapidly degraded by exo- and endonucleases, which can significantly limit their utilization in antisense technology *(62,63)*. Previous studies have confirmed that the presence of simple 3′ or 3′ plus 5′ modifications may provide protection from degradation by exonucleases *(64,65)*. However, the action of intracellular endonucleases is sufficient to degrade the end-modified oligomers; uniform modification throughout the oligomers has been suggested. Interestingly, previous studies *(41)* have shown that unmodified ODN is more efficacious in vivo and in vitro than modified ODN.

The affinity of the oligonucleotides depends on their length and base composition. An increase in ODN length also increases its affinity; however, after a particular oligonucleotide length has been reached, its affinity decreases. The affinity also increases as the number of guanosine-cytidine pairs increase *(66)*. The effect of ODN is believed to be highly specific owing to complementary base pairing between the antisense DNA and the target mRNA, but it does not prevent frequent nonspecific effects described earlier *(42)*.

## DELIVERY SYSTEMS FOR ANTISENSE OLIGONUCLEOTIDES

One of the most important technical problems in the clinical applicability of antisense technology is the development of an efficient and suited delivery system for oligonucleotides. Local drug delivery was designed to bring the antisense agent to the coronary artery during the period of time corresponding to peak-injury response. The earliest attempts to deliver antisense agents to prevent restenosis involved a rat carotid artery model using adventitial *(49)* or surgical application *(50)*. The initial clinically applicable devices were catheter-based and provided local delivery as a bolus injection, at which time the catheter was withdrawn. The combination of antisense targeting to c-Myc with catheter-based delivery to coronary arteries of pigs for prevention of restenosis began with phosphorothioate oligonucleotides *(29)*. The bolus injection of phosphorothioate oligomers produced a reduction in heart rate, blood pressure, and cardiac output in primate models that was sometimes lethal *(67–70)*.

Modified angioplasty balloons have been designed and developed for local delivery of genes or drugs into the vascular wall *(71)*. Some examples of modified angioplasty balloons are the double balloon catheter, in which the agent is infused into a closed compartment between the balloons and can diffuse with minimal pressure onto the vessel wall; perforated balloon, in which the agent is infused under pressure through pores in the balloon wall and onto vessel tissue; and the hydrogel-coated balloon, in which the agent is mixed in hydrogel, which dissolves in the bloodstream when the balloon is inflated and pressed against the vessel wall (the agent can then diffuse into the luminal cells). The limitation of these devices is pressure-driven delivery that causes additional vessel damage and low efficacy. Viral vectors or different lipid carriers may increase efficacy of delivery. Fibrin meshwork is an alternative vehicle for sustained release of antisense, a factor that may be important in the case of stent implantation. Polymer-coated stents have been used successfully to deliver micromolar concentrations of c-Myc antisense phosphorodiamidate morpholino oligomers (PMO) into the vessel wall *(72)*. This experience showed that ultimate success will require polymers that are capable of rapid elution of the oligonucleotide with minimal capacity to inflame or otherwise cause additional injury to the vessel wall.

Perfluorobutane gas microbubbles with a coating of dextrose and albumin efficiently bind antisense oligomers *(73)*. These 0.3–10 μm particles bind to sites of vascular injury. Furthermore, perfluorobutane gas is an effective cell membrane fluidizer. The potential advantages of microbubble carrier delivery include minimal additional vessel injury from delivery; no resident polymer to degrade, leading to eventual inflammation; rapid bolus delivery; and the high likelihood of repeated delivery. In addition, the potential for PGMC to deliver to vessel regions both proximal and distal to stents in vessels suggests that this mode of delivery will serve as an excellent adjuvant to a variety of catheter and coated-stent delivery techniques.

## CLINICAL IMPLICATIONS AND FIRST EXPERIENCE OF ANTISENSE THERAPY IN THE TREATMENT OF VASCULAR PROLIFERATIVE DISEASE

The clinical applicability of antisense technology remains limited by a relative lack of specificity, slow uptake across the cell membrane, and rapid degradation of oligonucleotides. Promising results emerged from the PREVENT trial *(74)*, which showed efficacy of ex-vivo gene therapy of human vascular bypass grafts with an antisense oligonucleotide to E2F transcription factor, which is essential for VSMC proliferation in lowering the incidence of venous bypass graft failure. Recently reported results of another clinical trial (ITALICS) in Rotterdam *(75)* that examined the effectiveness of antisense compound directed against c-Myc, however, were disappointing. The authors considered several reasons for the observed lack of effect of the antisense compound. Among them, the local concentration of antisense compound achieved may not have been high enough to show a significant effect. Also, the single administration of the antisense compound might not be effective in suppressive c-Myc, which showed biphasic response to the vessel injury. The authors also used a self-expanding stent, which can cause chronic injury of stented arteries. Under these circumstances, a single injection of antisense may not be adequate to reduce myointimal response.

Optimistic results have been obtained with the newly introduced AVI-4126, which belongs to a family of molecules known as the PMO (28). These oligomers include (dimethylamino) phosphinylideneoxy-linked morpholino subunits, which contain a heterocyclic base recognition moiety of DNA attached to a substituted morpholine ring system. In general, PMOs are capable of binding to RNA in a sequence-specific fashion with sufficient avidity to be useful for the inhibition of the translation of mRNA into protein in vivo.

Although PMOs share many similarities with other substances that are capable of producing antisense effects (e.g., DNA, RNA, and their analogous oligonucleotide analogs, such as the phosphorothioates, there are several critical differences. Most importantly, PMOs are uncharged and resistant to degradation under biological conditions, exceptionally stable at temperature extremes, and resistant to degradation in plasma and to the nucleases found in serum and liver extracts (76). They also exhibit a high degree of specificity and efficacy, both in vitro and in cell culture (77), which averts a variety of potentially significant limitations observed in phosphorothioates chemistry. The antisense mechanism of action appears to be through the PMO hybrid duplex with mRNA to inhibit translation. Finally, PMOs have demonstrated antisense activity against c-Myc pre-mRNA in living human cells (78). The combined efficacy, potency, and lack of nonspecific activities of PMO chemistry has compelled us to re-examine the approach of antisense therapy in the prevention of restenosis following balloon angioplasty.

PMOs have been evaluated for adverse effects after intravenous bolus injections in both primates (GLP studies by Sierra Biomedical) and man (GCP studies at MDS Harris). No alterations in heart rate, blood pressure, or cardiac output were observed. In summary, bolus injections of PMO by local catheter-based delivery devices are feasible.

The studies with endoluminal delivery of advanced c-Myc antisense PMO into the area of PTCA (Transport Catheter™; rabbit iliac artery model) (79) and into coronary arteries following stent implantation (Infiltrator™ delivery system; pig model) (80) demonstrated complete inhibition of c-Myc expression and a significant reduction of the neointimal formation in the treated vessels in a dose-dependent fashion whereas allowing for complete vascular healing. Similar results were obtained after implantation of advanced c-Myc antisense PMO-eluting phosphorylcholine-coated stents in the porcine coronary restenosis model (72). Less inflammation was also observed after implantation of the antisense-loaded stent. This favorable influence on hyperplasia (a 40% reduction of intima) in the absence of endothelial toxicity may represent an advantage of antisense PMO over more destructive methods, such as brachytherapy (81) or cytotoxic inhibitors (82).

Novel perfluorocarbon gas microbubble carriers were also tested for site-specific delivery of AVI-4126 to the injured vessel wall and obtained encouraging results (83). The most robust of observations to date by multiple investigators is the finding that AVI-4126 is safe and effective in vascular application in a number of species. Different methods for local delivery have also been tested, but these observations fall short of proof that AVI-4126 will be effective in the treatment of human restenosis. Efficacy in animal models has also been encouraging. Furthermore, all of these studies with AVI-4126 indicated that the agent is safe. The last remaining question is if AVI-4126 will

## Avail clinical events

| Event | Control (%) | 3 mg (%) | 10 mg (%) |
|---|---|---|---|
| TVR-PCI | 3 (27.3) | 6 (33.3) | 1 (6.7) |
| TLR-PCI | 3 (27.3) | 4 (22.2) | 1 (6.7) |
| PCI with angina | 1 (9.1) | 5 (27.8) | 1 (6.7) |
| Q-wave MI | 0 (0) | 0 (0) | 0 (0) |
| Non Q-wave MI | 0 (0) | 0 (0) | 1 (6.7) |
| Death | 0 (0) | 0 (0) | 0 (0) |

**Fig. 1.** AVAIL study, associated clinical events. TVR-PCI, transvascular revascularization at the previous percutaneous coronary intervention; TLR-PCI, transluminal revascularization at the previous percutaneous coronary intervention.

## QCA follow-up, 6-mo In-stent

|  | Control | 3 mg | 10 mg |
|---|---|---|---|
| Ref Diameter (mm) | 2.63 ± 0.40 | 2.79 ± 78 | 2.77 ± 0.46 |
| MLD pre | 0.65 ± 0.40 | 0.94 ± 0.71 | 1.10 ± 0.50 |
| MLD post | 2.81 ± 0.38 | 3.00 ± 0.63 | 2.84 ± 0.71 |
| MLD @FU | 1.55 ± 0.64 | 1.69 ± 0.99 | 2.00 ± 0.74 |
| DS (%): |  |  |  |
| Pre | 71.10 ± 18.04 | 68.35 ± 19.80 | 60.58 ± 15.50 |
| Post | 6.85 ± 8.94 | 8.82 ± 7.49 | 9.71 ± 9.58 |
| Follow-up | 39.45 ± 22.03 | 41.91 ± 24.86 | 22.23 ± 21.23 |
| Late loss | 1.26 ± 0.19 | 1.45 ± 0.19 | 0.74 ± 0.16* |
| Binary restenosis: |  |  |  |
| Number | 3/9 | 4/12 | 1/12 |
| Percent | 33.3 | 33.3 | 83 |

*ANOVA significant difference, $p < 0.03$

**Fig. 2.** AVAIL study, 6-mo follow-up by QCA, in-stent changes/restenosis. QCA, quantitative coronary analysis; DS, diameter stenosis; MLD, minimal luminal diameter; FU, follow-up.

find a place in future therapeutic regimens for the prevention of restenosis; this answer might be found in the results of phase II clinical studies currently completed, such as AVAIL. The results (Figs. 1 and 2) indicate that antisense (AVI-4126) was safe and effective in the prevention of restenosis in patients with denovo and restenotic lesions when delivered through local delivery catheter.

## CONCLUSION

Proof of principle has been established that the inhibition of several cellular proto-oncogenes including: DNA binding protein c-myb, nonmuscle myosin heavy chain PCNA, platelet-derived growth factor, basic fibroblast growth factor, and c-myc, inhibit SMC proliferation in vitro and in several animal models. The first clinical study (ITALICS) demonstrated the safety and feasibility but not efficacy of local delivery of antisense in the treatment and prevention of restenosis. Another randomized clinical trial with local delivery of a third generation antisense: c-myc morpholino compound in patients with coronary artery disease demonstrated safety and trend in the reduction of restenosis. Further identification of new transcriptional factors and signaling mediators would be an important step in the development of new, potential targets for therapy for vascular restenosis.

## ACKNOWLEDGMENTS

The authors wish to thank Cathy Kennedy for editorial assistance on this manuscript.

## REFERENCES

1. Simonsen M. Changing role for cardiac surgery as use of stents continues growth. Cardiovasc Device Update 2003;9:1–7.
2. Topol EJ, Serruys PW. Frontiers in interventional cardiology. Circulation 1998;98:1802–1820.
3. Serruys PW, Foley DP, Suttorp M-J, et al. A randomized comparison of the value of additional stenting after optimal balloon angioplasty for long coronary lesions. J Am Coll Cardiol 2002;39:393–399.
4. Van den Brand M, Rensing J, Morel MM, et al. The effect of completeness of revascularization on event-free survival at one-year in the ARTS trial. J Am Coll Cardiol 2002;39:559–564.
5. Nakatani M, Takeyama Y, Shibata M, et al. Mechanisms of restenosis after coronary intervention. Difference between plain old balloon angioplasty and stenting. Cardiovasc Pathol 2003;12:40–48.
6. Goldberg SL, Loussararian A, De Gregorio J, Di Mario C, Albierro R, Colombo A. Predictors of diffuse and aggressive intrastent restenosis. J Am Coll Cardiol 2001;37:1019–1025.
7. Yla-Herttuala S, Martin JF. Cardiovascular gene therapy. Lancet 2000;355:213–222.
8. Libby P, Schwartz D, Bogi E, Tanaka H, Clinton SK. A cascade model for restenosis: special case of atherosclerosis progression. Circulation 1992;86:47–52.
9. Clowes AW, Clowes MM, Fingerle J, Reidy MA. Regulation of smooth muscle cell growth in injured artery. J Cardiovasc Pharmacol 1989;S12–S15.
10. Fingerele J, Johnson R, Clowes AW, Majesky MW, Reidy MA. Roles of platelets in smooth muscle cell proliferation and migration after vascular injury in rat carotid artery. Proc Natl Acad Sci USA 1989;86:8412–8416.
11. Nikkari ST, Clowes AW. Restenosis after vascular reconstruction. Ann Med 1994;26:95–100.
12. Schwartz SM, DeBlois D, O'Brien ERM. The intima—soil for restenosis and atherosclerosis. Circ Res 1997;77:445–465.
13. Agata J, Zhang JJ, Chao L, Chao L. Adrenomedullin gene delivery inhibits neointima formation in rat artery after balloon angioplasty. Regul Rep 2003;112:115–120.
14. Kipshidze N, Moses J, Shankar LR, et al. Perspectives on antisense therapy for the prevention of restenosis. Curr Opin Mol Therap 2001;3;265–277.
15. Kipshidze N, Iversen P, Keane E, et al. Complete vascular healing and sustained suppression of neointimal thickening after local delivery of advanced c-myc antisense at six months follow-up in a rabbit balloon injury model. Cardiovasc Radiat Med 2002;3:26–30.
16. George SJ, Andelini GD, Capogrossi MC, et al. Wild-type p53 gene transfer inhibits neointima formation in human saphenous vein by modulation of smooth muscle cell migration and induction of apoptosis. Gene Therap 2001;8:668–676.
17. Murakami H, Yayama K, Miao RQ, et al. Kallikrein gene delivery inhibits vascular smooth muscle cell growth and neointima formation in the rat artery after balloon angioplasty. Hypertension 1999;34:164–170.

18. Steg GP, Tahlil O, Aubailly N, et al. Reduction of restenosis after angioplasty in an atheromatous rabbit model by suicide gene therapy. Circulation 1997;96:408–411.
19. Harell RL, Rajanayagam S, Doanes AM, et al. Inhibition of vascular smooth muscle cell proliferation and neointimal accumulation by adenovirus-mediated gene transfer of cytosine deaminase. Circulation 1997;96:621–627.
20. Zoldheliy P, McNatt J, Shelat H, et al. Thromboresistance of balloon-injured porcine carotid arteries after local gene transfer of human tissue factor pathway inhibitor. Circulation 2000;101:289–295.
21. Van Belle E, Tio FO, Chen D, et al. Passivation of metallic stents after arterial gene transfer of phVEGF 165 inhibits thrombus formation and intimal thickening. J Am Coll Cardiol 1997;29: 1371–1379.
22. Yoon J, Wu CJ, Homme J, et al. Local delivery of nitric oxide from an eluting stent to inhibit neointimal thickening in a porcine coronary injury model. Yonsei Med J 2002;43:242–251.
23. Feldman MD, Bo Sun, Koci B, et al. Stent-based gene therapy. J long term Eff Med Implants 2000;10:47–68.
24. Zamecnik P, Stephenson M. Inhibition of Rous sarcoma virus replication and cell transformation by a specific deoxyoligonucleotide. Proct Natl Acad Sci 1978,75;280–284.
25. Wang A, Creasy A, Lardner M, et al. Molecular cloning of the complementary DNA for human tumor necrosis factor. Science 1985, 228:149–154.
26. Morishita R, Kaneda Y, Ogihara T. Therapeutic potential of oligonucleotide-based therapy in cardiovascular disease. Bio Drugs 2003;17:383–389
27. Helene C, Toulme JJ. Specific regulation of gene expression by antisense, sense and antigene nucleic acids. Biochem Biophys Acta 1990;1049:99–125.
28. Stein CA, Cheng YC. Antisense oligonucleotides as therapeutic agents -Is the bullet really magical? Science 1993;261:1004–1012.
29. Shi Y, Fad A, Galleon A, et al. Transcatheter delivery of c-myc antisense oligomers reduced neointimal formation in a porcine model of coronary artery balloon injury. Circulation 1994;90:944–951.
30. Bennett MR, Schwartz SM. Antisense therapy for Angioplasty restenosis: Some critical considerations. Circulation 1995;92:1981–1993.
31. Stein CA, Tokinson JL, Yakubov L. Phosphorothioate Oligodeoxynucleotides antisense inhibitors of gene expression? Pharmacol Ther 1991;52:365–384.
32. Bolziau C, Kurfirst R, Cazenave C, Roig V, Thoung NT, Toulme JJ. Inhibition of translation initiation by antisense oligonucleotides via an RNAase independent mechanism. Nucleic Acid Res 1991;19:1113–1119.
33. Goodchild J. Inhibition of gene expression by oligonucleotides. In: Cohen J ed. Oligonucleotides: Antisense Inhibitors of Gene Expression. London, Mac Mil press, 1989, pp. 53–77.
34. Kozak M. Influences of mRNA secondary structure on inhibition by eucaryotic ribosome. Proc Natl Acad Sci USA 1996;83:2850–2854.
35. Wagner R, Nishikura K. Cell cycle expression of RNA duplex unwinding activity in cells. Mol Cell Biol 1988;8:770–777.
36. Dash P, Lotan L, Knapp M, Kandel ER, Goelet P. Selective elimination of mRNA in vivo: Complementary oligodeoxynucleotides promote RNA degradation by RNAse-H like activity. Proc Natl Acad Sci 1987;84:7896–7900.
37. Dagle JM, Walder JA, Weeks DL. Target degradation of mRNA in Xenopus oocytes and embryos directed by modified oligonucleotides: studies of An2 and cyclin in embryogenesis Nucleic Acid Res 1990;18:4751–4757.
38. Mc Mannaway ME, Neckers LM, Loke SL, et al. Tumor-specific inhibition of lymphoma growth by an antisense oligodeoxynucleotide. Lancet 1990;335:808–811.
39. Burgess TL, Fisher EF, Ross SL, et al. The antiproliferative effect of c-myb and c-myc antisense oligonucleotides in smooth muscle cells is caused by a non antisense mechanism. Proc Natl Acad Sci USA 1995;92:4051–4055.
40. Simons M, Rosenburg RD. Antisense non-muscle, myosin, heavy chain and c-myb oligonucleotides suppress smooth muscle cell proliferation in vitro. Circ Res 1992;70:835–843.
41. Gunn J, Holt CM, Francis SE, et al. The effect of oligonucleotides to c-myb on vascular smooth muscle cell proliferation and neointima formation after porcine coronary angioplasty. Circ Res 1997;80:520–531.
42. Speir E, Epstein SE. Inhibition of smooth muscle cell proliferation by an antisense deoxyoligonucleotide targeting the mRNA coding proliferating cell nuclear antigen. Circulation 1992;86:538–547.

43. Simons M, Edelman ER, Rosenberg RD. Antisense PCNA oligonucleotides inhibit neointimal hyperplasia in a rat carotid artery injury model. J Clin Invest 1994;93:2351–2356.

44. Sugiki H. Suppression of vascular smooth muscle cell proliferation by an antisense oligonucleotide against PDGF receptor. Hokkaido Igaku Zasshi 1995;70:485–495.

45. Hanna AAK, Fox JC, Neschis DG, Safford SD, Swain JL. Golden MA. Antisense basic fibroblast growth factor gene transfer reduces neointimal thickening after arterial injury. J Vasc Surg 1997;25:320–325.

46. Mandiyan S, Schumacher C, Cioffi C, et al. Molecular and cellular characterization of baboon C-Raf as target for antiproliferative effects of antisense oligonucleotides. Antisense Nucleic Acid Drug Dev 1997;7:539–548.

47. Biro S, Fu YM, Yu ZX, Epstein SE. Inhibitory effects of oligodeoxynucleotides targeting c-myc RNA on smooth muscle cell proliferation and migration. Proct Natl Acad Sci USA 1993;90:654–658.

48. Daum T, Engels JW, Mag M, et al. Antisense deoxynucleotide: Inhibitor of splicing of mRNA of Human immunodeficiency virus. Intern Virol 1992;89:7031–7035.

49. Simons M, ER, Dekeyser J-L, Langer R, Rosenberg RD. Antisense c-myb oligonucleotides inhibits intimal arterial smooth muscle cell accumulation in vivo. Nature 1992;359:67–70.

50. Morshita R, Gibbons GH, Ellison KE, et al. Single intraluminal delivery of antisense cdc kinase PCNA results in chronic inhibition of neointimal hyperplasia. Proc Natl Acad Sci USA 1993;90: 8474–8478.

51. Bayever E, Iversen PL, Bishop MR, et al. Systemic administration of a phosphorothioate oligonucleotide with a sequence complementary to p53 for acute myelogenous leukemia and myelodysplastic syndrome: initial results of a phase I trial. Antisense Res Dev 1993;4:383–390.

52. Summerton J, Stein D, Huang B, Matthews P, Welder D, Partridge M. Morpholino and phosphorothioate antisense oligomers compared in cell-free and in-cell systems. Antisense Nucleic Acid Drug Div 1997;7:63–70.

53. Abe J, Zhou W, Taguchi J. Suppression of neointimal smooth muscle cell accumulation in vivo by antisense cdc2 and cdk2 oligonucleotides in rat carotid artery. Biochem Biophys Commun 1994;198:16–24.

54. Robinson KA, Chronos NAF, Schieffer E, et al. Endoluminal local delivery of PCNA/cdc2 antisense oligonucleotides by porous balloon catheter does not affect neointima formation or vessel size in the pig coronary artery model of post angioplasty restenosis. Cathet Cardiovasc Diagn 1997;41:348–353.

55. Schmidt A, Sindermann J, Peyman A, et al. Sequence specific antiproliferative effects of antisense and end-capping modified antisense oligodeoxynucleotides targeted against the 5′-terminus of Basic-fibroblast growth factor mRNA in coronary smooth muscle cells. Eur J Biochem 1997;248:543–549.

56. Tanaka S, Amling M, Neff L, et al. c-cbl downstream of c-src in a signaling pathway necessary for bone resorption. Nature 1996;383:528–531.

57. Peyman A, Helsberg M, Kretzschmar G, Mag M, Ryte A, Uhlmann E. Nuclease stability as dominant factor in the antiviral activity of oligonucleotides directed again HSV-1 IE I 10. Antiviral Res 1997;33:135–139.

58. Stein D, Foster E, Huang SB, Weller D, Summerton J. A specificity comparison of four antisense types: Morpholino, 2′-O methyl RNA, DNA and Phosphorothioate DNA. Antisense Nucleic Acid Drug Dev 1997;7:151–157.

59. Holt JT, Redner RL, Nelhus AW. An oligomer complementary to c-myc RNA inhibits proliferation of HL-60 promyelocytic cells and induces differentiation. Mol Cell Biol 1988;8:963–973.

60. Villa AE, Guzman LA, Poptic EJ, et al. Effects of antisense c-myb oligonucleotides on vascular smooth muscle cell proliferation and response to vessel wall injury. Circ Res 1995;76:505–513.

61. Muler DWM. The role of proto-oncogenes in coronary restenosis. Pro Cardiovasc Ids 1997; 40:117–128.

62. Wickstrom E. Antisense c-myc inhibition of lymphoma growth. Antisense Nucleic Acid Drug Dev 1997;7:225–228.

63. Cazenave C, Loreau N, Thuong NT, Toulme JJ. Enzymatic amplification of translation inhibition of rabbit beta-globin mRNA mediated by anti-messenger oligodeoxynucleotides covalently linked to intercalating agents. Nucleic Acid Res 1995;15:4717–4736.

64. Shaw JP, Kent K, Bird J, Fishback J, Froehler BF. Modified deoxyoligonucleotide stable to exonuclease degradation in serum. Nucleic acids Res 1991;19:747–750.

65. Ott J, Eckstein F. Protection of oligonucleotide primers against degradation by DNA polymerase I. Biochem 1987;26:8237–8241.

66. Hoke GD, Draper K, Freier SM, et al. Effect of phosphorothioate capping on Antisense oligonucleotide stability, hybridization and antiviral efficacy versus Herpes simplex virus infection. Nucleic Acid Res 1991;20:5743–5748.

67. Cornish KG, Iversen PL, Smith L, Arneson M, Bayever E. Cardiovascular effects of a phosphorothioate oligonucleotide with sequence antisense to p53 in the conscious rhesus monkey. Pharmacol Commun 1993;3:239–247.

68. Galbraith WM, Hobson WC, Giclas PC, Schechter PJ, Agrawal S. Complement activation and hemodynamic changes following intravenous administration of phosphorothioate oligonucleotides in the monkey. Antisense Res Dev 1994;4:201–206.

69. Henry, SP, Bolte H, Auletta C, Kornburst DJ. Evaluation of the toxicity of ISIS 2302 a phosphorothioate oligonucleotide, in a four week study in cynomolgus monkeys. Toxicology 1997;120:145–155.

70. Iversen PL, Cornish KG, Iversen LJ, Mata JE, Bylund DB. Bolus intravenous injection of phosphorothioate oligonucleotides causes hypotension by acting as a1-adrenergic receptor antagonists. Toxicol Appl Pharmacol 1999;160:289–296.

71. Hedin U, Wahlberg E. Gene therapy and vascular disease: potential applications in vascular surgery. Eur J Vasc Endovasc Surg 1997;13:101–111.

72. Kipshidze NN, Iversen P, Kim HS, et al. Advanced c-myc antisense (AVI-4126)-eluting phosphorylcholine-coated stent implantation is associated with complete vascular healing and reduced neointimal formation in the porcine coronary restenosis model. Catheter Cardiovasc Interv 2004;61: 518–527.

73. Porter TR, Iversen PL, Li S, Xie F. Interaction of Diagnostic Ultrasound with Synthetic Oligonucleotide-Labeled Perfluorocarbon-Exposed Sonicated Dextrose Albumin Microbubbles. J Ultrasound Med 1996;15:577–584.

74. Mann MJ, Whittemore AD, Donaldson MC, et al. Ex-vivo gene therapy of human vascular bypass grafts with E2F decoy: the PREVENT single-centre, randomised, controlled trial. Lancet 1999;354:1493–1498.

75. Kutryk MJ, Foley DP, van den Brand M, et al. Local intracoronary administration of antisense oligonucleotide against c-myc for the prevention of in-stent restenosis: results of the randomized investigation by the Thoraxcenter of antisense DNA using local delivery and IVUS after coronary stenting (ITALICS) trial. J Am Coll Cardiol 2002;39:281–287.

76. Hudziak RM, Barofsky E, Barofsky DF, et al. Resistance of morpholino phosphorodiamidate oligomers to enzymatic degradation. Antisense Nucl Acid Drug Dev 1996;6:267–272.

77. Hudziak RM, Summerton J, Weller DD, Iversen PL. Antiproliferative effects of steric blocking phosphorodiamidate Morpholino antisense agents directed against c-myc. Antisense Nucleic Acid Drug Dev 2000;10:163–176.

78. Dani C, Blanchard JM, Piechaczyk M, El Sabouty S, Marty L, Jeanteur P. Extreme instability of myc mRNA in normal and transformed human cells. Proc Natl Acad Sci USA 1984;81:7046–7050.

79. Kipshidze N, Keane E, Stein D, et al. Local Delivery of c-myc Neutrally Charged Antisense Oligonucleotides with Transport Catheter Inhibits Myointimal Hyperplasia and Positively Affects Vascular Remodeling in the Rabbit Balloon Injury Model. Catheter Cardiovasc Interv 2001;54:247–256

80. Kipshidze NN, Kim H-S, Iversen, et al. Intramural Delivery of Advanced Antisense Oligonucleotides with Infiltrator Catheter Inhibits c-myc Expression and Intimal Hyperplasia in the Porcine. J Am Coll Cardiol 2002;39:1686–1691.

81. Sheppard R, Eisenberg MJ. Intracoronary radiotherapy for restenosis. N Engl J Med 2001;344: 295–297.

82. Herdeg C, Oberhoff M, Baumbach A, et al. Local paclitaxel delivery for the prevention of restenosis: biological effects and efficacy in vivo. J Am Coll Cardiol 2000;35:1969–1976.

83. Kipshidze NN, Porter TR, Dangas G, et al. Systemic targeted delivery of antisense with perflourobutane gas microbubble carrier reduced neointimal formation in the porcine coronary restenosis model. Cardiovasc Radiat Med 2003;4:152–159.

# 26 Cell Cycle Approaches to the Treatment of In-Stent Restenosis

*Elizabeth G. Nabel, MD*

## CONTENTS

INTRODUCTION
THE CELL CYCLE: CYCLINS, CDKs, AND CDK INHIBITORS
P27$^{Kip1}$ AND P21$^{Cip1}$ FUNCTION
THE CDKs AND CKIs IN VASCULAR REMODELING
CLINICAL APPLICATION OF THE CKIs
REFERENCES

## INTRODUCTION

Effective tissue remodeling is essential to the function of blood vessels. Many of the signaling pathways that control vascular remodeling are regulated by nuclear interactions of cell cycle proteins. The cyclin-dependent kinases (CDKs) and the cyclin-dependent kinase inhibitors (CKIs) are a new class of therapeutic agents, which target tissue remodeling in multiple organ systems, particularly the cardiovascular system including restenosis. Understanding their function in the vasculature is leading to the development of exciting new therapies for in-stent restenosis and other cardiovascular diseases.

Tissue repair is critical to the maintenance of blood vessel function following vascular injury. Effective vascular remodeling required the coordinated expression of cellular proteins to repair the injured blood vessel without excessive scar tissue formation. Cell cycle proteins, located within the nucleus of smooth muscle cells, endothelial cells, and inflammatory cells, play a central and critical role in the process of vascular remodeling. Understanding the basic biology of how these cell cycle proteins work is essential to the rationale design of new therapies. The concept of molecular targeting is important in this regard. Therapeutic agents can be precisely targeted to the molecular pathways in a disease, providing specificity to the therapy. In this chapter, the normal components of the cell cycle will be reviewed and the molecular pathogenesis of restenosis will be outlined. These concepts provide a rationale for the molecular targeting of cell cycle proteins to treat restenosis and other cardiovascular diseases.

From: *Contemporary Cardiology: Essentials of Restenosis: For the Interventional Cardiologist*
Edited by: H. J. Duckers, E. G. Nabel, and P. W. Serruys © Humana Press Inc., Totowa, NJ

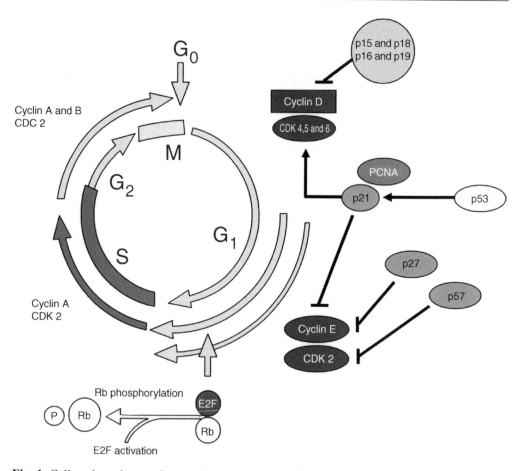

**Fig. 1.** Cell cycle pathways. Progression through the cell cycle is regulated by the CDKs whose activities are controlled by CDK inhibitors (CKIs). CKIs have been assigned to two families based on their structure, the INK4 proteins (p15, p16, p18, p19) and the Cip/Kip proteins (p21, p27, p57). Adapted with permission *(50)*. (Please *see* insert for color version.)

## THE CELL CYCLE: CYCLINS, CDKs, AND CDK INHIBITORS

Vascular smooth muscle cells and endothelial cells in adult blood vessels are normally quiescent, nonproliferative, and are in G0 phase of the cell cycle. When blood vessels are injured, growth factors stimulate the proliferation of these cells. Cell proliferation is a tightly regulated series of events, which occur through the cell cycle. There are four phases of the cell cycle, G0 or a quiescent phase, G1 or gap 1 phase, S or synthetic phase in which DNA replication occurs, and M or mitosis when the cell divides into two daughter cells (Fig. 1). A critical checkpoint occurs in the transition between G1 and S phases, called the G1 checkpoint, in which a commitment to DNA replication and mitosis occurs. Growth factor-stimulated progression through G1 phase of the cell cycle and initiation of DNA replication in S phase are coordinated by proteins called the CKIs or CDKs *(1)*.

The CDKs include Cdk 2, 4, and 6. These CDKs, in turn, bind with specificity to the cyclins, including cyclin-D, -E, and -A. Coordinated progression through the G1 and G2 phases of the cell cycle occurs through the phosphorylation of the cyclins by the

CDKs. The activities of the CDKs, in turn, are regulated by CDK inhibitors termed the CKIs (Fig. 1) *(2)*. There are two families of CKIs based on their structures and CDK targets. The Cip/Kip proteins are inhibitors of cyclin D-, E-, and A-dependent kinases. This family includes p21$^{Cip1}$, p27$^{Kip1}$, and p57$^{Kip2}$. All three of these CKIs contain similar binding regions that bind cyclin and CDK substrates. The INK4 family of proteins (inhibitors of Cdk4) consists of p16$^{INK4a}$, p15$^{INK4b}$, p18$^{INK4c}$, and p19$^{INK4d}$. These CKIs contain multiple similar ankyrin repeats, bind only to Cdk4 and Cdk6 and not to other CDKs, and specifically inhibit the catalytic subunits of Cdk4 and Cdk6.

A complex series of biochemical events take place between the CDKs and their inhibitors *(3)*. The CDKs are enzyme complexes that contain cyclin regulatory and cdk catalytic subunits. Progression through G1 phase and transition through the G1 checkpoint into S phase is mediated by two families of enzymes, the cyclin D- and E-dependent kinases. The D-type cyclins (D1, D2, D3) interact with two catalytic partners, Cdk4 and Cdk6, to yield at least six different enzyme complexes that are expressed in tissue-specific patterns. Cyclin E enters into a complex with its catalytic partner Cdk2 and collaborates with the cyclin D-dependent kinases to complete phosphorylation of the retinoblastoma (*Rb*) gene product, Rb, at the G1 to S transition. Rb phosphorylation releases repression of E2F family members and activates genes required for S phase entry, including the cyclins E and -A.

## p27$^{Kip1}$ AND p21$^{Cip1}$ FUNCTION

The Cip/Kip proteins p27$^{Kip1}$ p21$^{Cip1}$ are important growth regulators of vascular smooth muscle cells and endothelial cells. p27$^{Kip1}$ was discovered as a Cdk inhibitor, which was stimulated by antigrowth signals *(4)*. The *p27$^{Kip1}$* gene in mouse and humans consists of two coding exons; there is also a third noncoding exon 3′ to the translation stop codon *(5)*. The p27$^{Kip1}$ promoter is transactivated by two Sp1-binding sites *(6)*. The 27-kDa protein has a CDK-binding domain in the N-terminal region, a nuclear localization signal in the C-terminal, and three phosphorylation sites at serine 10 (S10), serine 178 (S178), and threonine 187 (T187) *(7)*. p27$^{Kip1}$ is regulated by transcriptional *(8)*, translational *(9)*, and proteolytic mechanisms. Two proteolytic pathways act in sequence during the cell cycle to control p27$^{Kip1}$ abundance. The first pathway functions during G0/G1 and is triggered by growth factors *(10)*. Phosphorylation of p27$^{Kip1}$ on S10 by a kinase called kinase-interacting stathmin occurs early in G0 following growth factor stimulation and leads to p27$^{Kip1}$ export from the nucleus to the cytoplasm *(11)*. The second pathway operates in late G$_1$, S, and G$_2$ phases when Cdk2 phosphorylates p27$^{Kip1}$ on T187, leading to completion of nuclear export of degradation of p27$^{Kip1}$ by proteasomes *(12)*. These sequentially acting pathways that inactivate p27$^{Kip1}$ are molecular targets to regulate p27$^{Kip1}$ function and cell cycle transition.

p27$^{Kip1}$ inhibits cell division. An increase in p27$^{Kip1}$ causes proliferating cells to exit from the cell cycle and prevents their proliferation. Likewise, a decrease in p27$^{Kip1}$ is necessary for quiescent cells to resume division. Knockout of the *p27$^{Kip1}$* gene in mice results in benign hyperplasia of multiple organs, including the adrenals, the thyroid, the retina, and the thymus *(13–15)*. Deletion of p27$^{Kip1}$ is associated with increased tissue inflammation as a result of proliferation of neutrophils, monocytes, and T and B cells in the bone marrow followed by maturation in the thymus (T cells) and the spleen (B cells) *(16)*.

p21$^{Cip1}$ has many functions associated with cell proliferation and cell survival. p21$^{Cip1}$ inhibits CDKs and the proliferating-cell nuclear antigen (PCNA). As a transcriptional target of p53, p21$^{Cip1}$ is also a downstream target of p53 and mediates apoptosis or cell death following DNA damage. p21$^{Cip1}$ also plays a role cell senescence when cells complete differentiation. p21$^{Cip1}$-deficient mice undergo normal development, but their fibroblasts fail to undergo G1 arrest following DNA damage *(17)*. p21$^{Cip1}$ null mice develop tumors late in life *(18)*.

p27$^{Kip1}$ and p21$^{Cip1}$ have a similar or conserved amino-terminal domain that is associated with binding to cyclin–Cdk complexes and inhibition of CDK activity. However, these proteins have different C-terminal regions, which diversify their functions. For example, p21$^{Cip1}$ binds PCNA in the carboxy-terminal and inhibits PCNA activity *(19)*. The Cip/Kip inhibitors can also be distinguished by their responses to growth and antigrowth signals. p21$^{Cip1}$ expression increases in a p53-dependent manner in cells containing, damaged DNA, and a p53-independent manner in postmitotic, terminally differentiated cells *(20)*. In contrast, p27$^{Kip1}$ expression increases primarily in response to extracellular antigrowth signals. Normal cells express elevated levels of p27$^{Kip1}$ protein *(21)*, and cells exposed to antigrowth factors like rapamycin also express high levels of p27$^{Kip1}$ protein *(22)*.

## THE CDKs AND CKIs IN VASCULAR REMODELING

Vascular injury leads to a remodeling process that is adaptive in normal conditions but maladaptive in vascular diseases, such as restenosis. In response to physiological stimuli, vascular smooth muscle cells proliferate and migrate in or within the intima to form a thickened neointima. Normally, this self-limited process results in a well-healed vascular wound and preservation of blood flow. However, in vascular diseases, such as restenosis and vein-graft occlusion, vascular smooth muscle cell proliferation becomes excessive leading to a pathological lesion in the blood vessel, which in turn produces clinical symptoms, termed in-stent restenosis. In-stent restenosis is also characterized by systemic and/or local inflammation, which exacerbates the smooth muscle cell proliferation.

Studies in the laboratory have demonstrated that p27$^{Kip1}$ and p21$^{Cip1}$ regulate modeling following vascular injury. As stated earlier, vascular smooth muscle cells in the media of arteries are normally quiescent G0 phase of the cell cycle, and they proliferate at very low rates, less than 0.05% *(23)*. Following vascular injury, growth factors are released by multiple cells, and vascular smooth muscle cells are stimulated to divide. After several rounds of cell division, a small neointima is formed, and the blood vessel is "healed." p27$^{Kip1}$ and p21$^{Cip1}$ have very distinct patterns of expression during this normal wound healing. p27$^{Kip1}$ is expressed in vascular smooth muscle cells of normal arteries, but is quickly downregulated after vascular injury when vascular smooth muscle cells are stimulated to divide *(24)*.

Vascular smooth muscle cells synthesize collagen and other extracellular matrix molecules, which signal back to vascular smooth muscle cells in autocrine and paracrine feedback loops produce an increase in p27$^{Kip1}$ protein and a decrease in cyclin E and Cdk2. p27$^{Kip1}$ protein is expressed in intimal vascular smooth muscle cells after the vascular wound is healed. In contrast, p21$^{Cip1}$ protein is not present in vascular smooth muscles of normal arteries. This protein is upregulated with p27$^{Kip1}$ during the completion of vascular repair. Interestingly, p16$^{INK4a}$ is not expressed at high levels in normal or injured arteries. It has been observed that these patterns of p27$^{Kip1}$ and p21$^{Cip1}$ expression are observed in several animal models of vascular disease, including rats and pigs *(25,26)*.

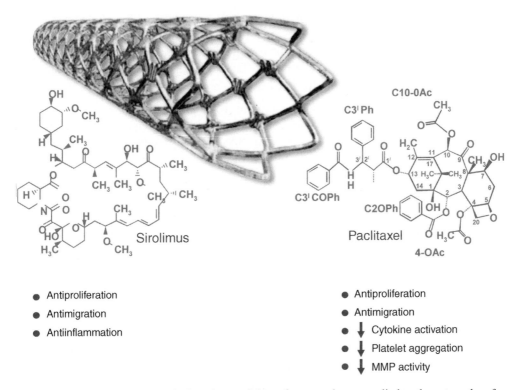

- ● Antiproliferation
- ● Antimigration
- ● Antiinflammation

- ● Antiproliferation
- ● Antimigration
- ● ↓ Cytokine activation
- ● ↓ Platelet aggregation
- ● ↓ MMP activity

**Fig. 2.** Drug-eluting stents permit the release of drugs from a polymer applied to the external surface of the stent. The drug enters the vascular wall, notably into endothelial and smooth muscle cells. Adapted with permission *(3)*.

In terms of human coronary arteries, p27$^{Kip1}$ expression was observed in vascular smooth muscle cells within the intima and media of nonatherosclerotic and atherosclerotic vessels. Interestingly, p27$^{Kip1}$ expression was also found within smooth muscle cells in new blood vessels forming within the intima, suggestive of angiogenesis. p21$^{Cip1}$ expression was present only in advanced atherosclerotic lesions *(24)*. The findings, then, support the relevance of molecular targeting to p27$^{Kip1}$ and p21$^{Cip1}$ in the treatment of vascular diseases.

Subsequently, these findings were confirmed by conducting gene-expression and gene-deletion experiments of these CKI proteins in mouse and pig blood vessels. Overexpression of p27$^{Kip1}$ and p21$^{Cip1}$ using gene-transfer vectors in balloon-injured arteries leads to a significant reduction in vascular smooth muscle cell proliferation and intimal lesion formation. The mechanism is cell cycle arrest in G1 phase *(25,26)*. Interestingly, deletion of *p27$^{Kip1}$* and *p21$^{Cip1}$* genes in mice accelerates cellular proliferation and impairs arterial wound repair following vascular injury *(16)*. In this model, the absence of p27$^{Kip1}$ within inflammatory cells also intensifies the immune response within injured blood vessels.

## CLINICAL APPLICATION OF THE CKIs

In-stent restenosis is a recurrence of an intimal lesion following an intra-arterial percutaneous coronary intervention because of a reduction in luminal area (Fig. 2). This process of wound healing occurs in every person undergoing percutaneous coronary intervention; however, the degree of luminal narrowing or severity of the intimal lesion varies considerably. Angiographic in-stent restenosis is defined as a reduction in the luminal size of more than 50% or more than 30% reduction from the initial postprocedure lumen size (27). The time-course of restenosis is typically 4–6 mo after balloon angioplasty and 6–9 mo following stenting. The stenting tends to delay the onset of clinical symptoms by several months because of:

1. The absence of elastic recoil, which is present following balloon angioplasty and
2. Possibly a slower growth rate of intimal cells. Typically, the incidence of restenosis following balloon angioplasty is approx 30–40%, whereas the in-stent restenosis rate is 20–25% (27).

In terms of the pathophysiology, restenosis results from the simultaneous action of at least four variables. Early elastic recoil of the blood vessel occurs in response to the mechanical dilation and is called the mechanical phase. Hemorrhage and formation of mural thrombi on denuded arterial intima is referred to as the thrombotic phase. Cell proliferation ensues leading to intimal lesion formation or the proliferative phase. Vascular remodeling results from chronic changes in the cellular content of the media, adventitia, and intima, often called the remodeling phase. Extracellular matrix proteins and matrix metalloproteinases play a major role in chronic vascular remodeling.

A number of therapies have attacked the four phases of restenosis. The scaffolding of arteries by stents has reduced the elastic recoil within arteries considerably (28). Several new antiplatelet agents, particularly the glycoprotein IIB/IIIA antagonists and aspirin, have satisfactorily addressed the potential thrombotic complications. However, until recently, cell proliferation has proceeded unabated without an effective therapy.

Molecular therapies that target the proliferative component of in-stent restenosis have played a major role in the revolutionary treatment of the disease. The concept of molecular targeting is based on the premise of site-specific gene or drug delivery. Although atherosclerosis is a diffuse process, the complications of the disease occur at focal sites in the circulation, particularly the coronary arteries. In order to effectively treat the local areas of plaque rupture, cell proliferation or thrombosis, as examples, balloon angioplasty catheters and stents can be used to dilate the artery and to deliver gene vectors or drugs directly to the disease site. This concept of site-specific gene delivery was used in the development of gene-transfer models of cell cycle inhibitors to prevent intimal lesion formation following coronary stenting (29–31). These studies demonstrated proof of principle for the concept of site-specific gene delivery. Further progress was hampered by the inability to deliver sufficient quantities of vectors into cells to achieve a persistent effect on cell proliferation. The benefit of these site-specific delivery studies, however, was that it created a new platform of technologies, which combined with stents, are now poised to prevent in-stent restenosis.

In-stent restenosis is now treated with the use of drug-eluting stents (Fig. 2) (32,33). These stents are coated with a polymer from which a drug elutes into the vessel wall following deployment of the stent. The approach is that of site-specific drug delivery, now using the deployed stent to deliver the drug precisely to the focal area of the artery with atherosclerotic complications. Two drug-eluting stents have been Food and Drug Administration (FDA) approved for use in the United States. Newer generation of drug-eluting stents are under development.

Taxol-eluting stents use the drug paclitaxel to prevent vascular cell proliferation following stent deployment. Taxol is the active component of paclitaxel (Fig. 3). This compound is a derivatized diterpenoid isolated from the bark of the Pacific yew, *Taxus*

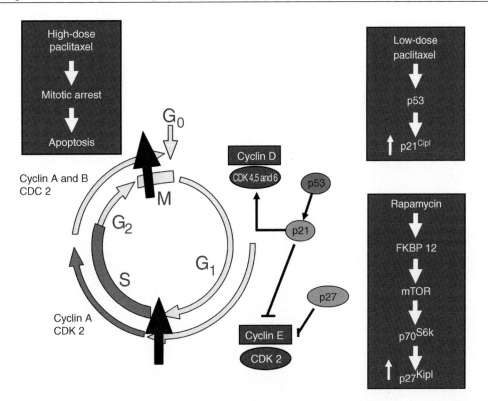

**Fig. 3.** Structure of sirolimus (left) and paclitaxel, along with their effects on the biology of the vasculature. (Please *see* insert for color version.)

*brevifolia (34).* The mechanism of action of Taxol is the induction of tubulin polymerization, which results in the formation of unstable microtubules *(35).* Microtubules are elements in the mitotic spindle that are required for cell division and maintenance of cell shape. Microtubules are also required for other cellular processes, such as motility, anchorage, transport between cellular organelles, extrasecretory processes, and intracellular signal transduction *(36).* The α- and β-tubulin heterodimers are protein subunits of microtubules and must be in equilibrium for cell division to occur. Taxol disrupts the equilibrium between the α- and β-tubulin heterodimers. Disruption of microtubule structure leads to altered function, including no cell division or motility (Figs. 3 and 4). Interesting, Taxol was initially developed as a therapeutic agent to prevent cell division in several malignancies, and perhaps is the most widely used in the treatment of breast cancer *(36).*

In a classic study, Taxol was shown to inhibit vascular smooth muscle cell proliferation and cell migration in tissue-culture studies. These observations were then extended to in vivo experiments in a rat carotid artery injury model in which administration of the drug prevented development of intimal hyperplasia following balloon angioplasty *(37).* Subsequent studies demonstrated the feasibility of administering Taxol from a polymer-coated stent, and these studies were quickly followed by a series of large animal investigators, which revealed the safety and efficacy of Taxol in these models of in-stent restenosis *(38).* Clinical trials quickly followed, which in turn, also demonstrated the safety and efficacy of Taxol to treat in-stent restenosis. Six Taxus clinical trials have been conducted:

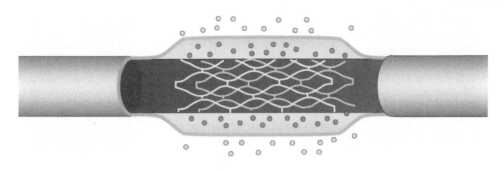

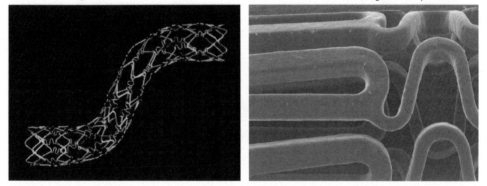

Balloon expandable stainless steel stent

Two polymers and sirolimus applied as a thin uniform coating at 5–10 µm thick

**Fig. 4.** Schematic representation of the mechanisms of action of paclitaxel and sirolimus in blocking the cell cycle and inhibiting cell proliferation.

1. Taxus I a randomized feasibility trial;
2. Taxus II an international efficacy trial;
3. Taxus III an in-stent restenosis feasibility trial;
4. Taxus IV a US pivotal trial;
5. Taxus V a US randomized *de novo* lesion pivotal expansion trial; and
6. Taxus IV a randomized international long-lesion trial *(39)*.

Results from the Taxus IV trial are representative of the efficacy trials: 9 mo target vessel revascularization (TVR) rate (primary end point) was reduced from 12% in the control group to 4.7% in the TAXUS Express stent group; and the TVR reduction was attributable to a lower TLR rate in the TAXUS Express group (3%) compared with the control group (11.3%). In addition, 9 mo MACE was reduced from 15% in the control group to 8.5% in the TAXUS Express group, and there were no significant differences in stent thrombosis between the groups. Taxol-eluting stents were approved by the FDA for treatment of in-stent restenosis in the United States in early 2004; this followed approval in Europe in 2003. Clinical investigations of Taxol-coated stents are underway. Taxol's antiproliferative properties and extraordinary success in clinical trials validate the concept of molecular targeting of a cell cycle inhibitor to treat in-stent restenosis.

A second antiproliferative drug has also been successfully used in the treatment of in-stent restenosis. Rapamycin is a natural product produced by fermentation from the bacteria *Streptomyces hygroscopicus* (Fig. 3). It was identified in 1964 from a soil sample taken from Easter Island by a Canadian medical research expedition *(40,41)*.

Rapamycin was initially developed as an antibiotic and antifungal agent, but it was found to have potent immunosuppressant activities, and its use to treat infectious disease was discontinued. Several decades later, its immunosuppressive properties were investigated and defined. Rapamycin binds a cytosolic receptor, FKBP12, leading to inhibition of a kinase called the target of rapamycin or TOR, elevation of nuclear p27[Kip1] protein, and G1 arrest *(42)*. FKBP12 is a FK506-binding protein and a member of the immunophilin family of proteins. FKBP12 has potent effects on T cells to inhibit T-cell proliferation, and accordingly, it was developed as an immunosuppressant to treat immune rejection following renal transplantation. The FDA approved rapamycin in 1999 for the treatment of acute rejection in renal transplantation.

Through the work of Andrew R. Marks, the molecular and cellular properties of rapamycin were examined with respect to vascular smooth muscle cells *(43–45)*. Dr. Mark's group found that rapamycin inhibits proliferation of vascular smooth muscle cells in tissue culture and in animal models *(43,46,47)* as well as disrupting smooth muscle cell migration *(44)*. His molecular and cellular studies suggest that rapamycin inhibits mitogen-dependent downregulation of p27[Kip1] and is one mechanism by which the drug inhibits vascular smooth muscle cell proliferation and migration (Figs. 3 and 4).

Clinical studies have also demonstrated the safety and efficacy of rapamycin-eluting stents for the treatment of in-stent restenosis. Phase III studies conducted in Europe, called RAVEL *(48)*, and in the United States, called SIRIUS *(49)*, have shown clinical efficacy that is similar to that of the TAXUS stent, with a restenosis rate of 0–9% in the CYPHER stent compared with 19–26% in the control group. The CYPHER stent was approved for the treatment of in-stent restenosis in the United States in 2003. The CYPHER and TAXUS stents are both in wide clinical use on multiple continents, again demonstrating the dramatic benefit of antiproliferative agents targeted to cell cycle proteins as an approach to treat in-stent restenosis.

## REFERENCES

1. Sherr CJ. Mammalian $G_1$ cyclins. Cell 1996;73:1059–1065.
2. Sherr CJ, Roberts JM. CDK inhibitors: positive and negative regulators of $G_1$-phase progression. Genes Dev 1999;13:1501–1512.
3. Nabel EG. CDKs, CKIs and tissue remodeling. Nat Rev Drug Discovery 2002;1:587–598.
4. Koff A, Ohtsuki M, Polyak K, et al. Negative regulation of G1 in mammalian cells: inhibition of cyclin E-dependent kinase by TGF-β. Science 1993;260:536–539.
5. Pietenpol J, Bohlander S, Sato Y, et al. Assignment of the human p27[Kip1] gene to 12p13 and its analysis in leukemias. Cancer Res 1995;55:1206–1210.
6. Zhang Y, Lin SC. Molecular characterization of the cyclin-dependent kinase inhibitor p27 promoter. Biochim Biophys Acta 1997;1353:307–317.
7. Ishida N, Kitagawa M, Hatakeyama S, et al. Phosphorylation at serine 10, a major phosphorylation site of p27[Kip1], increases its protein stability. J Biol Chem 2000;275:25,146–25,154.
8. Servant MJ, Coulombe P, Turgion B, et al. Differential regulation of p27[Kip1] expression by mitogenic and hypertrophic factors: involvement of transcriptional and posttranscriptional mechanisms. J Cell Biol 2000;148:543–556.
9. Hengst L, Reed SI. Inhibitors of the Cip/Kip family. Curr Top Microbiol Immunol 1996;227:25–41.
10. Malek NP, Sundberg H, McGrew S, et al. A mouse knock-in model exposes sequential proteolytic pathways that regulate p27[Kip1] in G1 and S phase. Nature 2001;413:323–327.
11. Boehm M, Yoshimoto T, Crook M, Nallamshetty S, True A, Nabel GJ, Nabel EG. A growth factor-dependent nuclear kinase phosphorylates p27[Kip1] and regulates cell cycle progression. EMBO J 2002;13:3390–3401.
12. Pagano M, Tam SW, Theodoras AM, et al. Role of the ubiquitin-proteasome pathway in regulating abundance of the cyclin-dependent kinase inhibitor p27. Science 1995;269:682–685.

13. Nakayama K, Ishida N, Shirane M, et al. Mice lacking p27[Kip1] display increased body size, multiple organ hyperplasia, retinal dysplasia, and pituitary tumors. Cell 1996;85:707–720.

14. Kiyokawa H, Kineman RD, Manova-Todorova KO, et al. Enhanced growth of mice lacking the cyclin-dependent kinase inhibitor function of p27[Kip1]. Cell 1996;85:721–732.

15. Fero ML, Rivkin M, Tasch M, et al. A syndrome of multiorgan hyperplasia with features of gigantism, tumorigenesis, and female sterility in p27[Kip1]-deficient mice. Cell 1996;85:733–744.

16. Boehm M, Olive M, True AL, et al. Bone marrow-derived immune cells regulate vascular disease through a p27[Kip1]–dependent mechanism. J Clin Invest 2004;114:419–426.

17. Brugarolas J, Chandrasekaran C, Gordon J, et al. Radiation-induced cell cycle arrest compromised by p21 deficiency. Nature 1995;377:552–557.

18. Deng C, Zhang P, Harper JW, et al. Mice lacking p21[CIP1/WAF1] undergo normal development but are defective in G1 checkpoint control. Cell 1995;82:675–684.

19. Waga S, Hannon G, Beach D, et al. The p21 inhibitor of cyclin-dependent kinases controls DNA replication by interaction with PCNA. Nature 1994;369:574–578.

20. Parker S, Eichele G, Zhang P, et al. p53-independent expression of p21Cip1 in muscle and other terminally differentiating cells. Science 1995;267:1024–1027.

21. Firpo E, Koff A, Solomon M, et al. Inactivation of a Cdk2 inhibitor during IL-2 induced proliferation of human T-lymphocytes. Mol Cell Biol 1994;14:4889–4901.

22. Nourse J, Firpo E, Flanagan M, et al. IL-2 mediated elimination of the p27[Kip1] cyclin-Cdk kinase inhibitor prevented by rapamycin. Nature 1994;372:570–573.

23. Gordon D, Reidy MA, Benditt EP, et al. Cell proliferation in human coronary arteries. Proc Natl Acad Sci USA 1990;87:4600–4604.

24. Tanner FC, Yang ZY, Duckers E, et al. Expression of cyclin-dependent kinase inhibitors in vascular disease. Circ Res 1998;82:396–403.

25. Tanner FC, Boehm M, Akyurek LM, et al. Differential effects of the cyclin-dependent kinase inhibitors p27[Kip1], p21[Cip1], and p16[Ink4] on vascular smooth muscle cell proliferation. Circulation 2000;101:2022–2025.

26. Yang ZY, Simari R, Perkins N, et al. Role of the p21 cyclin-dependent kinase inhibitor in limiting intimal cell proliferation in response to arterial injury. Proc Natl Acad Sci USA 1996;93:7905–7910.

27. Smith SC, Dove JT, Jacobs AK, et al. ACC/AHA guidelines of percutaneous coronary interventions (revision of the 1993 PTCA guidelines)–executive summary. A report of the American College of Cardiology/American Heart Association Task Force on Practice Guidelines. J Am Coll Cardiol 2001;37:2215–2238.

28. Sigwart U, Puel J, Mirkovitch V, et al. Intravascular stents to prevent occlusion and restenosis after transluminal angioplasty. N Engl J Med 1987;316:701–706.

29. Nabel EG, Plautz G, Boyce FM, Stanley JC, Nabel GJ. Recombinant gene expression in vivo within endothelial cells of the arterial wall. Science 1989;244:1342–1344.

30. Nabel EG, Plautz G, Nabel GJ. Site-specific gene expression in vivo by direct gene transfer into the arterial wall. Science 1990;249:1285–1288.

31. Ohno T, Gordon D, San H, et al. Gene therapy for vascular smooth muscle cell proliferation after arterial injury. Science 1994;265:781–784.

32. Sousa JE, Serruys PW, Costa MA. New frontiers in cardiology: Drug-eluting stents. Part I. Circulation 2003;107:2274–2279.

33. Sousa JE, Serruys PW, Costa MA. New frontiers in cardiology: Drug-eluting stents. Part II. Circulation 2003;107:2383–2389.

34. Wani MC, Taylor HL, Wall ME, et al. Plant antitumor agents. VI. The isolation and structure of taxol, a novel antileukemic and antitumor agent from Taxus brevifolia. J Am Chem Soc 1971;93:2325–2327.

35. Schiff PB, Horwitz SB. Taxol stabilizes microtubules in mouse fibroblast cells. Proc Natl Acad Sci USA 1980;77:1561–1565.

36. Rowinsky EK, Donehower RC. Paclitaxel (Taxol). N Engl J Med 1995;332:1004–1014.

37. Sollott SJ, Cheng L, Pauly RR, et al. Taxol inhibits neointimal smooth muscle cell accumulation after angioplasty in the rat. J Clin Invest 1995;95:1869–1876.

38. Heldman AW, Cheng L, Jenkins GM, et al. Paclitaxel stent coating inhibits neointimal hyperplasia at 4 weeks in a porcine model of coronary restenosis. Circulation 2001;103:2289–2295.

39. Boston Scientific, Inc. Taxus. Clinical trial summary. www.bostonscientific.com. Last accessed on January 17, 2007.

40. Vezina C, Kudelski A, Sehgal SN. Rapamycin (AY-22, 989), a new antifungal antibiotic. I: Toxoneme of the producing streptomycete and isolation of the active principle. J Antibiot (Tokyo) 1975;28: 721–726.
41. Sehgal SN, Baker H, Vezina C. Rapamycin (AY-22, 989), a new antifungal antibiotic. II: Fermentation, isolation and characterization. J Antibiot (Tokyo) 1995;28:721–726.
42. Marks AR. Cellular functions of the immunophilins. Physiol Rev 1996;76:631–649.
43. Marx SO, Jayaraman T, Go LO, et al. Rapamycin-FKBP inhibits cell cycle regulators of proliferation in vascular smooth muscle cells. Circ Res 1995;76:412–417.
44. Poon M, Marx SO, Gallo R, et al. Rapamycin inhibits smooth muscle cell migration. J Clin Invest 1996;98:2277–2283.
45. Bierer BE, Mattilia PS, Standaert R, et al. Two distinct signal transmission pathways in T lymphocytes are inhibited by complexes formed between an immunophilin and either FK506 or rapamycin. Proc Natl Acad Sci USA 1990;87:9231–9235.
46. Morris R, Cao W, Huang X, et al. Rapamycin (sirolimus) inhibits vascular smooth muscle cell DNA synthesis n vitro and suppresses narrowing in arterial allografts and in balloon-injured carotid arteries: evidence that rapamycin antagonizes growth factor action on immune ad nonimmune cells. Transplant Proc 1995;27:430–431.
47. Gallo R, Padurean A, Chesebro JH, et al. Inhibition of intimal thickening after balloon angioplasty n porcine coronary arteries by rapamycin. Circulation 1998;99:2164–2170.
48. Morice MC, Serruys PW, Sousa JE, et al. A randomized comparison of a sirolimus-eluting stent with a standard stent for coronary revascularization. N Engl J Med 2002;23:1773–1780.
49. Moses JW, Leon MB, Popma JJ, et al. Sirolimus-eluting stents versus standard stents in patients with stenosis in a native coronary artery. N Engl J Med 2003;349:1315–1323.
50. Boehm M, Nabel EG. Cell cycle and cell migration. Circulation 2001;103:2879–2881.

# 27 Local Gene and Cell Delivery Devices

## *Ravish Sachar, MD and Eric J. Topol, MD*

## INTRODUCTION

The concept of locally delivering therapy for the prevention of neointimal hyperplasia after arterial injury has received robust validation by the dramatic reduction in restenosis reported with the use of drug-eluting stents (DES) *(1,2)*. Interest in local delivery initially arose as a result of early studies in which therapeutic concentrations of systemically delivered antirestenotic therapies could only be achieved at the expense of unacceptable toxicity profiles. Locally, delivered therapies offer the distinct advantages of lower systemic side effects and toxicities, and enable a higher concentration of the therapeutic agent to be delivered where needed the most, at the site of intimal injury *(3–11)*. There has been considerable research over the last decade examining the possibility of genetic modulation for the prevention and treatment of restenosis. Local therapy is especially suited for delivering genetic material as systemic distribution can result in the permanent transfection of distant cells with long-term adverse consequences.

In order to successfully treat restenosis through genetic modulation of the cells responsible for neointimal hyperplasia, a three step approach is required:

1. The appropriate genes need to be targeted and/or the right gene products need to be translated to enable cell-cycle arrest or apoptosis of the cells responsible for restenosis;

From: *Contemporary Cardiology: Essentials of Restenosis: For the Interventional Cardiologist*
Edited by: H. J. Duckers, E. G. Nabel, and P. W. Serruys © Humana Press Inc., Totowa, NJ

2. The appropriate vectors, most commonly plasmids, liposomes, or viruses, must be utilized to maximize transfection efficiency and minimize the potential for systemic toxicity; and
3. The appropriate delivery device must be utilized. Failure of therapy can occur at any of the three steps in the treatment process.

The gene being targeted or gene product being introduced may be inappropriate, the genetic material may not reach the desired location in the arterial wall and, finally, even after successful delivery to the appropriate area in the arterial wall, the genetic material may be cleared before successful transfection of target cells. Identification of the gene targets to address and to prevent intimal hyperplasia, and utilization of the appropriate vector are topics that have been discussed elsewhere in this book. This chapter will focus on catheter-based devices used to percutaneously deliver local-gene therapy for the prevention of restenosis. Local delivery was initially validated as a form of treatment by the periadventitial application of polymeric matrices to suppress neointimal hyperplasia. Edelman and colleagues *(12)* applied polymeric matrices, containing heparin to rat carotid arteries, and demonstrated predictable pharmacokinetics and inhibition of smooth muscle cell (SMC) proliferation. Successful periadventitial application has also been reported using silicone polymers to deliver dexamethasone *(13)* and silicone capsules placed around the artery to deliver nuclear-targeted *lacZ (14)*. However, periadventitial application requires surgical isolation of the target vessel, and is therefore not a clinically viable strategy. Catheter-based devices are ideal for local gene delivery as they allow access to specific locations with transfection focused on the area of interest. There are number of characteristics, which must be taken into account in designing the ideal delivery device; the fact that none of the currently available devices possesses all these characteristics reflects the difficulty in designing the ideal device. These characteristics can be summarized as follows:

1. Deliverability of the device.
2. Minimal interaction of genetic material with blood.
3. Minimal vascular injury while delivering genetic material.
4. Rapid and efficient delivery of genetic material.
5. Simultaneous lesion treatment and therapeutic-agent delivery.
6. Minimal or no distribution of genetic material or vector systemically.
7. Homogeneous distribution of therapeutic agent to all three layers of the arterial wall.
8. Low cost.

Successful treatment of restenosis is contingent not only on delivery of genetic material to the appropriate location in the coronary artery, but also on the ability of the macromolecules to move across the internal elastic lamina (IEL) and target SMCs and fibroblasts in the media and adventitia. Transfection rates are the lowest with passive diffusion, and increase with strategies that employ active processes. Coronary arteries are lined with continuous endothelium, and molecules with an effective size of up to 6 nm can diffuse across the IEL. Larger molecules require a more active process to enable medial penetration *(15)*. As would be expected, lipophilic molecules tend to traverse the IEL and allow higher concentrations in the media than hydrophilic molecules *(16)*. Furthermore, once genetic material is introduced into the arterial wall, retention of the delivered material long enough to allow successful transfection is equally important. The pharmacokinetics governing clearance of locally delivered genetic material are dependent on several factors including permeability of the delivery vector and the proximity of the delivered material to the vasovasorum and intra-arterial lymphatics *(15,17)*.

Investigators have employed various markers to measure the depth of transmural penetration and transfection efficiency of therapeutic material in the arterial wall *(18,19)*. Horseradish peroxidase (HRP) has been found to be an ideal marker molecule for this purpose for a number of reasons. The peroxidase reaction of HRP in arterial tissue results in a characteristic brown stain, which can be readily identified under a light microscope *(20)*. Use of an image-processing system further allows accurate determination of spatial concentration. This technique preserves the structural integrity of cellular and extracellular tissue, enabling high-resolution localization of delivered material *(21)*.

Studies using HRP have shown that after local delivery to uninjured, nonatherosclerotic vessels, macromolecules and genetic material readily concentrate in the intima, but the IEL provides a strong barrier to further entry of the macromolecules into the media and adventitia *(20,22)*. As would be expected, the concentration of the macromolecules rapidly decreases radially as a function of the distance from the intima (Fig. 1) *(21)*. The transport of macromolecules through the arterial wall is a highly regulated process, and in addition to the passive resistance provided by the IEL to diffusion, there appear to be active processes that govern the movement of macromolecules in arterial tissue. Two other factors appear to be crucial in determining the permeability of genetic material into the arterial wall: endothelial cell injury and the presence of atherosclerosis.

Experimentally induced endothelial injury by lipopolysaccharide injection or by endotoxin increases the permeability of the IEL as compared with uninjured vessels (Fig. 2) *(23,24)*. Rangaswamy and colleagues *(25)* found a four- to fivefold increase in the HRP permeability coefficient in endothelium injured by oxidized low-density lipoprotein as compared with uninjured endothelium. Similarly, mechanical disruption by balloon angioplasty appears to increase IEL permeability enough to facilitate adenoviral and liposomal vector entry into the media and adventitia to allow successful transfection of SMCs *(26,27)*. Thus, endothelial disruption at the time of delivery is a double-edged sword. Although the risk of restenosis owing to injury is increased, the delivery of genetic material to the media and adventitia is enhanced.

The presence of atherosclerosis, on the other hand, appears to prevent the movement of macromolecules into the media, and thereby attenuates transfection efficiency. It has been hypothesized that the increased extracellular matrix and calcification in atherosclerotic arteries act as physical barriers to the diffusion of gene vectors deep into the media. This has been demonstrated by an increase in transfection seen in histological specimens adjacent to areas of plaque rupture and fissure after balloon angioplasty, but not in deeper areas of the media or in areas with an intact IEL and without evidence of plaque rupture *(28,29)*. Furthermore, Simari et al. *(28)* reported a seven-fold increase in transfection rates of medial SMCs in human pathological atherosclerotic specimens after treatment with collagenase and elastase, suggesting the extracellular matrix may have been retarding transfection.

Once genetic material has reached the appropriate location in the arterial wall, ensuring its presence there long enough to result in successful transfection poses a further challenge. Increased density of the vasovasorum in atherosclerotic vessels may reduce transfection rates by accelerating wash out of genetic material from the adventitia *(30)*. Sustained delivery systems have been proposed as they may improve transfection efficiency by providing prolonged exposure and higher concentration of genetic material to target cells *(10,11)*. Controlled release matrices employ a strategy of embedding drug or genetic material in microparticles, which are delivered to the target lesion. Hydrolysis of these microparticle matrices hypothetically results in the slow release of

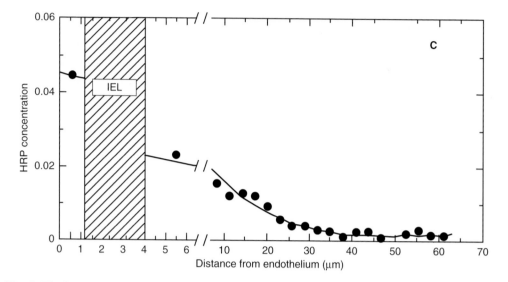

**Fig. 1.** The internal elastic lamina acts as a strong barrier to the entry of horseradish peroxidase into the media and adventitia. The concentration of horseradish peroxidase rapidly decreases radially as a function of the distance from the intima. (Reproduced with permission [21].)

encapsulated genetic material into the arterial wall. Guzman and colleagues (31) incorporated dexamethasone into poly-DL-lactide-co-glycolide (PLGA) nanoparticles and labeled them with rhodamine B as a fluorescent marker before delivery. Presence of the particles was demonstrated in all three arterial wall layers at 3 h with persistence for up to 14 d after a single short intraluminal delivery. Banai et al. (32) delivered nanoparticles, containing platelet-derived growth factor receptor tyrosine kinase blocker after balloon-induced injury, and demonstrated an inhibitory effect on the migration and proliferation of SMCs and a corresponding reduction intimal hyperplasia. Other investigators have similarly used PLGA nanoparticles to deliver drugs and antisense oligonucleotides to the arterial wall and demonstrated sustained presence of the nanoparticles in all three layers of the arterial wall (33,34). In addition to being hydrolyzed in the extracellular matrix, thereby releasing the entrapped material outside the target cells, the intracellular uptake of nanoparticles has recently been described (35,36). This can enable the release of encapsulated material directly into the cytosol, and may prove useful when the genetic material being delivered is in the form of naked plasmids, which do not have an inherent adenovirus type infective mechanism to cross the cellular membrane.

## LOCAL DELIVERY DEVICES

Catheter-based local delivery devices can broadly be classified into four categories (Table 1). The first generation devices, the prototype of which is the double balloon catheter, relied on simple diffusion for the transmural movement of therapeutic agent and are, in general, the least efficient. The second generation devices employed convection as the means of transmural penetration, and improved transfection rates. The Infiltrator® catheter (Boston Scientific, Nantick, MA) and Iontophoretic balloon (CorTrak Medical, St. Paul, MN) are third generation mechanical devices that go beyond convection to deliver genetic material by novel mechanisms. The final category stents represent an intuitive platform for the local delivery of genetic material.

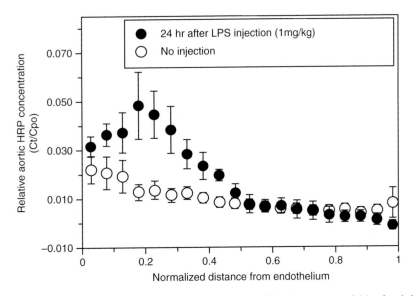

**Fig. 2.** Increased transmural penetration of horseradish peroxidase in rats seen 24 h after injection of 1 mg/kg of lipopolysaccharide. (Reproduced with permission [23].)

## DOUBLE BALLOON CATHETER

The double-balloon local delivery device consists of two sequential compliant urethane balloons at the distal end of a 3 French (Fr) polyethylene catheter. The distance between the balloons is 20 mm, and there are two infusion ports arising from the shaft of the catheter, one near the proximal balloon and one near the distal balloon (Fig. 3). Once the device is advanced to the area of interest, the balloons are simultaneously inflated distal and proximal to the treatment site, creating an isolated treatment compartment. After inflation of both balloons to approx 3 atm the compartment between the balloons is evacuated, followed by drug or genetic material administration through the infusion ports. The infusate is allowed to diffuse into the intima over a period of time. Theoretically, the drug diffuses from the intima and into the media, and is subsequently distributed into the adventitia through the vasovasorum.

This device has several limitations. The mechanism of delivery of genetic material into the vascular wall is diffusion, which is an inefficient means of delivery, and results in low-transfection rates of less than 1%. Although infusion pressures of 0.2 atm do not appear to result in endothelial damage, infusion pressures of more than 0.6 atm do result in endothelial trauma (37). Even low pressure inflation of the urethane balloons can injure the adjacent vascular endothelium, increasing the risk of restenosis. Additionally, diffusion of genetic material and drugs is a passive process, which can require prolonged dwell times, increasing the risk of symptomatic myocardial ischemia. Finally, the presence of side-branches, and leakage of infusate along the sides of the distal balloon can result in unintended systemic delivery of genetic material and transfection of endothelium distant from the treatment area. This device was first described by Wolinski, (37) and has since been used to locally deliver genetic material in animal models (38–42).

Table 1
Devices for Percutaneous Local Gene Delivery

| Device category | Device |
| --- | --- |
| Diffusion | Double balloon catheter |
| | Disptach catheter |
| Convective | Porous balloon |
| | Microporous balloon |
| | Channeled balloon |
| | InfusaSleeve catheter |
| | Hydrogel balloon |
| Facilitated diffusion | Ionotophoresis balloon |
| | Infiltrator catheter |
| Stents | Biodegradable polymer stents |
| | Polymer coated metallic stents |
| | Cell coated stents |

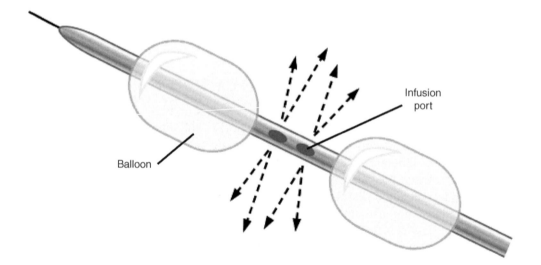

**Fig. 3.** The double-balloon local delivery device consists of two sequential compliant urethane balloons at the distal end of a 3 French polyethylene catheter. The distance between the balloons is 20 mm. After inflation of both balloons to approx 3 atm the compartment between the balloons is evacuated, followed by drug or genetic material administration through the infusion ports.

## DISPTACH™ CATHETER

In order to circumvent problems of prolonged ischemia, newer devices have been designed to allow continuous perfusion during drug or gene delivery. One such device is the Food Drug Administration approved Disptach catheter (Boston Scientific, Nantick, MA). This device consists of a 4.3 Fr over-the-wire shaft with a 20 mm polyolefin copolymer helical inflation balloon at its distal tip (Fig. 4). The helical balloon is wrapped around a urethane sheath. Inflation of the balloon to approx 8 atm to reach arterial diameter results in the creation of an inner lumen, allowing continuous distal blood flow. Infusate is then delivered through a separate sheath and exits the catheter through infusion openings,

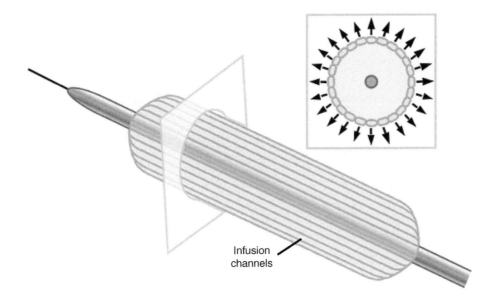

**Fig. 8.** The channeled balloon catheter. The lumen for infusate delivery leads to an a series of 24 distinct channels on the outer surface of the angioplasty balloon, each with several 100-μm holes through which infusate is delivered directly against the arterial wall.

compressed against the arterial wall. Infusate can then be delivered through a separate port directly against the vascular wall through infusion holes at the distal tip of the sheath (Fig. 9). Using HRP as a marker, it has been determined that inflating the underlying angioplasty balloon to 6 atm before infusion is optimal for delivery of infusate into the arterial media *(69)*. Although the striking advantage of this system is that it can be used with standard angioplasty equipment, a small randomized study has generated some caution. Tanguay and colleagues *(70)* investigated the efficacy of local heparin administration using the infusion sleeve catheter in dissected lesions after angioplasty and before bailout stenting. Local delivery of heparin with the infusion sleeve was associated with a nonsignificant increase in death, myocardial infarction, and coronary artery bypass surgery at 30 d (21% vs 0%, $p = 0.18$) and myocardial infarction at 6 mo (27% vs 10%, $p = 0.4$). Nevertheless, successful medial transfection of SMCs with *firefly luciferase* using a recombinant adenoviral vector has been reported with this device *(71)*.

## HYDRO-GEL ANGIOPLASTY BALLOON

The hydrogel angioplasty balloon represents an intuitive means for simultaneous lesion dilation and transmural delivery of therapeutic drugs or genes. A polyethylene angioplasty balloon is coated with the Hydro-Gel polymer (Boston Scientific, Nantick, MA) consisting of covalently linked polyacrylic-acid chains tethered to the balloon surface (Fig. 10). The Hydro-Gel polymer, when exposed to aqueous solution, absorbs the solution and swells radially outwards from the surface of the balloon. Any therapeutic materials in the solution are also absorbed into the Hydro-Gel. The balloon is then delivered to the desired location, and inflated. Compression of the balloon and Hydro-Gel against the arterial wall on inflation dilates the lesion and simultaneously reduces

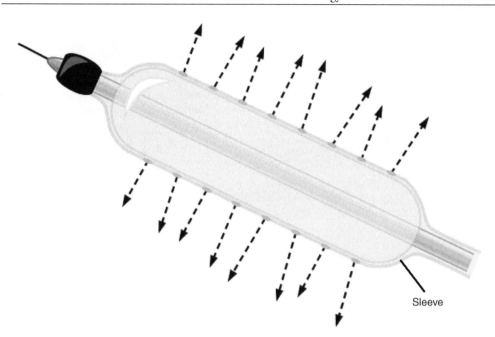

**Fig. 9.** The InfusaSleeve catheter. After advancing a standard angioplasty balloon over a guide wire to the lesion site, a retractable sheath is advanced over the balloon and aligned with the distal tip of the balloon. The sheath is equipped with four delivery lumens, each with nine 40-μm holes distally. After inflation of the angioplasty balloon, the delivery lumens are compressed against the arterial wall. Infusate can then be delivered through a separate port directly against the vascular wall through infusion holes at the distal tip of the sheath.

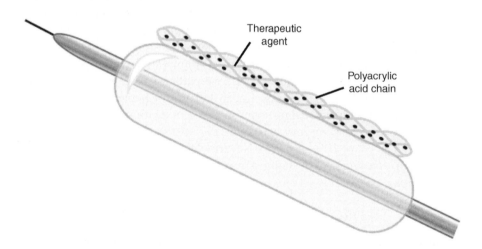

**Fig. 10.** The hydrogel balloon. A standard angioplasty balloon is coated with Hydro-Gel, which can absorb the therapeutic agent. When the balloon is expanded against the arterial wall, the therapeutic agent delivered transmurally.

the thickness of the Hydro-Gel, thereby increasing the concentration of the therapeutic agent in the Hydro-Gel and facilitating transmural diffusion. As would be expected, the efficiency of transfection is directly correlated with the duration and pressure of balloon inflation. High-pressure inflation not only compresses the Hydro-Gel more, but also serves to injure the IEL, thereby allowing deeper diffusion into the media and adventitia *(72)*. The biggest disadvantage to this system is the potential rapid wash-out of therapeutic agent from the hydrogel on exposure to blood in the guiding catheter and the artery *(73)*. Although rapid delivery may minimize the extent of loss, complex vascular anatomy may prohibit rapid deployment and thereby attenuate the efficacy of the device. Another potential disadvantage is that the absolute amount of material that can be delivered is small as compared with other delivery devices.

The hydrogel angioplasty balloon was first used to deliver intramural heparin in porcine peripheral arteries *(74)*, and has since been used to successfully deliver genetic material to the arterial wall *(75–77)*. Steg et al. *(77)* compared delivery of recombinant adenovirus to rabbit iliac arteries with the double balloon catheter vs the hydrogel angioplasty balloon, and found higher transfection rates with the hydrogel balloon (9.6% vs 2.2%, $p = 0.0001$). Furthermore, although transfection with the double balloon catheter was limited to the endothelial layer, the hydrogel balloon successfully transfected medial SMCs, supporting the contention that disruption of the IEL augments deeper transmural diffusion of therapeutic agent. Isner and colleagues *(78)* used the hydrogel angioplasty balloon to deliver naked plasmid DNA encoding for vascular endothelial growth factor to the arterial circulation of a patient with an ischemic lower extremity and subsequently documented angiogenesis using magnetic resonance angiography.

## INFILTRATOR CATHETER

All the devices described so far deliver therapeutic agent to the luminal side of the IEL and therefore depend on diffusion or convection for the transport of infusate into the arterial wall. As previously discussed, the IEL can act as a significant barrier to the movement of macromolecules from the intimal layer into the media and adventitia. The Infiltrator catheter has the unique advantage of being able to deliver genetic material directly into the arterial wall, and thereby bypass the IEL. The catheter consists of a 4.2 Fr, 132 cm, over-the-wire shaft with a 15 mm noncompliant balloon at the distal end (Fig. 11A,B). Although the rated burst pressure of the balloon is 8 atm, the nominal inflation pressure is 4 atm, and it is recommended that the balloon not be inflated to more than 6 atm. The device requires an 8 Fr sheath for delivery. There are two independent proximal ports on the device, one for balloon inflation and one for infusate delivery. The distal balloon has three equidistantly positioned longitudinal metallic strips at 120° to each other, and each has seven hair-sized injector ports for infusate delivery. All three metallic strips are connected to the same delivery lumen. When the balloon is in its deflated position, the injector ports are in a retracted state. On balloon inflation, the injector ports radially extend outwards and pierce the IEL, enabling the delivery of accurate quantities of infusate directly into the media *(79)*. The recommended delivery volume is 400 µL and larger delivery volumes carry the risk of hydraulic dissection. Although infusate delivery can be performed by hand injection, automatic injectors have been developed to ensure constant pressure delivery.

The Infiltrator catheter was first used in humans to deliver low-molecular weight heparin (LMWH) to patients after balloon angioplasty. Ten of seventeen patients required stent placement after angioplasty, but this decision was not influenced by the use of the Infiltrator catheter. All patients had a clinically uneventful course without any cases of cardiac enzyme elevation *(80)*. Since then, the catheter has been used successfully in the porcine balloon injury model to deliver several genes using a recombinant adenovirus

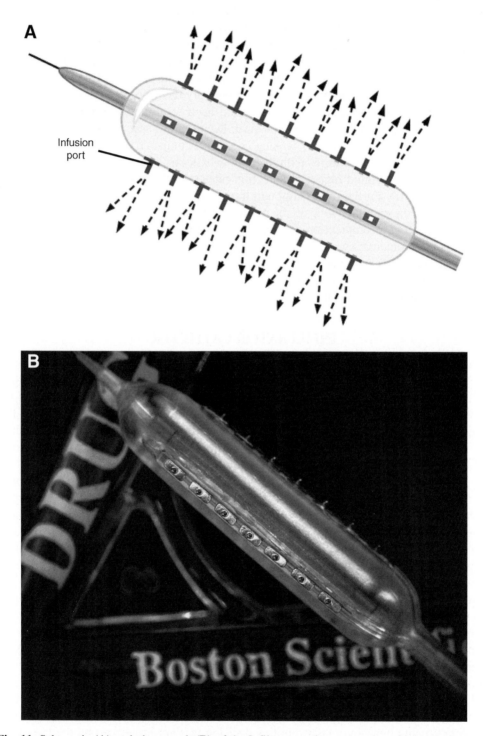

**Fig. 11.** Schematic **(A)** and photograph **(B)** of the Infiltrator catheter. A series of injection ports on the surface of a balloon pierce through the internal elastic lamina on balloon inflation and allow delivery of genetic material directly into the media. Figure 4B reproduced with permission from Boston Scientific.

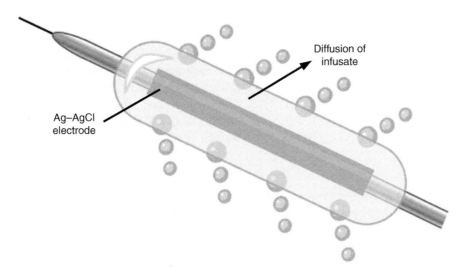

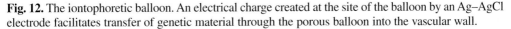

**Fig. 12.** The iontophoretic balloon. An electrical charge created at the site of the balloon by an Ag–AgCl electrode facilitates transfer of genetic material through the porous balloon into the vascular wall.

vector, including *endothelial nitric oxide synthase (81,82), plasminogen activator inhibitor-1 (83), C-type natriuretic peptide (84),* and *transforming growth factor β-1 (85).* The majority of these studies reported significant reductions in neointimal hyperplasia in treated animals. Histological analyses have shown that the injector ports result in minimal or no damage to the endothelium, and there appears to be homogeneous distribution of genetic material throughout the media and adventitia, with high-transfection rates. The device has also been used to deliver *endothelial nitric oxide synthase (82)* and *c-myc* antisense oligomers after balloon injury and before stent implantation *(86),* has been reported to reduce in-stent neointimal hyperplasia in porcine coronary arteries.

## IONTOPHORETIC BALLOON

One of the limitations of systems that use diffusion or convection for delivery of genetic material to the arterial wall is the low-transfection rate. Attempts to overcome this problem by delivering higher doses or by prolonging delivery times have been hampered by the side effects of larger systemic distribution of genetic material and ischemia owing to prolonged vessel occlusion, respectively. In order to overcome this problem, the Iontophoretic balloon was developed by CorTrak Medical. Iontophoresis refers to the use of electrical currents to facilitate the movement of charged particles across tissues and membranes. The device consists of a 7 Fr over-the-wire catheter shaft with a distal balloon, which is porous in its midportion and impermeable at its proximal and distal portions. An electrical charge is created at the site of the balloon by an Ag-AgCl electrode wrapped around the shaft of the catheter under the balloon (Fig. 12). Once a power source is attached, the balloon acts as the cathode, and an adhesive electrode attached to the patients skin serves as the anode, creating a constant-current density of approx 4–5 mA/cm$^2$ After low-pressure balloon inflation at the site of delivery at 1–2 atm, the drug or genetic material to be delivered is circulated through the balloon at 1–2 mL/min. using a pump for approx 5 min. The electrical charge at the site of the balloon facilitates transfer of drug or genetic material through the porous balloon into the vascular wall.

The Iontophoretic Balloon was first used to deliver [125]I-hirudin to porcine carotid arteries and resulted in 80-fold higher levels of drug in the vascular was as compared with passive diffusion (87). There was minimal damage to the endothelium at the delivery site with less than 10% denudation of the endothelium. This delivery system has subsequently been used to successfully deliver heparin (88) and antisense oligonucleotides (89) to porcine coronary arteries with high levels of distribution in the vascular wall as compared with passive diffusion. A potential disadvantage of this system; however, is that only negatively charged particles can be successfully delivered.

## STENTS

The concept of using stents as a platform for locally delivering therapeutic agent to the arterial wall has been validated by the dramatic success of DES. Although the use of stents for locally delivering of genes and cells may be viewed as a logical extension of the knowledge gained in the development of DES, the need for a genetic approach for the treatment of restenosis has come into question, especially on a stent platform. Nevertheless, there are data validating the use of stents as a potential delivery vehicle for genetic material as well as for genetically modified cells. Whether or not such a use for stents will find a place in clinical cardiology remains to be seen.

As compared with other gene delivery devices, stents offer several advantages. The lack of an infusate reduces the possibility of systemic spread of genetic material and potentially dangerous viral vectors. Furthermore, stents allow continuous exposure of the arterial wall to the therapeutic agent, with the theoretical benefit of higher transfection rates. In order to take advantage of the prolonged exposure time; however, the vector must demonstrate long-term biostability. Stents carry the disadvantages of smaller delivery volumes, and concentrations are limited by the physical properties of the polymer used. Furthermore, as only approx 10% of the arterial wall is in contact with the stent, inhomogeneous distribution of genetic material is a concern.

Gene delivery from polymer-coated stents can be accomplished by incorporating genetic material into a biostable polymer, biodegradable polymer, or through biodegradable stents made up of polymers with embedded genetic material. All three techniques have been described and successful gene transfer and expression have been demonstrated in animal models (90–92). The successful use of both recombinant adenovirus and naked plasmids as vectors has been described (90–92).

Klugherz and colleagues (90) incorporated plasmids encoding for green fluorescent protein into PLGA (a biodegradable polymer) coated stainless steel stents and demonstrated transfection of medial SMCs. The efficiency of transfection; however, was only 1%. In order to improve transfection efficiency, recombinant adenovirus encoding for green fluorescent protein was tethered to stainless steel stents using antiviral antibody, and transfection was rates of 5.9% were reported in porcine coronary arteries (91). Perlstein and colleagues (92) added denatured collagen to the polymer coating in order to control the rate of DNA release, and reported a dramatically higher 10.4% transfection rate. Although these findings are intriguing, they have not been reproduced by other investigators, and the mechanisms of higher transfection rates using denatured collagen are not well understood. A potential drawback of this technique is that biodegradable polymers have been reported to contribute to local inflammation and increased rates of restenosis as compared with nondegradable polymers (93,94). Further data are needed to verify this association.

The use of a polyurethane a nondegradable polymer for plasmid DNA delivery through a stainless steel stent was described recently by Takahashi et al. *(95)*. Transfection levels, while low, were found to be correlated with the concentration of plasmid DNA embedded in the stent polymer. Polymerase chain reaction analysis confirmed localized transfection only, with no evidence of spread to adjacent vascular tissue, lung, liver, and spleen. Additionally, transfection was noted not only in medial SMCs, but also in marcrophages. Ye and colleagues *(96)* investigated the use of bioresorbable microporous stents made up of poly-L-lactic acid/poly-epsilon-caprolactone (PLLA/PCL) to deliver recombinant adenovirus and demonstrated elution of infective virus from the stent in vitro, and successful in vivo transfection of the β-*Gal receptor* gene into rabbit carotid arteries. More research is needed to further define the role of bioresorbable stents as local delivery vehicles.

Some investigators have proposed coating stents with genetically modified cells, which secrete proteins designed to inhibit restenosis *(97,98)*. Dichek et al. *(97)* genetically modified sheep endothelial cells by transfecting them with adenovirus encoding human tissue-type plasminogen activator (t-PA). These cells were then used to seed stainless steel stents and allowed to grow until the stents were completely covered. After in vitro expansion of these stents, secretion of human t-PA from the endothelial cells was confirmed. This concept has yet to be studied in animal models, and the future application of this technology in the human clinical arena remains doubtful.

## COMPARISONS OF LOCAL DELIVERY DEVICES

There have been no comprehensive comparisons of all available local delivery devices utilizing standardized animal models, vectors, and genetic markers. However, there have been a few small studies, which have compared up with four devices. The results are, in general, consistent with those one would expect based on device mechanics (Table 2). One of the first comparisons performed was between the porous and microporous balloon designs, and confirmed that the slower delivery of infusate with the latter attenuated the endothelial damage associated with the former *(55)*. Willard and colleagues compared transfection rates in rabbit common carotid arteries using a recombinant adenovirus vector, encoding for *firefly luciferase* or β-*galactosidase*, delivered by one of four techniques:

1. Instilling vector in the artery after direct surgical isolation;
2. Through the double balloon catheter;
3. The porous catheter; or
4. The hydrogel angioplasty balloon.

Although transfection rates were higher with the surgical dwell technique and the double balloon catheter, the transfection was concentrated predominantly in the intima. They reported the highest transfection rates in the media using the hydrogel balloon and the porous catheter, but endothelial injury was the most pronounced with the porous catheter. The depth of transfection was correlated with the degree of IEL disruption *(99)*. This finding has been confirmed by other investigators *(71,100)*. As previously mentioned, IEL injury, although in itself a contributor to the restenotic process, enables transfection of the cells responsible for the initiation and propagation of restenosis, and may be a necessary precursor. The porous balloon does; however, in part owing to the larger volume and velocity of infusate delivery, result in a higher amount of systemic delivery of therapeutic agent as compared with other devices, such as the hydrogel balloon *(101)*.

Table 2
Studies Comparing Local Delivery Devices

| Authors | Animal model | Devices compared | Vector/marker used | Comments |
|---------|-------------|------------------|-------------------|----------|
| Lambert et al. (55) | Porcine coronary artery | 1. Porous balloon<br>2. Microporous balloon | Methylene blue | • Minimal endothelial trauma with the microporous balloon as compared with the porous balloon |
| Willard et al. (99) | New Zealand white rabbit common carotid artery and internal jugular vein | 1. Surgical isolation and dwell<br>2. Double balloon catheter<br>3. Porous balloon<br>4. Hydrogel balloon | Recombinant adenovirus encoding firefly luciferase and β-galactosidase | • Dwell and double balloon catheters transfected primarily intimal cells<br>• The porous and hydrogel catheters transfected primarily medial cells<br>• Endothelial injury was maximal with the porous balloon |
| Alfke et al. (100) | Postmortem porcine carotid artery | 1. Microporous balloon<br>2. Hydrogel balloon<br>3. Dispatch catheter | Biotin | • Postmortem study<br>• Hydrogel balloon delivered biotin mainly to the intimal layer<br>• The microporous balloon and Dispatch catheter delivered biotin deeper into the media |
| Varenne et al. (71) | Porcine coronary artery<br><br>3. InfusaSleeve catheter | 1. Remedy balloon (channeled)<br>2. Crescendo balloon (microporous)<br><br>4. Infiltrator catheter | Recombinant adenovirus encoding firefly luciferase | • The Infiltrator, Crescendo, and InfusaSleeve catheters had higher transfection rates than the remedy balloon<br>• Degree of intimal injury was positively correlated with higher transfection rates |

| Reference | Model | Catheter/Balloon | Agent | Findings |
|---|---|---|---|---|
| Dick et al. (*101*) | Porcine Iliac artery | 1. Porous balloon<br>2. Hydrogel balloon | HRP | • Delivery efficiency for porous balloon vs hydrogel balloon was 0.3% vs 1.7%<br>• Higher systemic levels of HRP with the porous balloon |
| Mitchel et al. (*102*) | Porcine coronary artery | 1. Hydrogel balloon<br>2. Infiltrator catheter | Heparin | • Delivery efficiency for Infiltrator catheter vs hydrogel balloon was 4.5% vs 0.8%<br>• No excessive vessel wall trauma with the Infiltrator catheter |
| Panyam et al. (*48*) | Porcine coronary artery | 1. Dispatch catheter<br>2. Infiltrator catheter | Nanoparticles with fluorescent marker | • Delivery to the media and adventitia was higher with the Dispatch catheter<br>• The infusion pores of the Infiltrator catheter did not result in excessive endothelial damage as assessed by transmission electron microscopy |

437

The Infiltrator catheter, by virtue of its design, bypasses the IEL and allows direct delivery of therapeutic agent directly into the media. Head to head comparisons of the Infiltrator catheter with the hydrogel balloon and the channeled balloon have confirmed the benefit of such a strategy *(71,102)*, although one study found the Disptach catheter enabled higher delivery of nanoparticles into the media and adventitia *(48)*. The injector ports of the Infiltrator catheter do not appear to result in excessive endothelial damage as compared with other local delivery devices *(48,102)*.

## CONCLUSION

There have been dramatic advances in the ability to locally deliver therapeutic material to the vascular wall during the last 15 yr. Devices, such as the double balloon catheter, employing simple diffusion have led to second generation convective devices, such as the porous, microporous, and channeled balloons, the hydrogel balloon, and the InfusaSleeve catheter. More recently, complex delivery systems, such as the Dispatch™ catheter, Infiltrator catheter, and Iontophoretic balloon have further increased the ability to successfully deliver therapeutic material to the media and adventitia. As moving forward, the challenge now is to find the ideal target gene or gene product, the most efficient vector, and combine these with the most suitable local delivery device.

The field of interventional cardiology; however, has been revolutionalized by the advent of DES. Once the Achilles heel of percutaneous interventions, restenosis, and target lesion -revascularization rates have now been dramatically reduced across all patient and lesion subsets. It is conceivable and likely that as newer generations of DES continue to address deliverability issues and further reduce restenosis rates, research addressing local gene therapy for restenosis is further warranted. Whether or not genetic modulation of intimal-medial SMCs, fibroblasts, and macrophages for preventing and treating restenosis ultimately finds a place in everyday clinical cardiology remains to be seen. It has been suggested that in the future, gene therapy for restenosis may eliminate the need for stents after angioplasty *(3)*. At the current time; however, the promise of gene therapy for restenosis remains to be realized.

## REFERENCES

1. Morice MC, Serruys PW, Sousa JE, et al. A randomized comparison of a sirolimus-eluting stent with a standard stent for coronary revascularization. N Engl J Med 2002;346:1773–1780.
2. Stone GW, Ellis SG, Cox DA, et al. A polymer-based, paclitaxel-eluting stent in patients with coronary artery disease. N Engl J Med 2004;350:221–231.
3. Dzau VJ. Predicting the future of human gene therapy for cardiovascular diseases: what will the management of coronary artery disease be like in 2005 and 2010? Am J Cardiol 2003;92:32N–35N.
4. Baek S, March KL. Gene therapy for restenosis: getting nearer the heart of the matter. Circ Res 1998;82:295–305.
5. Reis ED, Skladany M. Update on gene therapy for intimal hyperplasia. Bratisl Lek Listy 1999;100:417–421.
6. Riessen R, Isner JM. Prospects for site-specific delivery of pharmacologic and molecular therapies. J Am Coll Cardiol 1994;23:1234–1244.
7. Brieger D, Topol E. Local drug delivery systems and prevention of restenosis. Cardiovasc Res 1997;35:405–413.
8. Rutanen J, Markkanen J, Yla-Herttuala S. Gene therapy for restenosis: current status. Drugs 2002;62:1575–1585.
9. Ettenson DS, Edelman ER. Local drug delivery: an emerging approach in the treatment of restenosis. Vasc Med 2000;5:97–102.

10. Sriram V, Patterson C. Cell cycle in vasculoproliferative diseases: potential interventions and routes of delivery. Circulation 2001;103:2414–2419.

11. Lincoff AM, Topol EJ, Ellis SG. Local drug delivery for the prevention of restenosis. Fact, fancy, and future. Circulation 1994;90:2070–2084.

12. Edelman ER, Adams DH, Karnovsky MJ. Effect of controlled adventitial heparin delivery on smooth muscle cell proliferation following endothelial injury. Proc Natl Acad Sci USA 1990;87:3773–3777.

13. Villa AE, Guzman LA, Chen W, Golomb G, Levy RJ, Topol EJ. Local delivery of dexamethasone for prevention of neointimal proliferation in a rat model of balloon angioplasty. J Clin Invest 1994; 93:1243–1249.

14. Hiltunen MO, Turunen MP, Turunen AM, et al. Biodistribution of adenoviral vector to nontarget tissues after local in vivo gene transfer to arterial wall using intravascular and periadventitial gene delivery methods. Faseb J 2000;14:2230–2236.

15. Opanasopit P, Nishikawa M, Hashida M. Factors affecting drug and gene delivery: effects of interaction with blood components. Crit Rev Ther Drug Carrier Syst 2002;19:191–233.

16. Baumbach A, Herdeg C, Kluge M, et al. Local drug delivery: impact of pressure, substance characteristics, and stenting on drug transfer into the arterial wall. Catheter Cardiovasc Interv 1999; 47:102–106.

17. Chorny M, Fishbein I, Golomb G. Drug delivery systems for the treatment of restenosis. Crit Rev Ther Drug Carrier Syst 2000;17:249–284.

18. Bell FP, Gallus AS, Schwartz CJ. Focal and regional patterns of uptake and the transmural distribution of 131-I-fibrinogen in the pig aorta in vivo. Exp Mol Pathol 1974;20:281–292.

19. Duncan LE, Jr., Cornfield J, Buck K. The effect of blood pressure on the passage of labeled plasma albumin into canine aortic wall. J Clin Invest 1962;41:1537–1545.

20. Penn MS, Koelle MR, Schwartz SM, Chisolm GM. Visualization and quantification of transmural concentration profiles of macromolecules across the arterial wall. Circ Res 1990;67:11–22.

21. Penn MS, Saidel GM, Chisolm GM. Relative significance of endothelium and internal elastic lamina in regulating the entry of macromolecules into arteries in vivo. Circ Res 1994;74:74–82.

22. Rome JJ, Shayani V, Flugelman MY, et al. Anatomic barriers influence the distribution of in vivo gene transfer into the arterial wall. Modeling with microscopic tracer particles and verification with a recombinant adenoviral vector. Arterioscler Thromb 1994;14:148–161.

23. Penn MS, Chisolm GM. Relation between lipopolysaccharide-induced endothelial cell injury and entry of macromolecules into the rat aorta in vivo. Circ Res 1991;68:1259–1269.

24. Penn MS, Saidel GM, Chisolm GM. Vascular injury by endotoxin: changes in macromolecular transport parameters in rat aortas in vivo. Am J Physiol 1992;262:H1563–H571.

25. Rangaswamy S, Penn MS, Saidel GM, Chisolm GM. Exogenous oxidized low-density lipoprotein injures and alters the barrier function of endothelium in rats in vivo. Circ Res 1997;80:37–44.

26. Todaka T, Yokoyama C, Yanamoto H, et al. Gene transfer of human prostacyclin synthase prevents neointimal formation after carotid balloon injury in rats. Stroke 1999;30:419–426.

27. Yonemitsu Y, Kaneda Y, Tanaka S, et al. Transfer of wild-type p53 gene effectively inhibits vascular smooth muscle cell proliferation in vitro and in vivo. Circ Res 1998;82:147–156.

28. Simari RD, San H, Rekhter M, et al. Regulation of cellular proliferation and intimal formation following balloon injury in atherosclerotic rabbit arteries. J Clin Invest 1996;98:225–235.

29. Rekhter MD, Simari RD, Work CW, Nabel GJ, Nabel EG, Gordon D. Gene transfer into normal and atherosclerotic human blood vessels. Circ Res 1998;82:1243–1252.

30. Barger AC, Beeuwkes R 3rd, Lainey LL, Silverman KJ. Hypothesis: vasa vasorum and neovascularization of human coronary arteries. A possible role in the pathophysiology of atherosclerosis. N Engl J Med 1984;310:175–177.

31. Guzman LA, Labhasetwar V, Song C, et al. Local intraluminal infusion of biodegradable polymeric nanoparticles. A novel approach for prolonged drug delivery after balloon angioplasty. Circulation 1996;94:1441–1448.

32. Banai S, Wolf Y, Golomb G, et al. PDGF-receptor tyrosine kinase blocker AG1295 selectively attenuates smooth muscle cell growth in vitro and reduces neointimal formation after balloon angioplasty in swine. Circulation 1998;97:1960–1969.

33. Fishbein I, Chorny M, Banai S, et al. Formulation and delivery mode affect disposition and activity of tyrphostin-loaded nanoparticles in the rat carotid model. Arterioscler Thromb Vasc Biol 2001;21:1434–1439.

34. Cohen-Sacks H, Najajreh Y, Tchaikovski V, et al. Novel PDGFbetaR antisense encapsulated in polymeric nanospheres for the treatment of restenosis. Gene Ther 2002;9:1607–1616.

35. Panyam J, Labhasetwar V. Biodegradable nanoparticles for drug and gene delivery to cells and tissue. Adv Drug Deliv Rev 2003;55:329–347.
36. Panyam J, Labhasetwar V. Dynamics of endocytosis and exocytosis of poly(D,L-lactide-co-glycolide) nanoparticles in vascular smooth muscle cells. Pharm Res 2003;20:212–220.
37. Goldman B, Blanke H, Wolinsky H. Influence of pressure on permeability of normal and diseased muscular arteries to horseradish peroxidase. A new catheter approach. Atherosclerosis 1987;65:215–225.
38. Nabel EG, Plautz G, Nabel GJ. Site-specific gene expression in vivo by direct gene transfer into the arterial wall. Science 1990;249:1285–1288.
39. Nabel EG, Shum L, Pompili VJ, et al. Direct transfer of transforming growth factor beta 1 gene into arteries stimulates fibrocellular hyperplasia. Proc Natl Acad Sci USA 1993;90:10,759–10,763.
40. Nabel EG, Yang Z, Liptay S, et al. Recombinant platelet-derived growth factor B gene expression in porcine arteries induce intimal hyperplasia in vivo. J Clin Invest 1993;91:1822–1829.
41. Rome JJ, Shayani V, Newman KD, et al. Adenoviral vector-mediated gene transfer into sheep arteries using a double-balloon catheter. Hum Gene Ther 1994;5:1249–1258.
42. Oberhoff M, Herdeg C, Al Ghobainy R, et al. Local delivery of paclitaxel using the double-balloon perfusion catheter before stenting in the porcine coronary artery. Catheter Cardiovasc Interv 2001;53:562–568.
43. Camenzind E, Kint PP, Di Mario C, et al. Intracoronary heparin delivery in humans. Acute feasibility and long-term results. Circulation 1995;92:2463–2472.
44. Groh WC, Kurnik PB, Matthai WH Jr, Untereker WJ. Initial experience with an intracoronary flow support device providing localized drug infusion: the Scimed Dispatch catheter. Cathet Cardiovasc Diagn 1995;36:67–73.
45. Kerensky RA, Franco EA, Bertolet BD, Thomas G, Wargovich TJ. Lysis of intravascular thrombus prior to coronary stenting using the dispatch infusion catheter. Cathet Cardiovasc Diagn 1996;38:410–414.
46. McKay RG, Fram DB, Hirst JA, et al. Treatment of intracoronary thrombus with local urokinase infusion using a new, site-specific drug delivery system: the Dispatch catheter. Cathet Cardiovasc Diagn 1994;33:181–188.
47. Tahlil O, Brami M, Feldman LJ, Branellec D, Steg PG. The Dispatch catheter as a delivery tool for arterial gene transfer. Cardiovasc Res 1997;33:181–187.
48. Panyam J, Lof J, O'Leary E, Labhasetwar V. Efficiency of Dispatch and Infiltrator cardiac infusion catheters in arterial localization of nanoparticles in a porcine coronary model of restenosis. J Drug Target 2002;10:515–523.
49. Ahn YK, Kook H, Jeong MH, et al. Local RAD50 gene delivery induces regression of preformed porcine coronary in-stent neointimal hyperplasia. J Gene Med 2004;6:93–104.
50. Buchwald AB, Wagner AH, Webel C, Hecker M. Decoy oligodeoxynucleotide against activator protein-1 reduces neointimal proliferation after coronary angioplasty in hypercholesterolemic minipigs. J Am Coll Cardiol 2002;39:732–738.
51. Ma X, Glover C, Miller H, Goldstein J, O'Brien E. Focal arterial transgene expression after local gene delivery. Can J Cardiol 2001;17:873–883.
52. Suzuki T, Hayase M, Hibi K, et al. Effect of local delivery of L-arginine on in-stent restenosis in humans. Am J Cardiol 2002;89:363–367.
53. Numaguchi Y, Okumura K, Harada M, et al. Catheter-based prostacyclin synthase gene transfer prevents in-stent restenosis in rabbit atheromatous arteries. Cardiovasc Res 2004;61:177–185.
54. Wolinsky H, Thung SN. Use of a perforated balloon catheter to deliver concentrated heparin into the wall of the normal canine artery. J Am Coll Cardiol 1990;15:475–481.
55. Lambert CR, Leone JE, Rowland SM. Local drug delivery catheters: functional comparison of porous and microporous designs. Coron Artery Dis 1993;4:469–475.
56. Wolinsky H, Lin C. Use of the perforatged balloon catheter to infuse marker substances into diseased coronary artery walls after experimental postmortem angioplasty. J Am Coll Cardiol 1991;17:174B–178B.
57. Kimura T, Miyauchi K, Yamagami S, Daida H, Yamaguchi H. Local delivery infusion pressure is a key determinant of vascular damage and intimal thickening. Jpn Circ J 1998;62:299–304.
58. Stadius ML, Collins C, Kernoff R. Local infusion balloon angioplasty to obviate restenosis compared with conventional balloon angioplasty in an experimental model of atherosclerosis. Am Heart J 1993;126:47–56.
59. Santoian EC, Gravanis MB, Schneider JE, et al. Use of the porous balloon in porcine coronary arteries: rationale for low pressure and volume delivery. Cathet Cardiovasc Diagn 1993;30:348–354.

60. Flugelman MY, Jaklitsch MT, Newman KD, Casscells W, Bratthauer GL, Dichek DA. Low level in vivo gene transfer into the arterial wall through a perforated balloon catheter. Circulation 1992; 85:1110–1117.

61. French BA, Mazur W, Ali NM, et al. Percutaneous transluminal in vivo gene transfer by recombinant adenovirus in normal porcine coronary arteries, atherosclerotic arteries, and two models of coronary restenosis. Circulation 1994;90:2402–2413.

62. Feldman LJ, Steg PG, Zheng LP, et al. Low-efficiency of percutaneous adenovirus-mediated arterial gene transfer in the atherosclerotic rabbit. J Clin Invest 1995;95:2662–2671.

63. Hong MK, Wong SC, Farb A, et al. Feasibility and drug delivery efficiency of a new balloon angioplasty catheter capable of performing simultaneous local drug delivery. Coron Artery Dis 1993;4:1023–1027.

64. Hong MK, Wong SC, Farb A, et al. Localized drug delivery in atherosclerotic arteries via a new balloon angioplasty catheter with intramural channels for simultaneous local drug delivery. Cathet Cardiovasc Diagn 1995;34:263–270; discussion 271.

65. Kalinowski M, Alfke H, Hamann C, et al. Effects of altering infusion parameters on intimal hyperplasia following local catheter-based delivery into the rabbit iliac artery. Atherosclerosis 2004;172: 71–78.

66. Hong MK, Wong SC, Barry JJ, Bramwell O, Tjurmin A, Leon MB. Feasibility and efficacy of locally delivered enoxaparin via the Channeled Balloon catheter on smooth muscle cell proliferation following balloon injury in rabbits. Cathet Cardiovasc Diagn 1997;41:241–245.

67. Kalinowski M, Alfke H, Bergen S, Klose KJ, Barry JJ, Wagner HJ. Comparative trial of local pharmacotherapy with L-arginine, r-hirudin, and molsidomine to reduce restenosis after balloon angioplasty of stenotic rabbit iliac arteries. Radiology 2001;219:716–723.

68. Van Belle E, Tio FO, Couffinhal T, Maillard L, Passeri J, Isner JM. Stent endothelialization. Time course, impact of local catheter delivery, feasibility of recombinant protein administration, and response to cytokine expedition. Circulation 1997;95:438–448.

69. Gottsauner-Wolf M, Jang Y, Penn MS, et al. Quantitative evaluation of local drug delivery using the InfusaSleeve catheter. Cathet Cardiovasc Diagn 1997;42:102–108.

70. Tanguay JF, Cantor WJ, Krucoff MW, et al. Local delivery of heparin post-PTCA: a multicenter randomized pilot study. Catheter Cardiovasc Interv 2000;49:461–467.

71. Varenne O, Gerard RD, Sinnaeve P, Gillijns H, Collen D, Janssens S. Percutaneous adenoviral gene transfer into porcine coronary arteries: is catheter-based gene delivery adapted to coronary circulation? Hum Gene Ther 1999;10:1105–1115.

72. Fram DB, Aretz T, Azrin MA, et al. Localized intramural drug delivery during balloon angioplasty using hydrogel-coated balloons and pressure-augmented diffusion. J Am Coll Cardiol 1994;23: 1570–1577.

73. Nunes GL, Hanson SR, King SB 3rd, Sahatjian RA, Scott NA. Local delivery of a synthetic antithrombin with a hydrogel-coated angioplasty balloon catheter inhibits platelet-dependent thrombosis. J Am Coll Cardiol 1994;23:1578–1583.

74. Azrin MA, Mitchel JF, Fram DB, et al. Decreased platelet deposition and smooth muscle cell proliferation after intramural heparin delivery with hydrogel-coated balloons. Circulation 1994;90: 433–441.

75. Landau C, Pirwitz MJ, Willard MA, Gerard RD, Meidell RS, Willard SE. Adenoviral mediated gene transfer to atherosclerotic arteries after balloon angioplasty. Am Heart J 1995;129:1051–1057.

76. Riessen R, Rahimizadeh H, Blessing E, Takeshita S, Barry JJ, Isner JM. Arterial gene transfer using pure DNA applied directly to a hydrogel-coated angioplasty balloon. Hum Gene Ther 1993;4: 749–758.

77. Steg PG, Feldman LJ, Scoazec JY, et al. Arterial gene transfer to rabbit endothelial and smooth muscle cells using percutaneous delivery of an adenoviral vector. Circulation 1994;90:1648–1656.

78. Isner JM. Arterial gene transfer of naked DNA for therapeutic angiogenesis: early clinical results. Adv Drug Deliv Rev 1998;30:185–197.

79. Barath P, Popov A, Dillehay GL, Matos G, McKiernan T. Infiltrator Angioplasty Balloon Catheter: a device for combined angioplasty and intramural site-specific treatment. Cathet Cardiovasc Diagn 1997;41:333–341.

80. Pavlides GS, Barath P, Maginas A, Vasilikos V, Cokkinos DV, O'Neill WW. Intramural drug delivery by direct injection within the arterial wall: first clinical experience with a novel intracoronary delivery-infiltrator system. Cathet Cardiovasc Diagn 1997;41:287–292.

81. Varenne O, Pislaru S, Gillijns H, et al. Local adenovirus-mediated transfer of human endothelial nitric oxide synthase reduces luminal narrowing after coronary angioplasty in pigs. Circulation 1998;98:919–926.

82. Wang K, Kessler PD, Zhou Z, et al. Local adenoviral-mediated inducible nitric oxide synthase gene transfer inhibits neointimal formation in the porcine coronary stented model. Mol Ther 2003;7:597–603.

83. Varenne O, Sinnaeve P, Gillijns H, et al. Percutaneous gene therapy using recombinant adenoviruses encoding human herpes simplex virus thymidine kinase, human PAI-1, and human NOS3 in balloon-injured porcine coronary arteries. Hum Gene Ther 2000;11:1329–1339.

84. Morishige K, Shimokawa H, Yamawaki T, et al. Local adenovirus-mediated transfer of C-type natri-uretic peptide suppresses vascular remodeling in porcine coronary arteries in vivo. J Am Coll Cardiol 2000;35:1040–1047.

85. Chung IM, Ueno H, Pak YK, et al. Catheter-based adenovirus-mediated local intravascular gene delivery of a soluble TGF-beta type II receptor using an infiltrator in porcine coronary arteries: efficacy and complications. Exp Mol Med 2002;34:299–307.

86. Kipshidze NN, Kim HS, Iversen P, et al. Intramural coronary delivery of advanced antisense oligonu-cleotides reduces neointimal formation in the porcine stent restenosis model. J Am Coll Cardiol 2002;39:1686–1691.

87. Fernandez-Ortiz A, Meyer BJ, Mailhac A, et al. A new approach for local intravascular drug delivery. Iontophoretic balloon. Circulation 1994;89:1518–1522.

88. Mitchel JF, Azrin MA, Fram DB, Bow LM, McKay RG. Localized delivery of heparin to angioplasty sites with iontophoresis. Cathet Cardiovasc Diagn 1997;41:315–323.

89. Robinson KA, Chronos NA, Schieffer E, et al. Pharmacokinetics and tissue localization of antisense oligonucleotides in balloon-injured pig coronary arteries after local delivery with an iontophoretic balloon catheter. Cathet Cardiovasc Diagn 1997;41:354–359.

90. Klugherz BD, Jones PL, Cui X, et al. Gene delivery from a DNA controlled-release stent in porcine coronary arteries. Nat Biotechnol 2000;18:1181–1184.

91. Klugherz BD, Song C, DeFelice S, et al. Gene delivery to pig coronary arteries from stents carrying antibody-tethered adenovirus. Hum Gene Ther 2002;13:443–454.

92. Perlstein I, Connolly JM, Cui X, et al. DNA delivery from an intravascular stent with a denatured collagen-polylactic-polyglycolic acid-controlled release coating: mechanisms of enhanced transfec-tion. Gene Ther 2003;10:1420–1428.

93. De Scheerder IK, Wilczek KL, Verbeken EV, et al. Biocompatibility of biodegradable and non-biodegradable polymer-coated stents implanted in porcine peripheral arteries. Cardiovasc Intervent Radiol 1995;18:227–232.

94. De Scheerder IK, Wilczek KL, Verbeken EV, et al. Biocompatibility of polymer-coated oversized metallic stents implanted in normal porcine coronary arteries. Atherosclerosis 1995;114:105–114.

95. Takahashi A, Palmer-Opolski M, Smith RC, Walsh K. Transgene delivery of plasmid DNA to smooth muscle cells and macrophages from a biostable polymer-coated stent. Gene Ther 2003;10:1471–1478.

96. Ye YW, Landau C, Willard JE, et al. Bioresorbable microporous stents deliver recombinant aden-ovirus gene transfer vectors to the arterial wall. Ann Biomed Eng 1998;26:398–408.

97. Dichek DA, Neville RF, Zwiebel JA, Freeman SM, Leon MB, Anderson WF. Seeding of intravascu-lar stents with genetically engineered endothelial cells. Circulation 1989;80:1347–1353.

98. Kutryk MJ, van Dortmont LM, de Crom RP, van der Kamp AW, Verdouw PD, van der Giessen WJ. Seeding of intravascular stents by the xenotransplantation of genetically modified endothelial cells. Semin Interv Cardiol 1998;3:217–220.

99. Willard JE, Landau C, Glamann DB, et al. Genetic modification of the vessel wall. Comparison of surgical and catheter-based techniques for delivery of recombinant adenovirus. Circulation 1994;89:2190–2197.

100. Alfke H, Wagner HJ, Calmer C, Klose KJ. Local intravascular drug delivery: in vitro comparison of three catheter systems. Cardiovasc Intervent Radiol 1998;21:50–56.

101. Dick A, Kromen W, Jungling E, et al. Quantification of horseradish peroxidase delivery into the arte-rial wall in vivo as a model of local drug treatment: comparison between a porous and a gel-coated balloon catheter. Cardiovasc Intervent Radiol 1999;22:389–393.

102. Mitchel JF, Fram DB, Gillam LD, Giri S, Waters DD, Kiernan FJ. Enhanced Local Intracoronary Delivery of Heparin with the Infiltrator feminine Catheter: A Comparative Study. J Invasive Cardiol 1999;11:463–470.

# INDEX